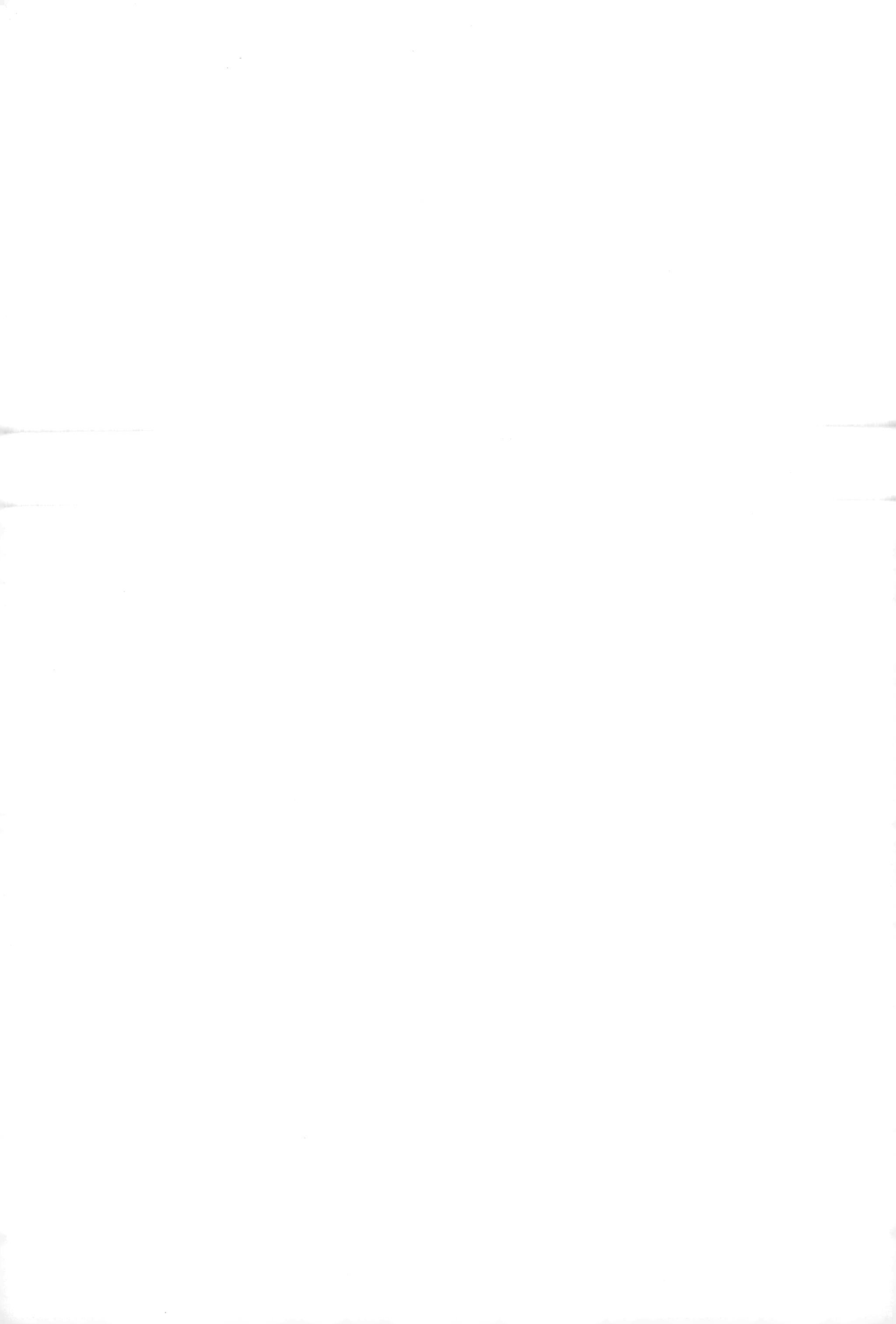

STRENGTH AND POWER IN SPORT

STRENGTH AND POWER IN SPORT

VOLUME III OF THE ENCYCLOPAEDIA OF SPORTS MEDICINE

AN IOC MEDICAL COMMISSION PUBLICATION

IN COLLABORATION WITH

THE INTERNATIONAL FEDERATION OF SPORTS MEDICINE

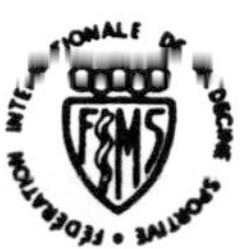

EDITED BY

PAAVO V. KOMI

SECOND EDITION

Blackwell
Science

Published by Blackwell Science Ltd
a Blackwell Publishing Company
Editorial Offices:
Blackwell Science Ltd, Osney Mead, Oxford OX2 0EL, UK
Blackwell Science, Inc., 350 Main Street, Malden, MA 02148-5018, USA
Blackwell Science Asia Pty Ltd, 550 Swanston Street, Carlton South, Victoria 3053, Australia
Blackwell Wissenschafts Verlag, Kurfürstendamm 57, 10707 Berlin, Germany

First published 1991
Reissue in paperback 1993
Reprinted 1994, 1998
German translation 1994
Second edition 2003

ISBN 0-632-05911-7

Library of Congress Cataloging-in-Publication Data

Strength and power in sport / edited by Paavo V. Komi.—
2nd ed.
p. cm. — (The Encyclopaedia of sports medicine ; v. 3)
'An IOC Medical Commission publication in collaboration with the International Federation of Sports Medicine'
ISBN 0-632-05911-7
1. Sports—Physiological aspects. 2. Muscle strength.
3. Physical education and training. I. Komi, Paavo V.
II. IOC Medical Commission. III. International Federation of Sports Medicine. IV. Series.
RC1235 .S76 2002
612'.044—dc21
2002005028

A catalogue record for this title is available from the British Library

Set in 9/12pt Palatino by Graphicraft Ltd, Hong Kong

Commissioning Editor: Andy Robinson
Production Editor: Alice Emmott
Production Controller: Kate Wilson

For further information on Blackwell Science, visit our website:
http://www.blackwellpublishing.com

Contents

List of Contributors

R. AIT-HADDOU, PhD, *Human Performance Laboratory, Faculty of Kinesiology, University of Calgary, 2500 University Drive, N.W. Calgary, AB T2N 1N4, Canada*

B.A. ALKNER, MD, *Department of Physiology and Pharmacology, Karolinska Institute, Huddinge University Hospital, SE-17177, Stockholm, Sweden*

R. BILLETER, PhD, *School of Biomedical Sciences, University of Leeds, Worsley Building, Leeds LS2 9JT*

V. DIETZ, FRCP, *Paracare, Swiss Paraplegic Centre, University Hospital Balgrist, Forchstrasse 340, CH-8008 Zürich, Switzerland*

J. DUCHATEAU, PhD, *Laboratory of Biology, Université Libre de Bruxelles, 28, av. P. Heger, CP 168 1000, Brussels, Belgium*

G.A. DUDLEY, PhD, *Department of Exercise Science, 115 M Ramsey Student Center, The University of Georgia, 300 River Road, Athens, GA 30602, USA*

V.R. EDGERTON, PhD, *Department of Physiological Science, Neurobiology, and Brain Research Institute, University of California, Los Angeles, 695 Charles E. Young Drive, Los Angeles, CA 90095-1761, USA*

K.A.P. EDMAN, PhD, *University of Lund, Department of Physiological Sciences, The Biomedical Centre, F11 S-221 84, Lund, Sweden*

S.J. FLECK, PhD, *Sports Science Department, Colorado College, Colorado Springs, CO 80903, USA*

J. GARHAMMER, PhD, *Biomechanics Laboratory, Department of Kinesiology, California State University, Long Beach, CA 90840, USA*

G. GOLDSPINK, PhD, *Basic Biomedical Sciences, Royal Free Campus, Royal Free and University College Medical School, Rowland Hill Street, London NW3 2PF, UK*

A. GOLLHOFER, PhD, *Institut für Sport und Sportwissenschaft, Universität Freiburg, Schwarzwaldstr. 175 D-7800, Freiburg, Germany*

K. HAINAUT, PhD, *Laboratory of Biology, Université Libre du Bruxelles 28, av. P. Heger, CP 168 1000, Brussels, Belgium*

S. HARRIDGE, PhD, *Wellcome Research Fellow, Department of Physiology, Royal Free and University College Medical School, Rowland Hill Street, London NW3 2PF, UK*

W. HERZOG, PhD, *Human Performance Laboratory, Faculty of Kinesiology, University of Calgary, 2500 University Drive, N.W. Calgary, AB T2N 1N4, Canada*

H. HOPPELER, MD, *Institute of Anatomy, University of Bern, Bühlstrasse 26, CH-3000 Bern 9, Switzerland*

K. HÄKKINEN, PhD, *Neuromuscular Research Center, Department of Biology of Physical Activity, University of Jyväskylä, P.O.Box 35, FIN-40351, Jyväskylä, Finland*

H.G. KNUTTGEN, PhD, *Harvard University, Spaulding Rehabilitation Hospital, 125 Nashua Street, Boston, MA 02114-1198, USA*

C. KARATZAFERI, PhD, *Department of Biochemistry/Biophysics, University of California at San Francisco, P.O. Box 0448, San Francisco, CA 94143, USA*

P.V. KOMI, PhD, *Neuromuscular Research Center, Department of Biology of Physical Activity, University of Jyväskylä, P.O.Box 35, FIN-40351, Jyväskylä, Finland*

W.J. KRAEMER, PhD, *Department of Kinesiology, Unit 1110, The Human Performance Laboratory, The University of Connecticut, Storrs, CT 06269-1110, USA*

A.M. LAI, MD, *927 Westwood Boulevard, Suite 650, Box 957087, Los Angeles, CA 90095-7087, USA*

B. LOITZ-RAMAGE, PhD, *University of Calgary, McCaig Centre for Joint Injury and Arthritis Research, 3330 Hospital Drive, N.W. Calgary, AB T2N 1N4, Canada*

J.D. MACDOUGALL, PhD, *Professor Emeritus, Department of Kinesiology, McMaster University, Hamilton, ON L8S 4K1, Canada*

S.A. MAZZETTI, MS, *School of Physical Education, Ball State University, Muncie, IN, 47304, USA*

J. MESTER, PhD, *Deutsche Sporthochschule, Köln, Carl-Diem-Weg 6, D-50933, Köln, Germany*

R.J. MONTI, PhD, *Brain Research Institute, 1320 Gonda Neuroscience and Genetics Building, University of California Los Angeles, 695 Charles E. Young Drive, Los Angeles, CA 90095-1761, USA*

T. MORITANI, PhD, *Kyoto University, Laboratory of Applied Physiology, Graduate School of Human and Environmental Studies, Sakyo-Ku, Kyoto, 606-850, Japan*

C. NICOL, PhD, *UMR 6559, Movement and Perception CNRS, Université de la Méditerranée, Faculty of Sports Science, 163, Avenue de Luminy CP 910, F-13288, Marseille, Cedex 9, France*

N.A. RATAMESS, MS, *Department of Kinesiology, Unit 1110, The Human Performance Laboratory, The University of Connecticut, Storrs, CT 06269-1110, USA*

R.R. ROY, PhD, *Brain Research Institute, 1320 Gonda Neuroscience and Genetics Building, University of California Los Angeles, 695 Charles E. Young Drive, Los Angeles, CA 90095-1761, USA*

D.G. SALE, PhD, *Department of Kinesiology, McMaster University, Hamilton, ON L8S 4K1, Canada*

P. SPITZENPFEIL, PhD, *Technische Universität München, Connollystr. 32, D-80809, München, Germany*

S. STEVENSON, PhD, *Department of Kinesiology and Health Promotion, California State Polytechnic University, Pomona, CA 91768, USA*

M.H. STONE, PhD, *Department of Sport Physiology, USOC, One Olympic Plaza, Colorado Springs, CO 80909, USA*

B. TAKANO, *Senior International Coach, USA Weightlifting Federation, c/o Van Nuys High School, 6535 Cedros Avenue, Van Nuys, CA 91, USA*

P.A. TESCH, PhD, *Department of Physiology and Pharmacology, Karolinska Institute, Huddinge University Hospital, SE–17177, Stockholm, Sweden*

Z. YUE, PhD, *Deutsche Sporthochschule, Köln, Carl-Diem-Weg 6, D-50933, Köln, Germany*

V.M. ZATSIORSKY, PhD, *Pennsylvania State University, Department of Kinesiology, Biomechanics Laboratory, 39 Recreation Building, University Park, PA 16802, USA*

R.F. ZERNICKE, PhD, *University of Calgary, Faculty of Kinesiology, Medicine and Engineering, 2500 University Drive, N.W. Calgary, AB T2N 1N4, Canada*

Forewords

In 1991, the IOC Medical Commission published Vol. III of the Encyclopaedia of Sports Medicine series, on the topic *Strength and Power in Sport*. Professor Paavo V. Komi, as editor, recruited a team of 29 internationally renowned scientific colleagues to produce a reference volume that constituted an important contribution to scientific literature in an area which arrived relatively late in the study of exercise and sports science.

Since the publication of the first edition of *Strength and Power in Sport*, a large volume of research literature has appeared both to reinforce the information contained and to expand the body of literature relative to the training and performance of strength and highest power. The popularity of the first edition and the availability of such a large amount of new information led the IOC Medical Commission to decide that a second edition of this important volume was both justified and essential.

I would like to thank the IOC Medical Commission for yet another valuable contribution to literature in sports medicine and the sport sciences.

Dr Jacques Rogge
IOC President

Extensive research started appearing in the literature of the 1950s concerning aerobic metabolism and the importance of cardiopulmonary function to relative long periods of physical activity. Additional research subsequently appeared on the subject of sprint events and team sports. The physical expression of explosive movements and the training of strength relative to sport were, however, neglected. 'Strength training' in earlier times prompted unjustified fears of the athlete becoming 'muscle bound' with a resultant loss of flexibility. These mistaken beliefs discouraged athletes from training with free weights and high-resistance exercise machines now associated with the training of strength and highest power.

This second edition adds valuable information concerning the basic science and provides additional information that can result in better performance, the prevention of injuries, and greater enjoyment of sports participation by the elite athlete, the recreational athlete, the young athlete and the veteran athlete.

Strength and Power in Sport will certainly continue to be the most frequently cited source of information on this topic area and, in its new and expanded second edition, will make an even greater contribution to the health, well-being and success of athletes of all ages.

I would like to thank Professor Komi for having again gathered a team of authoritative scientists from around the world as co-authors to produce this all-new second edition.

Prince Alexandre de Merode
Chairman, IOC Medical Commission

Preface

It was a rewarding pleasure to follow the success of the first volume of *Strength and Power in Sport*. Since its publication in 1991, the volume has been reprinted several times. In addition, it has been translated into German (1994). Despite the continuous interest in this first volume, it became obvious that the material had to be updated before any additional printing or translating could be planned. During the last 10 years, a considerable amount of knowledge has become available through an increasing number of studies performed both on basic mechanisms and applied aspects of strength and power training. Thus, it was necessary to produce a new volume with the latest possible information.

The editorial work of the first volume was a challenge, but the second volume of *Strength and Power in Sport* was perhaps an even more motivating experience. We were fortunate to receive acceptance of most of the previous authors to revise their chapters, but new contributions from other authors were also included in this second volume. The recruited team now consists of 39 contributing authors representing the most prominent scientists and clinicians, all of whose interest have involved the various problems related to strength and power training. But more importantly, they have all established themselves as world leaders in their particular research or applied area.

Several books have been published related to strength and power which have advanced our understanding of the subject area. In the present volume, we have made an effort to take a slightly different approach to the problem. While it is very easy to demonstrate improvement of muscle strength with almost any method (if sufficiently intensive), the present volume, *Strength and Power in Sport*, examines the basic mechanisms and reasons for beneficial strength exercises. In order to give state-of-the-art information – as is the purpose of the Encyclopaedia of Sports Medicine – a great portion of the book is devoted to the basics of strength and power and their adaptation. The material is divided into five sections.

1 Definition of fundamental terms and concepts.
2 A comprehensive coverage of the biological basis for strength and power including the structural, hormonal, neural and mechanical aspects. This material is presented in 10 different chapters.
3 A detailed examination of the reasons (mechanisms) leading to the adaptations of the organism when subjected to various strength and power exercises. This section covers nine different topics ranging from cellular and neural adaptation to endocrine and cardiovascular responses.
4 Special problems of strength and power training including age-related changes, the potential use of electrical stimulation, and clinical aspects.
5 The volume finishes with a more applied and solely sports-orientated section where three chapters cover the current knowledge of the practical strength and power training principles, as based on available scientific knowledge.

The way the material has been presented varies slightly among the chapters. In some cases, considerable depth and detail were necessary while, on the other hand, a few chapters have been written in a more readable and overview-type format. Whatever the writing style has been, the material should be accessible to readers with a background in the biological aspects of sport sciences. Because of the wide coverage of the basic mechanistic features of strength and power training, it is expected that this volume will become required reading for many graduate programmes in the medicine and science of sport. The study of strength and power is one of the major components of sports science and an understanding of the relationships among neural, hormonal, muscular and mechanical factors is central to athletic performance as well as to strength and power needs of other human populations. Thus, it is believed that this second volume of *Strength and Power in Sport* fulfills well the major objectives established by the IOC Medical Commission for this material: Importance of understanding the basic problems in various aspects of Strength and Power in order to analyze different sport events and to plan objectively training and conditioning not only of athletes but other groups as well.

Paavo V. Komi
Jyväskylä, Finland

Units of Measurement and Terminology*

Units for quantifying human exercise

Mass	kilogram (kg)
Distance	metre (m)
Time	second (s)
Force	newton (N)
Work	joule (J)
Power	watt (W)
Velocity	metres per second ($m \cdot s^{-1}$)
Torque	newton-metre (N·m)
Acceleration	metres per second^2 ($m \cdot s^{-2}$)
Angle	radian (rad)
Angular velocity	radians per second ($rad \cdot s^{-1}$)
Amount of substance	mole (mol)
Volume	litre (l)

Terminology

Muscle action: The state of activity of muscle.

Concentric action: One in which the ends of the muscle are drawn closer together.

Isometric action: One in which the ends of the muscle are prevented from drawing closer together, with no change in length.

Eccentric action: One in which a force external to the muscle overcomes the muscle force and the ends of the muscle are drawn further apart.

Force: That which changes or tends to change the state of rest or motion in matter. A muscle generates force in a muscle action. (SI unit: newton.)

Work: Force expressed through a displacement but with no limitation on time. (SI unit: joule; note: 1 newton × 1 metre = 1 joule.)

Power: The rate of performing work; the product of force and velocity. The rate of transformation of metabolic potential energy to work or heat. (SI unit: watt.)

Energy: The capability of producing force, performing work, or generating heat. (SI unit: joule.)

Exercise: Any and all activity involving generation of force by the activated muscle(s). Exercise can be quantified mechanically as force, torque, work, power, or velocity of progression.

Exercise intensity: A specific level of muscular activity that can be quantified in terms of power (energy expenditure or work performed per unit of time), the opposing force (e.g. by free weight or weight stack) isometric force sustained, or velocity of progression.

Endurance: The time limit of a person's ability to maintain either an isometric force or a power level involving combinations of concentric and/or eccentric muscle actions. (SI unit: second.)

Mass: The quantity of matter of an object which is reflected in its inertia. (SI unit: kilogram.)

Weight: The force exerted by gravity on an object.

* Compiled by the Sub-commission on Publications in the Sports Sciences, IOC Medical Commission.

(SI unit: newton; traditional unit: kilogram of weight.) (Note: mass = weight/acceleration due to gravity.)

Free weight: An object of known mass, not attached to a supporting or guiding structure, which is used for physical conditioning and competitive lifting.

Torque: The effectiveness of a force to overcome the rotational inertia of an object. The product of force and the perpendicular distance from the line of action of the force to the axis of rotation. (SI unit: newton-metre.)

Strength: The maximal force or torque a muscle or muscle group can generate at a specified or determined velocity.

PART 1

DEFINITIONS

Chapter 1

Basic Considerations for Exercise

HOWARD G. KNUTTGEN AND PAAVO V. KOMI

The performance of sport as for all physical exercise is the result of a coordinated activation of the appropriate skeletal muscles. These muscles, acting through the lever systems of the body skeleton, provide the forces and the power that can be translated into skilled movement. The assessment and quantification of such physical performance is accomplished by use of the International System of Measurement (the SI) for force (newtons); energy, work and heat (joules); torque (newton-metres); and power (watts). If the term *exercise* is defined as any and all activity involving force generation by activated muscles (Knuttgen & Komi 1992; Knuttgen & Kraemer 1987), the resultant physical performance must be described in these terms.

Force is that which changes or tends to change the state of rest or motion in matter. *Work* is equivalent to a force expressed through a displacement with no limitation on time. *Torque* is the effectiveness of a force to produce rotation of an object about an axis. *Power* is the rate at which work is performed or the rate of the transformation of metabolic potential energy to work and/or heat.

The exercise intensity can therefore be quantified in various situations as: the opposing force in dynamic exercise (e.g. provided by a free weight, exercise machine or ergometer); isometric force sustained; power (energy expenditure or work performed per second or force times velocity); or velocity of progression (e.g. running, cycling, rowing). Endurance is the time limit of a person's ability to maintain either an isometric force or a power level of dynamic exercise—the basic SI unit of time is the second (s).

Power can be determined for a single body movement, a series of movements or, as in the case of aerobic exercise, a large number of repetitive movements. Power can be determined instantaneously at any point in a movement or averaged for any portion of a movement or bout of exercise.

Energy, power and endurance

The relationship of the ability to continue exercise to power is presented in Fig. 1.1 where endurance time to exhaustion is plotted against metabolic power during steady state for an average-sized male athlete. In Fig. 1.2, the relative

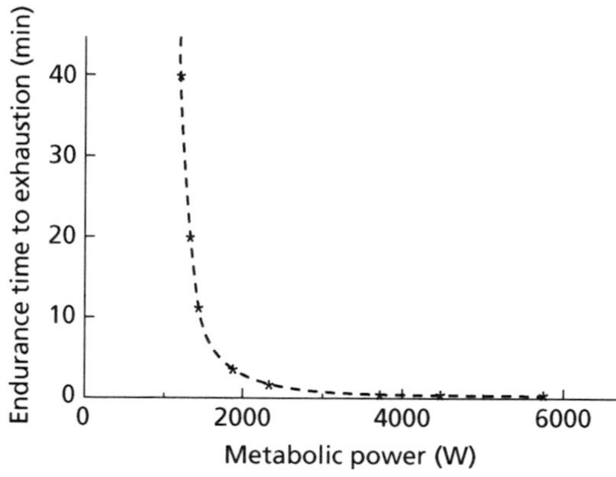

Fig. 1.1 The relationship of endurance time to human metabolic power production for an 80-kg athlete with a maximal oxygen uptake of 2.7 $mmol \cdot s^{-1}$.

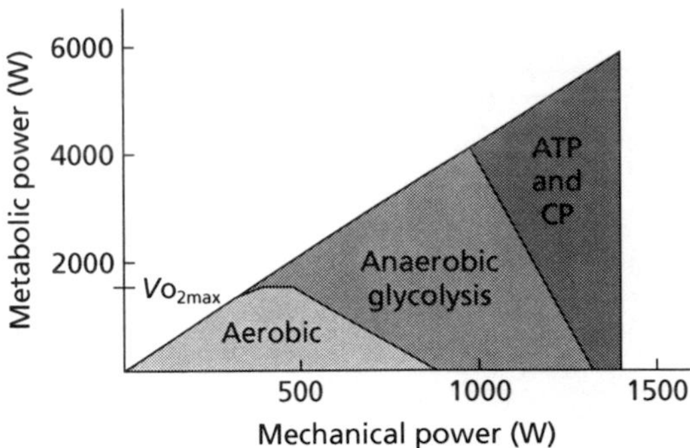

Fig. 1.2 The sources of energy (aerobic metabolism, anaerobic glycolysis and the high-energy phosphates) when metabolic power is related to mechanical power production.

contributions of aerobic metabolism, anaerobic glycolysis (leading to lactic acid formation), and the combination of adenosine triphosphate (ATP) and creatine phosphate (CP) being considered as an energy store are presented when metabolic power is plotted against mechanical power.

The final biochemical carrier of energy to the myofilaments for the development of force by muscles is the high-energy phosphate compound, ATP. A second high-energy phosphate compound, CP, can provide energy for immediate resynthesis of ATP during high-intensity exercise when other sources of energy are not available. Under conditions of the very highest intensities of exercise (i.e. power development), ATP is not only the final carrier of energy but, as the sole source brought into play, it could be considered to have an important role as an energy store as well. Similarly, ATP continues to be the final step in energy transfer at slightly lower intensities of exercise (e.g. 5–10 s until exhaustion), but ATP together with CP constitute the energy storage employed.

As exercise intensity is lowered and ability to continue is increased, anaerobic glycolysis can provide energy for resynthesis of ATP and CP. At much lower intensities of exercise, muscle cells depend upon the oxidation (aerobic metabolism) of fat (fatty acids), carbohydrate (glucose and glycogen) and, to a very limited extent, protein (amino acids) as the sources of energy to resynthesize both ATP and CP.

Power in sport

The metabolic power for such events as throwing and jumping in track and field, weightlifting, and springboard and platform diving is obtained solely from the high-energy phosphate compounds. Events lasting approximately 10 s or somewhat longer (e.g. 100-m run) utilize anaerobic glycolysis for energy in ATP resynthesis. The lower the intensity and the longer the event, the better is the mechanism of anaerobic glycolysis able to contribute energy. In events that last at least 60 s, the aerobic metabolism of carbohydrate and fat begin to contribute energy. The longer lasting the event (lasting minutes and hours), the greater is the aerobic contribution.

For the male athlete described in Fig. 1.1, metabolic power production higher than 5000 W can be obtained solely from ATP. Between 3500 and 5000 W, CP is utilized to resynthesize ATP from adenosine diphosphate (ADP) and CP and the total energy required is obtained from these two high-energy phosphates. In the range of 1500–3500 W, anaerobic glycolysis constitutes the major source of energy for ATP resynthesis. When the power requirement becomes less than 2000 W, aerobic metabolism begins to make a small contribution to ATP resynthesis and the lower the power requirement is from that point on the greater is the contribution of the aerobic metabolism of carbohydrate and fat. Below 1000 W for this athlete, ATP resynthesis during exercise is accomplished totally by the aerobic metabolism and the athlete can continue to run, swim, cycle, row, ski, etc. for extended periods, as can be assessed from the endurance time to exhaustion.

The authors of the various chapters in this volume will consider only the highest levels of force development and the highest levels of mechanical and metabolic power production. Anaerobic glycolysis will contribute energy at intensities lower than are totally accommodated by the high-energy phosphates by themselves but at intensities much higher than those that elicit peak oxygen uptake. Aerobic metabolism will be considered to play no role in the performance of such high-intensity exercise but, on completion of any such conditioning activity or competitive event, aerobic metabolism will assume its role as the sole source of energy for recovery.

Muscle actions

The interaction of the force developed by muscle groups with the external forces presented by the mass of the body parts, gravity, sports objects (e.g. ball, discus, javelin, shot), or opponents in body contact sports will result in muscle actions that produce static exercise (no movement about the related joints) or dynamic exercise (involving either a decrease or an increase in joint angles). Static exercise of activated muscle is traditionally described as an *isometric* action. Force is developed but, as no movement occurs, no work is performed. The other muscle actions involve movement and therefore are designated as dynamic. The term *concentric* is used to identify a shortening action and the term *eccentric* is used to identify a lengthening action (see Table 1.1).

Isometric and dynamic actions can be assessed at any particular length of the muscle and/or positioning of the related body parts in terms of: directly measured force from the muscle or its tendon; force at a particular point on the related body parts; or torque about the axis of rotation. A dynamic action must be further described in terms of directionality (shortening or lengthening) and the velocity of muscle length change or body part movement.

Table 1.1 Classification of exercise and muscle action types.

Exercise	Muscle action	Muscle length
Dynamic	Concentric	Decreases
	Eccentric	Increases
Static	Isometric	No change

The definitions given in Table 1.1 refer, however, to the entire muscle–tendon complex. As will be discussed in Chapter 9, and especially in Chapter 10, the fascicle and tendon may not follow each other (and the entire muscle–tendon complex) in various measures of muscle mechanics, such as force–length and force–velocity relationships. It will further be demonstrated in Chapter 10 that in natural movements involving several joints, these relationships are not only effort dependent, but also muscle and joint dependent.

Because of the variation in mechanical advantages as a joint angle is changed, as well as the differences in maximal force capability of a muscle through its range of length, no dynamic action of a muscle in exercise and sport performance involves constant force development. Therefore, the term 'isotonic', implying uniform force throughout a dynamic muscle action, is inappropriate for the description of human exercise performance and should not be employed. Equally inappropriate is the older practice of identifying all muscle force development as a contraction, thereby leading to 'eccentric contraction' signifying a lengthening shortening and 'isometric contraction' signifying a no-change-in-length shortening. Certain authors contributing to this volume have been granted leeway as regards continuation of this practice.

Furthermore, a variation in linear movement occurs with muscles during both sport skill performance and exercise on mechanical devices. For this reason, the term 'isokinetic' to denote constant velocity should not be employed to describe a muscle action. Although the controlled movement of an exercise machine or ergometer may be at constant velocity and described as being isokinetic, this provides no guarantee that the muscles that are providing force in the movement are acting at constant velocity.

Human locomotion seldom involves pure forms of isolated concentric, eccentric or isometric actions. This is because the body segments are periodically subjected to impact forces, as in running or jumping, or because some external force such as gravity causes the muscle to lengthen.

In many situations, the muscles first act eccentrically with a concentric action following immediately. The combination of eccentric and concentric action forms a natural type of muscle function called a *stretch–shortening cycle* or SSC (Norman & Komi 1979; Komi 1984). A SSC is an economical way to cause movement and, consequently, the performance of the muscle can be enhanced. Chapter 10 in this volume has been especially devoted to muscle performance in SSC.

Strength and high levels of power production

The term *strength* will be employed to identify the maximal force or torque that can be developed by the muscles performing a particular joint movement (e.g. elbow flexion, knee extension). However, the muscles may perform at maximal effort as either isometric, concentric or eccentric actions and the two dynamic actions may be performed at a wide range of velocities. An infinite number of values for the strength of muscle(s) may be obtained either for an isolated muscle preparation or for a human movement as related to the type of action, the velocity of the action, and the length of the muscle(s) when the measurement is accomplished.

Therefore, strength is not the result of an assessment performed under a single set of conditions. Because of the number of variables or conditions involved, *strength* of a muscle or muscle group must be defined as the maximal force generated at a specified or determined velocity (Knuttgen & Kraemer 1987). For a particular exercise performance with free weights (e.g. military press in power lifting, clean and jerk in Olympic weightlifting), the combination of strengths employed to complete the manoeuvre is assessed as the largest mass lifted.

Strength assessment and strength exercise prescription

Increases in maximal force production (strength) and maximal power of the muscles are brought about through exercise programmes of very high opposing force (routinely termed 'resistance') that limit repetitions to approximately 20 or fewer and therefore a duration of less than 30 s. Exercise programmes based on higher repetitions (e.g. 30–50 repetitions leading to exhaustion in a 'set') develop local muscular endurance but are not conducive to strength development. Exercise involving a very large number of repetitions in a set (e.g. 400–1000 repetitions) brings about physiological adaptations that result in enhanced aerobic performance that can be especially counterproductive to the development and expression of strength and high levels of power.

Mechanical power will be discussed extensively in Chapter 9 with regard to the force–velocity relationships obtained with constant activation either with isolated muscles or even in human muscle. The obtained force–velocity curves (and consequently power–velocity curves) are not, however, representative of naturally occurring muscle function, in which the activation is continuously variable. In these situations the terms instantaneous force–velocity and power-velocity relationship are more appropriate (see also Chapter 10).

'Resistance training' is performed with a variety of exercise machines, free weights, or even the use of gravity acting upon the athlete's body mass. Most resistance training (strength) programmes are based on a system of exercise to a *repetition maximum* (RM) as presented in the mid-1940s by T.L. De Lorme (De Lorme 1945) for use in physical medicine and rehabilitation. Every time the athlete performs a particular exercise, the bout (or 'set') is performed for the maximum number of repetitions possible (repetition maximum or RM) and this number is recorded along with the mass lifted or opposing force imposed by an exercise machine. Repeated testing at increasingly higher opposing force will eventually lead to the determination of a 1 RM, in which the athlete can perform the movement only once and not repeat it. In this system, the mass lifted or opposing force for the 1 RM is described as the athlete's strength at that particular point in time and for the particular movement (see example presented in Fig. 1.3).

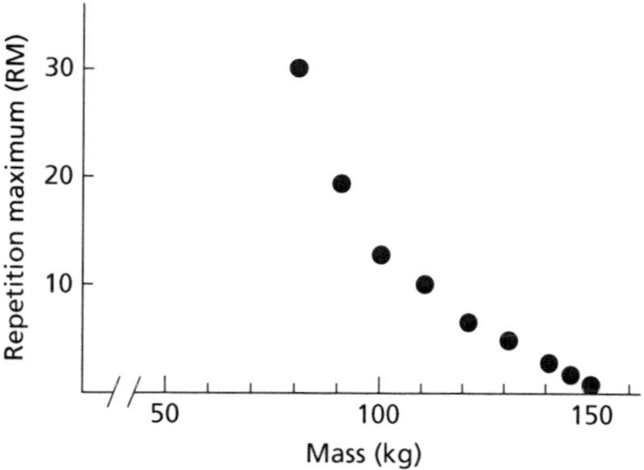

Fig. 1.3 The relationship of endurance capability in repetition maximum (RM) to the mass of the free weights being employed for an athlete performing a particular exercise (in this case, a bench press)

Bouts of strength exercise and the daily programme can be based on percentages of 1 RM or, preferably, within heavy (3–5) medium (9 or 10), and light (15–18) RM zones (Fleck & Kraemer 1997). The number of bouts performed in a set, the number of sets performed per day and the number of daily workouts per week are then prescribed for each movement or muscle group as based on the point in time in the competitive season, the physical condition of the athlete, programme variation for both physiological and psychological considerations, and programme objectives.

The principal adaptation of the athlete's body is the increase in size (commonly termed hypertrophy) of Type II muscle cells. It is generally held that no interchange takes place between Type I and Type II fibres as the result of specific conditioning programmes.

Summary

The performance of sport and all exercise can be assessed and described in terms of force, work, torque, power and endurance time, and presented in the units of the International System of Measurement (the SI). The human body is capable of power production over a wide range from low-intensity aerobic exercise, to exercise eliciting peak oxygen uptake for the muscles involved, high-intensity anaerobic exercise emphasizing anaerobic glycolysis as the main energy source, and the highest power productions which rely solely on the high-energy phosphates as the energy source. The chapters of this volume will concentrate on the highest expressions of power which involve predominantly the high-energy phosphates, with the possible contribution of anaerobic glycolysis when the short, intense exercise performance lasts for periods somewhat longer than a few seconds.

References

De Lorme, T.L. (1945) Restoration of muscle power by heavy resistance exercises. *Journal of Bone and Joint Surgery* **27**, 645.

Fleck, S.J. & Kraemer, W.J. (1997) *Designing Resistance Training Programs.* Human Kinetics, Champaign, IL.

Knuttgen, H.G. & Komi, P.V. (1992) Basic definitions for exercise. In: *Strength and Power in Sport* (ed. P.V. Komi), pp. 3–6. Blackwell Scientific Publications, Oxford.

Knuttgen, H.G. & Kraemer, W.J. (1987) Terminology and measurement in exercise performance. *Journal of Applied Sports Science Research* **1**(1), 1.

Komi, P.V. (1984) Physiological and biomechanical correlates of muscle function: effects of muscle structure and stretch–shortening cycle on force and speed. In: *Exercise and Sport Sciences Reviews*, Vol. 12 (ed. R.L. Terjung), pp. 81–121. The Collamore Press, Lexington, MA.

Norman, R.W. & Komi, P.V. (1979) Electromyographic delay in skeletal muscle under normal movement conditions. *Acta Physiologica Scandinavica* **106**, 241.

Suggested reading

Bureau International des Poids et Mésures (1977) *Le Système International d'Unités (SI)*, 3rd edn. Sèvres, France.

Cavanagh, P.R. (1988) On 'muscle action' vs. 'muscle contraction.' *Journal of Biomechanics* **22**(1), 69.

Komi, P.V. & Knuttgen, H.G. (1996) Sport science and modern training. In: *Sports Science Studies*, Vol. 8, pp. 44–62. Verlag Karl Hofmann, Schorndorf.

PART 2

BIOLOGICAL BASIS FOR STRENGTH AND POWER

Chapter 2

Neuronal Control of Functional Movement

VOLKER DIETZ

Summary

This chapter deals with the neuronal control of functional movements including the interactions between central programmes and afferent input. The issue is centred around the performance of posture and locomotion as a paradigm for human motor control. The chapter will review those electrophysiological investigations that have addressed the neuronal mechanisms underlying gait. The aims of the review are to provide further insights into the underlying physiological mechanisms of locomotion. Biologically useful behaviour does not consist of the isolated action of single neurones, muscles or limbs. A wide range of sources of afferent activity acts at several levels within the nervous system to produce functionally integrated patterns of muscle activity. This complexity necessitates an eclectic approach in studies of the function of the nervous system and has to be supplemented by data gained from animal experiments. Discussions of the relative significance of reflexes on central rhythms and programming in locomotion were present from the beginning of these investigations and they continue. Here the current state of research in this field will be established.

The central mechanisms involved in locomotion are reflected as a di- or triphasic pattern of leg muscle activation following displacement of the feet. The basic structure of this pattern is thought to be programmed. Close similarities with the triphasic electromyographic (EMG) pattern described for ballistic voluntary movements suggest that there is an analogous neuronal mechanism controlling locomotion. The EMG pattern is assumed to be a consequence of multisensory afferent input and generated by spinal interneuronal circuits that are closely connected with spinal locomotor centres. The extent to which the timing of the pattern can be modified by afferent input has yet to be determined. A basic requirement of bipedal locomotion is that both legs act in a cooperative manner, i.e. each limb affects the timing and strength of muscle activation of the other. Some evidence has shown that this interlimb coordination is mediated by spinal interneuronal circuits, which are themselves under supraspinal (i.e. cerebral and cerebellar) control.

With respect to the reflex mechanisms, short-latency stretch reflexes in leg extensor muscles are profoundly modulated during gait. This occurs mainly by presynaptic inhibition of group Ia input and to a lesser extent by fusimotor influences. However, this reflex might predominantly be involved in the compensation of small surface irregularities during distinct phases of gait. Compensation of foot displacements during gait is provided by polysynaptic spinal reflexes. This includes activation of synergistic muscle groups of both legs. These EMG responses are thought to be modified predominantly by peripheral input from group II afferents converging (along with different peripheral and supraspinal inputs) onto common spinal interneurones within a spinal pathway. These reflexes modulate the basic motor pattern of spinal interneuronal circuits underlying the motor task.

Recent evidence has emphasized the crucial importance of load receptor input in the control of bipedal stance and gait. Yet we still do not fully understand its nature nor its interaction with other afferent inputs and control mechanisms. Vestibular and visual functions are mainly context dependent and only become essential when afferent input from other sources is reduced.

Introduction

In the 18th century, the investigation of movement was based on the premise that upright stance and gait, and also differentiation of hand movements, represented a basic requirement for human cultural development (Herder 1785). This necessitates that the nervous system must function to automatically balance the body's centre of mass over the feet during all motor activities. In other words, every movement must begin and end with a postural adjustment.

Analysis of human gait first became possible towards the end of the 19th century with the development of photographic recording of running movements (Marey 1894). Later, Bernstein (1936) extended the analysis techniques by making biomechanical recordings. Finally, the techniques to record electrophysiological responses during locomotion were developed and were first demonstrated in cats (Engberg & Lundberg 1969; Grillner 1972).

Basic requirements

The relative significance of reflexes on central rhythms and programming in locomotion has been addressed. Hoffmann (1922) described the monosynaptic pathway as the simplest spinal feedback system and emphasized that in humans, the so-called 'Eigenreflexapparat' is responsible for the adaptation of muscle innervation to unexpected stress. Förster (1927) suggested that slow stretch reflexes and 'adaptational reflexes' were an essential contribution to motor coordination. However, in cats, the locomotor pattern was found to be preserved following complete deafferentation (Bickel 1897; Hering 1897) and as a result the 'reflex chain' theory as the basis for the generation of the rhythmic alternating movements, and therefore locomotion, was rejected. Many years later it was suggested that a spinal generator was responsible for locomotion (Lundberg 1975). This proposal was extended further when Grillner (1981) proposed that the spinal locomotor centre was activated and controlled by the brainstem and was also influenced by peripheral feedback mechanisms.

Central generators and programmes interacting with peripheral reflexes represent only a portion of the mechanisms involved in the control of locomotion. Afferent information from a variety of sources within the visual, vestibular and proprioceptive systems contributes toward the overall control. The convergence of spinal reflex pathways and descending tracts onto common spinal interneurones appears to be the rule rather than the exception, implying that the interneurones play an integrative role (for review see Schomburg 1990). The shortcoming of studying human locomotion is reflected in the fact that the function of human motor control mechanisms can only be determined by indirect methods. Therefore, the findings must be largely interpreted with respect to animal experiments. Although there are clearly some common features between the pattern of activity and the underlying neuronal mechanisms during quadrupedal locomotion in cats and that seen during bipedal gait in humans (Grillner 1981; Nilsson *et al.* 1985; MacPherson *et al.* 1989; Dietz 1992, 1997), distinct differences do exist which are necessary to maintain the body in an upright position during bipedal locomotion.

Irrespective of the conditions under which gait is investigated, the neuronal pattern evoked during a particular task is always directed towards maintaining the body's centre of mass over the base of the support. One consequence is that the selection of afferent input by central mechanisms must correspond to the requirements for body stabilization. As neuronal signals indicating muscle stretch and/or length are by themselves insufficient to fully control upright posture, all sensory information is considered in order for body equilibrium to be controlled.

However, it is generally accepted that locomotor movements in mammals depend primarily upon neuronal mechanisms in the spinal cord that can act in the absence of any afferent input (for review see Grillner 1981). Afferent information results in the modification of the spinal locomotor pattern according to the external requirements (Duysens & Pearson 1980; Forssberg *et al.* 1977; for review see Grillner 1981, 1986). Both the spinal locomotor centres and the reflex mechanisms are under the control of the brainstem and supraspinal motor centres (see Fig. 2.1). Further refinement is achieved from supraspinal areas, namely the cerebellum (Arshavsky *et al.* 1972; Armstrong 1988).

In several aspects the neurophysiology of normal human gait must be viewed with respect to the neuronal basis of animal locomotion. For more detailed information about this field the reader is referred to Grillner (1981) and Baldissera *et al.* (1981). The biomechanical aspects of posture and gait will be discussed only with respect to corresponding neuronal events, although neuronal mechanisms clearly cause biomechanical changes while at the same time being constrained by the body's biomechanics (see Thorstensson *et al.* 1984). The neurophysiology of human gait will be assumed to be centred around central programming and reflex behaviour during locomotion. The feedforward control offered by the visual system and the role of the vestibular system during locomotion will only be touched upon in connection with the interactions between different systems.

During control of gait afferent information is selected from a variety of sources which then interacts with central programmes resulting in a modification of the movement to the actual requirements. Although a predominant working range exists for each receptor system, considerable overlap between systems is present. Thus, under normal conditions, stepping movements are little affected in the absence of one of the main systems, e.g. the visual, proprioceptive or labyrinthine systems. To separate the relative significance of each of these systems is difficult due to the close interaction between the systems, in particular that between central mechanisms and proprioceptive reflexes, in maintaining the body's centre of mass over the feet.

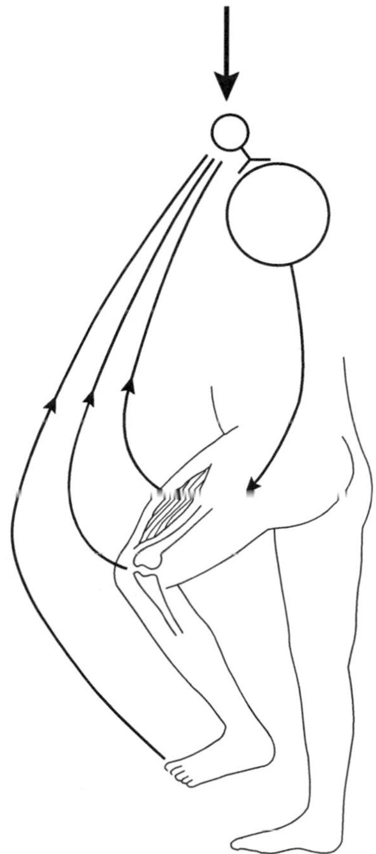

Fig. 2.1 Schematic drawing of the neuronal mechanisms involved in human gait. Leg muscles become activated by a programmed pattern generated within spinal interneuronal circuits. This pattern is modulated by a multisensory afferent input, which adapts the pattern to the actual requirements. Both the programmed pattern and the reflex mechanisms are under supraspinal control. (From Jankowska & Lundberg 1981.)

Besides the leg movements, swinging of the arms is essential to stabilize the body during locomotion (Elftman 1939). On the basis of the locomotor pattern induced in patients with complete para- or tetraplegia, it is suggested that the neuronal circuits responsible for the control of locomotion are coupled with those responsible for arm movements during locomotion (Dietz *et al.* 1999). It was found that the higher the level of spinal cord lesion the more 'normal' was the locomotor pattern. This suggests that neuronal circuits underlying locomotor 'pattern generation' in humans are *not* restricted to any specific level(s) of the spinal cord, but that an intricate neuronal network contributing to bipedal locomotion extends from thoracolumbal to cervical levels.

Central programming

A 'motor programme' has been variously defined in the literature as 'communications in the CNS that are based on past experience and that can generate postural adjustments and movements' (Brooks 1979) or as 'a set of muscle commands that are structured before a movement sequence begins and that allows the entire sequence to be carried out uninfluenced by peripheral feedback' (Keele 1968). However, in human gait, neither definition is totally accurate. With respect to the first definition, programmes are not based solely upon experience but are also innate. Steplike movements are present at birth, spontaneously initiated or triggered by peripheral stimuli. A central origin of these movements is implied, as the EMG bursts precede the actual mechanical events (Forssberg 1986). Infant stepping also occurs in anencephalic children (Forssberg 1986), which suggests that a spinal mechanism coordinates the movement. More generally, central programming in the context of gait generates a complex and widespread pattern of muscle activation triggered by external or internal events.

With regard to the second definition of central programming, it is known that 'programmed' movements can be influenced by sensory input under some circumstances (Brooks 1979). This again is illustrated by infant stepping. Although rhythmic alternating leg movements are coordinated by a central generator, the infant is unable to maintain body equilibrium. These children lack the appropriate afferent input to be integrated into the programmed leg muscle EMG pattern that is needed to achieve modulation and adaptation to the actual needs.

To achieve functional movement it is reasonable to assume that afferent information would influence the central pattern and, conversely, that the central pattern generator would select the appropriate afferent information. Recently, the effect of changing stance conditions on anticipatory postural adjustments (APA) and reaction time (RT) to voluntary arm movement was studied (Dietz *et al.* 2000). It was found that both the RT and the duration of APA can be modified by a translation of the support surface in a functionally appropriate way by updating the internal representation of actual stance condition within the central nervous system.

In addition, the programmed motor response in humans can be altered by instruction or by expectation. This 'set'-dependent aspect of muscle responses (see Prochazka 1989) is thought to depend on cerebellar integrity (Hore & Vilis 1985). Voluntary commands have to interact with the spinal locomotor generator in order to change, for example, the direction of gait or to avoid an obstacle. The significance of corticospinal input upon the gait pattern has recently been investigated using transcranial magnetic stimulation of the motor cortex during locomotion (Schubert *et al.* 1997). Only in the tibialis anterior was there an extrafacilitation of the evoked motor response prior to and during the swing phase of the stride cycle (see Fig. 2.2). This phase-linked facilitation was proposed to ensure postural stability in case there was corticospinal intervention during locomotion.

A characteristic of human standing posture and gait is that a high centre of gravity is maintained over a relatively small base of support, i.e. the feet. To maintain this constant vertical stance postural adjustments are required. To investigate the mechanisms underlying the equilibrium control, perturbations of balance were elicited. For example, by using a treadmill the surface underneath the supporting leg can be translated

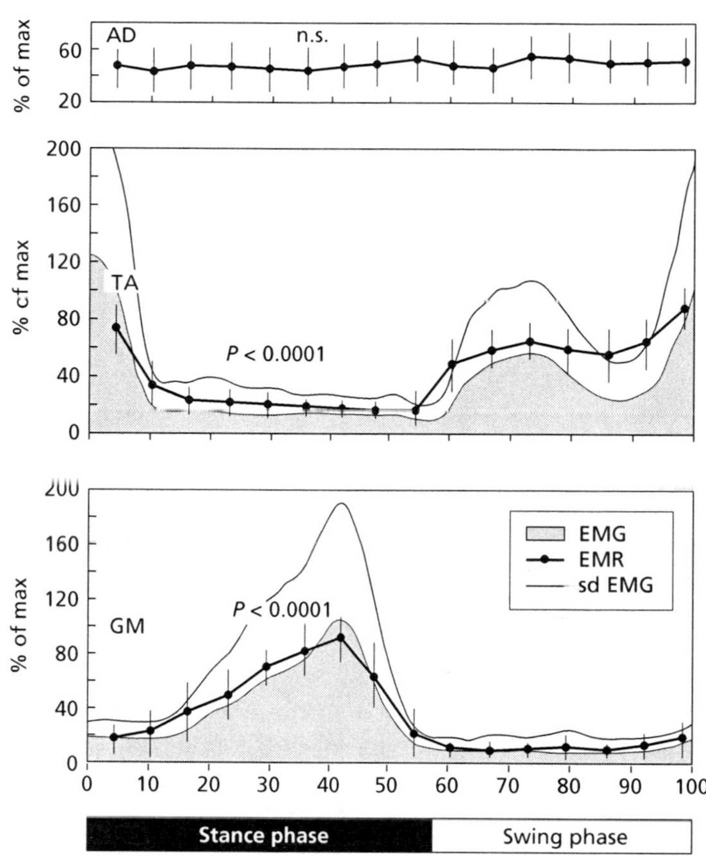

Fig. 2.2 Modulation of the corticospinal input during gait. Grand averages from all subjects ($n = 10$) of the motor response evoked by transcranial magnetic brain stimulation (EMR) in the tibialis anterior (TA) and gastrocnemius (GM) muscles during gait. The EMR amplitudes (root mean square values) were normalized with respect to the individual 95-percentile values. Means, standard deviations (bars) and the P-levels of an analysis of variance (ANOVA, repeated measurements design) are indicated. The rectified and averaged ($n = 45$) EMG pattern underlying one stride cycle is shown for the TA and GM (shaded areas). Stance/swing phases are indicated by the bar at the bottom. There is a significant modulation of the EMG with the TA and GM background EMG activity (shaded area) during step cycle, while no modulation is seen in the adductor digiti minimi (AD) muscle (control). An extrafacilitation of EMR amplitude occurs in the TA before the onset and at the end of the swing phase of gait. (From Schubert *et al.* 1997.)

backwards or forwards. Alternatively the swing phase of the non-supporting leg can be blocked. Directionally specific compensatory responses are induced in synergistic muscles of both legs following such perturbations.

The activity pattern to such perturbations is thought to be largely programmed, although a reflex contribution affecting the duration of the first burst of the pattern has been demonstrated (Angel 1974). The muscle response to a given displacement differs according to the actual conditions of gait. For example, an obstruction of leg movement can be introduced at the beginning or the end of the swing phase (Dietz *et al.* 1986b) or a displacement of the feet can be induced during stance on a narrow support (Nashner & McCollum 1985). For the selection of the appropriate postural movement strategy, studies done on subjects with somatosensory or vestibular loss indicate that both modes of sensory information can play an important role (Horak *et al.* 1990).

The assumption that the various response patterns to perturbations of stance and gait are programmed in their basic structure (presumably on a spinal level) and appropriately selected (i.e. triggered), is based on the complexity of the patterns which themselves cannot be explained by local afferent input and the dependence of the response pattern on the actual conditions (i.e. the phase of the step cycle).

Further evidence for the release of a fixed central programme in these compensatory postural patterns has been provided by the observation that when a second perturbation impulse in the

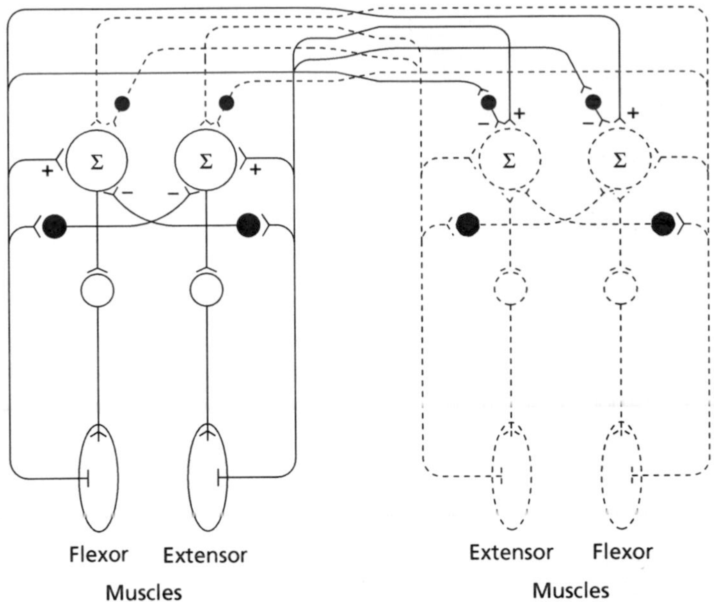

Fig. 2.3 Interlimb coordination of the legs during stance and gait. The excitatory and inhibitory pathways found to be involved in the coordination are schematically drawn. (From Dietz *et al.* 1989a.)

opposite direction was applied shortly after the first, the initial compensatory response was unchanged in neither amplitude nor timing. The remainder of the response pattern evoked by the second disturbance appeared time-locked to the second stimulus. This part was identical in form to the corresponding part of the response obtained when the second displacement was applied in isolation (Dietz *et al.* 1986a).

Regulation of human locomotion is based on the finely tuned coordination of muscle activation between both legs. The normal automatic coordination of the legs requires that adequate neuronal mechanisms exist to achieve task-directed coupling of bilateral leg muscle activation. Interlimb coordination is necessary to keep the body's centre of gravity over the feet (Dietz *et al.* 1989a). During unilateral displacements, a bilateral activation of corresponding leg muscles occurs (Fig. 2.3). The rapid, automatic coaction of muscles of the non-displaced leg provides a base from which to compensate for the perturbation and to keep the body's centre of gravity over the feet. Also, unilateral tactile stimuli evoke a bilateral response pattern, which is modulated in a phase-dependent manner (Tax *et al.* 1995).

Interlimb coordination is thought to be based on a central mechanism and, in view of the short latencies of the bilateral responses, is likely to be mediated at a spinal level (Berger *et al.* 1984; Dietz *et al.* 1989a; Tax *et al.* 1995). A cerebellar contribution to interlimb coordination, via reticulospinal neurones, has also been suggested (Bonnet *et al.* 1976). Close interaction exists between those spinal interneuronal circuits responsible for interlimb coordination and peripheral afferent input. When displacements of different velocity are induced unilaterally, reflex responses in synergistic muscles of both legs are graded according to the size of the proprioceptive input from the displaced joint (Dietz *et al.* 1989a). Also during split-belt walking, interlimb coordination provides a quick adaptation to different velocities on the two sides (Jensen *et al.* 1998). In these experiments it could be shown that the actual afferent input influences this adaptation, i.e. that there exists an interaction between central and peripheral mechanisms. Body unloading or loading during the training period resulted in an improved adjustment of treadmill belt speed. This suggests that load receptor information plays a major role in the programming of a new walking pattern.

Reflex mechanisms

Several studies have demonstrated that the contribution of proprioceptive input to the regulation of stance and locomotion is not 'mild', as originally suggested by Sherrington (1906). These include studies on patients with postural instability (Marsden *et al.* 1984; Sanes & Evarts 1984; Sanes *et al.* 1985) or gait impairment (Lajoie *et al.* 1996) observed in deafferented humans or in patients following loss of proprioceptive input from the legs due to ischaemic nerve blockade (Mauritz & Dietz 1980; Diener *et al.* 1984). Feedback information from muscles, joints and associated tissues via proprioceptive reflex systems is required to adjust the motor programme to irregularities of the ground during walking or to respond if the leg encounters resistance. This proprioceptive input modulates muscle EMG activity in the legs during locomotion in connection with changes in tension. This closely correlates with the level of EMG activity during different speeds of locomotion (Gollhofer *et al.* 1984). Although proprioceptive information may be used to achieve servoregulation of, for example, muscle length during stabilization of posture, this still represents only one specific way in which the nervous system utilizes proprioceptive input. Spinal reflex responses are not stereotyped to a given sensory input but, depending upon the descending and segmental conditions, different available pathways are utilized (see Schomburg 1990). The following sections of this chapter discuss the action and possible significance of monosynaptic and polysynaptic spinal reflexes.

Significance of monosynaptic reflexes

The potential significance of group I afferent input to locomotion is based on the fact that its gain can be modulated by presynaptic inhibition and by changes of muscle spindle sensitivity via the fusimotor system (Matthews 1972; Stein 1978; Loeb & Hoffer 1985). Several studies using indirect methods have investigated the presynaptic inhibition of group I afferents during human gait (Morin *et al.* 1982; Capaday & Stein 1986, 1987). Both peripheral afferent inputs and supraspinal influences have been implicated in the modulation of presynaptic inhibition of transmission from primary afferents (for review see Baldissera *et al.* 1981). This modulation of reflex gain might take place on common spinal interneurones where a convergence of descending tracts and several different afferent systems occurs (Lundberg 1975; for review see Baldissera *et al.* 1981). For spinal motor systems, presynaptic inhibition provides a way to modulate the relative contribution of afferents to a given reflex response.

During locomotion, the threshold and amplitude of the soleus/gastrocnemius H-reflex is modulated over the entire step cycle. Maximal facilitation occurs at the end of the stance phase and maximal inhibition occurs during the swing and the beginning of the stance phases (Capaday & Stein 1986; Crenna & Frigo 1987). However, over the entire step cycle, the amplitude of the H-reflex of the leg extensor muscles was considerably smaller than that during stance (Morin *et al.* 1984; Capaday & Stein 1986, 1987; Stein & Capaday 1988).

Earlier studies have indicated that monosynaptic stretch reflexes are inhibited in much the same way as the H-reflex during gait (Berger *et al.* 1984; Burke 1983; Llewellyn *et al.* 1987; Dietz *et al.* 1990). This also implied that there was no dramatic change in the gamma motoneurone drive to the soleus/gastrocnemius muscle spindles. Recent experiments in humans have indicated that modulation of the short-latency stretch reflex occurs during the step cycle with a significant reflex contribution being observed during the transition from stance to swing and also during the early stance phase. In the latter experiments (Sinkjaer *et al.* 1996) a rotational displacement which induced foot dorsiflexion was applied during different phases of the step cycle.

However, a qualitatively different response pattern with a small or absent short-latency stretch reflex response was obtained for similar stretches of the triceps surae than when a backward translation was induced during stance and gait (Berger *et al.* 1984; Gollhofer *et al.* 1989). The discrepancy between these different approaches investigating the contribution of short-latency stretch reflexes to leg muscle activation during gait may be due to the mode of displacement. The possibility exists that different extensor load receptor input occurs between translational and rotational displacements (Dietz *et al.* 1992). This may account for the differing strength of monosynaptic stretch reflex activity between the two modes of perturbation (see also 'Significance of load receptor input' below).

The functional implications of modulation of group I afferent input during locomotion have been suggested to be twofold. Firstly, facilitation of the gastrocnemius/soleus stretch reflex at the end of the stance phase contributes towards the compensation of ground irregularities and assists during the push-off phase (Nichols & Houk 1976; Capaday & Stein 1986, 1987; Sinkjaer *et al.* 1996). Secondly, the depression of leg extensor Ia input during the swing phase prevents the occurrence of the extensor stretch reflex during ankle dorsiflexion (Capaday & Stein 1986).

The functional significance of monosynaptic stretch reflexes during gait remains obscure for the following reasons. According to the properties of the monosynaptic stretch reflex (Sanes & Evarts 1984; for review see Matthews 1972) with a high sensitivity for small inputs, its use during gait should be restricted to compensation for ground irregularities. Furthermore, during postural tasks only polysynaptic EMG responses show direction-specific effects. This is not the case for short-latency EMG responses (Woollacott *et al.* 1984).

Significance of polysynaptic reflexes

Although rapid stretches of triceps surae occur during translational perturbations of gait, no significant EMG responses are elicited within the range of a monosynaptic transmission, whereas strong EMG responses appear with longer latency. Further investigations have indicated that primary afferent input from leg and foot muscles is not likely to play a dominant role in mediating compensatory leg muscle EMG responses to translational perturbations (Berger *et al.* 1984; Dietz *et al.* 1985).

It has been suggested that compensatory polysynaptic responses in the leg muscles evoked in response to translational perturbations during gait are mediated predominantly by muscle proprioceptive input from group II (see Berger *et al.* 1984; Matthews 1984; Lundberg *et al.* 1987; Nardone *et al.* 1996) and even group III (see Hasan & Stuart 1984) afferent fibres. However, it should be stressed that those studies provided no direct, positive evidence for this assumption.

A polysynaptic pathway probably mediates the effects of flexion reflex afferents (FRA; for review see Lundberg 1979) as there are several similarities to the phasic modulation of flexion reflexes observed during locomotion in humans (Duysens & Pearson 1980; Kanda & Sato 1983; Belanger & Patla 1984; Duysens *et al.* 1990, 1996a,b; Yang & Stein 1990). Because this pathway is polysynaptic it allows the integration of input from muscle, joint and cutaneous afferents with commands from supraspinal centres. In addition, these reflexes have excitatory and inhibitory connections to both extensors and flexors, respectively (Duysens *et al.* 1990, 1996a,b).

Clearly the polysynaptic reflex system does not behave as a simple stretch reflex mechanism as its function depends on both multisensory afferent information and supraspinal influences. However, the behaviour of these reflexes during locomotion must still result in a defined pattern of activity (see Gurfinkel *et al.* 1979; Ito 1982; Loeb *et al.* 1989). Based on the findings that the covariation of muscle activity across several joints cannot be explained simply by differences in stretch input from local muscles, a close interaction between a central programme and muscle proprioceptive input may occur to generate the appropriate pattern (Gurfinkel & Latash 1979;

Dietz *et al.* 1989a; for review see Dietz 1992, 1996; see also Gurfinkel *et al.* 1979; Matthews 1988; Macpherson *et al.* 1989). Sensory input during postural tasks may determine the direction, velocity and amplitude of the adjustment that is needed to restore the subject's centre of gravity over the feet.

However, this influence occurs in a continuous interaction with other afferent input and central mechanisms. For example, a modulation of cutaneous reflexes was shown to occur by changes of load receptor input during walking (Bastiaanse *et al.* 2000). In the latter study reflex amplitudes increased with body unloading and decreased with body loading. However, the reflex responses were not a simple function of the level of background activity. For example, in gastrocnemius and soleus, the largest reflex responses occurred during walking with body unloading, when background activity was decreased. Hence, stable ground conditions (body loading) yielded smaller reflexes. It was suggested that load receptors are involved in the regulation of cutaneous reflex responses in order to adapt the locomotor pattern to the environmental conditions.

Significance of load receptor input

To study the relative contribution of a given mechanism to motor control during human posture and gait, Nashner (1976) introduced the following experimental paradigm. Subjects stood on a moveable platform that could be activated on command to slide horizontally forwards or backwards or tilt 'toes up' or 'toes down'. The EMG pattern induced by dorsiflexing rotation of the feet was basically different from that induced by backward platform translations even though the triceps surae were stretched at a similar velocity in both conditions.

Following dorsiflexing *rotations* of the feet a small, short-latency response in the gastrocnemius was followed by a stronger activation of the tibialis anterior. The latter activity was required to compensate for the backward sway of the body induced by the rotation. In contrast, backward *translation* was followed only by strong, long-latency (about 80 ms) gastrocnemius activity. This EMG activity resulted in the restoration of a stable, vertical position over the feet. It was suggested that the difference in the EMG pattern between the two conditions was due to a *reflex adaptation* based upon the assumption that postural stabilization is the product of diminishing muscular destabilization (Nashner 1976). This adaptation was assumed to be achieved through a selection of appropriate postural reflexes. If the input is 'inappropriate' for a functionally directed tibialis anterior (rotational) or gastrocnemius (translational) activation, successive 'adaptation' of the reflex response occurs within two to four trials.

However, subsequent experiments failed to support this concept of adaptation of the response pattern. Rather they have shown that there is an immediate change within the first trial following the perturbation (Hansen *et al.* 1988; Gollhofer *et al.* 1989). Therefore, the neuronal mechanisms are directed towards maintaining the body's centre of mass over the feet. Depending upon the stance condition, muscle stretch need not necessarily result in a compensatory stretch reflex response but may instead result in activation of antagonistic muscles. The generation of an appropriate compensatory response pattern was suggested to be achieved by the integration of multiple divergent sensory inputs on a spinal level (Hansen *et al.* 1988; Gollhofer *et al.* 1989).

The question of how the position of the body's centre of mass relative to the feet is reported has been neglected in most investigations of postural control (for exceptions see Clément *et al.* 1985; Mittelstaedt 1995). Indeed we are just beginning to appreciate the influence that gravity has on sensory information and motor behaviour. For appropriate gain control of postural reflexes, peripheral information is required that determines the influence of 'gravity' as well as the inputs from muscle stretch receptors and the vestibular system.

A basic aspect of the neuronal control of quadrupedal locomotion of the cat and of bipedal stance and gait of humans concerns the antigravity function of leg extensors (for review see Dietz & Duysens 2000). In humans proprioceptive reflexes involved in the maintenance of body equilibrium depend on the presence of contact forces opposing gravity. Extensor load receptors are thought to signal changes of the projection of body's centre of mass with respect to the feet. According to observations in the cat, this afferent input probably arises from Golgi tendon organs and represents a newly discovered function of these receptors in the regulation of stance and gait. From these experiments it can be concluded that during locomotion there is a closing of Ib inhibitory and an opening of Ib extensor facilitatory paths. In humans evidence for a significant contribution of load receptor contribution to leg muscle activation came from immersion experiments. Compensatory leg muscle activation depends on the actual body weight. Also during gait the strength of leg extensor activation during the stance phase is load dependent.

The effect of reduced weight, induced by water immersion, upon those receptors involved in signalling changes in the position of the body's centre of mass has been studied (Dietz *et al.* 1989b; Dietz & Colombo 1996). The advantage of this particular technique compared with postural reactions during space flights (Clément *et al.* 1985) is that it does not affect vestibular function yet still allows manipulation of body mass. If a gravity dependence of the compensatory EMG responses exists then manipulation of the force between the feet and the support platform should affect the responses to destabilizing platform movements.

During immersion, postural reactions were qualitatively similar to those seen under normal conditions and also during space flights (Clément *et al.* 1985). There was a close relationship between actual body weight and the magnitude of the EMG responses after both backward and forward displacements (Dietz *et al.* 1989b). However, no correlation existed between loading and the EMG responses when the subject was not submerged. This saturation of the response out of water might represent a natural limitation of muscle activation to prevent possible injury (e.g. rupture) of the musculoskeletal system.

In order to define both the type and properties of the receptor that signals the projection of the centre of body's mass relative to the feet, rotational and quasi-'translational' feet dorsiflexing displacements were induced during horizontal body posture and also with different loads applied to the body (Dietz *et al.* 1992). It was observed that only during translational displacements were different torques induced by loading which resulted in compensatory activation of the leg extensor muscles. The rotational impulses were followed by a small, short-latency EMG response (Fig. 2.4). The translational impulses were followed by a stronger gastrocnemius response of longer latency compared to the rotational response. Application of a load to the body acting against the moveable platform had a significant effect only on the magnitude of the long-latency gastrocnemius response following translational perturbation. Increased loading of the body against the support area augments the torque only in the translational displacement condition. The magnitude of the torque during translational impulses is directly proportional to the amount of the loading, according to the formula

$$T = L \times r$$

where T is torque, L is load and r is translation distance. Therefore it was assumed that load receptors in the leg extensors were mainly responsible for the different EMG patterns and thus explained their antigravity function (Dietz *et al.* 1992).

A potentially excitatory function of load receptors during locomotion has been described for the extensor muscles of the cat (Duysens & Pearson 1980; Conway *et al.* 1987; Pearson & Collins 1993; Gossard *et al.* 1994). Accordingly, the function of those reflexes known to be involved in the stabilization of human posture (e.g. muscle proprioceptive and vestibulospinal reflexes) might depend on the activity of receptors within the body that indicate deviations of the body's centre of mass from a certain neutral

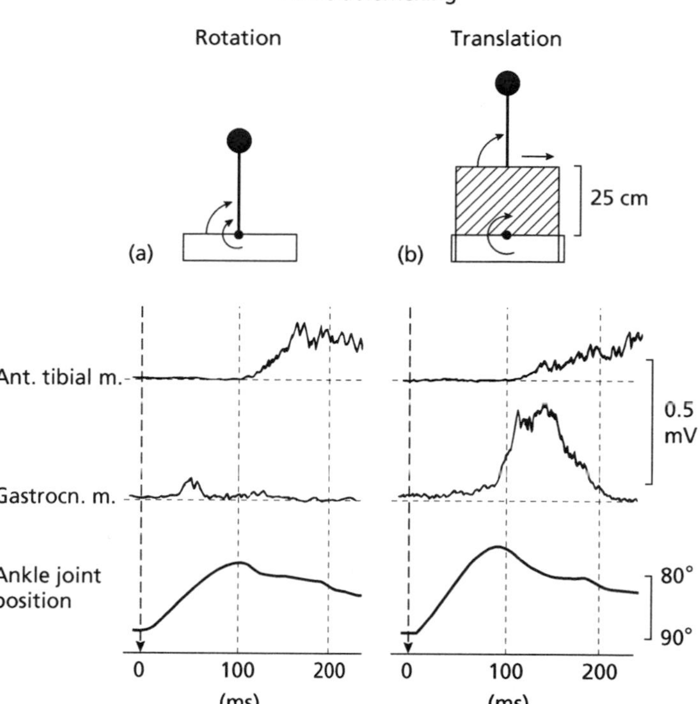

Fig. 2.4 Mean of rectified and averaged (n = 10) leg muscle EMG responses together with the ankle joint position of 10 subjects following a dorsiflexing rotation of the platform colinear with the ankle joint, and with the ankle joints 25 cm above the rotational axis during upright stance. The schematic illustrations indicate the movement induced by the two impulse modalities. (After Dietz *et al.* 1992.)

position. Similarly to the cat, human extensor load receptor input could provide such essential information. In the cat experiments it was suggested that these receptor signals arise from Golgi tendon organs and are mediated by Ib afferents to the spinal locomotor generator.

Vestibular and visual function

The contribution of the *vestibular* system to the destabilization of stance and gait is debatable. Several observations indicate that this system is involved in the stabilization of the head and in the compensation of body sway by vestibulospinal reflexes. The vestibular system is believed to be essential for balance whenever other sources of information (e.g. from the proprioceptive and visual systems) are irregular or reduced (Horak *et al.* 1990). The contribution of the vestibular system to compensatory reactions during stance and gait is obviously of minor significance. For example, during situations where horizontal displacement of the feet occurs leg muscle EMG activity attributed to vestibulospinal reflexes is small compared with that induced by proprioceptive reflexes (Dietz *et al.* 1988a,b; Fitzpatrick *et al.* 1994; Horak *et al.* 1994). Patients who had lost vestibular function as infants had near-normal trunk and leg responses to head displacement, suggesting that substitution of upper trunk and neck somatosensory input for missing vestibular inputs had occurred during development (Horak *et al.* 1994).

During locomotion the *visual* system was found to be essential for feedforward control of postural adjustments, and thus maximal stability, when afferent input from other sources was reduced (Fitzpatrick *et al.* 1994). Visual information is used to regulate locomotion on a local level (step-by-step basis) and a global level (route planning) and is related to the feedforward control of foot positioning in order to circumvent obstacles (Patla *et al.* 1991; for review see Patla 1997).

Not only does vision contribute to body sway stabilization in the low-frequency range but it can also influence postural stability, especially when it is contradictory to other sensory input. In these situations stabilization of posture is achieved by rapid adaptation to the new situation. This is related to an altered weighting of the afferent inputs (Nashner & Berthoz 1978; Harris 1980).

The influence of supraspinal mechanisms on this weighting of afferent information was studied by magnetically evoked motor responses in a precision stepping task (Schubert *et al.* 1999). There was increased facilitation of gastrocnemius (GM) evoked motor potentials (EMPs) during the swing phase of a visual task, prior to heel strike and prior to plantarflexion, which was the moment when the target was hit. Thus, the effect of visual input upon EMP in the tibialis anterior and GM was differential and reciprocal according to the respective functional state. The results support the hypothesis of a conditioning effect of visual, or alternatively volitional, drive on EMPs during stepping.

The motor cortex is obviously one of the principal structures involved in the control of such anticipatory gait modifications (Beloozerova & Sirota 1998; for reviews see Drew 1993).

Interaction between central programmes and afferent input

There is general agreement that the control of gait is not based on local reflex responses but that a selection and integration of peripheral and supraspinal inputs occurs to generate an appropriate response pattern (for review see Baldissera *et al.* 1981).

For example, in many leg muscles the stimulation of cutaneous afferents from the foot elicits reflex responses with an amplitude and sign dependent on the phase of the step cycle during gait (Pijnappels *et al.* 1998). This is functionally meaningful since reflexes may be useful in some phases but unwanted in others. For example, a flexor reflex is appropriate at the onset of the swing phase when the leg is flexed, but the same reflex is not convenient at end swing when the foot is ready to take up body weight. Some of the modulation may be provided by the locomotor pattern generator, but it is also possible that interaction between afferent inputs is important (for a review see Brooke *et al.* 1997) or that supraspinal sources play a role.

Recently, the cortical convergence on sural nerve reflex pathways was investigated by means of transcranial magnetic stimulation (TMS) of the cortex during the step cycle during human walking on a treadmill (Pijnappels *et al.* 1998). For both tibialis anterior (TA) and biceps femoris (BF) muscles, the data showed a significant facilitation mainly in the swing phase of the step cycle. This indicates a facilitation of corticospinal input onto cutaneous reflex pathways at distinct phases of the step cycle.

These observations have led to the question as to how so much information can be processed within a short time. Some interesting hypotheses concerning this problem have been proposed. All are based on the premise that error detection occurs by comparison of the ongoing movement with a central reference pattern, i.e. by the divergence from the anticipated movements by the actual stepping movements (Nashner 1980). In 1950 von Holst and Mittelstaedt proposed the 'Reafferenzprinzip' as the organizational principle of neuronal motor control, an idea subsequently extended by Held (1961). According to this theory, each efferent central command is accompanied by an 'efference copy' in the central pattern generator. The actual movement is signalled back as the reafference and compared with the efference copy. Deviations from this copy determine the compensatory reaction. A similar organization for the adjustment of an ongoing movement to a central body representation (the 'body scheme') for postural stabilization was put forward by Gurfinkel *et al.* (1988).

Although these hypotheses have still to be substantiated by experimental findings there is increasing support in favour of such control mechanisms. The fusimotor system may be acting not to report what is actually occurring at the spindles but rather whether or not what is happening differs from that which was expected to happen (Loeb 1984). Indicative of such control is the similarity between the response patterns of the obstruction of a limb movement (Dietz *et al.* 1986b) and limb displacement (Berger *et al.* 1984) during locomotion. Following a stumble, the corrective antagonist muscle command could in theory be computed on the basis of reafference from the agonist muscle command from an efference copy in the cerebellum (see Hore & Vilis 1985). This is a process by which appropriate compensatory patterns could be rapidly generated.

References

Angel, R.W. (1974) Electromyography during voluntary movement: the two-burst pattern. *Electroencephalography and Clinical Neurophysiology* **36**, 493–498.

Armstrong, D.M. (1988) The supraspinal control of mammalian locomotion. *Journal of Physiology (London)* **405**, 1–37.

Arshavsky, Y.I., Berkinblit, M.B., Gelfand, I.M., Orlovsky, G.N. & Fukson, O.I. (1972) Activity of the neurons of the dorsal spinocerebellar tract during locomotion. *Biophysics* **17**, 506–514.

Baldissera, F., Hultborn, H. & Illert, M. (1981) Integration in spinal neuronal systems. In: *Handbook of Physiology*, Sect. 1, Vol. II, Part 1. *The Nervous System. Motor Control* (eds J.M. Brookhart & V.B. Mountcastle), 12: pp. 509–595. American Physiological Society, Washington DC.

Bastiaanse, C.M., Duysens, J. & Dietz, J. (2000) Modulation of cutaneous reflexes by load receptor input during walking. *Experimental Brain Research* **135**, 189–198.

Belanger, M. & Patla, A.E. (1984) Corrective responses to perturbation applied during walking in humans. *Neuroscience Letters* **49**, 291–295.

Beloozerova, I.N. & Sirota, M.G. (1988) Role of motor cortex in control of locomotion. In: *Stance and Motor, Facts and Concepts* (eds V.S. Gurfinkel, M.E. Joffe, J. Massion & J.P. Roll), pp. 163–176. Plenum Press, New York.

Berger, W., Dietz, V. & Quintern, J. (1984) Corrective reactions to stumbling in man: neuronal coordination of bilateral leg muscle activity during gait. *Journal of Physiology (London)* **357**, 109–125.

Bernstein, N.A. (1936) Die kymozyclographische Methode der Bewegungsuntersuchung. In: *Handbuch der Biologischen Arbeitsmethoden*, Sect. 5, Part 5A (ed. E. Abderhalden), pp. 629–680. Urban Schwarzenberg, Wien.

Bickel, A. (1897) Über den Einfluss der sensiblen Nerven und der Labyrinthe auf die Bewegungen der Tiere. *Pflügers Archiv Gesamte Physiologie der Menschen Tiere* **67**, 299–344.

Bonnet, M., Gurfinkel, S., Lipchits, M.J. & Popov, K.E. (1976) Central programming of lower limb muscular activity in the standing man. *Agressologie* **17** (Suppl. B), 35–42.

Brooke, J.D. *et al.* (1997) Sensori-sensory afferents conditioning with leg movement: gain control in spinal reflex and ascending paths. *Progress in Neurobiology* **51**, 393–421.

Brooks, V.B. (1979) Motor programs revisited. In: *Posture and Movement* (eds R.E. Talbott & D.R. Humphrey), pp. 13–49. Raven Press, New York.

Burke, D. (1983) Critical examination of the case for or against fusimotor involvement in disorders of muscle tone. In: *Advances in Neurology Motor Control: Mechanisms in Health and Disease*, Vol. 39 (ed. J.E. Desmedt), pp. 133–150. Raven, New York.

Capaday, C. & Stein, R.B. (1986) Amplitude modulation of the soleus H-reflex in the human during walking and standing. *Journal of Neuroscience* **6**, 1308–1313.

Capaday, C. & Stein, R.B. (1987) Difference in the amplitude of the human soleus H-reflex during walking and running. *Journal of Physiology (London)* **392**, 513–522.

Clément, G., Gurfinkel, S., Lestienne, F., Lipchits, M.I. & Popov, K.E. (1985) Changes of posture during transient perturbations in microgravity. *Aviation Space and Environmental Medicine* **56**, 666–671.

Conway, B.A., Hultborn, H. & Kiehn, O. (1987) Proprioceptive input resets central locomotor rhythm in the spinal cat. *Experimental Brain Research* **68**, 643–656.

Crenna, P. & Frigo, C. (1987) Excitability of the soleus H-reflex arc during walking and stepping in man. *Experimental Brain Research* **66**, 49–60.

Diener, H.C., Dichgans, J., Guschlbauer, B. & Mau, H. (1984) The significance of proprioception on postural stabilization as assessed by ischemia. *Brain Research* **296**, 103–109.

Dietz, V. (1992) Human neuronal control of automatic functional movements: interaction between central programs and afferent input. *Physiological Reviews* **72**, 33–69.

Dietz, V. (1997) Neurophysiology of gait disorders: present and future applications. *Electroencephalography and Clinical Neurophysiology* (Review) **103**, 333–355.

Dietz, V. (1996) Interaction between central programs and afferent input in the control of posture and locomotion. *Journal of Biomechanics* **29**, 841–844.

Dietz, V. & Colombo, G. (1996) Effects of body immersion on postural adjustments to voluntary arm movements in humans: role of load receptor input. *Journal of Physiology (London)* **497**, 849–856.

Dietz, V. & Duysens, J. (2000) Modulation of reflex mechanisms by load receptors. *Gait and Posture* **11**, 102–110.

Dietz, V., Quintern, J., Berger, W. & Schenk, E. (1985) Cerebral potentials and leg muscle EMG responses associated with stance perturbation. *Experimental Brain Research* **57**, 348–354.

Dietz, V., Quintern, J. & Berger, W. (1986a) Stumbling reactions in man: release of a ballistic movement pattern. *Brain Research* **362**, 355–357.

Dietz, V., Quintern, J., Boos, G. & Berger, W. (1986b) Obstruction of the swing phase during gait: phase-dependent bilateral leg muscle coordination. *Brain Research* **384**, 166–169.

Dietz, V., Horstmann, G.A. & Berger, W. (1988a) Fast head tilt has only a minor effect on quick compensatory reactions during the regulation of stance and gait. *Experimental Brain Research* **73**, 470–476.

Dietz, V., Horstmann, G.A. & Berger, W. (1988b) Involvement of different receptors in the regulation of human posture. *Neuroscience Letters* **94**, 82–87.

Dietz, V., Horstmann, G.A. & Berger, W. (1989a) Interlimb coordination of leg muscle activation during perturbation of stance in humans. *Journal of Neurophysiology* **62**, 680–693.

Dietz, V., Horstmann, G.A., Trippel, M. & Gollhofer, A. (1989b) Human postural reflexes and gravity: an underwater simulation. *Neuroscience Letters* **106**, 350–355.

Dietz, V., Discher, M., Faist, M. & Trippel, M. (1990) Amplitude modulation of the human quadriceps tendon jerk reflex during gait. *Experimental Brain Research* **82**, 211–213.

Dietz, V., Gollhofer, A., Kleiber, M. & Trippel, M. (1992) Regulation of bipedal stance: dependence on 'load' receptors. *Experimental Brain Research* **89**, 229–231.

Dietz, V., Nakazawa, K., Wirz, M. & Erni, Th. (1999) The level of spinal cord lesions determines the locomotor activity in spinal man. *Experimental Brain Research* **128**, 405–409.

Drew, T. (1993) Motor cortical activity during voluntary gait modifications in the cat. I. Cells related to forelimbs. *Journal of Neurophysiology* **79**, 179–199.

Duysens, J. & Pearson, K.G. (1980) Inhibition of flexor burst generation by loading extensor muscles in walking cats. *Brain Research* **187**, 321–332.

Duysens, J., Trippel, M., Horstmann, G.A. & Dietz, V. (1990) Gating and reversal of reflexes in ankle muscles during human walking. *Experimental Brain Research* **82**, 351–358.

Duysens, J., Tax, A.A.M., Murrer, L. & Dietz, V. (1996a) Backward and forward walking use different patterns of phase-dependent modulation of cutaneous reflexes in humans. *Journal of Neurophysiology* **76**, 301–310.

Duysens, J., van Wezel, B.M.H., Prokop, T. & Berger, W. (1996b) Medial gastrocnemius is more activated than lateral gastrocnemius in sural nerve induced reflexes during human gait. *Brain Research* **727**, 230–232.

Elftman, H. (1939) The function of the arm during walking. *Human Biology* **11**, 529–535.

Engberg, I. & Lundberg, A. (1969) An electromyographic analysis of muscular activity in the hindlimb of the cat during unrestrained locomotion. *Acta Physiologica Scandinavica* **75**, 614–630.

Fitzpatrick, R., Rogers, D.K. & McCloskey, D.I. (1994) Stable human standing with lower-limb muscle vestibular and visual proprioceptive afferents providing the only sensory input. *Journal of Physiology (London)* **480**, 395–403.

Forssberg, H. (1986) A developmental model of human locomotion. In: *Wenner-Gren International Symposium Series. Neurobiology of Vertebrate Locomotion*, Vol. 45 (eds S. Grillner, P.S.G. Stein, D.G. Stuart, H. Forssberg & R.M. Herman), pp. 485–501. Macmillan, London.

Forssberg, H., Grillner, S. & Rossignol, S. (1977) Phasic gain control of reflexes from the dorsum of the paw during spinal locomotion. *Brain Research* **132**, 121–139.

Förster, O. (1927) Schlaffe und Spastische Lähmung. In: *Handbuch der Normalen und Pathologischen Physiologie*, Vol. 10 (eds A. Bethe, G. Bergmann, G. von Embden & A. Ellinger), pp. 893–972. Springer, Berlin.

Gollhofer, A., Schmidtbleicher, D. & Dietz, V. (1984) Regulation of muscle stiffness in human locomotion. *International Journal of Sports Medicine* **5**, 19–22.

Gollhofer, A., Horstmann, G.A., Berger, W. & Dietz, V. (1989) Compensation of translational and rotational perturbations in human posture: stabilization of the centre of gravity. *Neuroscience Letters* **105**, 73–78.

Gossard, J.P., Brownstone, R.M., Barajon, I. & Hultborn, H. (1994) Transmission in a locomotor-related group Ib pathway from hindlimb extensor muscles in the cat. *Experimental Brain Research* **98**, 213–228.

Grillner, S. (1972) The role of muscle stiffness in meeting the changing postural and locomotor requirements for force development by ankle extensors. *Acta Physiologica Scandinavica* **86**, 92–108.

Grillner, S. (1981) Control of locomotion in bipeds, tetrapods, and fish. In: *Handbook of Physiology*, Sect. 1, Vol. II, Part 2. *The Nervous System. Motor Control*, 26 (eds M. Brookhart & V.B. Mountcastle) pp. 1179–1236. American Physiological Society, Washington DC.

Grillner, S. (1986) Interaction between sensory signals and the central networks controlling locomotion in lamprey, dogfish and cat. In: *Neurobiology of Vertebrate Locomotion*, Vol. 45 (eds S. Grillner, P.S.G. Stein, D.G. Stuart, H. Forssberg. & R.M. Herman), *Wenner-Gren International Symposium Series*, pp. 505–512. Macmillan, London.

Gurfinkel, V.S. & Latash, M.L. (1979) Segemental postural mechanisms and reversals of muscle reflexes. *Agressologie* **20** (Suppl. B), 145–146.

Gurfinkel, S., Lipchits, M.I. & Popov, K.E. (1979) On the origin of short-latency muscle responses to postural disturbances. *Agressologie* **20** (Suppl. B), 153–154.

Gurfinkel, S., Levik, Y.S., Popov, K.E. & Sme-Tanin, B.N. (1988) Body scheme in the control of postural activity. In: *Stance and Motion Facts and Concepts* (eds S. Gurfinkel, M.E. Joffe, J. Massion & J.P. Roll), pp. 185–193. Plenum, New York.

Hansen, P.D., Woollacott, M.H. & Debu, B. (1988) Postural responses to changing task conditions. *Experimental Brain Research* **73**, 627–636.

Harris, C.S. (1980) Insight or out of sight? Two examples of perceptual plasticity in the human adult. In: *Visual Coding and Adaptability* (ed. C.S. Harris), pp. 95–149. Erlbaum and Hillsdale, NJ.

Hasan, Z. & Stuart, D.G. (1984) Mammalian muscle receptors. In: *Handbook of the Spinal Cord*, Vol. 3 (ed. R.A. Davidoff), pp. 559–607. Dekker, New York.

Held, R. (1961) Exposure history as a factor in maintaining stability of perception and coordination. *Journal of Nervous and Mental Diseases* **132**, 26–32.

Herder, J. G. (1785) *Ideen zur Philosphie der Geschichte der Menschheit*, Vol. I. Hartknoch, Leipzig.

Hering, H.E. (1897) Ueber Bewegungsstörungen nach centripetaler Lähmung. *Archiv der Experimentellen Pathologie und Pharmakologie* **38**, 266–283.

Hoffmann, P. (1922) *Die Eigenreflexe (Sehnenreflexe) Menschlicher Muskeln*. Springer, Berlin.

Horak, F.B., Nashner, L.M. & Diener, H.C. (1990) Postural strategies associated with somatosensory and vestibular loss. *Experimental Brain Research* **82**, 167–177.

Horak, F.B., Shupert, C.L., Dietz, V. & Horstmann, G. (1994) Vestibular and somatosensory contributions to responses to head and body displacements in stance. *Experimental Brain Research* **100**, 93–106.

Hore, J. & Vilis, T. (1985) A cerebellar-dependent efference copy mechanism for generating appropriate muscle responses to limb perturbations. In: *Proceedings in Life Sciences: Cerebellar Functions* (eds J.R. Bloedel, J. Dichgans & W. Precht), pp. 1–23. Springer, Heidelberg.

Ito, M. (1982) The CNS as a multivariable control system. *Behavioral Brain Science* **5**, 552–553.

Jankowska, E. & Lundberg, A. (1981) Interneurones in the spinal cord. *Trends in Neuroscience* **4**, 230–233.

Jensen, L., Prokop, T. & Dietz, V. (1998) Adaptational effects during human split belt walking: influence of afferent input. *Experimental Brain Research* **118**, 126–130.

Kanda, K. & Sato, H. (1983) Reflex responses of human thigh muscles to non-noxious sural stimulation during stepping. *Brain Research* **288**, 378–380.

Keele, S.W. (1968) Movement control in skilled motor performance. *Psychological Bulletin* **70**, 387–403.

Lajoie, Y., Teasdale, N., Cole, J.D. *et al.* (1996) Gait of a deafferented subject without large myelinated sensory fibers below the neck. *Neurology* **47**, 109–115.

Llewellyn, M., Prochazka, A. & Vincent, S. (1987) Transmission of human tendon jerk reflexes during stance and gait. *Journal of Physiology (London)* **382**, 82P.

Loeb, G.E. (1984) The control and responses of mammalian muscle spindles during normally executed motor tasks. *Exercise and Sport Sciences Reviews* **12**, 157–204.

Loeb, G.E. & Hoffer, J.A. (1985) Activity of spindle afferents from cat anterior thigh muscles. II. Effects of fusimotor blockade. *Journal of Neurophysiology* **54**, 565–577.

Loeb, G.E., He, J. & Levine, W.S. (1989) Spinal cord circuits: are they mirrors of musculoskeletal mechanics? *Journal of Motor Behaviour* **21**, 473–491.

Lundberg, A. (1975) Control of spinal mechanisms from the brain. In: *The Nervous System*, Vol. 1 (ed. D. B. Tower), pp. 253–265. Raven. New York.

Lundberg, A. (1979) Multisensory control of spinal reflex pathways. In: *Progress in Brain Research*, Vol. 50. *Reflex Control of Posture and Movement* (eds R. Granit & O. Pompeiano), pp. 12–28. Elsevier, Amsterdam.

Lundberg, A., Malmgren, K. & Schomburg, E.D. (1987) Reflex pathway from group I muscle afferents. 3. Secondary spindle afferents and the FRA: a new hypothesis. *Experimental Brain Research* **65**, 294–306.

MacPherson, J.M., Horak, F.B., Dunbar, D.C. & Dow, R.S. (1989) Stance dependence of automatic postural adjustments in humans. *Experimental Brain Research* **78**, 557–566.

Marey, E.J. (1894) *Le Mouvement*. Masson, Paris.

Marsden, C.D., Rothwell, J.C. & Day, B.L. (1984) The use of peripheral feedback in the control of movement. *Trends in Neuroscience* **7**, 253–257.

Matthews, P.B.C. (1972) *Mammalian Muscle Receptors and Their Central Actions*. Arnold, London.

Matthews, P.B.C. (1984) Evidence from the use of vibration that the human long-latency stretch reflex depends upon spindle secondary afferents. *Journal of Physiology (London)* **348**, 383–415.

Matthews, P.B.C. (1988) Proprioceptors and their contribution to somatosensory mapping: complex messages require complex processing. *Canadian Journal of Physiology and Pharmacology* **66**, 430–438.

Mauritz, K.H. & Dietz, V. (1980) Characteristics of postural instability induced by blocking of leg afferents by ischaemia. *Experimental Brain Research* **38**, 117–119.

Mittelstaedt, H. (1995) The formation of the visual and the postural vertical. In: *Multisensory Control of Pos-*

ture (eds T. Mergner & F. Hlavacka), pp. 147–155. Plenum, New York.

Morin, C., Katz, R., Mazières, L. & Pierrot-Deseilligny, E. (1982) Comparison of soleus H-reflex facilitation at the onset of soleus contractions produced voluntarily and during the stance phase of human gait. *Neuroscience Letters* **33**, 47–53.

Morin, C., Pierrot-Deseilligny, E. & Hultborn, H. (1984) Evidence for presynaptic inhibition of muslce spindle Ia afferents in man. *Neuroscience Letters* **44**, 137–142.

Nardone, A., Grasso, M., Giordano, A. & Schieppati, M. (1996) Different effect of height on latency of leg and foot short- and medium-latency EMG responses to perturbation of stance in humans. *Neuroscience Letters* **206**, 89–92.

Nashner, L.M. (1976) Adapting reflexes controlling the human posture. *Experimental Brain Research* **26**, 59–72.

Nashner, L.M. (1980) Balance adjustments of humans perturbed while walking. *Journal of Neurophysiology* **44**, 650–664.

Nashner, L.M. & Berthoz, A. (1978) Visual contribution to rapid motor responses during postural control. *Brain Research* **150**, 403–407.

Nashner, L.M. & McCollum, G. (1985) The organization of human postural movements: a formal basis and experimental synthesis. *Behavioral Brain Science* **8**, 135–172.

Nichols, T.R. & Houk, J. (1976) Improvement in linearity and regulation of stiffness that results from actions of stretch reflex. *Journal of Neurophysiology* **39**, 119–142.

Nilsson, J., Thorstensson, A. & Halbertsma, J. (1985) Changes in leg movements and muscle activity with speed of locomotion and mode of progression in humans. *Acta Physiologica Scandinavica* **123**, 457–475.

Patla, A.E. (1997) Understanding the roles of vision in the control of human locomotion (review article). *Gait and Posture* **5**, 54–69.

Patla, A.E., Prentice, S.D., Robinson, C. & Neufeld, J. (1991) Visual control of locomotion: strategies for changing direction and for going over obstacles. *Journal of Experimental Psychology: Human Perception and Performance* **17**, 603–634.

Pearson, K.G. & Collins, D.F. (1993) Reversal of the influence of group Ib-afferents from plantaris on activity in medial gastrocnemius muscle during locomotor activity. *Journal of Neurophysiology* **70**, 1009–1017.

Pijnappels, M., van Wezel, B.M.H., Colombo, G., Dietz, V. & Duysens, J. (1998) Cortical facilitation of cutaneous reflexes in leg muscles during human gait. *Brain Research* **787**, 149–153.

Prochazka, A. (1989) Sensorimotor gain control: a basic strategy of motor systems? *Progress in Neurobiology* **33**, 281–307.

Sanes, J.N. & Evarts, E.V. (1984) Motor psychophysics. *Human Neurobiology* **2**, 217–225.

Sanes, J.N., Mauritz, K.H., Dalakas, M.C. & Evarts, E.V. (1985) Motor control in humans with large-fiber sensory neuropathy. *Human Neurobiology* **4**, 101–114.

Schomburg, E.D. (1990) Spinal sensorimotor systems and their supraspinal control. *Neuroscience Research* **7**, 265–340.

Schubert, M., Curt, A., Jensen, L. & Dietz, V. (1997) Corticospinal input in human gait: modulation of magnetically evoked motor responses. *Experimental Brain Research* **115**, 234–246.

Schubert, M., Curt, A., Colombo, G., Berger, W. & Dietz, V. (1999) Voluntary control of human gait: conditioning of magnetically evoked responses in a precision stepping task. *Experimental Brain Research* **126**, 583–588.

Sherrington, C.S. (1906) On the proprioceptive system, especially its reflex aspect. *Brain* **29**, 476–482.

Sinkjaer, T., Anderson, J.B. & Larsen, B. (1996) Soleus stretch reflex modulation during gait in humans. *Journal of Neurophysiology* **76**, 1112–1120.

Stein, P.S.G. (1978) Motor systems, with specific reference to the control of locomotion. *Annual Review of Neuroscience* **1**, 61–81.

Stein, R.B. & Capaday, C. (1988) The modulation of human reflexes during functional motor tasks. *Trends in Neuroscience* **11**, 328–332.

Tax, A.A.M., van Wezel, B.M.H. & Dietz, V. (1995) Bipedal reflex coordination to tactile stimulation of the sural nerve during human running. *Journal of Neurophysiology* **73**, 1947–1964.

Thorstensson, A., Nillson, J., Carlson, H. & Zomlefer, M.R. (1984) Trunk movements in human locomotion. *Acta Physiologica Scandinavica* **121**, 9–22.

Woollacott, M.H., Bonnet, M. & Yabe, K. (1984) Preparatory process for anticipatory postural adjustments: modulation of leg muscles reflex pathways during preparation for arm movements in standing man. *Experimental Brain Research* **55**, 263–271.

Yang, J.F. & Stein, R.B. (1990) Phase-dependent reflex reversal in human leg muscles during walking. *Journal of Neurophysiology* **63**, 1109–1117.

Chapter 3

Motor Unit and Motoneurone Excitability during Explosive Movement

TOSHIO MORITANI

Introduction

The human neuromuscular system has evolved to cope with such a great diversity of internal and external demands and constraints. These include the regulation of force output for extremely powerful dynamic and static movements, locomotion, precise manipulation, upright posture, and even our repertoire of gestures. As it is impossible to describe all the specific control features of the various neuromuscular control systems in isolation, an attempt will be made to delineate the basic principles of motor control which play the major role in the control of force and explosive movements in humans.

Factors affecting motor unit activities and contractile characteristics

Neural control mechanism

There are a variety of specialized receptors located in the muscles, tendons, fascia and skin that provide information to appropriate parts of the central nervous system (CNS) concerning the length and force characteristics of the muscles during movements. The simplest functional element of the motor activity is the so-called 'stretch reflex'. Reflexes are mostly automatic, consistent and predictable reactions to sensory stimuli. A typical example of this stretch reflex can be demonstrated by a physician tapping a patient's knee, which will result in leg extension, regardless of the patient's intention. Figure 3.1 schematically represents the basic components involved in this stretch reflex.

Within each muscle fibre there are numerous sensory receptors called muscle spindles. Muscle spindles can provide information to the nervous system regarding the absolute length of the muscle and the rate of change of the length (velocity). The tap stretches the muscle and the resultant stretch is then detected by the muscle spindle and conveyed directly to a spinal motoneurone via a sensory afferent (Ia afferent). This leads to excitation of the motoneurone and efferent impulses that cause action of the corresponding muscle. In this way, the muscle is shortened, the stretching of the muscle spindles is removed and their Ia afferent activity diminishes. In this process, only one synapse is involved: a sensory Ia afferent to motoneurone. The term monosynaptic is therefore typically used to describe the stretch reflex. Although the stretch reflex is termed monosynaptic, the sensory afferent from the spindle also contacts interneurones, sensory neurones and neurones that send ascending projections to higher centres such as the thalamus. From there, processed messages return to the motoneurones, closing a longer parallel reflex arc. The stretch reflex therefore also has polysynaptic components (i.e. involving more than one synapse). Note that all reflexes, no matter how simple, can be modified by signals from the brain.

Muscle spindles are composed of intrafusal fibres, sensory endings and motor axons. Each spindle contains several muscle fibres and

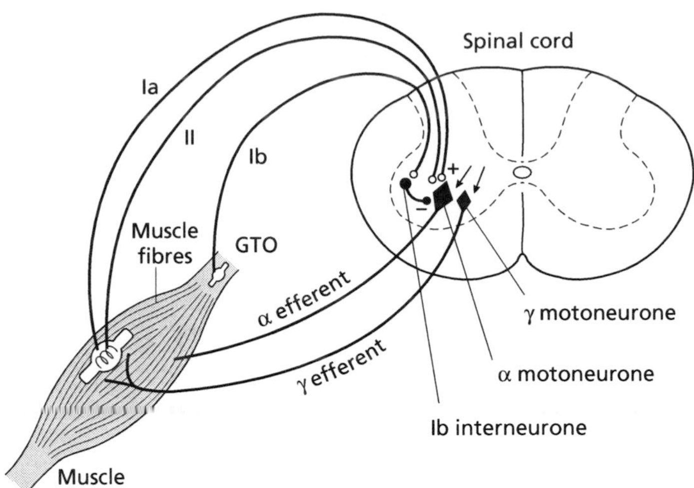

Fig. 3.1 A simplified schematic representation of basic neural components involved in the stretch reflex.

sensory endings and is innervated by fusiomotor neurones or gamma (γ) motoneurones (see Fig. 3.1). The main function of fusiomotor neurones is to control the sensitivity of muscle spindle afferents to dynamic stretches by innervating intrafusal muscle fibres. Some fusiomotor neurones (beta (β) motoneurones) innervate both extrafusal (skeletal) and intrafusal (muscle spindle) muscle fibres so as to adjust their length for optimizing sensitivity.

As just described, muscle spindles are only one type of receptor that provides information necessary for movement. Control of dynamic movements and posture requires monitoring not only of muscle length, but also of muscle tension. We do possess another specialized receptor called the Golgi tendon organ (GTO). GTOs are specialized sensory receptor organs located primarily in the musculotendinous junction. GTOs provide information regarding the amount of force, or tension, being generated within the muscle. Thus, the functioning of these peripheral receptors (muscle spindles and GTOs) is absolutely essential to the control of muscle action. GTOs have a low threshold (i.e. they tend to respond to small changes) for contraction-induced changes in muscle tension, and a higher threshold for stretch-induced tension.

The sensory information detected by the GTO receptors is conveyed via group Ib sensory afferents (see Fig. 3.1). Group Ib afferents from GTOs play a critical role in non-reciprocal inhibition. Non-reciprocal inhibition, also termed autogenic inhibition, refers to inhibitory input to an agonist (i.e. the prime mover) and its synergists concomitant with an excitatory input to opposing (antagonist) muscles. The inhibition of agonist motoneurone pools and the excitation of antagonist motoneurones are accomplished by Ib interneurones. This type of inhibition assists with the matching of muscle forces to the requirements of a motor task (Leonard 1998). Ib interneurones can be either facilitatory or inhibitory. GTO activation therefore results in many other responses in addition to non-reciprocal inhibition.

Now one should realize that smooth coordinated movement relies not only on muscle activation, but also on muscle deactivation. When you are trying to extend the arm by activating the triceps brachii muscle, it would be impossible if muscles that opposed that movement (i.e. the biceps brachii muscle) were contracting. As previously described, the Ia afferents that convey stretch reflex information branch when they enter the spinal cord (see Fig. 3.2).

Some of these branches synapse on interneurones. One type of interneurone that is contacted is the Ia inhibitory interneurone. So when you try to extend the arm, the muscle spindles of the arm extensor will be stimulated and cause stretch

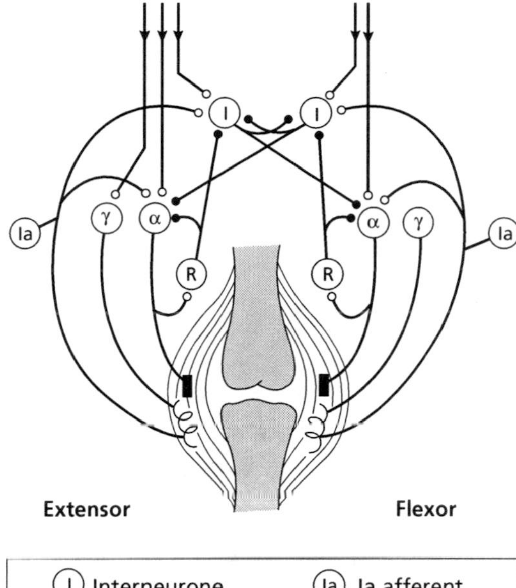

Fig. 3.2 Stretch reflex neural circuitry and neural–mechanical coupling between antagonistic pairs of limb musculature. (Modified from Moore & Hutton 1980.)

reflex together with excitation of this Ia inhibitory interneurone, which will have an inhibitory effect on motoneurones innervating muscles that are antagonists to the stretched muscle, in this case the arm flexor muscles. This process is referred to as reciprocal innervation (inhibition) or disynaptic inhibition because two synapses are involved in the inhibitory pathway. The Ia inhibitory interneurone receives rich convergent inputs from many other sources and processes in such a way that the appropriate amount of antagonist muscle inhibition is achieved. Obviously different motor tasks including explosive and static actions require varying degrees of antagonist muscle inhibition and synergist muscle activation.

Finally, inhibition of antagonists and other muscle groups can also be accomplished by Renshaw cell-mediated inhibition, Ib-mediated inhibition (discussed earlier in the GTO description), and presynaptic inhibitory mechanisms. Renshaw cells are interneurones that directly synapse on α motoneurones and Ia inhibitory interneurones (see Fig. 3.2). The Renshaw cell will inhibit the α motoneurone of a contracting muscle and its synergists. In addition, it will inhibit the antagonist muscle's Ia inhibitory interneurone (disinhibition). This aids in grading muscle actions and assisting task-appropriate agonist/antagonist coaction (Leonard 1998).

Motor unit

Figure 3.3 illustrates a simplified schematic diagram representing the central motor system and the concept of a motor unit (MU). As you already know, the central nervous system is organized in a hierarchical fashion. Motor programming takes place in the premotor cortex, the supplementary motor area and other association areas of the cortex. Inputs from these areas, from the cerebellum and, to some extent, from the basal ganglia converge to the primary motor cortex and excite or inhibit the various neurones of the primary motor cortex. The outputs from the primary motor cortex have a very powerful influence upon interneurones and motoneurones of the brainstem and of the spinal cord. There exists a link between the corticospinal tract and alpha (α) motoneurones, providing direct cortical control of muscle activity.

An MU consists of an α motoneurone in the spinal cord and the muscle fibres it innervates. The α motoneurone is the final point of summation for all the descending and reflex inputs, and the net membrane current of this motoneurone determines the discharge (motoneurone firing rate) pattern of the motor unit and thus the muscle activity. The number of MUs per muscle in humans may range from about 100 for a small hand muscle to 1000 or more for large limb muscles (Henneman *et al.* 1981). It has also been shown that different MUs vary greatly in force-generating capacity, i.e. a 100-fold or more difference in twitch force (Stephens & Usherwood 1977; Garnett *et al.* 1979).

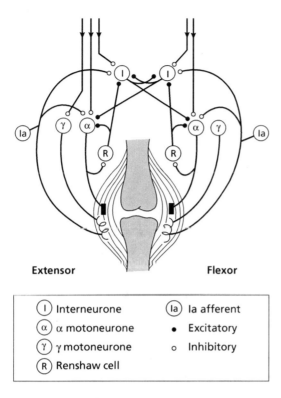

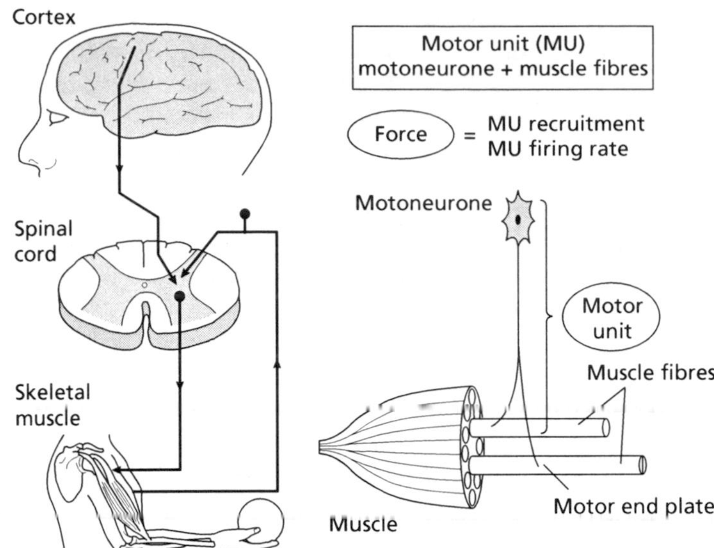

Fig. 3.3 A schematic representation of a motor unit and its basic components. (Modified from Sale 1981.)

Earlier studies (Burke 1981) identified three types of motor units based on physiological properties such as speed of action and fatigability (sensitivity to fatigue). According to Burke (1981) three types of motor units can be distinguished: (i) fast-twitch, fatigable (FF); (ii) fast-twitch, fatigue-resistant (FR); and slow-twitch (S), which is most resistant to fatigue. The FF type motor units are predominantly found in pale muscle (high ATPase content for anaerobic energy utilization, low capillarization, less haemoglobin, myoglobin and mitochondria for oxidative energy supply), while red muscle (low ATPase, high capillarization, abundant haemoglobin, myoglobin and mitochondria for oxidative energy supply) such as the soleus is predominantly composed of type S motor units.

The wide variation in the morphological and electrophysiological properties of the individual motoneurones comprising a motoneurone pool is matched by an equally wide range in the physiological properties of the muscle units they innervate. Interestingly, the muscle fibres that are innervated by a particular motoneurone manifest nearly identical biochemical, histochemical and contractile characteristics. Thus muscle fibre types can also be classified into three types: fast-twitch, glycolytic (FG or human equivalent of Type IIb); fast-twitch, oxidative glycolytic (FOG, Type IIa); and slow-twitch, oxidative (SO, Type I) fibres.

Motor unit recruitment and firing frequency (rate coding)

In voluntary actions, force is modulated by a combination of MU recruitment and changes in MU activation frequency (rate coding) (Milner-Brown *et al.* 1973; Kukulka & Clamann 1981; Moritani & Muro 1987). The greater the number of MUs recruited and their discharge frequency, the greater the force will be. It is generally accepted that common information from higher brain centres to the motoneurones is coded in the firing intervals at which the motoneurones are made to fire. In other words, information transmission in our nervous system is accomplished through frequency modulation. During MU recruitment the muscle force, when activated at any constant MU firing frequency, is approximately 2–5 kg·cm^{-2}, and in general is relatively independent of species, gender, age and training status (Ikai & Fukunaga 1970; Alway *et al.* 1990).

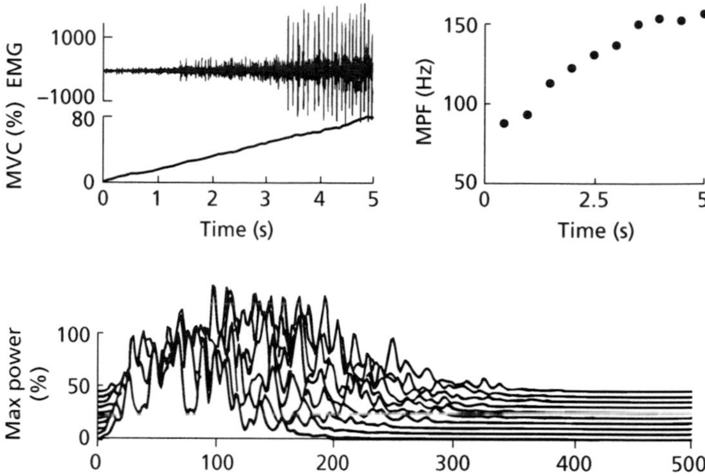

Fig. 3.4 A typical set of computer outputs showing the changes in raw EMG signal recorded from the biceps brachii muscle and the corresponding frequency power spectra during linearly force-varying isometric muscle action.

Our current understanding of MU recruitment is based on the pioneer work of Henneman and colleagues in the 1960s, who proposed that MUs are always recruited in order of increasing size. Since this 'size principle' of Henneman *et al.* (1965) was first proposed based upon results from cat motoneurones, strong evidence has been presented that in muscle action there is a specific sequence of recruitment in order of increasing motoneurone and MU size (Milner-Brown *et al.* 1973; Kukulka & Clamann 1981; De Luca *et al.* 1982). Goldberg and Derfler (1977) have also shown positive correlations among recruitment order, spike amplitude and twitch tension of single MUs in human masseter muscle. Because of the great wealth of data supporting this size-based recruitment order in a variety of experimental conditions, it is often referred to as the 'normal sequence of recruitment' or 'orderly recruitment' (Heckman & Binder 1993). Recent data provide further support for this 'size principle', demonstrating that transcortical stimulation generates normal orderly recruitment (Bawa & Lemon 1993).

It is well documented that MU recruitment and firing frequency (rate coding) depend primarily upon the level of force and the speed of action. When low-threshold MUs are recruited, this results in a muscular action characterized by low force-generating capabilities and high fatigue resistance. With requirements for greater force and/or faster action, high-threshold fatigable MUs are recruited (Freund *et al.* 1975; Henneman & Mendell 1981). Figure 3.4 represents a typical set of data showing the changes in neural activation level (surface electromyograph (EMG) recording) of the biceps brachii and the corresponding frequency power spectra (frequency components of the action potentials) obtained from a highly trained power lifter during linearly force-varying isometric action. Note that large 'spike-like' potentials probably originating from fast-twitch MUs could be observed even with surface EMG recording at higher force levels (see Fig. 3.4).

The technical difficulties associated with single MU recordings at high forces in humans and the difficulty in generating controlled forces in animal preparations limit the accuracy with which the precise MU recruitment and rate coding can be established. However, Kukulka and Clamann (1981) and Moritani *et al.* (1986a) demonstrated in the human adductor pollicis that for a muscle group with mainly Type I fibres, MU firing rate plays a more prominent role in force modulation. For a muscle group composed of both Type I and II fibres, MU recruitment seems to be the major mechanism for generating

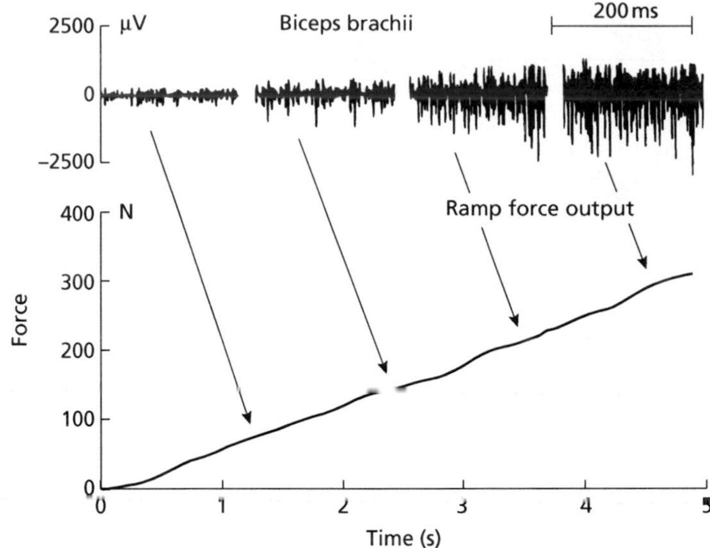

Fig. 3.5 Intramuscular spike recordings obtained from the biceps brachii muscle during linearly force-varying isometric muscle action.

extra force above 40–50% of maximal voluntary contraction (MVC). Thus, in the intrinsic muscles of the hand in humans, MU recruitment appears to be essentially complete at about 50% of maximal force, but MU recruitment in the biceps, brachialis and deltoid muscles may continue until more than 80% of maximal force is attained (Kukulka & Clamann 1981; De Luca *et al.* 1982; Moritani *et al.* 1986a; Moritani & Muro 1987) (see Fig. 3.5).

As movement speed increases, the force supplied by slow-twitch MUs decreases much more rapidly than that supplied by type F units because of differences in their force–velocity relations. As a consequence, it has been proposed that rapid movements may be accomplished by selective recruitment of fast-twitch MUs. This selective recruitment of either slow or fast ankle extensor muscles has been documented during a variety of locomotor tasks in cats (Smith *et al.* 1980; Hodgson 1983). For example, Smith *et al.* (1980) demonstrated selective recruitment of the fast lateral gastrocnemius (LG) muscle during rapid paw shaking without concomitant recruitment of the slow soleus (SOL) muscle, possibly due to the time constraints imposed by the rapid movements during which the recruitment of slow muscle would be incompatible with the demands of the movement. Studies in humans have generally not supported this idea. Moritani *et al.* (1991a,b), however, reported some evidence of phase-dependent and preferential activation of the relatively 'fast' gastrocnemius muscle (as compared to 'slow' soleus) with increasing demands of force and speed during different types of hopping in humans.

Catchlike properties of muscle

Burke *et al.* (1970) demonstrated a very interesting muscle contractile phenomenon called 'catchlike' property, i.e. force enhancement induced by addition of an extra pulse (catchlike property) during constant-frequency stimulation for whole-muscle or single MU preparations. The original findings of Burke *et al.* (1970) together with our human data are displayed in Fig. 3.6. These data clearly indicated that just one extra high-frequency impulse given during constant-frequency stimulation could enhance subsequent force output that continued for a period of time during which the original stimulation frequency resumed (see Fig. 3.6).

We have investigated this catchlike property of force enhancement mechanisms in terms of electrophysiological and metabolic responses in human skeletal muscles by means of surface

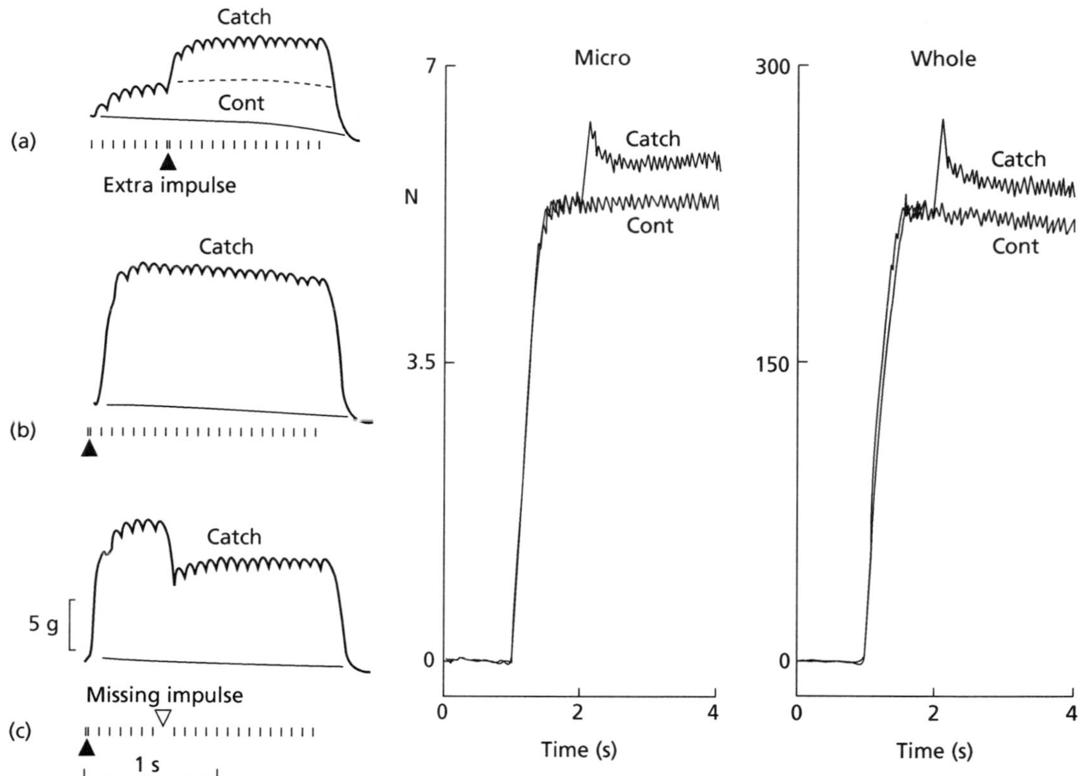

Fig. 3.6 Catchlike property (force enhancement) of a single isolated motor unit stimulation in animals (Burke *et al.* 1970) and intramuscular and nerve stimulations in humans (Moritani & Yoshitake 1998). Force curves obtained during constant-frequency stimulation (CONT) or with an extra high-frequency pulse (CATCH).

and intramuscular EMG recordings and near-infrared spectroscopy (NIRS), respectively (Moritani & Yoshitake 1998). In this study, two different stimulation methods were employed: (i) the posterior tibial nerve was stimulated supramaximally to induce maximal actions of triceps surae muscle; and (ii) intramuscular microstimulation was performed to study the catchlike property of single muscle fibres. Measurements were made continuously for force and electromyographic signals (M-wave) together with the measurement of muscle oxygenation level during constant electrical stimulation with (CATCH) or without (CONT) one extra 50-Hz pulse. The results indicated that the total force output during CATCH was significantly greater than that of CONT. However, when the averaged peak-to-peak amplitude of M-wave obtained during CONT was compared with that obtained during CATCH at the same period, no statistically significant difference could be observed. Moreover, there was no significant difference in the total changes of muscle oxygenation between CONT and CATCH stimulation.

In the present study, a significant enhancement of the force output induced by only one additional high-frequency extra pulse was found in both micro- and whole-muscle stimulation in the human triceps surae muscles (see Fig. 3.6). Despite the significant difference in the developed force, there were no significant differences between two different stimulation patterns in the electrophysiological and the metabolic characteristics (see Fig. 3.7).

Our data are consistent with previous findings that neural factors largely accounted for the

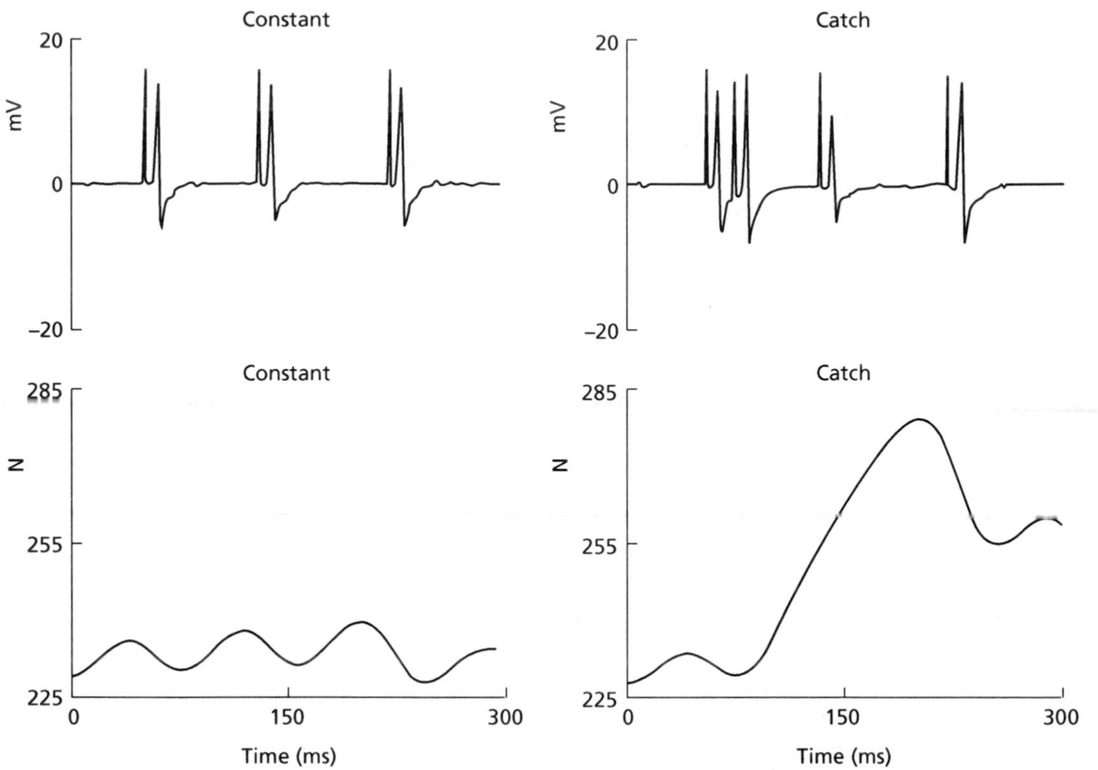

Fig. 3.7 Changes in the force curves and evoked mass action potentials (M-waves) recorded during constant-frequency stimulation and with an extra high-frequency pulse (CATCH).

strength increment during the initial stage of strength training (Moritani & deVries 1979; Komi 1986; Moritani 1993). Our data also provide some interesting neurophysiological prospectives for muscle training as one can induce this catchlike property by training-induced changes in the MU firing patterns at the initiation of muscular actions.

Common drive of motor units in regulation of muscle force

Several previous studies (Milner-Brown *et al.* 1973; Tanji & Kato 1973) all demonstrated that the firing rates of active MUs increased proportionally with increasing force output. This may imply that increased excitation to the active muscle motoneurone pool increases the firing rates of all the active MUs. De Luca *et al.* (1982) investigated this commonality in the behaviour of the MU firing rates of up to eight concurrently active MUs during various types of isometric muscle action: attempted constant force, ramp force increase and force reversals. Their results strongly indicated that there was a unison behaviour of the firing rates of motor units, as a function of both time and force. This property has been termed the *common drive*. The existence of this common drive implies that the nervous system does not control the firing rates of MUs individually. Instead, it modulates the pool of motoneurones in a uniform fashion; i.e. a demand for force modulation can be achieved by modulation of excitation and/or inhibition on the motoneurone pool.

Joint analysis of the time course changes in the firing rate of concurrently active MUs revealed that they acted in a highly interdependent fashion. In other words, the firing rates of all MUs vary simultaneously, with an increase (or decrease) in a particular MU firing rate being accompanied by similar changes in the firing rates of other MUs. Cross-correlation analysis between the firing rates of all possible pairs of MUs studied indicated a high level of correlation, attesting the existence of neural modulation for simultaneous MU firing rate control strategy (De Luca & Erim 1994). Since this common drive phenomenon occurs even in the muscle that has no muscle spindles, e.g. the orbicularis oris inferior muscle of the lip, and in isometric muscle action where muscle spindle activity is minimal, the observed common fluctuations in MU firing rates could most likely stem from the central nervous system.

On the other hand, if the neuromuscular system was designed to maximize the force output, the higher-threshold MUs would be driven to fire at higher rates, as these MUs require greater firing rates to tetanize and produce their maximal force. But in reality, this is not the case. De Luca and Erim (1994) have shown that the firing rates of earlier-recruited MUs are *greater* than those later-recruited MUs. One possible explanation for the higher-threshold MUs being driven at lower firing rates is that they are fatigued more quickly than lower-threshold MUs and would be quickly exhausted. Thus, under voluntary control, the neuromuscular system might have a reserve capacity for generating unusual levels of force for brief periods of time. In extraordinary circumstances including emergency, competition, etc. and/or as a result of prolonged high-intensity muscular training, it is quite conceivable that the higher-threshold MUs might be activated briefly with dramatically greater firing rates that tetanize and contribute even more to the muscle force capability. It is generally believed that the so-called MU firing doublets, which might have a potential catchlike property described earlier, can be more frequently seen in a group of highly trained athletes.

Based upon the above-mentioned MU recruitment and firing rate modulation, De Luca and Erim (1994) have proposed a simple hydraulic model to summarize the basic principles governing the regulation of MUs during muscle action. Figure 3.8 shows such a model. According to this model, the water flow into the tank corresponds to the drive to the motoneurone pool, while the outflow from the individual spouts, and the distance it travels, corresponds to the recruitment of a given MU and its firing rate. The length of each spout is representative of the initial MU firing rate, and the net accumulation of the water in the tank corresponds to the common drive (excitation–inhibition). Figure 3.8(a) represents the behaviour of firing rates when the central drive is only enough to recruit three MUs. Figure 3.8(b) demonstrates the situation when the recruitment of a new MU and the increase in the firing rates of already active MUs take place as the neural drive to the motoneurone pool is further increased. Finally the convergence of the firing rates to the same value at maximal firing rates is shown in Fig. 3.8(c) in the case of an extreme drive where the differences between the individual spout heights become negligible compared with the water level. In this model, the control of the MUs within a muscle presents a functional elegance that relates the specifics of the hierarchical grading to the local size-related excitation of the MUs. Although the applicability of this model to ballistic and non-isometric conditions remains to be investigated at the present time, such a neural organization would free the central nervous system to provide a global input to the motoneurone pool corresponding to the intended output of the muscle.

Motor unit activation patterns during explosive movement

Maximal power development

The maximal hopping movement is considered to be one of the most powerful movements that humans can perform, exceeding nearly 30 $W \cdot kg^{-1}$ (Moritani *et al.* 1991a). Figure 3.9 shows such hopping movements (top) with different heights together with neural activation patterns recorded from the medial gastrocnemius (MG) and soleus

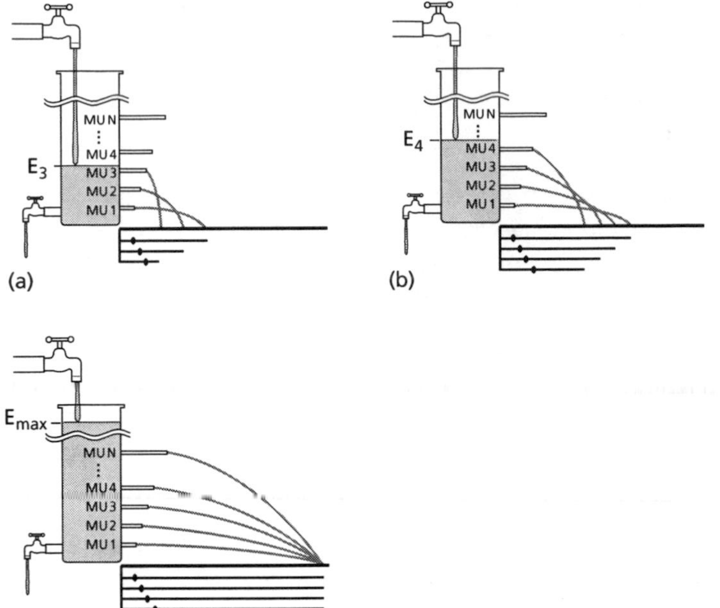

Fig. 3.8 A model of motor unit recruitment and firing rate regulation during muscle contraction proposed by De Luca and Erim (1994).

(SOL) muscles, respectively. The averaged EMG data clearly indicate that the greater increase in the relative activation levels of MG as compared to SOL during the maximal height hopping (MAX) trials in preactivation (before ground contact) and eccentric (lengthening) phases. During the intermediate (2 Hz) and MAX hopping trials, with peak ground reaction forces roughly equivalent to 5.3 and 6.4 times body mass, the MG was selectively (precontact phase) and predominantly (eccentric phase) activated (see Fig. 3.3). Note that the preactivation of MG occurred about 200 ms prior to ground contact during which the SOL was for a large part inactive. Unlike the fastest hopping (FAST, mean height of hopping being less than 1 cm) in which both the MG and SOL displayed an almost simultaneous phase-shifted preactivation, the MAX hopping would require not only a high speed of action, but also a considerable amount of force. For such extreme mechanical and time constraints, the greater reliance of the fast synergist MG should be more compatible with the demands of the movement while the neural activation level of slow SOL MUs might have been saturated during this powerful movement.

Evidence for such differential neural control of fast and slow MUs in the decerebrate cat was reported by Kanda *et al.* (1977). Their findings, that slow synergist SOL and slow-twitch fibres of the MG were inhibited when fast-twitch fibres of the MG were preferentially facilitated during sural nerve stimulation, suggest that complex neuronal interactions within the motoneurone pool may modify the excitability of motoneurones (Burke 1971). The observed greater reliance on MG muscle during the preactivation and eccentric action phases of maximal hopping (see Fig. 3.9) may thus suggest that such complex neuronal interactions play an important role in the selective activation of fast muscle within a synergy in humans. During the rapid and enormously powerful MAX hopping, the recruitment of slow synergist SOL may be incompatible with the demands of the movement.

On the other hand, the extent to which stretch reflexes contribute to the explosive movements in humans is still somewhat controversial. The

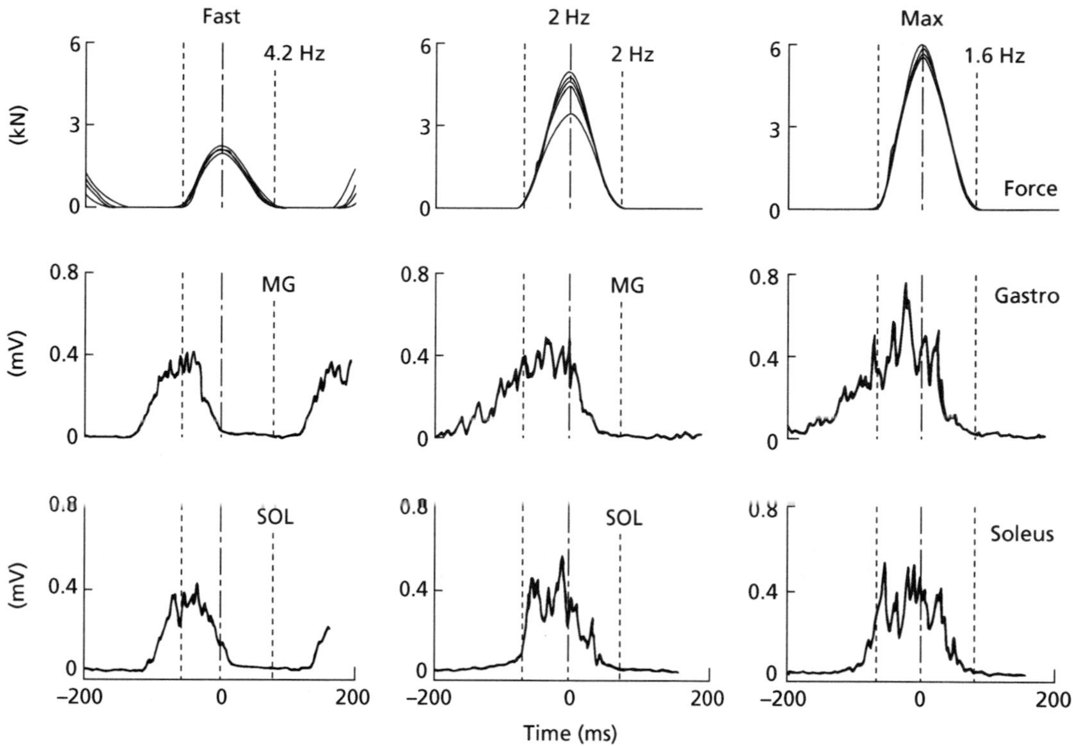

Fig. 3.9 Changes in ground reaction force and EMGs recorded from the gastrocnemius (MG) and soleus (SOL) during three different modes of hopping requiring varying degrees of force and speed of contraction.

data presented by Dietz *et al.* (1979), however, have clearly demonstrated that spinal reflexes could play an important role and be mechanically effective during running, even at very high speeds with a ground contact time of approximately 120 ms. They found that the maximal muscle activation level recorded immediately after the ground contact was considerably higher than the neural drive that can be exerted during maximal voluntary contraction. Thus, stretching of the active muscles during eccentric or lengthening action phases may evoke segmental reflexes which in turn could potentiate muscle activation and contribute to the increase of muscle stiffness in meeting the enormous force requirements (Dietz *et al.* 1979; Grillner 1981). Preactivation therefore appears to be a preparatory necessity both for enhancement of stretch reflex and for advancing the onset of muscular action in time with respect to ground contact during this highly powerful movement. Otherwise, the contribution of the stretch reflex and the peak force of each motor unit would appear too late to be effective (Moritani *et al.* 1991b).

Maximal power training and neural adaptations

The development of muscular power is of great importance in sports events requiring a high level of force and speed. Muscle power is the product of muscle force and action velocity, each of which is influenced by intrinsic muscle properties. The primary intrinsic properties governing muscle force development are the force–length and force–velocity relationships and the kinetics of muscle activation and deactivation.

Significant correlations have been demonstrated among the force–velocity characteristics, muscle mechanical power and muscle fibre composition in human knee extensor muscles (Thorstensson *et al.* 1976; Tihanyi *et al.* 1982). Faulkner *et al.* (1986) studied the contractile properties of bundles of muscle fibres from human skeletal muscles and found that the peak power output of fast-twitch fibres was fourfold that of slow-twitch fibres due to a greater shortening velocity for a given afterload. When the composite power curve for the mixed muscle was studied, the fast-twitch fibres contributed 2.5 times more than the slow-twitch fibres to the total power.

There have been many studies demonstrating the specificity of different types of muscle training upon neural and mechanical adaptations (Komi & Viitasalo 1977; Komi *et al.* 1978). The specificity of power training effects on the force–velocity relationship and maximal power output in human muscles was extensively studied by Kaneko and colleagues (Kaneko 1970, 1974; Kaneko *et al.* 1983). Kaneko (1974), for example, studied the time course of changes in the force–velocity characteristics and the resultant maximal power output with respect to different training loads (e.g. 0, 30, 60, 100% F_0 (maximal voluntary contraction force)) for a period of 20 weeks. This study showed significantly large initial improvements in the force–velocity curve and the corresponding mechanical power outputs as a result of muscle power training. Kaneko *et al.* (1983) also demonstrated the 'specificity' of muscle power training effect; i.e. the training by maximal actions with 0% F_0 was found to be most effective for improving the maximal velocity tested with no external load, while 100% F_0 training improved maximal strength most. It was concluded that different training loads could bring about specific modifications of the force–velocity relationship, and that the 30% F_0 load was most effective in improving maximal mechanical power output (Fig. 3.10).

In these and the other studies (Caiozzo *et al.* 1981; Coyle *et al.* 1981), no EMG recordings were made so that it was not possible to determine the effects of muscle power training on maximal muscle activation level and other possible neural adaptations. We therefore investigated the effects of short-term 30% F_0 muscle power training upon the force–velocity curve, power and electrophysiological parameters (Moritani *et al.* 1987). The right biceps brachii muscle was trained by pulling the load equivalent to 30% F_0 with maximal effort, 30 times a day, 3 times a week for a period of 2 weeks. The surface and intramuscular EMGs from the long and short heads were recorded simultaneously and analysed by means of frequency power spectrum and MU amplitude frequency histogram techniques, respectively (Moritani *et al.* 1985, 1986b). Results indicated that the level of muscle activation as determined by RMS (root mean square) EMG amplitude values increased dramatically at any given load after training. On the other hand, MPF (mean power frequency), which reflects the frequency component of the recorded action potentials, markedly shifted toward lower frequency bands as a result of large, low-frequency EMG oscillations, due possibly to better summation (synchronization) of the underlying action potentials.

To further elucidate the possibility of synchronous muscle activation patterns or of an association in the time and frequency domains, cross-power spectra and cross-correlation coefficients were obtained between the action potentials recorded from the biceps brachii short- and long-head muscles in the pre- and post-training periods. Figures 3.11 & 3.12 represent the typical changes observed. It seems apparent that two action potential waveforms have little association in the amplitude and waveform patterns at pretraining, revealing a maximal cross-correlation coefficient (R_{xy}) of 0.40 (see Fig. 3.11). However, very similar action potential waveforms with much higher amplitude were obtained after the training, increasing R_{xy} to 0.91 (Fig. 3.12). This suggests a greater muscle activation and more synchronous MU activities after training (Milner-Brown & Stein 1975) and/or greater 'common drive' resulting in negligible MU firing rate differences among the active MUs at this extremely high neural drive (De Luca & Erim 1994). This may lead to an increased oscillation in the surface EMG which may theoretically

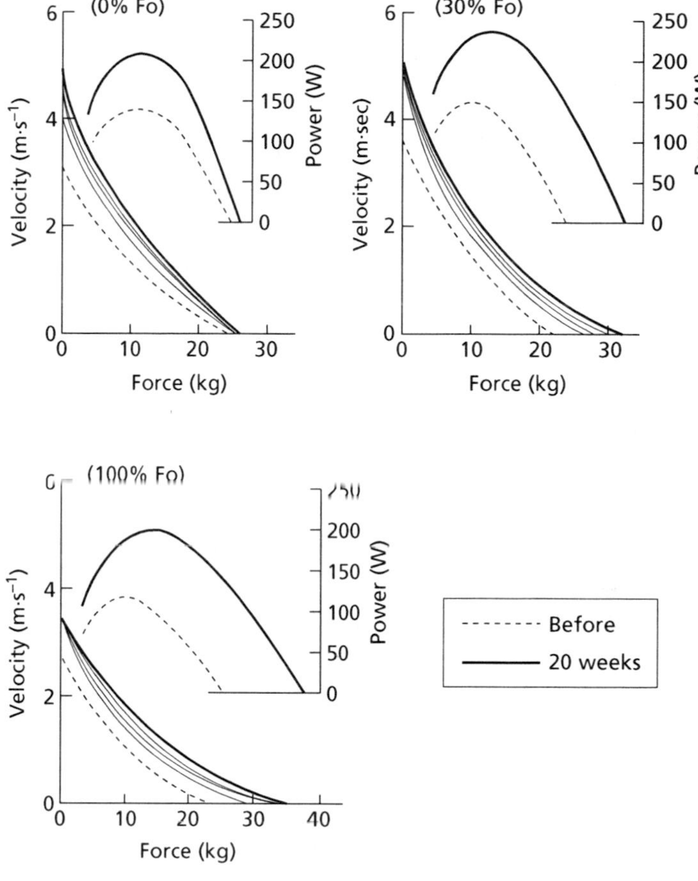

Fig. 3.10 The time course of changes in the force–velocity (concave) and force–power (convex) relationships during 20 weeks of muscle power training with different loads. Power = force × distance (work) ÷ time (velocity) = force × velocity. (Based on Kaneko 1974.)

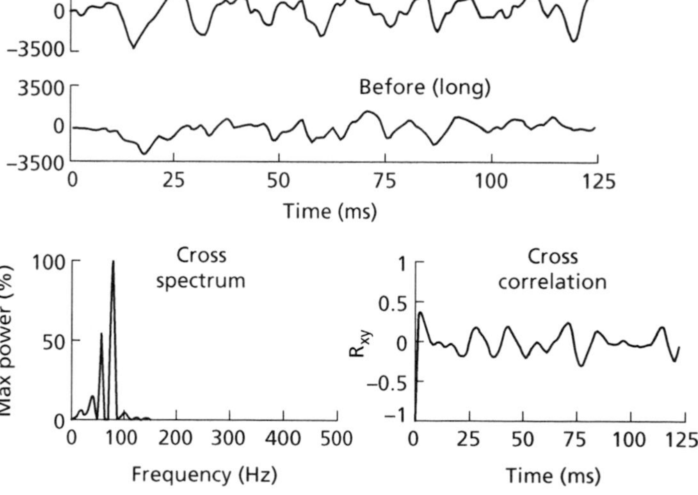

Fig. 3.11 A typical set of action potential recordings from the biceps brachii short- and long-head muscles and the corresponding cross-spectra and cross-correlation coefficients obtained before training. (Based on Moritani *et al.* 1987.)

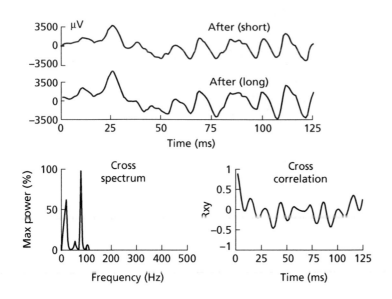

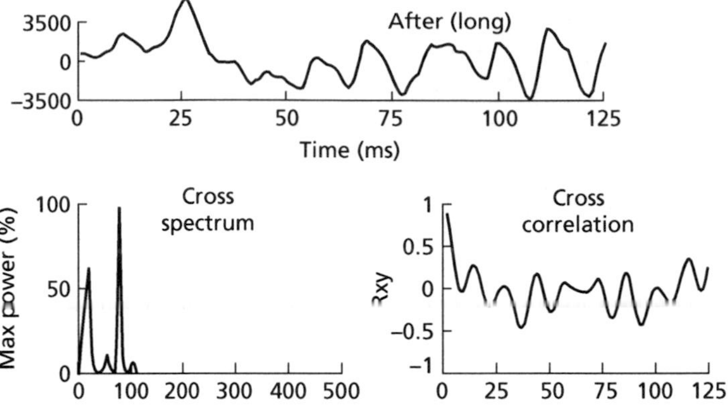

Fig. 3.12 A typical set of action potential recordings from the biceps brachii short- and long-head muscles and the corresponding cross-spectra and cross-correlation coefficients obtained after training. (Based on Moritani *et al.* 1987.)

approach the level of the maximally evoked M-waves (mass action potential), indicating that all MUs are now fully synchronized (Bigland-Ritchie 1981). Group data indicated that there were highly significant increases in the maximal power output, RMS and R_{xy}, together with a significant decrease in MPF, after training in all load conditions. These data strongly suggest that the short-term training-induced shifts in force–velocity relationship and the resultant mechanical power output might have been brought about by the neural adaptations in terms of greater muscle activation levels and more synchronous activation patterns.

Maximal ballistic movement

Previous studies attempting to analyse central mechanisms for the initiation and execution of ballistic movements have mainly dealt with qualitative and quantitative aspects of the early EMG bursts of the agonist muscles (Hallett & Marsden 1979; Lestienne 1979). The triphasic muscle activation patterns of agonist and antagonist muscles have also been intensively studied during rapid movements (Garland & Angel 1971; Sanes & Jennings 1984). Interestingly, it has been shown that the earliest manifestation of rapid movements is not an activation, but rather a depression or silencing of EMG activity (called the premovement silent period, SP), which has been described for both antagonist and agonist muscles (Yabe 1976; Conrad *et al.* 1983; Kawahatsu & Miyashita 1983; Mortimer *et al.* 1984; Aoki *et al.* 1989). The definite functional role of the SP and its neurophysiological mechanisms remains to be determined. Conrad *et al.* (1983) have suggested that in high-speed movements where a maximal number of motor units have to be recruited, those motoneurones that are already tonically active have to be released from tonic activity for optimal synchrony.

Moritani and Shibata (1994) have investigated the possible neurophysiological mechanisms of SP preceding a ballistic voluntary movement in young subjects. The subjects were asked to respond to a flashing light signal by performing a plantar flexion as strongly and quickly as possible. The EMG signals from the agonists (lateral gastrocnemius, LG and soleus, SOL) and antagonist (tibialis anterior, TA) were simultaneously recorded together with the force signal. Figure 3.13 shows a typical set of data demonstrating the appearance of an SP period prior to a ballistic movement. Note the disappearance of intramuscularly recorded MU spikes and the correspond-

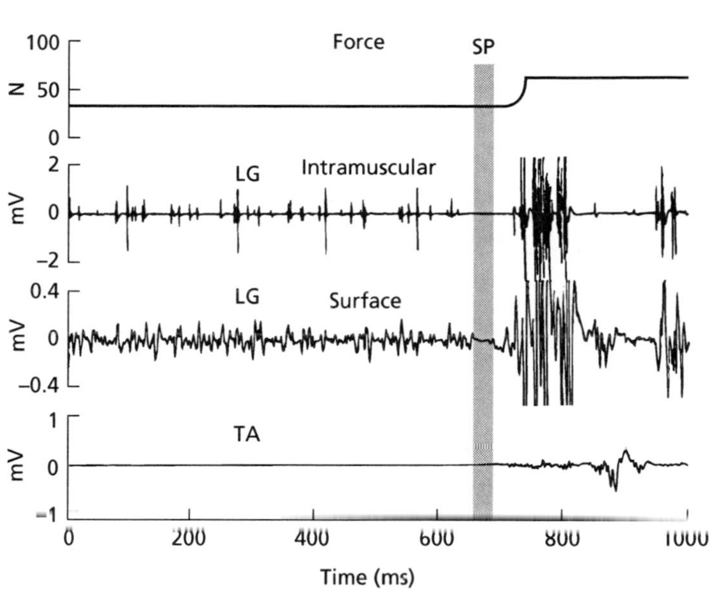

Fig. 3.13 A typical set of data showing force curve, intramuscular and surface EMG recordings from gastrocnemius (LG) muscle and antagonist tibialis anterior (TA) muscle during a ballistic plantar flexion. Note the complete silence in LG MU activity and surface EMG. Since electromechanical delay time (EMD) for relaxation is much longer than contraction-induced EMD, force could be sustained in the absence of muscle activation. (For more details see Moritani & Shibata 1994.)

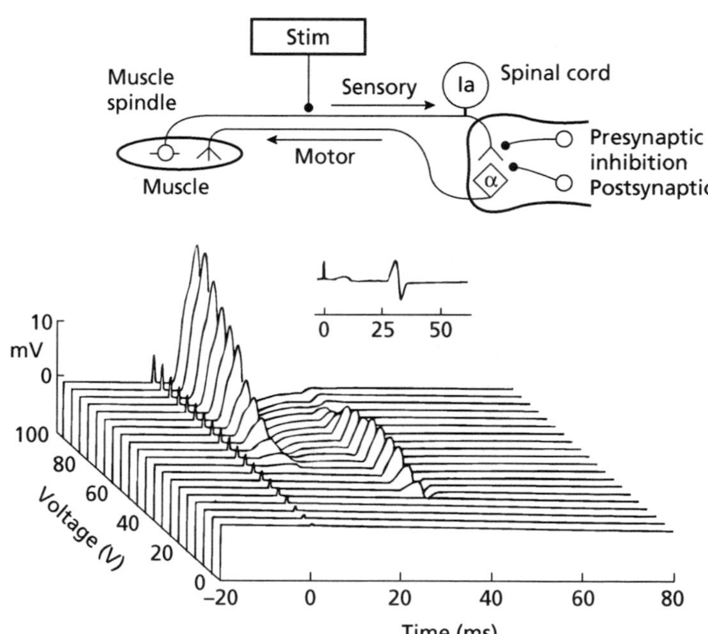

Fig. 3.14 A typical set of evoked muscle action potentials as a function of stimulus intensity during H-reflex testing.

ing surface EMG activity in the absence of force and the antagonistic TA muscle activity.

The excitability of spinal α motoneurone pools by means of H-reflex analysis was also determined at various phases of the movement. Figure 3.14 represents our method for eliciting H-reflex. A single electrical stimulation to the posterior tibial nerve elicits two discrete muscle action potentials in the calf muscles. The first evoked action potential is referred to as the M-wave, which results from the direct stimulation of motor axons, whereas the second action potential or H-wave results from stimulation of the largest sensory axons (group Ia afferents

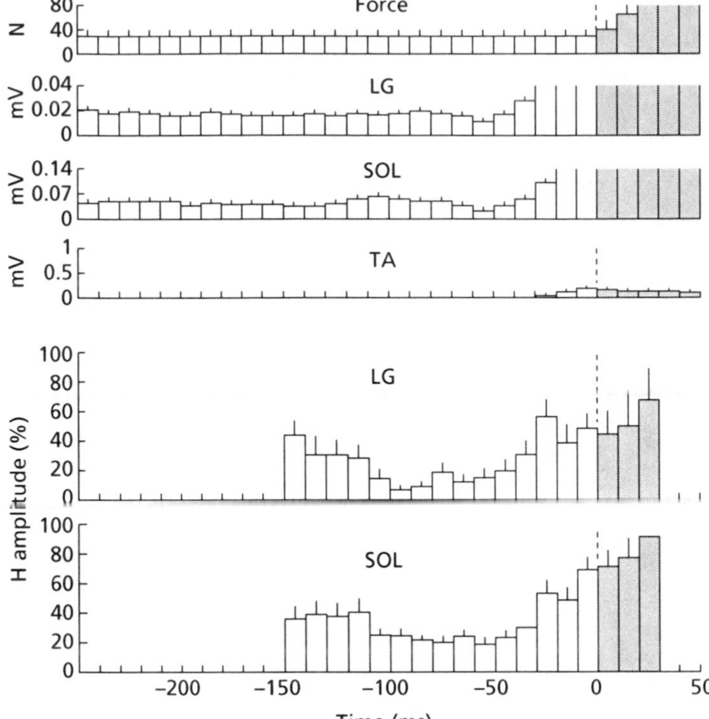

Fig. 3.15 Group data (mean + SE, $n = 5$) on force, rectified EMG mean amplitude for lateral gastrocnemius (LG), soleus (SOL) and tibialis anterior (TA) (top four traces) together with H-reflex amplitude changes for LG and SOL during ballistic plantar flexion accompanying premotion EMG silent period. H-reflexes elicited at different phases of movement were grouped in 10-ms bins and averaged with reference to the onset of force production denoted as 0 time.

arising from the muscle spindle) which have a strong monosynaptic connection to α motoneurones. The H-reflex therefore provides a useful means of testing spinal reflex modulation during motor behaviour as the change in H-wave amplitude would reflect the corresponding change in the monosynaptic reflex excitability in the spinal cord (Stein & Capaday 1988).

Our results indicated that: (i) the SP occurred in some, but not all, trials within single subjects and had a variable duration from trial to trial; (ii) the maximal rate of force development (d_F/d_t) was significantly greater in the trials with the SP than in those without the SP; and (iii) the significant decrease in H-wave amplitude was observed approximately 40 ms prior to the appearance of the SP which precedes the force development by about 50–60 ms (see Fig. 3.15). Several physiological mechanisms that may explain the occurrence of the SP have been suggested by Mortimer *et al.* (1984): (i) inhibition by supraspinal centres producing disfacilitation of tonically active motoneurones; (ii) postsynaptic inhibition by spinal interneurones; and (iii) presynaptic inhibition by primary afferent depolarization. Reciprocal inhibition could not be responsible since the SP occurs in the absence of any EMG burst in antagonists. Furthermore, SP latencies are much shorter than the fastest premotor times in pretensed muscles. Ward (1978) argues against postsynaptic inhibition via spinal interneurones activated in parallel with the motoneurones.

One may, on the other hand, speculate that the SP could serve to increase the synchrony of the motoneurone pool; many of the tonically active motoneurones would be refractory when the command of rapid action reaches this motoneurone pool. On this basis, Conrad *et al.* (1983) have suggested that the SP would bring all motoneurones into a non-refractory state, enabling all available motoneurones to be ready to fire at the same time. This could be achieved, for example, by inhibition of the α motoneurone via spinal inhibitory interneurones known to be activated monosynaptically by the corticospinal tract. Our findings of decreased H-reflex amplitude and complete disappearance of motor unit firings during the SP thus seem to support this hypothesis, although the possible inhibitory mechanisms acting on supraspinal centres disfacilitating tonic activity could not be ruled out.

The fact that the SP manifests a variable duration from trial to trial and that some subjects appear to be more capable of producing the SP than others suggests that the SP may be a learned motor response rather than an automatic component of the movement programme. In this regard, it may be worth noting that top world athletes (sprinters and high jumpers) demonstrated considerably shorter SP duration than a group of physical education students (Kawahatsu 1981). Furthermore, in the movement of shooting an arrow, Nishizono *et al.* (1984) observed a SP prior to release in world-class archers and the appearance rate of the SP was also found to be significantly higher in the group of highly skilled archers than that of the less skilled archers (Nishizono & Kato 1987).

Our surface EMG and H-reflex data also argue against postsynaptic inhibition via spinal interneurones since the period of depressed H-reflex amplitude was not accompanied by any significant decreases in either LG and SOL surface EMG records in our experiments. If there were postsynaptic inhibition taking place, simultaneous decreases in both H-reflex and surface EMG activity would have been seen. We however, did not observe such parallel decreases. This leaves presynaptic inhibition and disfacilitation as the most likely mechanisms involved in the SP preceding a ballistic movement.

Modulation of motoneurone excitability during explosive movement

Spinal reflexes are often viewed as stereotyped motor patterns with limited scope for modification. However, recent evidence suggests that even short-latency, largely monosynaptic reflexes show a high degree of modulation during simple human motor activities such as walking and standing, and that the pattern of modulation can be specifically altered for the different functional requirements of each activity (Capaday & Stein 1987; Stein & Capaday 1988; Yamashita & Moritani 1989; Moritani *et al.* 1990). For example, Capaday and Stein (1987) have demonstrated that H-reflex amplitude of the soleus increases progressively during the stance phase and reaches its peak amplitude late in the stance phase during walking. During running, however, the H-reflex is found to be significantly smaller than during walking, suggesting a modified spinal reflex gain for the different functional requirements of the motor behaviour. Our subsequent studies have also confirmed these findings (Moritani *et al.* 1990; Moritani & Shibata 1994).

In the previous section on maximal power development, we described such a high power output during maximal height hopping together with some evidence of preferential activation of the gastrocnemius muscle, since this type of maximal hopping would require not only a high speed of action, but also a tremendous amount of force. For such extreme mechanical and time constraints, the greater reliance of the fast synergist gastrocnemius muscle should be more compatible with the demands of the movement while the neural activation level of slow soleus muscle might be suppressed during this powerful movement. We therefore examined the underlying spinal level neural modulation of the two functionally specialized muscles (gastrocnemius and soleus) within the ankle extensors during different types of hopping movements by using spinal H-reflex paradigms (Moritani *et al.* 1990). In order to determine the H-reflex amplitude at various phases of hopping, a 'phase-dependent' averaging technique was employed by a computerized data processing system (Moritani *et al.* 1991a,b; Moritani & Shibata 1994). Single rectangular pulses were delivered at 36 different phases of hopping so as to obtain fine time resolution of the H-reflex changes during the entire hopping cycle. To achieve these measurements, the subject performed more than 360–720

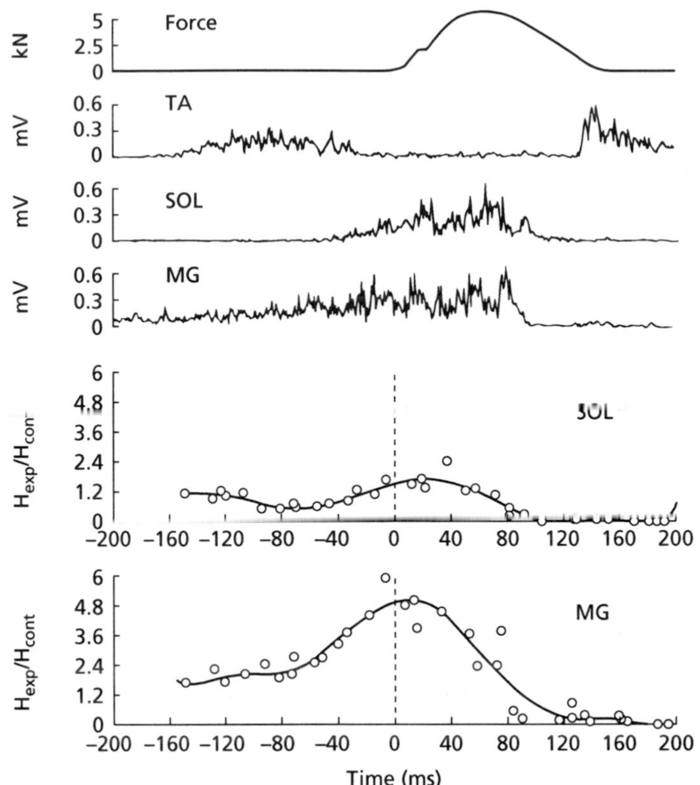

Fig. 3.16 A typical set of computer outputs for maximal hopping trials (height 27 cm, power 2010 W) showing the time course changes of force, tibialis anterior (TA), soleus (SOL) and medial gastrocnemius (MG) rectified EMGs together with the SOL and MG H-reflex changes (H_{exp}) being normalized by the standing rest control value (H_{cont}). Zero time indicates onset of ground contact (cf. force curve on top). Each data point represents an average of 20 trials. (Based upon Moritani *et al.* 1990.)

hops for each of the three types of hopping on three different occasions (one type of hopping experiment per day). Furthermore, the temporal relationships between H-reflex changes and force developed during hopping were also determined by a computer-implemented cross-correlation routine.

Figure 3.16 represents a set of computer outputs showing the force, tibialis anterior (TA), soleus (SOL) and medial gastrocnemius (MG) rectified EMGs and the corresponding SOL and MG H-reflex amplitude changes during various phases of maximal height (MAX) hopping. Results indicated that the H-reflex amplitude (H_{exp}) from the MG showed marked increases over the resting control (H_{cont}) during preground contact and eccentric (lengthening) phases of muscular action, i.e. the peak H-reflex amplitude increased progressively from SMALL (4 Hz), LIGHT (2 Hz) and MAX (1.6 Hz) amplitude hopping. The corresponding SOL H-amplitudes were actually decreased. Thus, the spinal reflex gain appeared to be modulated, i.e. a decrease for the slow SOL and an increase for the relatively fast MG with increasing demands of force and speed. Cross-correlation analyses revealed that the time course changes of the H-reflex amplitude preceded the force curves by an average of 45, 58 and 67 ms for the MG and 39, 59 and 54 ms for the SOL during SMALL, LIGHT and MAX hopping. Our data are in agreement with these results and suggest that spinal reflexes are not stereotyped motor patterns, but can be specifically modulated for different functional requirements of the muscles during the execution of highly powerful movements.

Movement-related cortical potentials during maximal action

Potentials occurring immediately preceding and following a voluntary movement have been

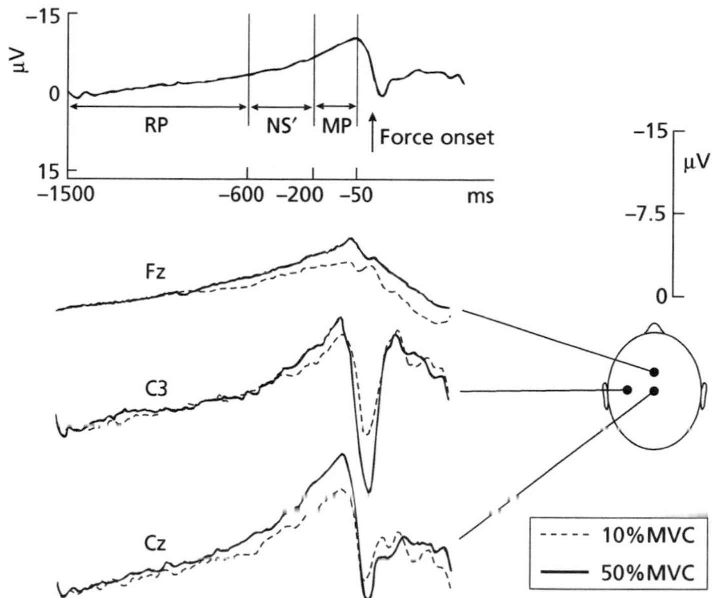

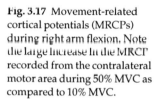

Fig. 3.17 Movement-related cortical potentials (MRCPs) during right arm flexion. Note the large increase in the MRCP recorded from the contralateral motor area during 50% MVC as compared to 10% MVC.

defined as movement-related cortical potentials (MRCPs) (Neshige *et al.* 1988b). Human MRCPs have been studied in normals (Deecke *et al.* 1969; Shibasaki *et al.* 1980; Neshige *et al.* 1988a,b) and in patients (Neshige *et al.* 1988b; Singh & Knight 1990). The fact that MRCPs onset up to 1.5 s prior to movements suggest that these potentials are generated by neural circuits involved in motor preparation and initiation.

MRCPs recorded from chronically implanted subdural electrodes in patients have indicated discrete MRCP sources in pre- and postcentral gyrus with additional contributions from supplementary and premotor cortices (Neshige *et al.* 1988a,b). Most investigators agree that the motor potential (MP) has its major neural source in the primary motor area (Shibasaki *et al.* 1980; Singh & Knight 1990). Direct intracranial data in humans (Neshige *et al.* 1988a,b) also indicate that the sensorimotor cortex is a major contributor to the earlier MRCP components (readiness potential, RP; and late portion of the RP, termed negative shift, NS′).

Figure 3.17 represents examples of MRPs recorded from scalp electrodes using the international 10–20 system so as to investigate the relationship between MRCPs and force output amplitude during force-varying isometric actions corresponding to 10 and 50% MVC. In this figure, only Fz (mid-frontal gyrus near superior frontal cortex), C3 and Cz recordings are shown for clarity. In order to observe the EEG activity before and after right arm flexion, an average electroencephalogram (EEG), time-locked to the onset of force production, was prepared using special computer programs developed in our laboratory. The RP, which corresponds to the previously described Bereitschaftspotential (Deecke *et al.* 1969), started at least 1000 ms prior to the force output and slowly increased in amplitude. Approximately 500 ms before the force onset, the slope of this negative potential became steeper (negative slope NS′ according to the terminology used by Shibasaki *et al.* 1980). These data clearly indicate that NS′ and MP are maximal over scalp sites contralateral to movements which in turn suggests that sensorimotor areas and the supplementary motor area participate in the preparation of movements, but that mainly the contralateral cortex generates the discharges

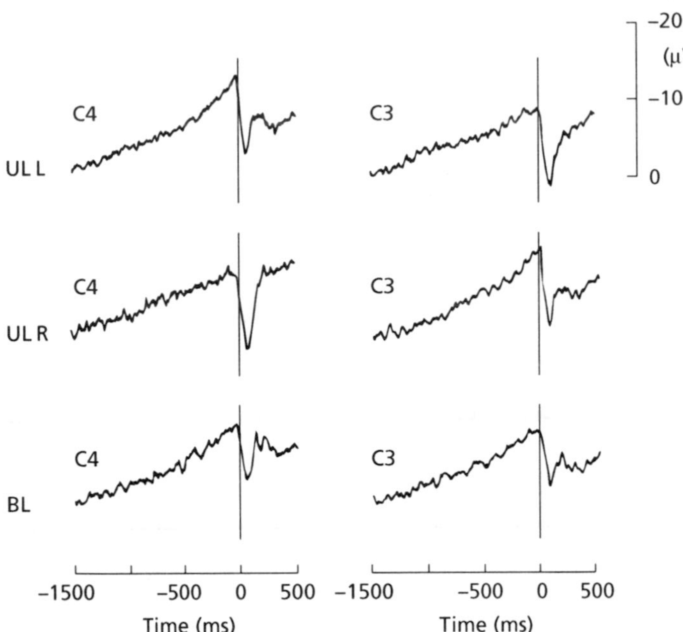

Fig. 3.18 The grand averages of MRCP data during unilateral (UL) and bilateral (BL) contractions for the left (L) and right (R) hand (see Oda & Moritani 1994, 1995).

necessary to produce the actual movement (Neshige *et al.* 1988b; Singh & Knight 1990; Oda & Moritani 1996a,b; Oda *et al.* 1996; Shibata *et al.* 1997). The significant increase of MP corresponding to the exerted force level (10% vs. 50% MVC) might indicate the relative increase of the pyramidal tract cell discharge.

Interestingly, many investigators have reported a reduction in maximal voluntary strength induced by simultaneous bilateral (BL) exertion as compared with unilateral (UL) exertion (Koh *et al.* 1993; Oda & Moritani 1994, 1995). However, the neurophysiological mechanism producing the BL strength and EMG deficits remains unknown. We have investigated MRCPs from left and right motor cortex areas (C3 and C4, respectively) and isometric force and EMG activity in association with maximal BL and UL handgrip action in eight right-handed subjects (Oda & Moritani 1995). The BL grip exhibited significant deficits in maximal force and EMG compared with the UL grip. In the UL actions, the amplitudes of MRCPs were also significantly greater in the contralateral hemisphere. For the BL actions, the asymmetry of the larger potentials for the contralateral side disappeared and lower symmetrical potentials were observed (see Fig. 3.18).

Muscle action is controlled mainly by the contralateral cerebral hemisphere and thus the BL action is generated by the simultaneous activation of both hemispheres. Therefore, one explanation for the BL strength and EMG deficits that has been given is that it could be neural interaction between the two hemispheres connected by commissural nerve fibres (Otsuki 1983). Ferbert *et al.* (1992) have reported interhemispherical inhibition by magnetic stimulation to the motor cortex of the two hemispheres. We have therefore concluded that the BL deficit in force and EMG is associated with reduced MRCPs, suggesting that the bilateral force and EMG deficit compared with unilateral actions is caused, at least in part, by a mechanism of interhemispherical inhibition. This may also explain a common finding in strength training that many serious athletes seem to prefer unilateral muscle strength training over bilateral training, as maximal excitation from the motor cortex could be obtained during unilateral effort without suppression from the contralateral hemisphere.

References

Alway, S.E., Stray-Andersen, J., Grumbt, W.H. & Gonyea, W.J. (1990) Muscle cross sectional area and torque in resistance-trained subjects. *European Journal of Applied Physiology* **60**, 86–90.

Aoki, H., Tsukahara, R. & Yabe, K. (1989) Effects of pre-motion electromyographic silent period on dynamic force exertion during a rapid ballistic movement in man. *European Journal of Applied Physiology* **58**, 426–432.

Bawa, P. & Lemon, R.N. (1993) Recruitment of motor units in response to transcranial magnetic stimulation in man. *Journal of Physiology (London)* **471**, 445–464.

Bigland-Ritchie, B. (1981) EMG/force relations and fatigue of human voluntary contractions. *Exercise and Sport Sciences Reviews* **9**, 75–117.

Burke, R.E. (1971) Control systems operating on spinal reflex mechanisms. *Neuroscience Research Progress Bulletin* **9**, 60–85.

Burke, R.E. (1981) Motor units. Anatomy, physiology and functional organization. In: *Handbook of Physiology. The Nervous System* (ed. V.D. Brooks), pp. 345–422. American Physiological Society, Bethesda.

Burke, R.E., Rundomin, P. & Zajac, F.E. (1970) Catch property in single mammalian motor units. *Science* **168**, 122–124.

Caiozzo, V.J., Perrine, J.J. & Edgerton, V.R. (1981) Training-induced alterations of the in vivo force velocity relationship of human muscle. *Journal of Applied Physiology* **51**, 750–754.

Capaday, C. & Stein, R.B. (1987) Difference in the amplitude of the human soleus H reflex during walking and running. *Journal of Physiology (London)* **392**, 513–522.

Conrad, B., Benecke, R. & Goehmann, M. (1983) Premovement silent period in fast movement initiation. *Experimental Brain Research* **51**, 310–313.

Coyle, E.F., Feiring, D.C., Rotkis, T.C., Cote, R.W. III & Wilmore, J.H. (1981) Specificity of power improvements through slow and fast isokinetic training. *Journal of Applied Physiology* **51**, 1437–1442.

De Luca, C.J. & Erim, Z. (1994) Common drive of motor units in regulation of muscle force. *Trends in Neuroscience* **17**, 299–305.

De Luca, C.J., LeFever, R.S., McCue, M.P. & Xenakis, A.P. (1982) Behavior of human motor units in different muscles during linearly varying contractions. *Journal of Physiology (London)* **329**, 113–128.

Deecke, L., Scheid, P. & Kornhuber, H.H. (1969) Distribution of readiness potential, pre-motion positivity, and motor potential of the human cerebral cortex preceding voluntary finger movements. *Experimental Brain Research* **7**, 158–168.

Dietz, V., Schmidtbleicher, D. & Noth, J. (1979) Neural mechanisms of human locomotion. *Journal of Neurophysiology* **42**, 1212–1222.

Faulkner, J.A., Claflin, D.R. & McCully, K.K. (1986) *Power output of fast and slow fibers from human skeletal muscles*. In: *Human Muscle Power* (eds N.L. Jones, N. McCartney & A.J. McComas), pp. 81–94. Human Kinetics, Illinois.

Ferbert, A., Priori, A., Rothwell, J.C., Day, B.L., Colebatch, H.G. & Marsden, C.D. (1992) Interhemispheric inhibition of the human motor cortex. *Journal of Physiology (London)* **453**, 525–546.

Freund, H.J., Budingen, H.J. & Dietz, V. (1975) Activity of single motor units from human forearm muscles during voluntary isometric contractions. *Journal of Neurophysiology* **38**, 993–946.

Garland, H. & Angel, R.W. (1971) Spinal and supraspinal factors in voluntary movement. *Experimental Neurology* **33**, 343–350.

Garnett, R.A.F., O'Donovan, M.J., Stephens, J.A. & Taylor, A. (1979) Motor unit organization of human medial gastrocnemius. *Journal of Physiology* **287**, 33–43.

Goldberg, L.J. & Derfler, B. (1977) Relationship among recruitment order, spike amplitude, and twitch tension of single motor units in human masseter muscle. *Journal of Neurophysiology* **40**, 879–890.

Grillner, S. (1981) *Control of locomotion in bipeds, tetrapods, and fish*. In: *Handbook of Physiology. The Nervous System* (ed. V.B. Brooks), pp. 1179–1236. American Physiological Society, Bethesda.

Hallett, M. & Marsden, C.D. (1979) Ballistic flexion movement of the human thumb. *Journal of Physiology (London)* **294**, 33–50.

Heckman, C.J. & Binder, M.D. (1993) Computer simulation of the effects of different synaptic input system on motor unit recruitment. *Journal of Neurophysiology* **70**, 1827–1840.

Henneman, E. & Mendell, L.M. (1981) *Functional organization of the motoneuron pool and its inputs*. In: *Handbook of Physiology. The Nervous System* (ed. V.B. Brooks), pp. 423–507. American Physiological Society, Bethesda.

Henneman, E., Somjem, G. & Carpenter, D.O. (1965) Functional significance of cell size in spinal motoneurons. *Journal of Neurophysiology* **28**, 560–580.

Hodgson, J.A. (1983) The relationship between soleus and gastrocnemius muscle activity in conscious cats —a model for motor unit recruitment? *Journal of Physiology (London)* **337**, 553–562.

Ikai, M. & Fukunaga, T. (1970) A study on training effect on strength per unit cross-sectional area of muscle by means of ultrasonic measurements. *Internationale Zeitschrift fur Angewandte Physiologie Einschliesslich Arbeitsphysiologie* **28**, 173–180.

Kanda, K., Burke, R.E. & Walmsley, B. (1977) Differential control of fast and slow twitch motor units in the decerebrate cat. *Experimental Brain Research* **29**, 57–74.

Kaneko, M. (1970) The relationship between force, velocity and mechanical power in human muscle. *Research Journal of Physical Education Japan* **14**, 141–145.

Kaneko, M. (1974) *The Dynamics of Human Muscle*. Kyorinshoin Book Company, Tokyo [in Japanese].

Kaneko, M., Fuchimoto, T., Toji, H. & Suei, K. (1983) Training effect of different loads on the force–velocity relationship and mechanical power output in human muscle. *Scandinavian Journal of Sports Sciences* **5**, 50–55.

Kawahatsu, K. (1981) *Switching mechanism of neuromuscular activity in top world athletes*. In: *Biomechanics VIII-A* (eds H. Matsui & K. Kobayashi), pp. 289–293. Human Kinetics, Illinois.

Kawahatsu, K. & Miyashita, M. (1983) Electromyogram premotion silent period and tension development in human muscle. *Experimental Neurology* **82**, 287–302.

Koh, T.J., Grabiner, M.D. & Clough, C.A. (1993) Bilateral deficit is larger for step than ramp isometric contractions. *Journal of Applied Physiology* **74**, 1200–1205.

Komi, P.V. (1986) Training of muscle strength and power: Interaction of neuromotoric, hypertrophic and mechanical factors. *International Journal of Sports Medicine* **7**, 10–15.

Komi, P.V. & Viitasalo, J.T. (1977) Changes in motor unit activity and metabolism in human skeletal muscle during and after repeated eccentric and concentric contractions. *Acta Physiologica Scandinavica* **100**, 246–256.

Komi, P.V., Viitasalo, J.T., Rauramaa, R. & Vihko, V. (1978) Effect of isometric strength training on mechanical, electrical and metabolic aspects of muscle function. *European Journal of Applied Physiology* **40**, 45–55.

Kukulka, C.G. & Clamann, H.P. (1981) Comparison of the recruitment and discharge properties of motor units in human brachial biceps and adductor pollicis during isometric contractions. *Brain Research* **219**, 45–55.

Leonard, C.T. (1998) *The Neuroscience of Human Movement*. Mosby, St. Louis.

Lestienne, F. (1979) Effects of inertial load and velocity on the braking process of voluntary limb movements. *Experimental Brain Research* **35**, 407–418.

Milner-Brown, H.S. & Stein, R.B. (1975) The relation between the surface electromyogram and muscular force. *Journal of Physiology (London)* **246**, 549–569.

Milner-Brown, H.S., Stein, R.B. & Yemm, R. (1973) Changes in firing rate of human motor units during linearly changing voluntary contractions. *Journal of Physiology (London)* **230**, 371–390.

Moore, M.A. & Hutton, R.S. (1980) Electromyographic investigation of muscle stretching techniques. *Medicine and Science in Sports and Exercise* **12**, 322–329.

Moritani, T. (1993) Neuromuscular adaptations during the acquisition of muscle strength, power and motor tasks. *Journal of Biomechanics* **26**, 95–107.

Moritani, T. & deVries, H.A. (1979) Neural factors versus hypertrophy in the time course of muscle strength gain. *American Journal of Physical Medicine* **58**, 115–130.

Moritani, T. & Muro, M. (1987) Motor unit activity and surface electromyogram power spectrum during increasing force of contraction. *European Journal of Applied Physiology* **56**, 260–265.

Moritani, T. & Shibata, M. (1994) Premovement electromyographic silent period and α-motoneuron excitability. *Journal of Electromyography and Kinesiology* **4**, 1–10.

Moritani, T. & Yoshitake, Y. (1998) The use of electromyography in applied physiology. *Journal of Electromyography and Kinesiology* **8**, 363–381.

Moritani, T., Muro, M., Kijima, A., Gaffney, F.A. & Persons, A. (1985) Electromechanical changes during electrically induced and maximal voluntary contractions: surface and intramuscular EMG responses during sustained maximal voluntary contraction. *Experimental Neurology* **88**, 484–499.

Moritani, T., Muro, M., Kijima, A. & Berry, M.J. (1986a) Intramuscular spike analysis during ramp force and muscle fatigue. *Electromyography and Clinical Neurophysiology* **26**, 147–160.

Moritani, T., Muro, M. & Nagata, A. (1986b) Intramuscular and surface electromyogram changes during muscle fatigue. *Journal of Applied Physiology* **60**, 1179–1185.

Moritani, T., Muro, M., Ishida, K. & Taguchi, S. (1987) Electromyographic analyses of the effects of muscle power training. *Journal of Medicine and Sports Sciences (Japan)* **1**, 23–32.

Moritani, T., Oddsson, L. & Thorstensson, A. (1990) Differences in modulation of the gastrocnemius and soleus H-reflexes during hopping in man. *Acta Physiologica Scandinavica* **138**, 575–576.

Moritani, T., Oddsson, L. & Thorstensson, A. (1991a) Phase dependent preferential activation of the soleus and gastrocnemius muscles during hopping in humans. *Journal of Electromyography and Kinesiology* **1**, 34–40.

Moritani, T., Oddsson, L. & Thorstensson, A. (1991b) Activation patterns of the soleus and gastrocnemius muscles during different motor tasks. *Journal of Electromyography and Kinesiology* **1**, 81–88.

Mortimer, J.A., Eisengerb, P. & Palmer, S.S. (1984) Premovement silence in agonist muscles preceding maximum efforts. *Experimental Neurology* **98**, 542–554.

Neshige, R., Luders, H., Friedman, L. & Shibasaki, H. (1988a) Recording of movement-related potentials from the human cortex. *Annals of Neurology* **24**, 439–445.

Neshige, R., Luders, H. & Shibasaki, H. (1988b) Recording of movement-related potentials from scalp and cortex in man. *Brain* **111**, 719–736.

Nishizono, H. & Kato, M. (1987) *Inhibition of muscle activity prior to skilled voluntary movement*. In: *Biomechanics* X-A (ed. B. Jonsson), pp. 455–458. Human Kinetics, Illinois.

Nishizono, H., Nakagawa, K., Suda, T. & Saito, K. (1984) An electromyographical analysis of purposive muscle activity and appearance of muscle silent period in archery shooting. *Journal of Physical Fitness Japan* **33**, 17–26.

Oda, S. & Moritani, T. (1994) Maximal isometric force and neural activity during bilateral and unilateral elbow flexion in humans. *European Journal of Applied Physiology* **69**, 240–243.

Oda, S. & Moritani, T. (1995) Movement-related cortical potentials during handgrip contractions with special reference to force and electromyogram bilateral deficit. *European Journal of Applied Physiology* **72**, 1–5.

Oda, S. & Moritani, T. (1996a) Interlimb co-ordination of force and movement-related cortical potentials. *European Journal of Applied Physiology* **74**, 8–12.

Oda, S. & Moritani, T. (1996b) Cross-correlation studies of movement-related cortical potentials during unilateral and bilateral muscle contractions in humans. *European Journal of Applied Physiology* **74**, 29–35.

Oda, S., Shibata, M. & Moritani, T. (1996) Force-dependent changes in movement-related cortical potentials. *Journal of Electromyography and Kinesiology* **6**, 247–252.

Otsuki, T. (1983) Decrease in voluntary isometric strength induced by simultaneous bilateral exertion. *Behavior and Brain Research* **7**, 165–178.

Sale, D.G. (1991) Neural adaptation to strength training. In: *Strength and Power in Sport* (ed P.V. Komi), pp. 249–265. Blackwell Scientific Publications, Oxford.

Sanes, J.N. & Jennings, V.A. (1984) Centrally programmed patterns of muscle activity in voluntary motor behavior of humans. *Experimental Brain Research* **54**, 23–32.

Shibasaki, H., Barrett, G., Halliday, E. & Halliday, A.M. (1980) Components of the movement-related cortical potential and the scalp topography. *Electroencephalography and Clinical Neurophysiology* **49**, 213–226.

Shibata, M., Oda, S. & Moritani, T. (1997) The relationship between movement-related cortical potentials and motor unit activity during muscle contraction. *Journal of Electromyography and Kinesiology* **7**, 79–85.

Singh, J. & Knight, R.T. (1990) Frontal lobe contribution to voluntary movements in humans. *Brain Research* **531**, 45–54.

Smith, J.L., Betts, B., Edgerton, V.R. & Zernicke, R.F. (1980) Rapid ankle extension during paw shakes: selective recruitment of fast ankle extensors. *Journal of Neurophysiology* **43**, 612–620.

Stein, R.B. & Capaday, C. (1988) The modulation of human reflexes during functional motor tasks. *Trends in Neurological Science* **11**, 328–332.

Stephens, J.A. & Usherwood, T.P. (1977) The mechanical properties of human motor units with special reference to their fatigability and recruitment threshold. *Brain Research* **125**, 91–97.

Tanji, J. & Kato, M. (1973) Firing rate of individual motor units in voluntary contraction of abductor digiti minimi in man. *Experimental Neurology* **40**, 771–783.

Thorstensson, A., Grimby, G. & Karlsson, J. (1976) Force–velocity relations and fiber composition in human knee extensor muscles. *Journal of Applied Physiology* **40**, 12–16.

Tihanyi, J., Apor, P. & Fekete, G. (1982) Force–velocity–power characteristics and fiber composition in human knee extensor muscles. *European Journal of Applied Physiology* **48**, 331–343.

Ward, T. (1978) Muscle state: reaction and movement time in elbow extension. *Archives of Physical Medicine and Rehabilitation* **59**, 377–383.

Yabe, K. (1976) Premotion silent period in rapid voluntary movement. *Journal of Applied Physiology* **41**, 470–473.

Yamashita, N. & Moritani, T. (1989) Anticipatory changes of soleus H-reflex amplitude during execution process for heel raise from standing position. *Brain Research* **490**, 148–151.

Chapter 4

Muscular Basis of Strength

R. BILLETER AND H. HOPPELER

Contractile machinery of skeletal muscle fibre types

The sarcomere

Muscle fibres, the cells of skeletal muscles, have one main function: to generate force. They are large cells, containing thousands of nuclei, about 50 μm wide and up to 10 cm long, filled to 80% by the contractile organelle, the myofibrils. These myofibrils are 1–2 μm in diameter. They often extend the whole length of the muscle fibre. They are built as a linear series of sarcomeres. Sarcomeres are the contractile units, consisting of longitudinal thick and thin filaments precisely arranged between the so-called Z-discs that are spaced about 2.5 μm apart (Fig. 4.1). Upon addition of calcium to isolated myofibrils in a test tube, the sarcomeres contract by sliding the thick and thin filaments past each other, pulling their Z-discs closer together, as shown in the electron micrographs of Fig. 4.2. The availability of calcium ions in the space around the myofibrils decides whether the thick and thin filaments can slide against each other. The simultaneous sliding of tens of thousands of sarcomeres in series generates considerable length changes and force development in this cell.

A consequence of the 'sliding filament' model is that the forces generated between actins and myosins are unidirectional, in the sense that they tend to shorten the sarcomere. Extension of an activated muscle (eccentric action) or of an inactive muscle (relaxation) has to be achieved by an

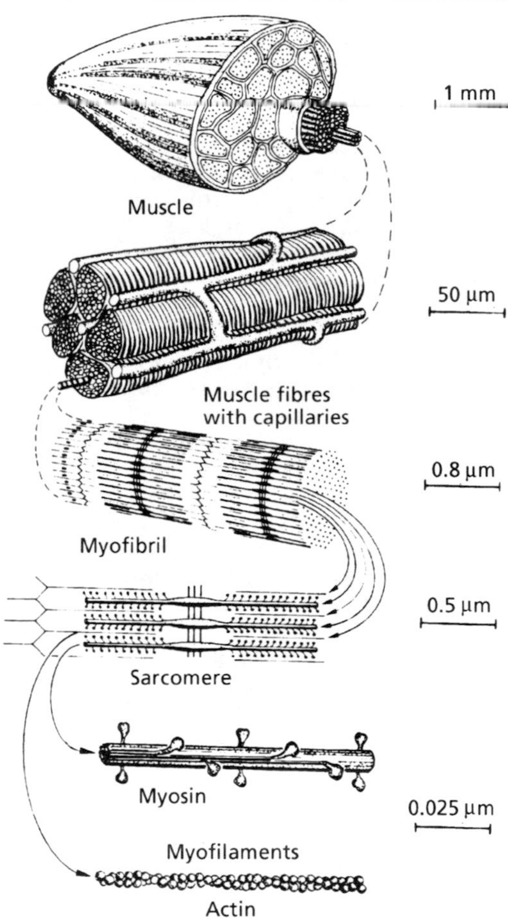

Fig. 4.1 Diagrammatic representation of the structural composition of skeletal muscle tissue. (From di Prampero 1985.)

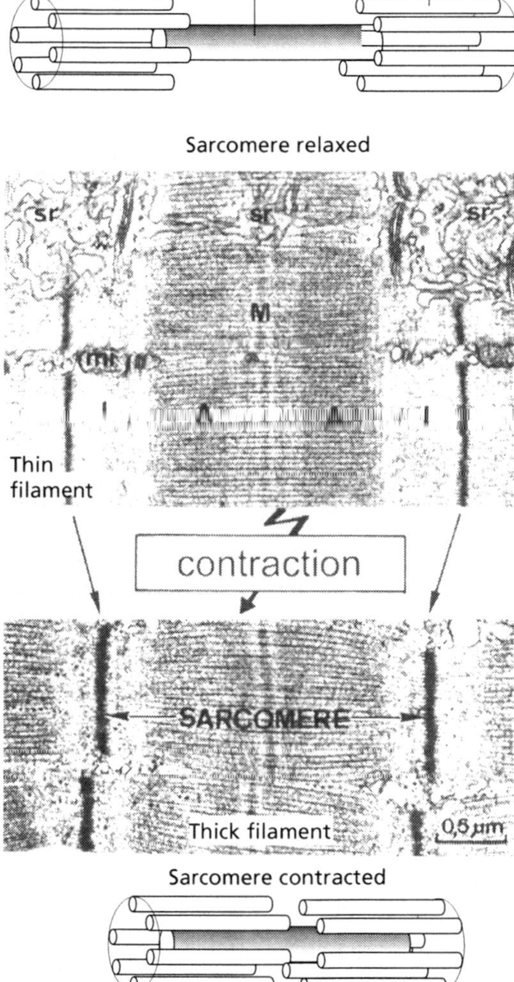

Fig. 4.2 Illustration of the 'sliding filament' theory of muscle contraction. In the relaxed extended state, the Z-lines are spaced about 2.5 µm apart. The thick and thin filaments overlap only partially. In the shortened state, the Z-lines have moved closer, and the thin and thick filaments overlap over most of their lengths. A, A-band; M, M-line; mi, mitochondria; sr, sarcoplasmic reticulum; Z, Z-line. (From Alberts *et al.* 1994.)

outside force. Every muscle in our body is therefore matched by another muscle that can counteract its action, a so-called antagonist. Skeletal muscles therefore work on the agonist–antagonist principle. For some muscles, gravity can take the function of the antagonist.

The thick filament: myosin

The principal protein of the thick filament is myosin. A single myosin molecule consists of two heavy chains with long intertwined tails connected to elongated heads with two light chains bound to each neck region (Fig. 4.3). Isolated myosin molecules can spontaneously form filaments because their tails aggregate spontaneously alongside each other. During the build-up of sarcomeres, this aggregation is thought to be controlled by accessory proteins, such as titin which has a ruler function. This arrangement leads to thick filaments with a bipolar structure composed of about 290 myosins with a bare zone in the middle of the filament, where the tails are packed in antiparallel fashion; no heads are found in this region (Fig. 4.4). The myosin heads are the force-generating sites in muscle. The energy for contraction is derived from the hydrolysis of adenosine triphosphate (ATP) to adenosine diphosphate (ADP) (see below). The ATP cleaving site, the ATPase activity, is located in the myosin head. This ATPase is activated several hundred-fold when the myosin head binds tightly to an actin molecule of the thin filament, as will be described below. An in-depth review of muscular contraction is Gordon *et al.* 2000.

The thin filament: actin with troponin and tropomyosin

The thin filaments (Fig. 4.5) consist of two intertwined strings of actin molecules. Each of the actin strands has a continuous string of adjoining tropomyosin molecules bound to it. These are long, rod-shaped molecules that span a length of seven actin residues each. Every tropomyosin molecule carries a troponin complex, consisting of one dumbbell-shaped protein troponin C, one more globular troponin I and one elongated troponin T, which stretches along the region where two adjoining tropomyosins overlap.

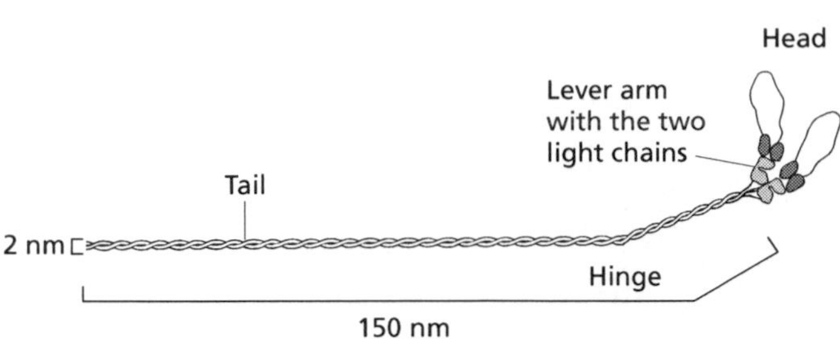

Fig. 4.3 A myosin molecule: myosin consists of a total of six protein chains, two intertwined heavy chains in each head and four light chains (grey), whose function is to stabilize the 'lever arm' at the base of the head. The ATPase activity is located in the heads. (Adapted from Alberts *et al.* 1994 and Geeves & Holmes 1999.)

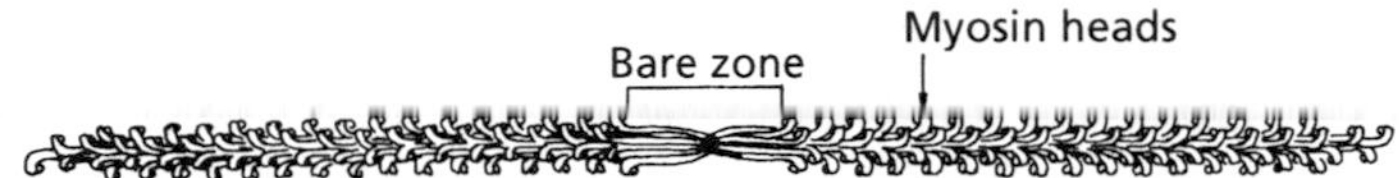

Fig. 4.4 Drawing of a thick filament, consisting of aligned myosin molecules. The myosins are aggregated with their tails, with the heads sticking out of the filament. The bare zone in the middle, where the myosin molecules change their orientation relative to the filament, is composed of tails. Its middle binds the M-line proteins. (From Alberts *et al.* 1994.)

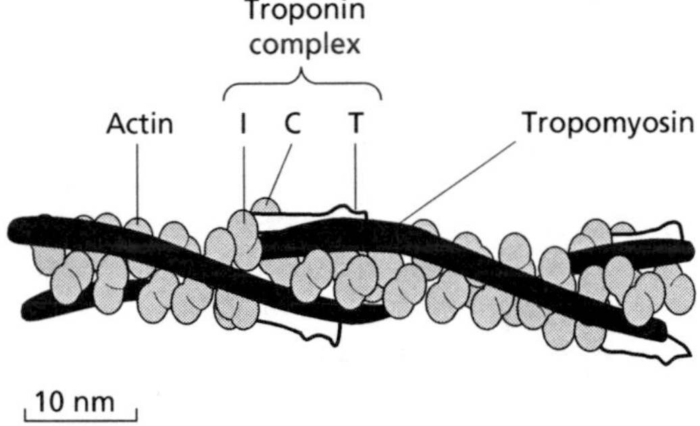

Fig. 4.5 Model of a section of a thin filament, indicating the positions of actin, tropomyosin and the troponin subunits (TnI, TnC and TnT). Each tropomyosin has seven evenly spaced regions of considerable homology, each of which are thought to bind a single actin residue. Since every tropomyosin has one troponin complex bound (consisting of one molecule each of troponin I, C and T), there is only one troponin complex per seven actin residues. The elongated troponin T stretches about a third along a tropomyosin molecule and covers the overlap region between two successive tropomyosins. (From Alberts *et al.* 1994.)

Troponin C does bind calcium ions, the triggers of contraction. Binding of calcium to troponin C induces a conformational change (the troponin C molecule 'opens up'). This motion triggers a series of molecular movements that lead to exposure of the greater part of the binding site for myosin on the actin molecules of the thin filament: Troponin C bends troponin I, which in turn moves troponin T, which moves the tropomyosin coil on the faces of the bound actins from the position covering most of their myosin binding sites to largely freeing them. The myosin heads can now bind to the actin and do so tightly, which moves the tropomyosin coil a little further and activates their ATPase (Fig. 4.6). A detailed model of the changes of the troponin/tropomyosins upon thin filament activation with calcium can be found on the internet under the address http://www.biochem.arizona.edu/classes/bioc462/462a/NOTES/contractile_protein/muscle_contraction.html and http://www.biochem.arizona.edu/classes/bioc462/462a/NOTES/contractile_protein/COMPLEX.GIF. One tropomyosin unit with its adjoining troponin complex forms a so-called 'regulatory unit'. A thin filament of 1 μm in length has 52 regulatory units and consists of about 360 actin molecules.

The cross-bridge cycle: myosin 'walks' along actin

In a muscle, force is generated by the concerted action of billions of myosin heads which bind to

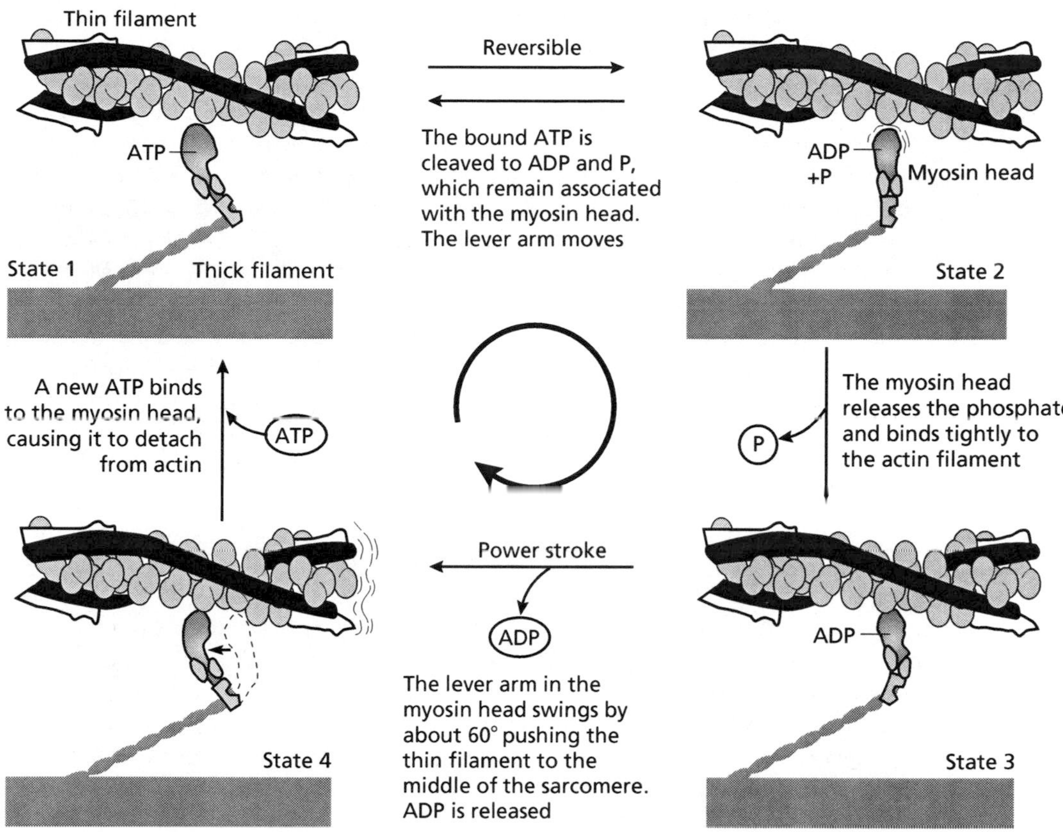

Fig. 4.6 Model of the cross-bridge cycle. Myosin binds ATP to detach from actin (state 1) and splits it into ADP and phosphate, which leads to a movement of the 'lever arm' in the myosin head. ADP and phosphate are still retained in the head, which is free or weakly bound to actin (state 2). Tight binding to actin is accompanied with the release of phosphate (state 3), which leads to release of ADP and a swing of the lever arm by about 60°. Since the myosin head is strongly attached to actin, this moves the whole thin filament (state 4). This is the step that generates force (powerstroke). The head is then detached from actin; it needs to take up a new ATP to do so. Only the transition between states 1 and 2 is reversible, the others are not. (Adapted from Alberts *et al.* 1994 and Geeves & Holmes 1999.)

actin, move, detach, interact with another actin, and so on. This repeated actin–myosin interaction (linked to the breakdown of ATP) is called the cross-bridge cycle (Fig. 4.6). The cross-bridge cycle can be subdivided into four different states of the myosin head. In state 1, the myosin head is not at all or just weakly bound to actin and has ATP bound in the 'pocket' of the ATPase enzyme site in the head. In state 2, the ATP is cleaved to ADP plus phosphate (P_i), but the products are not released; they stay bound at the ATPase site. The distal part of the myosin head, the so-called 'lever arm' stabilized by the two light chains, is twisted by about 60°. The reaction between state 1 and 2 is reversible. The myosin head then binds strongly to an actin residue in the thin filament, upon which the phosphate of the previous ATP is released (state 3). The strong binding and phosphate release is accompanied by a twist of the lever arm in the myosin head back by about 60° to the original position. With the actin bound strongly to the head, this shifts the thin filament towards the middle of the sarcomere (state 4). This step is called the 'powerstroke' of myosin. The step from state 2 (myosin not or weakly bound, ADP and phosphate bound in the head) to state 3 (strong binding and powerstroke) is the main regulatory step in this cycle. Only if the binding site (on the actin) for the myosin head is accessible can the head bind strongly and go into state 3. Accessibility to this binding site is regulated by the position of the tropomyosin on the thin filament. The binding site is accessible with calcium bound to troponin C; it is obstructed by tropomyosin when no calcium is bound to troponin C (see above). After the myosin head has performed its 'powerstroke', it detaches from the actin only after binding an ATP molecule. This brings the myosin back to state 1, but with the thin filament shifted by the distance of the powerstroke. With each thick filament having about 500 heads and each head going though the cycle from state 1 to 4 a few hundred times a second in the course of rapid shortening, thick and thin filaments can slide past each other at rates of up to 15 $mm \cdot ms^{-1}$.

Thus the step that requires ATP, namely the detachment of the myosin head from the actin filament after the powerstroke (state 4 back to state 1), is not the regulatory step that switches the cross-bridge cycle on and off. The regulation via calcium–troponin C–tropomyosin affects the step from state 2 to state 3. A muscle that is completely depleted of its ATP gets very stiff because the heads cannot be released from the actin filament. This is rigor mortis.

The sarcomere is built of many more proteins

While actin and myosin are clearly the most abundant proteins in the sarcomere, many more are necessary for its build-up, maintenance and function. Figure 4.7 locates a small number of the hundred or so different proteins thought to make up a sarcomere. Table 4.1 indicates their function. Structures or functions of many of the others are not well known yet. An in-depth review of thin filament proteins and their functions is Littlefield & Fowler 1998.

Titin is the largest protein so far isolated. It has a range of different functions. A titin molecule in a sarcomere stretches from the Z-disc all the way to the M-line, and thus spans half the sarcomere. The anchoring in the Z-line is strong; this part is thought to help determine the thickness (and thus the strength) of a fibre's Z-disc. Along the thin filament, titin is thought to bind weakly if at all; about in the middle of the thin filament, there is a region of great elasticity, while along the thin filament, titin binds tightly to elements in the aligned myosin tails. The elastic portions of titin are thought to be instrumental in keeping the thick filaments exactly centred in the middle of a sarcomere. The internet address http://www.leeds.ac.uk/bms/research/muscle/titin.htm shows an animated version of this concept. In sarcomeres stretched past the thick–thin filament overlap (i.e. loss of the contacts between thick and thin filaments through myosin heads), titin still holds the sarcomere together; without it, the sarcomere is thought to snap (Fig. 4.8). Titin is also thought to function as the principal measuring stick in the build-up of a sarcomere, functioning as central ruler in the mechanisms responsible for the precisely controlled lengths of thin and thick filaments (Gregorie *et al.* 1999).

In skeletal muscle fibres, the Z-discs of sarcomeres in neighbouring myofibrils are linked to each other via cytoskeletal proteins (e.g. desmin, Fig. 4.7), giving muscle fibres their characteristic 'striated' appearance. These lateral connections are extended to the fibre's membrane, where the links are anchored in large protein complexes (the so-called sarcoglycan complexes and costameres), from which there are connections into the fine mesh of connective tissue that surrounds each muscle fibre and is contiguous with the muscle's tendon. Thus, from every Z-disc, there is not just vertical force transmission along the myofibril, there is also (much weaker, but significant) lateral force transmission into the connective tissue scaffold of a muscle.

Excitation–contraction coupling

The large skeletal muscles in our body consist of up to a million muscle fibres. The exact coordination of the contraction of all these fibres and muscles is achieved by a subdivision of this huge

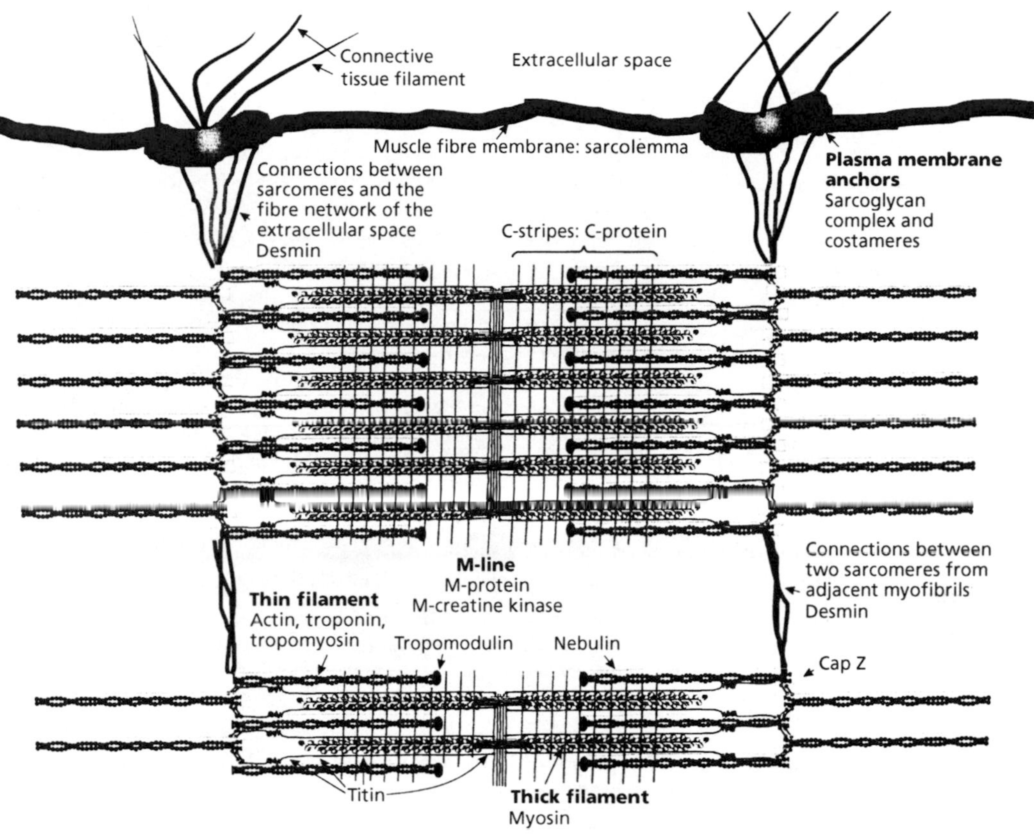

Fig. 4.7 Representation of additional sarcomeric proteins. Table 4.1 lists the known functions of the proteins indicated in this figure.

population of fibres into functional units—the motor units—that can be operated by the central nervous system.

The motor unit

Motor units consist of a motor nerve, which in the case of the limb muscles has its nerve body and nucleus located in the grey matter of the spinal cord and forms a long axon going all the way down the limb to the muscle, where it branches out and innervates several fibres (up to 2000 in large 'fast' motor units). Innervation of a given fibre is through one single nerve ending (synapse) located approximately in the middle of the muscle fibre (Fig. 4.9). When a motor unit is activated, impulses travel down the axon at a speed of several metres per second and are distributed to all the fibres in the motor unit. The excitation of the nerve is transferred by the synapse to the muscle fibre's membrane. The depolarization of the muscle cell membrane travels via the T-tubular system into the muscle fibre, where calcium is released from the sarcoplasmic reticulum stores. These calcium ions activate the troponin complex (by binding to troponin C), which in turn switches on the myosin cross-bridge cycle (see above). The whole activation process takes only a few milliseconds. Since all the fibres in a motor unit are contracting simul-taneously, they are of the same histochemical fibre type, and moreover have very similar metabolic and physiological properties (see below).

Table 4.1 Sarcomere proteins and their functions.

Element	Protein	Function
Z-line	α-Actinin	Holds thin filaments in place and in register. Z-lines of slow fibres have more α-actinin than those of fast ones
	Desmin	Forms the connection between adjacent Z-lines from different myofibrils. This keeps their sarcomeres in register. Desmin is thus responsible for the regular striated appearance of muscle fibres
Thin filament	Actin	Forms the core of the thin filament. Interacts with myosin
	Tropomyosin	Moves on the surface of the neighbouring actins upon calcium binding to the troponin complex, thereby freeing the site for strong binding of the myosin head
	Troponin	Troponin C binds calcium, changes upon binding, which induces the tropomyosin 'switch' that transforms the calcium signal into molecular signals, including cross-bridge cycling
	Cap Z	Caps the Z-line end of the actin strand in the thin filament
	Tropomodulin	Caps the inner end of the actin strand in the thin filament
	Nebulin	Located alongside thin filaments. Thought to be the 'ruler' that determines the precisely adjusted length of the thin filaments
Thick filament	Myosin	The 'motor' of muscle. Splits ATP. Generates force in the head
C-stripes	C-protein	Thought to increase the force of a sarcomere in situations of higher demand, by moving the myosin heads closer to the actin, thus increasing the chance of a greater number of heads binding at any one time
M-line	M-protein	Holds thick filaments in a regular array. Also anchoring point for titin
	M-creatine kinase (M-CK)	Provides ATP from creatine phosphate; located close to the myosin heads
Elastic filament	Titin	Keeps the thick filament in the middle between the two Z-discs during contraction and represents a security against overstretching the sarcomere; also thought to control the number of myosin molecules contained in the thick filament

The synapse

The site of transduction of the nerve electrical impulses from the motor nerve's membrane to the muscle fibre's membrane is the 'neuromuscular junction' (Fig. 4.10), the end of the axon or synapse, which in skeletal muscle has finger-like extensions indenting the fibre's surface. The membranes of these extensions are separated from the muscle fibre's membrane by a cleft of only 0.05 μm. When an electrical impulse arrives at the synapse, acetylcholine, a small molecule, is released by the nerve terminal and diffuses rapidly through the small cleft to the muscle membrane. There it is bound to an acetylcholine receptor, which in turn opens sodium channels giving rise to an electrical impulse travelling down the muscle cell's membrane. The acetylcholine is rapidly cleaved (and thus rendered non-functional) and taken back up by the nerve terminal. From the neuromuscular junction, the electrical impulse not only travels up and down the muscle fibre's membrane (at a speed exceeding 1 $m{\cdot}s^{-1}$), it also reaches the inside of the muscle fibre by way of the membranes of the T-tubular system (Fig. 4.11).

The sarcoplasmic reticulum regulates intracellular calcium

The T-tubules inside the fibre are connected by knob-like structures to the sarcoplasmic reticu-

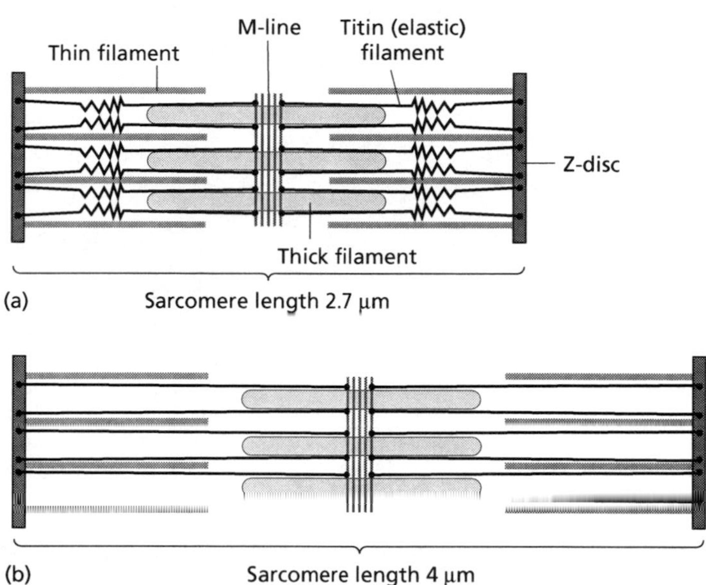

Fig. 4.8 Schematic illustration of titin (elastic) filament function. (a) Titin filaments link the M-lines of the thick filaments to the Z-discs. Titin is bound to the thick filament, but only weakly interacts with the thin filament. The jagged part of the line indicates the region with the greatest elasticity in titin. The action of these elastic elements on both sides keeps the thick filaments centred at rest. (b) An overstretched sarcomere is still kept together despite the loss of overlap between thin and thick filaments. (Adapted from Horowits & Podolsky 1987.)

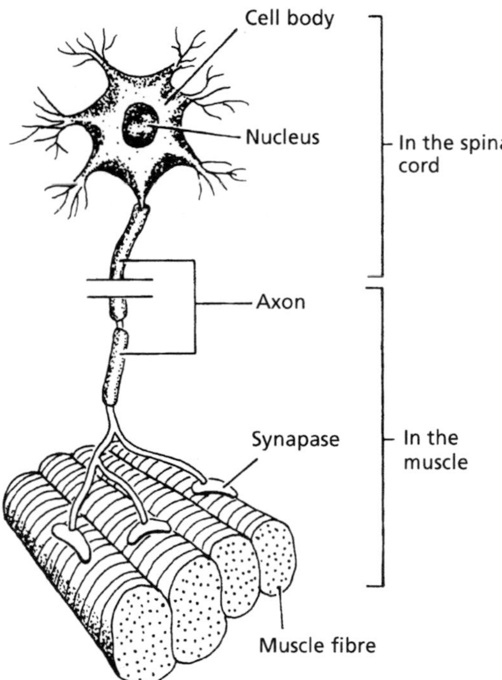

Fig. 4.9 A motor unit consists of its motor nerve, which branches out to form connections to many muscle fibres through synapses, called motor end plates. (From Brooks *et al.* 2000.)

lum, a sheet of anastomosing, flattened vesicles that surround each myofibril like a net stocking (Fig. 4.11). The sarcoplasmic reticulum is a calcium store. Inside, the calcium ion concentration is about 10 000-fold higher than in the sarcoplasm of the muscle fibre. The T-tubules are physically connected to their neighbouring part of the sarcoplasmic reticulum via protein complexes (so-called 'junctional feet') that provide contacts between the (sodium) channels that transmit the electrical impulses through the T-tubuli and the calcium channels of the sarcoplasmic reticulum (Fig. 4.12). These channel proteins are normally closed. With the electrical impulse going through the T-tubular channels, the connected sarcoplasmic reticulum calcium channels are opened and release a small quantity of calcium ions, enough to permit the calcium concentration inside the muscle fibre to rise about 100-fold. This calcium release is driven by the large concentration difference between the sarcoplasmic reticulum and the muscle fibre's sarcoplasm. If no other impulse comes along the T-tubules, the calcium ions are quickly pumped back by the calcium pumps of the sarcoplasmic reticulum membranes. These pumps are situated further away from the junctional feet. After a

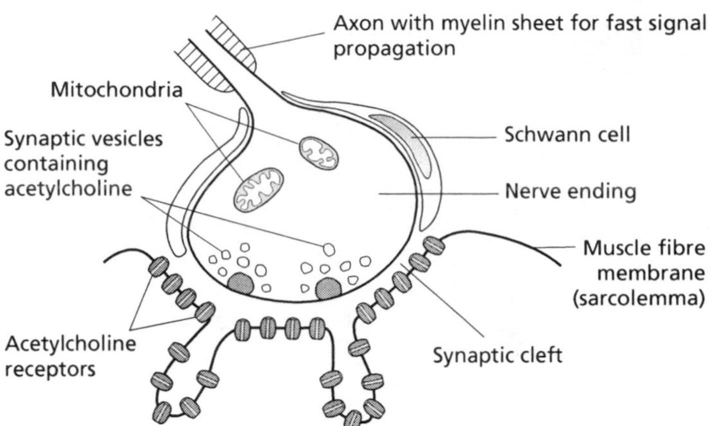

Fig. 4.10 The nerve ending on a skeletal muscle fibre has finger-like extensions that are lowered into the fibre's circumference. This illustration depicts a cross-section through such a 'finger' of a motor end plate. It is separated from the muscle fibre by a very small space, the synaptic cleft, which has further indentations in towards the muscle fibre. The motor end plate uses acetylcholine as transmitter substance. This is stored in synaptic vesicles. When an electrical impulse from the axon reaches the synapse, acetylcholine is released into the synaptic cleft and taken up by acetylcholine receptors that are located on the muscle side of the cleft in the fibre's membrane. The acetylcholine receptors then generate an electrical impulse that travels down the muscle membrane. On their 'exposed' side, the nerve's axon as well as the nerve ending (synapse) is covered by Schwann cells, which offer protection and tight control of the axons' ionic environment. (Adapted from Hall & Sanes 1993.)

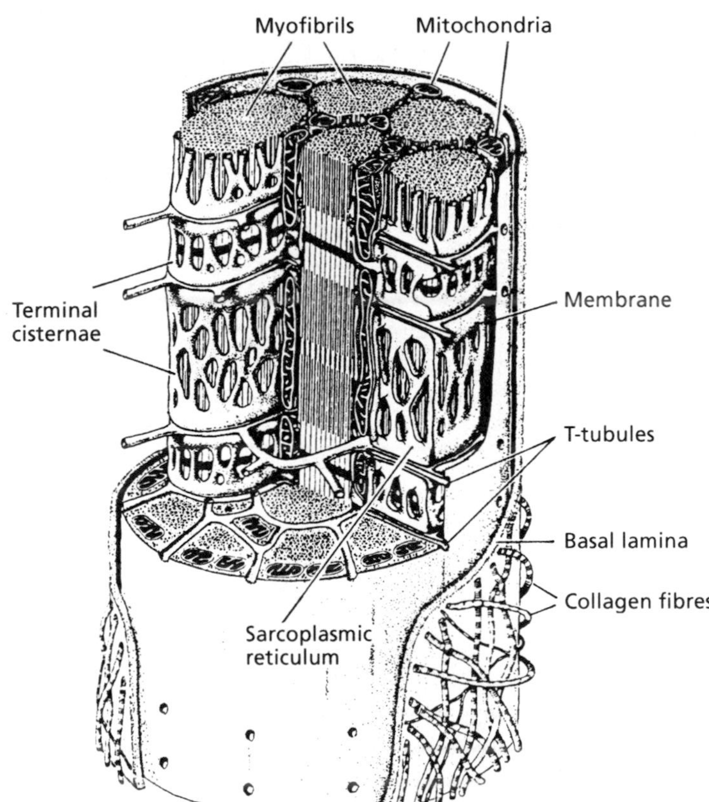

Fig. 4.11 Drawing of part of a skeletal muscle fibre, showing the relationship of sarcoplasmic reticulum, terminal cisternae, T-tubules and mitochondria to myofibrils. (From Krstic 1978.)

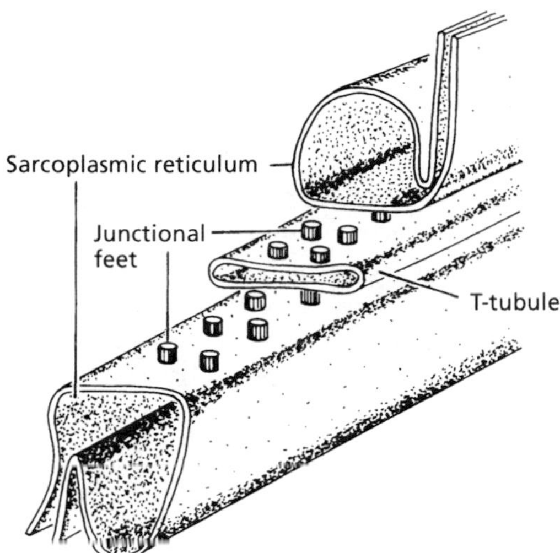

Fig. 4.12 Connection between T-tubules and the sarcoplasmic reticulum. The two structures are connected by large protein complexes, 'junctional feet'. In these junctional feet, the channels transmitting the impulse through the T-tubule make direct contact with calcium channels in the sarcoplasmic reticulum membrane. An impulse leads to opening of the sarcoplasmic reticulum channels, inducing release of calcium from the sarcoplasmic reticulum. (From Eisenberg 1983.)

single impulse, the calcium concentration in the cytosol is restored to resting levels, typically within 30 ms. The calcium pumps derive their energy to bring the ions back into the sarcoplasmic reticulum through splitting of ATP. Up to 30% of a muscle fibre's ATP used during contraction is accounted for by the sarcoplasmic reticulum calcium pumps. Inside the sarcoplasmic reticulum, excess calcium ions are bound to calsequestrin, a special calcium binding protein. When a muscle fibre is activated during a normal contraction, it generally does not receive just a single impulse, but rather a volley of several impulses; the calcium ions cannot be pumped back fast enough between these impulses. Calcium can thus accumulate to higher levels in the fibre's interior and has a better chance to activate the majority or all of the thin filaments in a given fibre. More regulatory units are activated and higher forces can be developed during such 'tetanic bursts' as compared to a single stimulus. The rise in intracellular calcium concentration also has a stimulating effect on the mitochondrial metabolism; thus ATP generation is enhanced at the same time that ATP use by the myofibrils is activated. Another possibility for regulating the force output of a given muscle is via modulation of the number of muscle fibres that are activated via motor units (see below).

Muscle fibre types

Isoforms of myofibrillar proteins

A majority of the proteins of the sarcomere and the sarcoplasmic reticulum exist in different molecular forms, so-called isoforms. Isoforms are different 'editions' of the same protein; they differ only slightly in their structures. Functional differences between isoforms include different reaction speeds, tighter binding to target proteins, etc.

The isoforms of myosin are the basis for the nomenclature of muscle fibre types. These myosin isoforms differ in the rate at which the ATPase in the myosin head operates. During an unloaded contraction in a fast human muscle fibre, a single head of fast myosin is estimated to split about 80 ATP per second. Slow myosins work at rates that are 3–5 times slower. The different ATPase reaction rates correspond to the contractile properties of the muscle fibres that contain different myosins: A human fast fibre is estimated to be able to shorten maximally in about a tenth of a second; a slow fibre needs about a third of a second. Since fibres with fast myosins have a faster cross-bridge cycle, they are optimally used in quick movements. Fibres with slow myosins, which have a slower cross-bridge cycle, are best suited for static (tonic) exercise and for the—relatively slow—everyday movements, as well as for posture. At these contraction speeds, fast fibres work less efficiently. The force that can be generated per head during a cross-bridge cycle does not vary between fast and slow myosins. Because fast myosins do split ATP faster (step 2 in the cross-bridge cycle above), the force generated per head over time is greater for fast than for slow myosins, because the fast myosins' cross-bridge cycle is shorter. This has been experimentally shown for isolated human fibres (He *et al.* 2000). The transfer of such data from isolated fibres to whole muscles is not straightforward, however: a majority of studies with human subjects have not been able to show a correlation between maximal strength and fibre type composition (determined from needle biopsies); the main factor determining maximal strength is the muscle's volume. This apparent contradiction could be due to the difficulty in simultaneously activating all muscle fibres to the maximum in a given muscle.

MUSCLE FIBRE TYPING IS BASED ON MYOFIBRILLAR ATPASE HISTOCHEMISTRY

The classical histochemical way of fibre typing relies on the recognition of the three distinct myosin isoforms, which can be distinguished on the basis of the sensitivity of their ATPase activity to acid and alkaline solutions (Fig. 4.13). When a muscle cryostat section (from a needle biopsy, for example) is incubated in a solution of pH 10.6 before the myosin ATPase reaction is performed, only fibres with predominantly fast myosin show the coloured reaction product and therefore ATPase activity. Such fibres are called fast, fast-twitch or Type II fibres. When a muscle

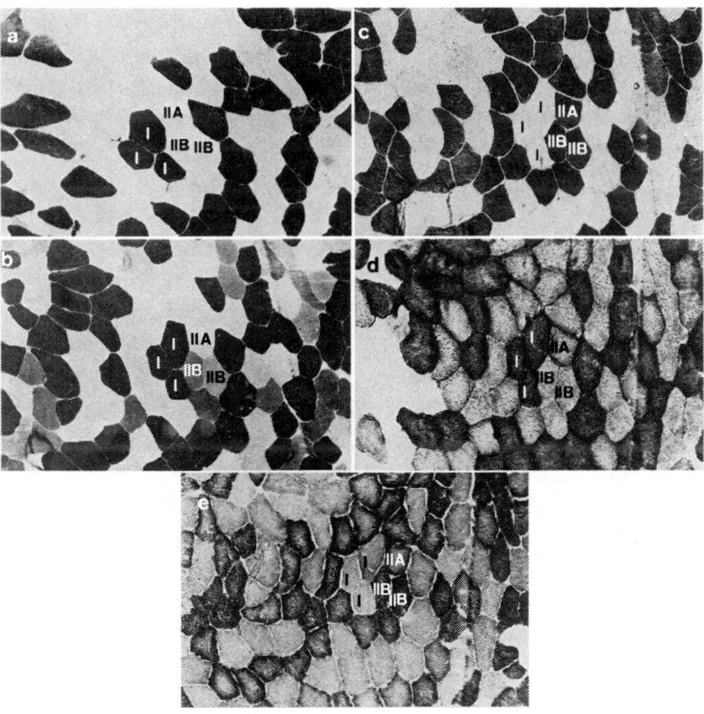

Fig. 4.13 Histochemical fibre typing in human *m. vastus lateralis*. (a) Myofibrillar ATPase reaction of a 10-µm cryostat section after preincubation at pH 4.3. The ATPase of Type I fibres is still active, Type II fibre ATPase is inactivated. (b) Myofibrillar ATPase reaction after preincubation at pH 4.6. The ATPase of Type I fibres is active, Type IIB fibre ATPase is moderately affected, Type IIA fibre ATPase is inactivated. (c) Myofibrillar ATPase reaction after preincubation at pH 10.6. The ATPase of Type II fibres is activated, Type I fibre ATPase is inactive. (d) Succinate dehydrogenase reaction. This stain indicates the oxidative capacities of the muscle fibres. Note the slightly higher activity of the IIA fibre compared to IIB. (e) α-Glycerolphosphate dehydrogenase reaction. It indicates the glycolytic (lactate-generating) capacities of the fibres. Note the variability in Type I fibres and slightly reduced reaction in some Type IIA fibres when compared to IIB.

cryostat section is incubated at pH 4.3 before the ATPase reaction, only the fibres containing the slow myosin show the reaction product and thus ATPase activity. These fibres are called slow, slow-twitch or Type I fibres. Preincubation at pH 4.6 reveals that the myosin ATPase of some of the Type II fibres shows resistance against this pH; the myosins of others do not. The fibres staining slightly after incubation at pH 4.6 are called Type IIB or, by some authors, IIX; the blank fibres are Type IIA.

As indicated by the differences in acid sensitivity of their ATPase reactions, the myosin isoforms of Type IIA and IIB fibres are different. In almost all human skeletal muscles, there are only two fast myosin isoforms (called IIA and IIB in this chapter). In rodent muscles, three fast myosin isoforms are found: IIA, IIB and IIX. The amino acid sequences of IIB and IIX myosins are very similar, but still different. Some authors argue that the myosin in human fibres staining intermediately after preincubation at pH 4.6 is closer in sequence to rodent IIX myosin than IIB, thus naming them IIX. The majority of the literature on human fibre types still uses the original nomenclature, typing these fibres as IIB. It is for this reason that we also use the original term IIB for this fibre for the time being.

Figure 4.13 also shows that these muscle fibre types have quite different metabolic capacities. Type I (slow-twitch) fibres stain stronger for succinate dehydrogenase than Type II (fast-twitch) fibres. They therefore have higher oxidative capacities, i.e. more mitochondria with more enzymes of the pathways of lipid and glucose oxidation. They generate their ATP mainly through the oxidation of glucose units and fatty acids (see below). Only when producing very high power output do they form lactate. They can also use lactate as an energy source. This is achieved by taking up lactate from the bloodstream or from the interstitial tissue between the fibres, turning it into pyruvate and oxidizing it in the mitochondria. As already mentioned, slow fibres have lower contraction velocities than fast fibres. Due to their oxidative metabolism and their higher efficiency, they show a much greater resistance to fatigue. Type II (fast-twitch) fibres stain weaker for succinate dehydrogenase than Type I, but they stain stronger for α-glycerolphosphate dehydrogenase. The α-glycerolphosphate dehydrogenase staining intensity indicates the glycolytic capacity of a muscle fibre. This is its ability to form lactate from the glycogen stores in the fibre. Type II fibres generate the ATP for force production chiefly through anaerobic glycolysis, which results in the production of lactate. They have smaller amounts of mitochondria, and their power output during repetitive activation could not be achieved through ATP produced in their mitochondria. They tend to fatigue quickly, because they accumulate the lactate produced (up to 30 fold the concentration in resting muscle). The low pH associated with this lactate accumulation as well as the corresponding rise in free phosphate inhibits the myosin ATPase, slowing contraction speed or stopping active contraction entirely. Type IIA fibres are intermediate to Type I and Type IIB fibres in their contractile and metabolic characteristics.

As previously mentioned, human Type II fibres have two- to fivefold faster shortening velocities than Type I. Within each fibre type, however, there is a considerable range of variation in the physiological parameters, such as velocity, relaxation time or fatigability. The distribution of these parameters among the fibres of a particular muscle is often continuous. 'Fine tuning' of a fibre's physiological property to its exact pattern of use is thought to involve appropriate isoform combinations of myofibrillar proteins other than myosin (e.g. troponin T, which occurs in a large number of forms). All of the fibres belonging to a given motor unit, however, have the same contractile and metabolic properties and should therefore also have identical protein isoform compositions.

Motor unit recruitment

In most voluntary everyday activity, slow (Type I) motor units are the first to be recruited. With increasing power output, more and more fast (Type II) units are activated. Trained people can

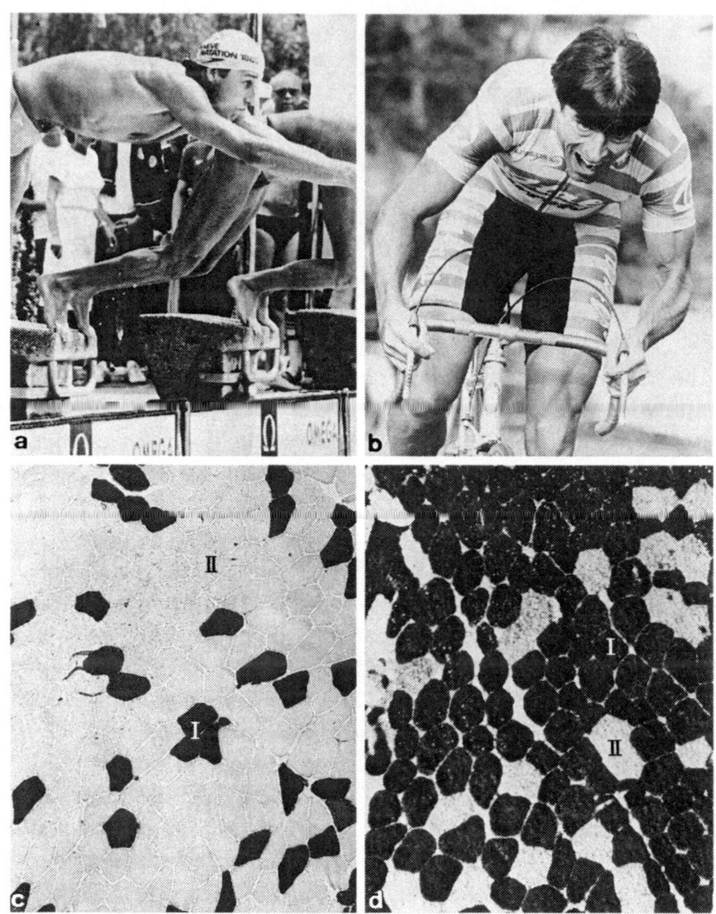

Fig. 4.14 Fibre type composition of two selected top athletes. (a) A swimmer whose speciality was the 50-m crawl sprint. (b) A professional cyclist of world-class 'roller' type. (c,d) Cryostat sections of the swimmer's and cyclist's *vastus lateralis* muscles, stained for ATPase after preincubation at pH 4.3. Type I fibres stain dark, Type II fibres remain unstained. (c) The vast majority of the swimmer's fibres are Type II (fast twitch). (d) The vast majority of the cyclist's fibres are Type I (slow twitch).

activate most if not all of the motor units in a large limb muscle during a static, maximal voluntary contraction, whereas this is not possible for untrained people. The 'fastest' (Type IIB) motor units are preferentially activated in fast corrective movements and reflexes. Explosive maximal contractions are thought to activate fast and slow motor units simultaneously. Slow motor units often contain only few fibres; fast motor units are larger and may contain up to 2000 fibres. For other details of motor unit recruitment see Chapter 2.

Athletes may have extreme fibre type distributions

It has been known for several decades that top athletes in sports requiring either high speed or very good endurance have very different fibre type compositions in their muscles. Figure 4.14 illustrates this, with muscle samples from a swimmer whose speciality was the 50-m crawl sprint; it is compared to a muscle sample from a professional cyclist. The swimmer has about 80% Type II (fast-twitch) fibres in his vastus lateralis muscle, the cyclist about 80% Type I (slow-twitch) fibres. Such extreme fibre type compositions can be a consequence of genetic predetermination as well as the consequence of the training of these athletes. Regular endurance training over periods of several months has been shown to induce fibre type conversions from Type IIB to IIA in most Type IIB fibres, and from Type IIA to Type I in a few per cent of the original Type IIA fibres. High volumes of endurance training over many years can transform a substantial number of Type II fibres in e.g. the vastus lateralis muscle to Type I. Recent data indicate that the response to a given dose of training can be quite different between individuals (Bouchard & Rankinen 2001), thus the ability to transform one's fibre types due to training could be an indirect effect of a person's own responsiveness to training.

Energy supply systems

The contractile machinery occupies some 80% of a muscle fibre's volume and thus represents about one-third of our body mass. The intricate network of T-tubules and sarcoplasmic reticulum cisternae that regulates actin–myosin interaction is comparatively compact and occupies only about 5% of a fibre's volume. However, both the process of muscle contraction as well as the maintenance of the necessary ion gradients within and around the muscle fibres are critically dependent on the energy status of the muscle cell. This section explores the pathways which channel energy into muscle force development.

Aerobic metabolism

When a muscle cell is not supplying external mechanical energy, but is simply ticking over, the comparatively small amount of energy it consumes is generated by cell respiration or 'oxidative phosphorylation'. In this process, foodstuff, primarily lipids, are being broken down in a sort of cellular furnace that is located in specific submicroscopic organelles called mitochondria (Fig. 4.15). These processes allow the capture of some 50% of the energy stored in the chemical bonds of the substrates. In the case of e.g. sucrose and fructose that we ingest when we eat an apple, this energy was derived from solar energy that served to bind atmospheric CO_2 at the time the fruit was ripening on the tree. Respiration can be considered a form of cellular combustion, which allows for the liberation of energy in a form that can be reused for the energy-requiring processes of the cell. The unused or waste energy is lost as heat and serves to maintain our body temperature.

It has been demonstrated that cellular combustion occurs at about the same efficiency in all mammals. Thus, the quantity of oxygen consumed is directly proportional to the power yield of the organism. The production of 1 W of metabolic power requires the consumption of 3 $ml \cdot min^{-1}$ of oxygen. At rest, a human consumes about 300 $ml \cdot min^{-1}$ of oxygen and therefore produces metabolic energy at a rate of approximately 100 W. The main oxygen consumers are the brain, heart, kidneys and intestinal organs. Despite its large size, the (inactive) musculature consumes less than 20% of the total energy at rest.

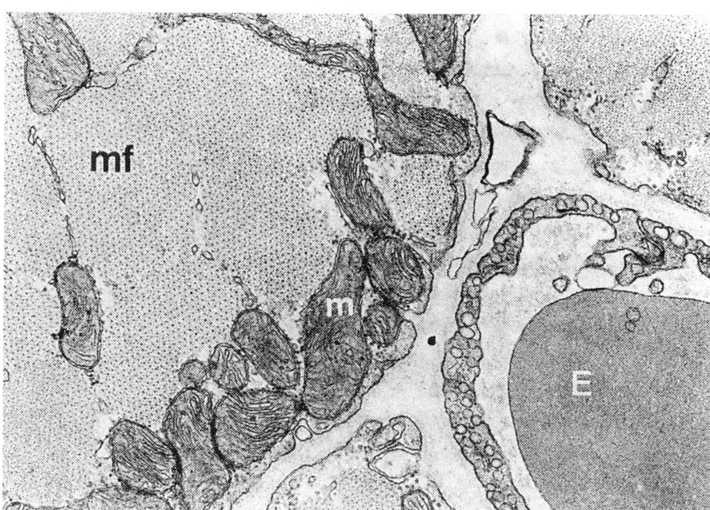

Fig. 4.15 Electron micrograph showing cross-sections of skeletal muscle fibre segments. A capillary contains an erythrocyte (E). In the muscle fibre, thin actin and thick myosin filaments (mf) are apparent, as well as mitochondria (m).

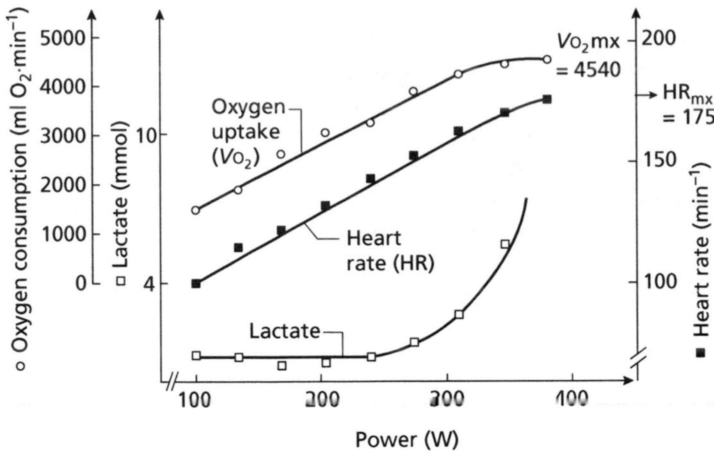

Fig. 4.16 Increase of oxygen consumption (○), heart rate (■) and plasma lactate concentration (□) during a typical bicycle ergometer performance test. Power was increased by 35 W every 2 min until the subject was exhausted.

This is different during mechanical work. With increasing workloads, e.g. in an aerobic performance test on a bicycle ergometer, oxygen consumption increases in proportion to the external load (Fig. 4.16). Eventually, oxygen consumption levels off and further energy for increased muscle contraction must be primarily supplied by anaerobic glycolysis. As a consequence, we observe a rapid increase in plasma lactate levels at these high power outputs. We will further explore the process of glycolysis below.

If we carry out the performance test with a large enough proportion of our total muscle mass, we will observe a plateau of oxygen consumption, beyond which it cannot be increased voluntarily. This plateau is called maximal oxygen consumption or $Vo_{2\,max}$. At $Vo_{2\,max}$, more than 90% of the oxygen taken up by the lungs goes to skeletal muscle mitochondria (Åstrand & Rodahl 1986). Thus, there is a large dynamic range of functional regulation of skeletal muscle cellular respiration, which by far surpasses the regulatory capacity of other organs. There has been a long lasting debate as to which of all the transfer steps from lungs to skeletal muscle mitochondria might be the limiting one, responsible for setting the pace of aerobic energy flow in humans. There is now considerable evidence that all the transfer steps add some resistance to oxygen flow into the periphery (Fig. 4.17). During exercise with a large muscle mass in

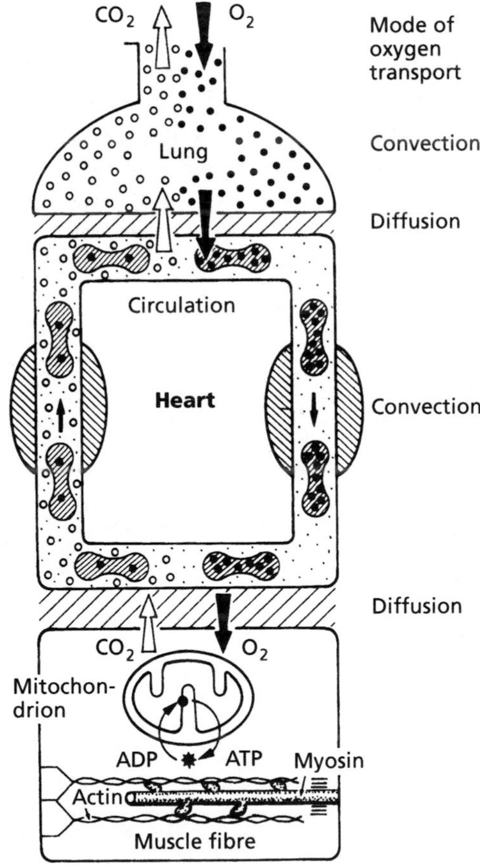

Fig. 4.17 Model of gas exchange in the human respiratory system.

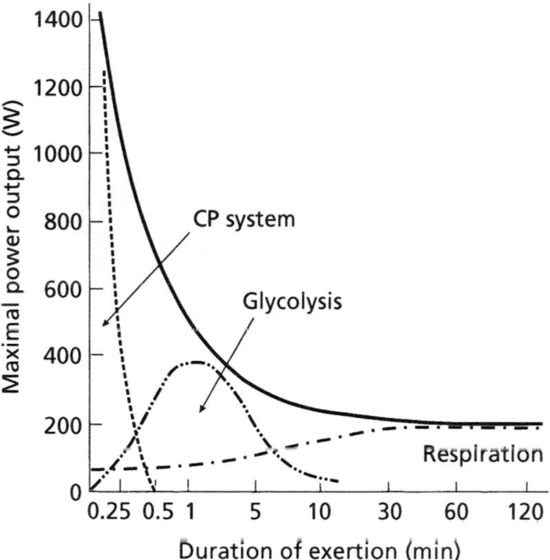

Fig. 4.18 Decrease of maximal mechanical power output on a bicycle ergometer as a function of the duration of exercise. The approximate contributions of the different cellular energy supply systems are indicated under the curve.

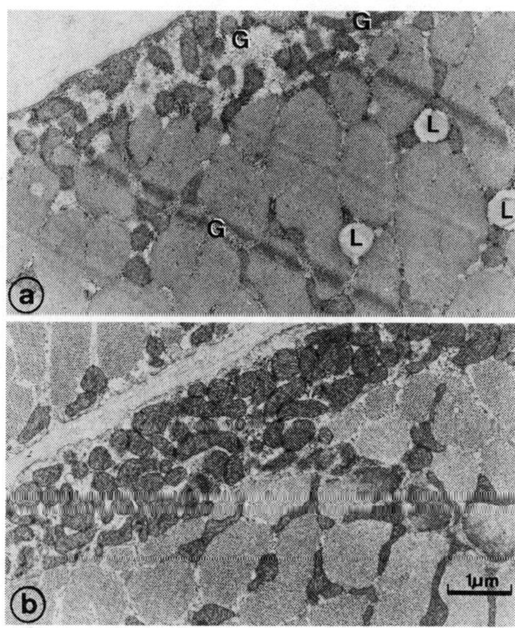

Fig. 4.19 Cross-sections of muscle fibres (a) before and (b) after running 100 km in 7 h. The cellular substrate stores of glycogen (G) and lipid (L) have almost completely disappeared after the long-distance run.

humans, cardiovascular transport is a major limiting factor (di Prampero 1985), but recent evidence highlights the importance of intracellular pH in the muscle fibres (Conley *et al.* 2001).

In order to maintain the highest possible power output for a prolonged period of time (e.g. over 30 min, Fig. 4.18), muscle cell respiration must be close to the value reached at $V\text{O}_{2max}$. An untrained, young man may be capable of maintaining a power output of 200 W, consuming just over 3 l·min^{-1} of oxygen. A highly trained professional bicyclist should be capable of a power output of just over 400 W, with a corresponding oxygen uptake of close to 6 l·min^{-1}. As discussed above, the limit for aerobic mechanical power production is not in the contractile machinery, it is rather given by the characteristics of an individual's entire respiratory system.

Energy storage and transfer

During aerobic exercise, oxygen must be supplied continuously to muscle fibres. The oxygen flow rate is therefore representative of the energy flux in active muscle cells. Oxygen must be constantly supplied from outside because only small quantities of oxygen can be stored in muscle tissue in humans.

This is not the case for the substrates of cellular combustion. Glucose (in its storage form glycogen) and lipids (in fat droplets) are stored intracellularly in muscle cells. Continuous, very long lasting exercise, such as a 100-km run, leads to almost complete depletion of these stores (Kayar *et al.* 1986, Fig. 4.19). Nutrient supply via the bloodstream through capillaries can, except for very low intensity exercise, only account for a fraction of the cellular substrate use. Active transport across the cell membrane is thought to be a bottleneck for the entry of both glucose and free fatty acids into the muscle cell. Energy can also be generated from amino acids, but this system is of minor importance for the energy budget of a working muscle cell in a well-nourished

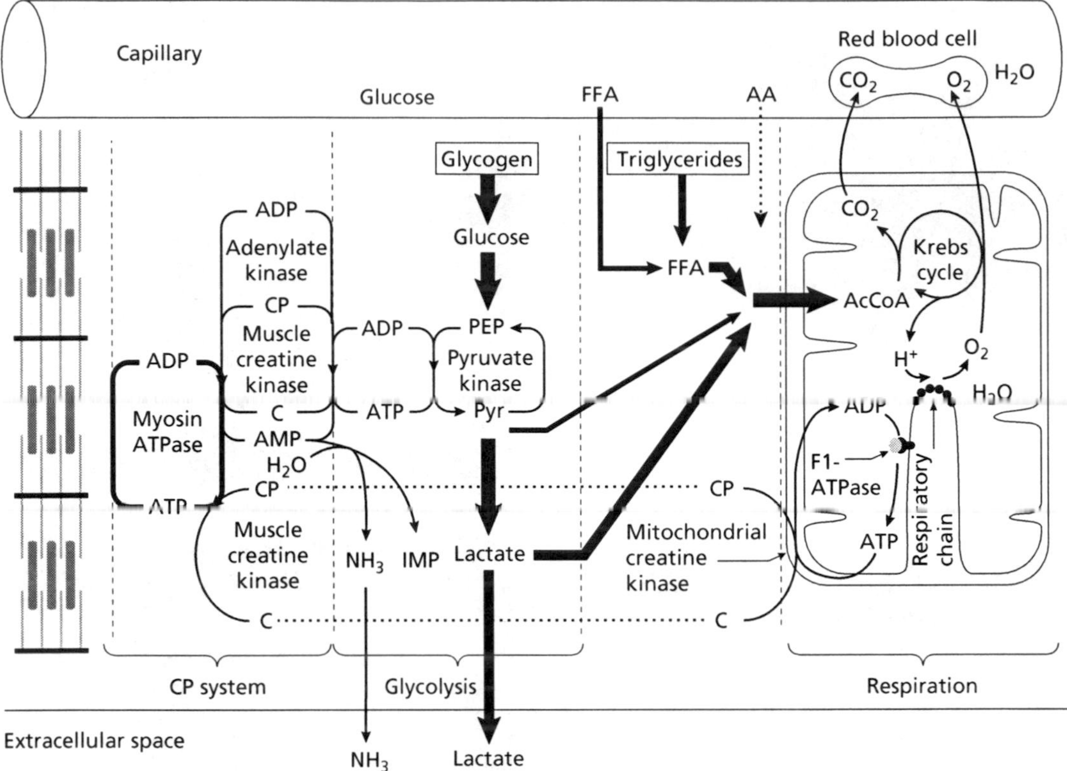

Fig. 4.20 Integrated, schematic view of the pathways of energy supply to the myofibrils. The thickness of the arrows indicates the relative importance of some of the substrate fluxes. The proportion of the produced lactate that is directly oxidized in a fibre's mitochondria is currently a matter of debate. AA, amino acids; AcCoA, acetyl coenzyme A; C, creatine; CP, creatine phosphate; FFA, free fatty acids; IMP, inosine monophosphate; PEP, phosphenolpyruvate; Pyr, pyruvate.

human. Certain amino acids have been implied in fatigue-related phenomena, however.

Degradation and terminal oxidation of substrates via the Krebs cycle and the respiratory chain in mitochondria results in H_2O and CO_2, both of which are innocuous and rapidly leave the muscle cells, being carried away by the capillary bloodstream (Fig. 4.20). Likewise, excess metabolic heat is dissipated and may, if heavy exercise is carried out in a hot environment, represent a serious hazard for the exercising subject.

The 'useful' energy is captured in a highly specialized chemical substance, ATP, which is composed of the purine base adenine and the sugar ribose, to which three phosphate residues are reversibly bound (Fig. 4.21). Enzymatic cleavage of these phosphate bonds yields the energy that is directly used in all energy-requiring processes of the muscle cell, such as contraction, ion pumping, biosynthesis and more. Most of this chemical energy is made available by splitting off the terminal phosphate from ATP (indicated by ~ in Fig. 4.21), liberating one ADP and one free phosphate. As indicated above, the remaining two phosphates of ADP can also be split off. The energy gain per bond is smaller, however, and different enzymatic systems are involved. Mitochondria maintain the energy charge of the muscle cell essentially by rephosphorylating ADP from ATP, keeping ATP at a relatively constant and high level.

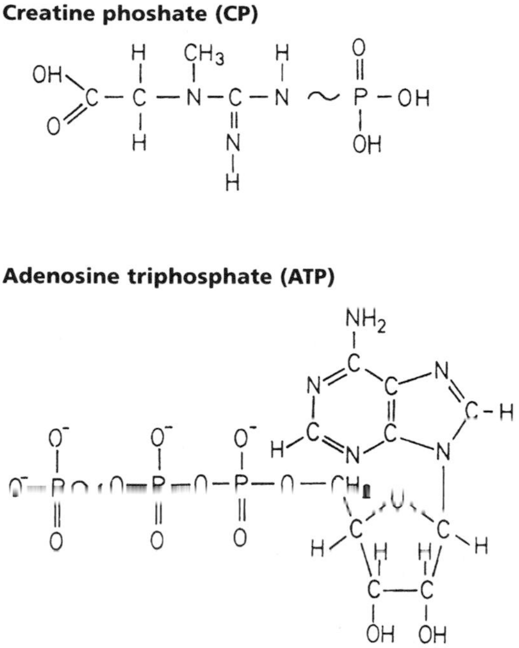

Creatine phoshate (CP)

Adenosine triphosphate (ATP)

Fig. 4.21 Molecular structure of ATP (adenosine triphosphate) and CP (creatine phosphate). ~ indicates the energy-rich bond. Cleavage of this bond in ATP yields the energy for energy-dependent enzymes in all organisms.

The creatine phosphate system

With the new technology of magnetic resonance spectroscopy (MR spectroscopy), muscle physiologists have obtained a tool by which the different phosphate pools, as well as the intracellular pH, in muscle cells can be monitored non-invasively (Fig. 4.22). It has thus become possible to evaluate the energy status of muscle cells while they develop force. These studies have revealed that a simple signalling system exists linking contractile ATP demand to aerobic ATP supply. At the heart of this system is creatine phosphate, the major storage form for energy in the cell, and the enzyme, creatine kinase (CK), which catalyses the transfer of the high-energy phosphate bond to ATP (Fig. 4.21). The equation for creatine kinase is written:

$$[\mathrm{PCr}] + [\mathrm{ADP}] + [\mathrm{H}^+] \leftrightarrow [\mathrm{ATP}] + [\mathrm{Cr}] \qquad (1)$$

The brackets [ ] indicate concentrations, i.e. [ADP] stands for the concentration of adenosine adenosine diphosphate and [Cr] stands for the concentration of free creatine. $[\mathrm{H}^+]$ is the concentration of protons, i.e. equivalent to pH. Increased ATP demand by muscle contraction is met by a shift in the creatine kinase reaction that drops creatine phosphate (PCr) without a change in ATP. This equilibrium shift keeps ATP (and the free energy of the ATP bond) relatively constant during a wide range of ATP fluxes in the cell. Thus PCr acts as a chemical capacitor for ATP that can be degraded at a very high rate for the myosin ATPase if need arises. During intensive exercise, such as sprinting, the PCr pool only lasts some 10 s (Fig. 4.18).

The buffering role of PCr that keeps ATP constant also causes a key signal for oxidative phosphorylation—ADP—to rise. The effect of a change in PCr on ADP via the CK equilibrium can be put into mathematical terms by rearranging eqn 1:

$$[\mathrm{ADP}] = ([\mathrm{ATP}]/[\mathrm{PCr}]) \cdot (1/(K_{eq} \cdot [\mathrm{H}^+])) \cdot ([\mathrm{Cr}] - [\mathrm{PCr}]) \qquad (2)$$

where K_{eq} is the creatine kinase equilibrium constant. The importance of [ADP] (the ADP concentration) lies in its role as the major factor regulating mitochondrial oxidative phosphorylation and therefore oxidative ATP supply. An elevation in [ADP] activates oxidative phosphorylation similarly in isolated mitochondria and in human muscle *in vivo*. This system therefore coordinates oxidative ATP supply to contractile demand via a simple feedback loop: in exercising muscle the net change in ATP flux causes [PCr] to drop and [ADP] to rise (the feedback signal). This elevation of [ADP] activates a rise in mitochondrial ATP supply. The drop in [PCr] with exercise continues until [ADP] rises enough to activate sufficient mitochondrial oxidative phosphorylation to balance ATP supply to ATP demand. Once an ATP balance is attained, [PCr] breakdown is no longer needed to meet ATP demands and [PCr] reaches a steady-state level. The changes in [ADP] from rest to the oxidative capacity of exercising

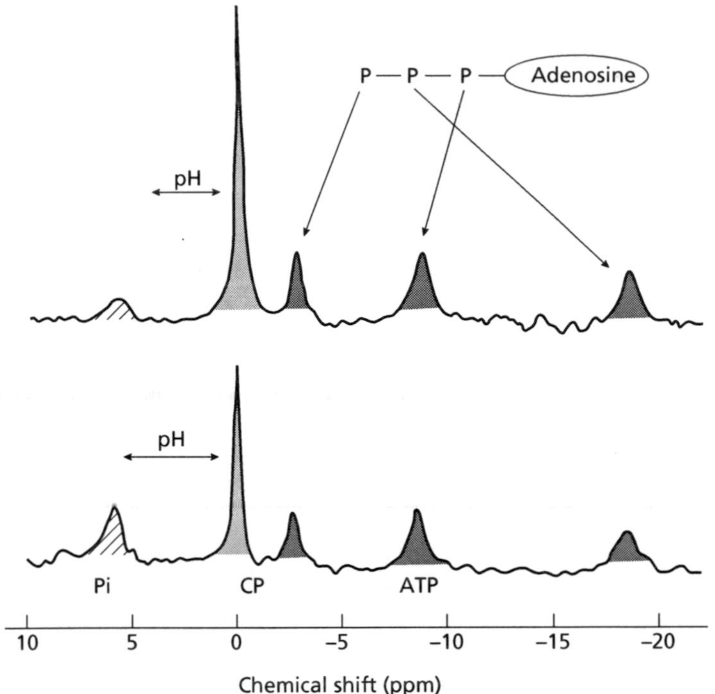

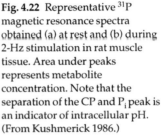

Fig. 4.22 Representative ^{31}P magnetic resonance spectra obtained (a) at rest and (b) during 2-Hz stimulation in rat muscle tissue. Area under peaks represents metabolite concentration. Note that the separation of the CP and P_i peak is an indicator of intracellular pH. (From Kushmerick 1986.)

skeletal muscle correspond with the changes seen in isolated mitochondria (see Conley *et al.* 2001 and Fig. 4.23). Thus, the shift in the creatine kinase equilibrium underlying the change in [PCr] buffers ATP levels to meet short-term energy demands and also raises the signal—[ADP]—for activating mitochondrial oxidative phosphorylation to meet the long-term needs of sustained oxidative ATP.

A specialized shuttle system has been suggested for the PCr–creatine kinase system for transferring energy from their mitochondria to the myofilaments. In this system, a specialized enzyme in the mitochondrial intermembrane space transfers the 'high-energy' phosphate from ATP to a creatine molecule (Fig. 4.21). A unidirectional shuttling of PCr to specialized CK isoforms located on the contractile elements is hypothesized to occur. However, PCr and ADP are freely diffusible and can provide sufficient high-energy phosphate flux without a specialized shuttle system. In addition, experiments with creatine kinase transgenic mice show little functional effect of switching the creatine kinase between mitochondria and contractile elements or knocking out specific isoenzymes altogether. Thus the simple buffering and signalling role of the PCr–creatine kinase system appears to be sufficient to explain the short-term maintenance of ATP levels and the long-term activation of mitochondrial ATP supply during exercise.

In recent years, a number of studies have investigated the effect of supplemental intake of creatine salts on exercise performance. In many individuals, additional intake of creatine leads to slightly increased CP pools in the muscle, which in turn can lead to slightly better sprinting performance. The effect manifests itself more clearly as improvement in repeated short sprinting exercises.

One limitation of the magnetic resonance technique for evaluating intracellular energetics is that the measurements can only be obtained from relatively large 'volumes' of muscle tissue, comprising hundreds of muscle fibres. The MR spectroscopy data therefore represent an average over many muscle fibres, which may be in different states of activation and fatigue.

Glycolysis

So far, we have considered respiration capable of furnishing a relatively low power output over a very long time period as well as the associated creatine phosphate system, which can be used for short bursts of very intense exercise (Fig. 4.18). Glycolysis represents an additional system of energy supply that may produce intermediate levels of power output for intermediate periods of time. Furthermore, glycolysis produces the metabolite pyruvate, which is a major fuel for mitochondrial oxidative phosphorylation (Fig. 4.20). During aerobic exercise, glycolysis furnishes pyruvate, which is transferred to mitochondria, where its carbon skeleton is entirely degraded to CO_2. This process of full oxidation of glucose in mitochondria yields 36 ATP for each glucose molecule degraded. Glycolysis of glucose to pyruvate or lactate yields only 2 ATP. Why then does the muscle cell bother about glycolysis? The reason is that glycolysis can proceed at a very high rate, indicated in Fig. 4.20 by the different thickness of the arrows. If glycolysis occurs at a rate exceeding the uptake capacity of mitochondria for pyruvate (and lactate, see below), there is a build-up of lactic acid in the muscle cells. Lactic acid lowers the intracellular pH, thus interfering with muscle contractile activity as previously mentioned. The pH of the muscle cell has to be restored if contractile activity is to proceed.

Recent data (Brooks 2000) have provided evidence that lactate does not have to be reconverted to pyruvate before it is taken up into a muscle fibre's mitochondria, but that mitochondria have transporters that allow them the direct uptake and metabolization of lactate produced by glycolysis in the sarcoplasm.

Glycolysis is also accompanied by activation of adenylate kinase. This enzyme converts 2 ADP (produced by the action of the myosin ATPase) into one ATP and one AMP (adenosine monophosphate). The ATP can be reutilized by the myosin ATPase. Some of the AMP generated this way is not rephosphorylated back to ADP and ATP but is rather transformed to IMP (inosine monophosphate) by the enzyme AMP deaminase. In this process, ammonia is produced, which is liberated to the bloodstream. Heavy muscle exercise with the activation of glycolysis is thus characterized by the appearance of lactate and ammonia in the bloodstream (Fig. 4.20).

Interdependence of muscle energetics and substrate choice

The different metabolic pathways are activated as a consequence of the intensity and duration of a particular type of exercise (Fig. 4.18). The CP system can be switched on immediately, because the energy is available in a directly degradable form. Glycolysis can be turned on quite rapidly as well, but it takes 2–3 min before oxidative phosphorylation is in full swing. The substrates and metabolites for the CP system and for glycolysis can be considered to be 'on board' the muscle cell. In contrast, stimulating respiration involves the activation of many processes throughout the entire body: The microcirculation must be increased in the exercising muscles, cardiac output must be stepped up via increased heart rate, and ventilation in the lungs must be augmented, so that a larger blood flow can be oxygenated. This takes some time. These steps are primarily regulated by the nervous system, but local metabolic and hormonal influences play a role as well.

In the course of an all-out sprint activity for 10 s, we are capable of lowering the CP levels to very low values, without much glycolysis occurring, i.e. we are incurring an alactic oxygen (energy) debt. If we then wait for a few minutes for respiration to reload the CP system, the same power output as before can be obtained. This is not the case when we run very hard for 800–1000 m. Glycolysis will be fully activated during this run, and plasma lactate levels may rise to very high levels (higher than 20 $mmol \cdot l^{-1}$ of blood in trained athletes). This will disturb acid–base balance and plasma pH may drop well below 6.9 (normal is 7.4). More importantly, because of the slow lactate removal from muscle cells, intracellular homeostasis is even more disturbed than what is apparent from the plasma concentrations of the relevant metabolites. When we stop such an exercise, it will take not just minutes but hours before the muscle cell has regained its equilibrium. It must be considered here that the CP system uses nucleotides that are shuttled around the muscle cell, but not used up in the process. This is different for glycolysis. If glycolysis were not switched off quickly by the accumulation of lactic acid in the muscle cell, it would be capable of breaking down all the available glycogen in only a few minutes. Reloading the glycogen stores from external (nutritional) sources can take a full day, even under optimal conditions of substrate supply.

If we engage in aerobic exercise that will last for a prolonged period of time, we know to pace ourselves, so that we do not accumulate high lactate levels at the beginning of the exercise. Despite this, glycolysis will have to energetically cover the time until respiration is fully activated. If we thus start to run at a pace of e.g. 75% of our maximal aerobic capacity, we will see an initial rise of lactate in the plasma, which later subsides when the muscle cells turn to oxidative phosphorylation.

The maximal rate at which we can exercise aerobically with a particular muscle or muscle group is essentially given by the quantity of mitochondria it contains, provided the capillary supply and cardiovascular oxygen delivery match mitochondrial oxidative capacity. Aerobic exercise not only augments all of these factors, it also helps to fine-tune all the energy transfer systems. In most mammals (muscle) cell respiration could theoretically proceed at higher rates than the maximal transport capacities of substrates (i.e. glucose and free fatty acids, FFA) across the cell membrane allow. High-intensity aerobic exercise thus necessarily leads to gradual depletion of the intracellular substrate stores. Once these are used up, respiration continues maximally at the rate of the membrane transport of the substrates. This is believed to be around 50% of the maximal rate of respiration or less. Thus in short- to medium-duration exercise, it is the mitochondrial oxidative capacity that limits aerobic work, while substrate supply becomes more and more important the longer a long-distance exercise lasts.

Structural basis of muscle training

For a given level of neural activation, muscle force is proportional to the total number of cross-bridges that can be formed in a given time period, as indicated in the first part of this chapter. As each myofilament contains the same number of myosin heads, the force in a healthy muscle is proportional to the total number of myofilaments on the muscle cross-section, or —roughly—to the muscle cross-sectional area. On the structural level, strength training acts through an increase of muscle cross-sectional area. Attempts to increase the CP pool of human muscle through training have shown to be unsuccessful; increased ingestion of creatine can lead to slightly increased CP pools, with small, but often measurable effects on sprint performance. Glycolysis can be significantly increased with high-intensity or interval-type training. Additionally, tolerance against acidosis and higher lactate levels is increased, both in the muscle fibres and on the systemic level, by these modes of training. The most malleable part of the muscle energy supply system is most likely respiration (Howald 1982). Both muscle capillarity and mitochondrial content can rapidly and largely increase with appropriate (endurance) training stimuli. Furthermore, the size of the heart and hence maximal cardiac output can also be increased under aerobic training conditions.

Perspective

A major challenge to basic muscle research is to uncover the mechanisms by which the precise molecular properties of the contractile, the regulatory and the energetic systems are controlled and adjusted to the patterns of use. Progress is likely to come from modern technologies, such as nuclear magnetic resonance (NMR) (e.g. Fig. 4.23), which allows *in vivo* measurements.

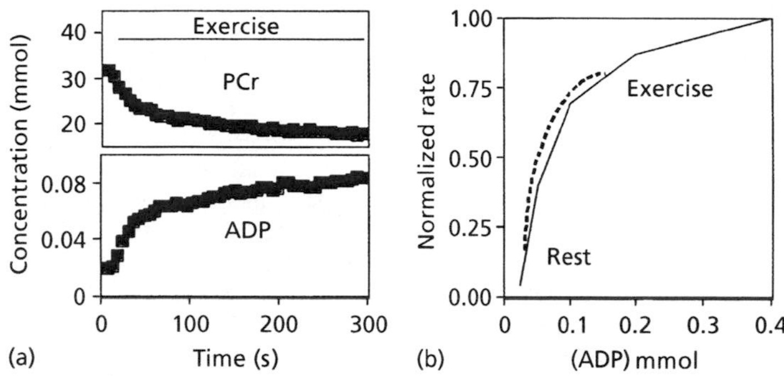

Fig. 4.23 (a) The changes in the contents of creatine phosphate (PCr) and ADP during exercise in human ankle dorsiflexor muscles, as determined by NMR spectroscopy. Note the relatively fast drop in PCr at the beginning of the exercise, which then changes to a near steady-state value. The concentration of ADP (the signal for mitochondrial oxidative phosphorylation) changes reciprocally. In (b), the values from experiment (a) are superimposed as a stippled line onto an oxidative phosphorylation activation curve that was determined from *in vitro* experiments using human heart mitochondria. Heart and skeletal muscle mitochondria are very similar in their properties. Note that the ADP concentrations reached during the exercise are in the steep part of the activation curve, i.e. a relatively small shift in concentration leads to a significant shift in oxidative phosphorylation. (Adapted from Conley *et al.* 2001.)

Further insights will come from *in vitro* techniques, which allow the simultaneous analysis of thousands of proteins (the so-called proteomics) or thousands of expressed genes (genomics, microarrays).

This will benefit not only athletes but all humans. This is because for all of us, the quality of our lives is largely dependent on an intact and fully functional locomotor system. We will better understand what to do to keep our muscles optimally functional and how we can get them back to function once they should fail.

Acknowledgements

The authors are indebted to Kevin Conley for the paragraph and the figure on the creatine kinase system. Both authors have been supported over many years by the Swiss National Science Foundation and the Swiss Sports Research Fund.

References

Alberts, B., Bray, D., Lewis, J., Raff, M., Roberts, K. & Watson, J.D. (1994) *Molecular Biology of the Cell*, 3rd edn. Garland Publishing, New York.

Åstrand, P.-O. & Rodahl, K. (1986) *Textbook of Work Physiology. Physiological Bases of Exercise*, 3rd edn. McGraw-Hill International Editions, New York.

Brooks, G.A. (2000) Intra- and extra-cellular lactate shuttles. *Medicine and Science in Sports and Exercise* **32**, 790–799.

Brooks, G.A., Fahey, T.D., White, T.P. & Baldwin, K.M. (eds) (2000) *Exercise Physiology: Human Bioenergetics and Its Applications*, 3rd edn. Mayfield Publishing Co, Mountain View.

Bouchard, C. & Rankinen, T. (2001) Individual differences in response to regular physical activity. *Medicine and Science in Sports and Exercise* **33** (Suppl.), S446–S451; discussion S452–S453.

Conley, K.E., Kemper, W.F. & Crowther, G.J. (2001) Limits to sustainable muscle performance: interaction between glycolysis and oxidative phosphorylation. *Journal of Experimental Biology* **204**, 3189–3194.

di Prampero, P.E. (1985) Metabolic and circulatory limitations to $\dot{V}O_{2\,max}$ at the whole animal level. *Journal of Experimental Biology* **115**, 319–332.

Eisenberg, G.R. (1983) Quantitative ultrastructure of mammalian skeletal muscle. In: *Handbook of Physiology. Skeletal Muscle* (eds L. D. Peachy, R. H. Adrian & S. R. Geiger), pp. 73–112. Williams & Wilkins, Baltimore.

Geeves, M.A. & Holmes, K.C. (1999) Structural mechanism of muscle contraction. *Annual Review of Biochemistry* **68**, 687–728.

Gordon, A.M., Homsher, E. & Reginer, M. (2000) Regulation of contraction in striated muscle. *Physiological Reviews* **80**, 854–924.

Gregorie, C.C., Granzier, H., Sorimachi, H. & Labeit, S. (1999) Muscle assembly: a titanic achievement? *Current Opinion in Cell Biology* **11**, 18–25.

Hall, Z.W. & Sanes, J.R. (1993) Synaptic structure and development: the neuromuscular junction. *Cell* **72** (Suppl.), 99–121.

He, Z.-H., Bottinelli, R., Pellegrino, M.A., Ferenczi, M.A. & Reggiani, C. (2000) ATP consumption and efficiency of human single muscle fibres with different myosin isoform composition. *Biophysical Journal* **79**, 945–961.

Horowits, R. & Podolsky, R.J. (1987) The positional stability of thick filaments in activated skeletal muscle depends on sarcomere length: evidence for the role of titin filaments. *Journal of Cell Biology* **105**, 2217–2223.

Howald, H. (1982) Training-induced morphological and functional changes in skeletal muscle. *International Journal of Sports Medicine* **3**, 1–12.

Kayar, S.R., Hoppeler, H., Howand, H., Claassen, H. & Oberholyer, F. (1986) Acute effects of endurance exercise on mitochondrial distribution and skeletal muscle morphology. *European Journal of Applied Physiology* **54**, 578–584.

Krstic, R.B. (1978) *Die Gewebe des Menschen und der Säugetiere*. Springer, Berlin.

Kushmerick, M.J. (1986) Spectroscopic applications of magnetic resonance to biomedical problems. *Cardiovascular and Interventional Radiology* **8**, 382–389.

Littlefield, R. & Fowler, V.M. (1998) Defining actin filament length in striated muscle. Rulers and caps or dynamic stability? *Annual Review of Cell Biology* **14**, 487–525.

Chapter 5

Hormonal Mechanisms Related to the Expression of Muscular Strength and Power

WILLIAM J. KRAEMER AND SCOTT A. MAZZETTI

Introduction

Heavy resistance exercise provides a specific set of stimuli, which innervates the body's musculature to produce force. The result of this activity sets into motion a variety of physiological mechanisms to support the acute and chronic demands of metabolism, recovery, repair and adaptation. Resistance training is the only natural stimulus that causes increases in lean tissue mass but dramatic differences exist among resistance training programmes in their ability to produce increases in muscle and connective tissue size. The endocrine system is a vital part of a homeostatic and adaptive set of strategies related to resistance exercise. Mechanisms are the sequences of molecular, biochemical and physiological events needed to produce a given physiological response or adaptation. Both acute and chronic mechanisms exist to mediate acute physiological function and chronic physiological adaptations. To date, a multitude of complex mechanisms exists in which hormones interact to provide such physiological support for resistance training's acute exercise demands and chronic adaptations.

Ultimately, the neuroendocrine system helps to mediate adaptations for enhanced strength and power. More importantly, the hormonal mechanisms involved are dependent upon the configuration of the exercise stimuli (i.e. characteristics of the training session) and the type of training programme used. The primary target for resistance training has been skeletal muscle. Therefore, interactions related to this target tissue have been of greatest interest. However, hormones interact with a multitude of other cells and tissues (e.g. immune cells, neurones), which directly affect the skeletal muscle's adaptation to heavy-resistance exercise stress (e.g. inflammatory process in repair).

The neuroendocrine system plays a crucial role as the primary communication network among physiological systems and target cells. Thus, a term such as 'neural–endocrine–immune–musculoskeletal system' starts to reflect the range of important interrelationships among physiological systems. It helps to mediate the interactions between activated skeletal muscle fibres (e.g. from exercise) and the genetic machinery responsible for signalling aspects of structural growth and remodelling. Here it can be observed that the classic definition of a hormone is implicated in such signalling where a molecule, upon its release into the blood by an endocrine gland, travels to target tissues and interacts with specific receptors to initiate a specific biological message resulting in a sequence of events (i.e. increased transcription/translation or activation of a protein). However, it is becoming increasingly evident that hormonal factors (related to growth) span an even wider variety of mechanisms beyond endocrine function. For example, cell-released factors can arise from nerve (e.g. norepinephrine, glial growth factor), immune (e.g. cytokines) and muscle cells (e.g. insulin-like growth factors) and can interact with proximal cells (e.g. paracrine) or with the same cell (autocrine) (McCusker & Clemmons 1994; Florini *et al.* 1996a,b; Frost *et al.* 1997). In addition, post-translational processing of some released hormones (e.g. growth hormone to prolactin prior to release into the capillary blood) can further alter the original message of the stimulatory signal. Major advancements made during the past 10 years have brought us to new boundaries in our theoretical paradigm for the adaptive influence of hormones and cell-released factors on target muscle cell development. This hormonal gestalt of influences affects the development of the muscle and mediates strength and power performances. Thus, the purpose of this chapter will be to describe some of the hormonal mechanisms related to such interactions with skeletal muscle leading to an influence on muscular strength and power performances.

System interactions

Complex cybernetic control networks exist among hormones because different circulating hormones are regulated by a variety of feedback mechanisms, as well as by other permissive factors which all contribute to the resultant hormonal milieu in which muscle cells grow (Fig. 5.1). In this regard, some hormones amplify the effects of other hormones and thus work synergistically to produce an effect (e.g. growth hormone influencing insulin-like growth factor I (IGF-I) release in cells). More commonly, however, different groups of hormonal factors elicit opposite biological effects (e.g. insulin and glucagon) in an attempt to maintain a tightly regulated homeostatic cellular environment. Hormones that can exert anabolic effects on skeletal muscle (e.g. testosterone, growth hormone, insulin-like growth factors and, under certain conditions, insulin) increase protein synthesis while catabolic hormones (e.g. cortisol, tumour necrosis factor α) can influence increases in protein degradation. This dynamic homeostatic balance between anabolic and catabolic metabolism will ultimately result in either an overall gain or loss of muscle mass. Furthermore,

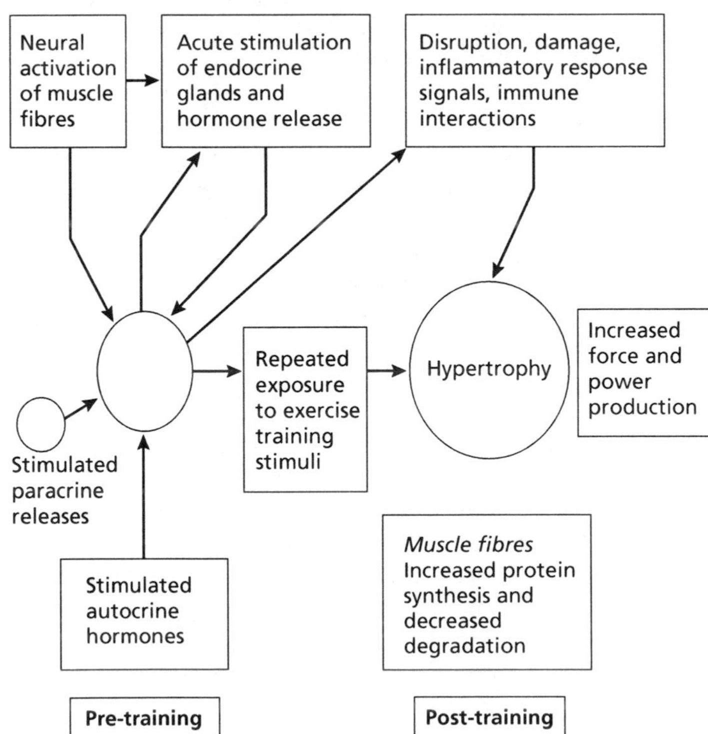

Fig. 5.1 Theoretical paradigm for the influence of resistance exercise and training on hormonal factors which influence muscle fibre hypertrophy and muscle strength and power performances.

target muscle cells themselves will vary in the manner they achieve hypertrophy (e.g. Type I and Type II muscle fibres differ in their reliance on synthesis vs. degradation to achieve net gains in muscle proteins). Obviously, increases in muscle size contribute largely to the enhancements in strength and power observed during long-term resistance training (for review see Fleck & Kraemer 1997). Ultimately, if a resistance training programme is effective (i.e. proper exercise prescription) in its ability to enhance strength and power performances, such adaptations are mediated through an optimal interaction with the neuroendocrine mechanisms.

Hormonal mechanisms that interact with skeletal muscle are a part of an integrated system that mediates the changes made in the metabolic and cellular processes of muscle as a result of resistance training. Remodelling of muscle involves the synthesis of new proteins and their orderly incorporation into or creation of new sarcomere. The most prominent resistance training adaptation in muscle is an increase in the amount of a muscle's contractile proteins, actin and myosin. Other changes in these proteins are also significant; for example, heavy chain myosin proteins can go through a change in their molecular structure from IIB to IIA heavy chain proteins. Furthermore, the prior synthesis of non-contractile proteins is needed for structural integrity and orientation of the contractile proteins within the sarcomere. Stimulation of protein synthesis by heavy-resistance training allows for both the quality and the quantity of muscle to be altered over a period of time.

The recovery phase after a workout is of vital importance. In general, the increase in protein synthesis and decrease in protein degradation are the first steps in muscle growth. Hormones are intimately involved with these mechanisms. The production of the contractile proteins actin and myosin, and ultimately the incorporation of these proteins into the sarcomere, is fundamental to the hypertrophy process at the molecular level. A multitude of hormones—including anabolic hormones (hormones that promote tissue building) such as insulin, insulin-like growth factors, testosterone and growth hormone—all contribute to various aspects of this anabolic process. Blocking the cell effects of catabolic hormones such as cortisol and progesterone that attempt to degrade cell proteins is also important. Thus, the remodelling of the muscle involves the changes in protein metabolism leading to the structural alterations and additions that take place after an exercise stress. The more muscle fibres involved with the performance of the exercise, the greater the extent of remodelling observed in the whole muscle, as only those muscle fibres that are stimulated will undergo an adaptive change. Such changes underlie the principle of 'specificity'. The hormonal interactions mediating the subsequent changes in structural and functional capabilities of muscle fibres provide the basis for the adaptive influence of hormones.

The role of receptors in mediating hormonal changes

Receptors are found in every cell, from muscle fibres to brain cells. One of the basic principles in neuroendocrinology is that a given hormone interacts with a specific receptor, a phenomenon classically known as the 'lock-and-key' theory. However, whereas only one hormone has exactly the right characteristics needed to interact with the receptor, there are cases of cross-reactivity, in which a certain receptor accepts hormones that are not specifically designed for it. When this occurs, the resulting biological actions can be different from those signalled by the primary hormone. Receptors can also have allosteric binding sites on them, at which substances other than hormones can enhance or reduce the cellular response to the primary hormone. Receptors may also have a number of domains. This means that part of the receptor may be outside the cell membrane, internalized within it (part inside the membrane, part outside), and/or within the cell membrane. Receptors are also observed in the nuclear portion of the cell for some hormones (e.g. steroid hormones). While hypothesized since the 1970s, recent evidence also suggests that some hormones (e.g. oestrogens) may have similar receptors on the cell membrane for rapid responses compared to the receptor on the DNA regulatory elements used for more permanent signal responses (Razandi *et al.* 1999). Thus, the location and redundancy of receptors is an expanding concept in the molecular aspects of hormonal signals.

It is usually the receptor or the hormone–receptor complex that transmits the message to the nucleus of the cell. The genetic material within the nucleus ultimately translates the hormonal message into either inhibition or facilitation of protein synthesis. When an adaptation is no longer possible (e.g. maximal amount of pain accretion in a fibre), receptors become non-responsive to the specific hormone that is trying to stimulate that response from the cell. This inability of a hormone to interact with a receptor has been called 'down-regulation' of receptor function. Therefore, receptors have the ability to increase or decrease their binding sensitivity, and or 'up-regulate' or 'down-regulate' the actual number of receptors available for binding. With resistive exercise training in rats, data indicate that the predominant mechanism has been to increase or decrease the maximum binding rather than affect binding sensitivity (Deschenes *et al.* 1994). Alterations in the receptor binding characteristics or changes in the number of receptors that can bind a hormone are adaptations often not considered in the construct of exercise-induced adaptations and may be quite dramatic. Important studies remain to be done at this level of adaptation consequent to resistance training. Obviously, if a receptor is not responsive to the hormone, little or no alteration in cell metabolism or signalling will result.

From a classic perspective, in terms of molecular structure there are two main categories of hormones, steroid and polypeptide hormones. Each interacts with muscle cells in different ways.

Steroid hormone interactions

Steroid hormones, which include the adrenal cortex hormones and those secreted by the gonads, are fat soluble and thus diffuse across the sarcolemma of a muscle fibre. Some scientists have hypothesized the presence of transport proteins in the sarcolemma that facilitate this movement. The location of steroid receptors in the cell has been controversial as they may be in the cytosol and/or bound to the nuclear membrane. Regardless of the location of the receptor, the basic series of events is the same. After diffusing across the sarcolemma, the hormone binds with its receptor to form a hormone–receptor complex (H-RC), causing a conformational shift in the receptor and activating it. The H-RC arrives at the genetic material in the cell's nucleus and 'opens' it in order to expose transcriptional units that code for the synthesis of specific proteins. The H-RC then recognizes specific enhancers, or upstream regulatory elements of the genes. RNA polymerase II then binds to the promoter that is associated with the specific upstream regulatory elements for the H-RC. The RNA polymerase II then transcribes the gene by coding for the protein dictated by the steroid hormone. Messenger RNA is processed and then moves into the sarcoplasm of the cell where it is translated into protein. Thus, the action of the steroid hormone is complete with its interaction at the genetic level of the cell. Figure 5.2 shows the standard steroid receptor sequence actions.

Polypeptide hormone interactions

Polypeptide hormones are made up of amino acids; examples are growth hormone and insulin. Polypeptide hormones bind to the receptors on the surface of the cell or to receptors that have domains integrated into the sarcolemma. Since polypeptide hormones are not fat soluble and thus cannot penetrate the sarcolemma, they rely on second messengers to get their message to the cell nucleus. Second messengers are activated by the conformational change in the receptor induced by the hormone. The second messenger directs its actions to specific areas in the cell, where the hormone's message is amplified. The subsequent cascade of intracellular events eventually leads up to the physiological response

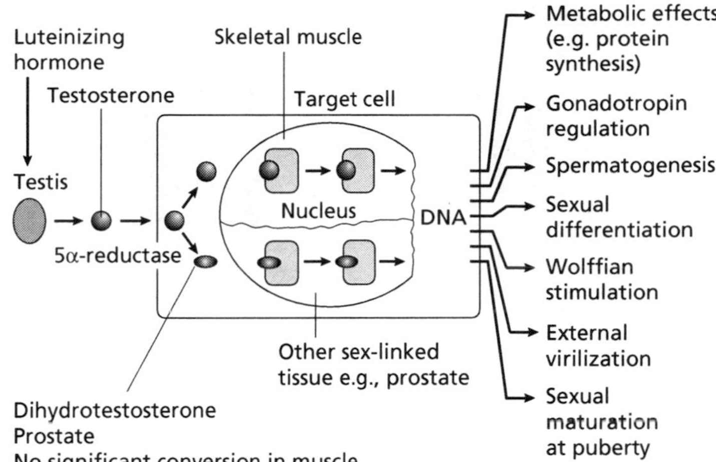

Fig. 5.2 Typical testosterone sequence of events in binding to the nuclear receptor in a cell.

ascribed to the hormone. Figure 5.3 gives an overview of two different polypeptide hormones and their cellular interactions.

In a muscle fibre, for example, a hormone arrives at the sarcolemma, forming a hormone–receptor complex. Adenyl cyclase, an enzyme bound to the cytoplasmic leaflet of the sarcolemma, is then activated, catalysing the formation of cyclic adenosine monophosphate (cAMP), which then activates a protein kinase (an enzyme involved in energy transfer). In turn, the protein kinase may phosphorylate and activate an enzyme that stimulates protein synthesis. This shows only one of the many second messenger systems that peptide hormones stimulate by binding to a receptor.

It is the nature of many hormones to play multiple roles in their physiological functions. However, some hormones have been identified as anabolic or catabolic mediators in protein metabolism in skeletal muscle.

Primary anabolic hormones

Growth hormone family

The pituitary gland is one of the most interesting endocrine glands and it secretes molecules that make up the growth hormone (GH) family of polypeptides in addition to many other important regulatory hormones. The main circulating isoform of GH (1–191 amino acids) is the 22-kDa polypeptide hormone derived from the GH-N gene on chromosome 17 and it is secreted by the anterior pituitary. Other spliced fragments are also released, including 20-kDa missing residues 32–46, residues 1–43 and 44–191 making 5- and 17-kDa GHs, respectively. In addition, hosts of other monomeric, dimeric, protein-bound GH, novel binding proteins, aggregates of GH and chemically altered molecules have been identified and make up the superfamily of GH. The biological roles of these different isoforms and aggregates are now the focus of new investigations as the GH family of polypeptides and binding proteins have been implicated in control of fat metabolism and growth-promoting actions, yet the mediating events at the molecular level remain speculative. To date, scientists have examined the concentrations in the blood, alterations with exercise or recombinant GH administration but scientific work is at the early stages of understanding the molecular heterogeneity of GH. A new era in GH research appears to be on the horizon as it relates to exercise stress (Hymer *et al.* 2000, 2001; McCall *et al.* 2000; Wallace *et al.* 2001). Thus, how the classic 22-kDa GH interacts with receptors, physiological mechanisms and integrated endocrine GH effects within the context of the superfamily of GH and

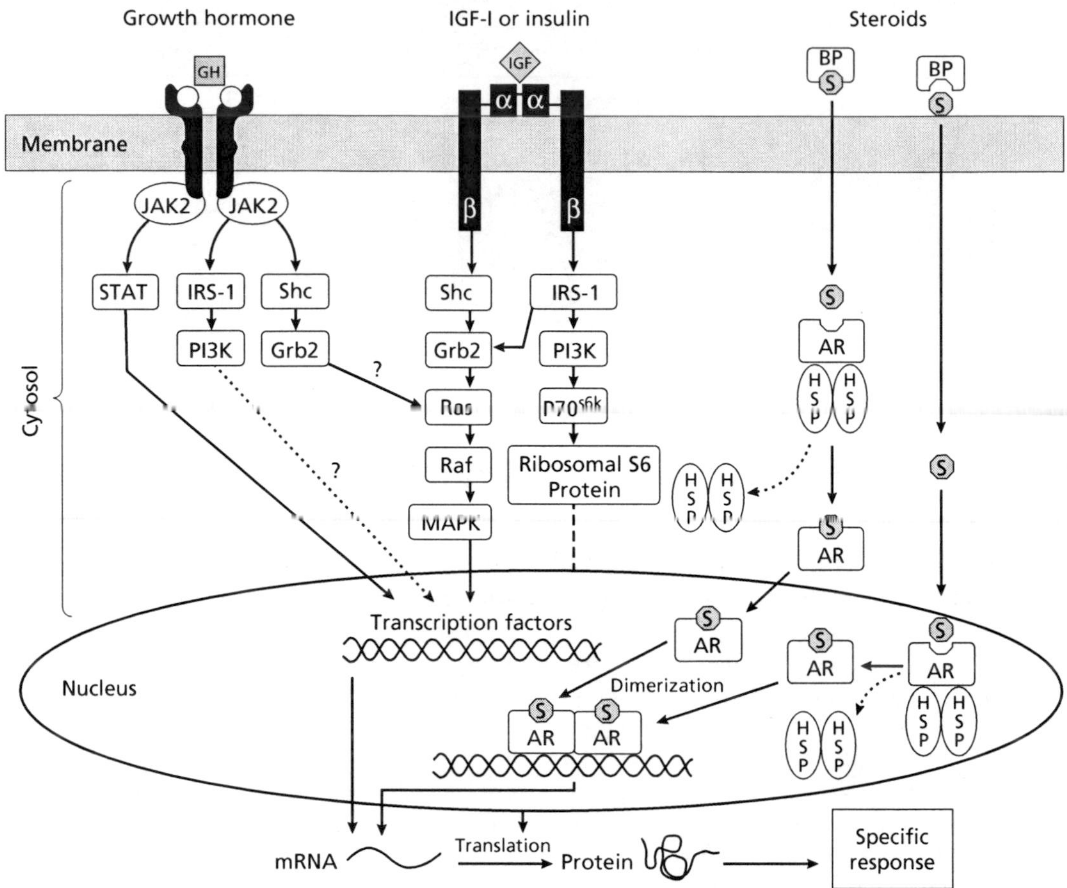

Fig. 5.3 Receptor signalling pathways. JAK2, janus kinase 2; STAT, signal transduction and activation of transcription signalling molecules; IRS-1, insulin receptor substrate 1; PI3-K, phosphatidyl-inositol-3 kinase; Shc, SRC homology-containing proteins; Grb2, growth factor receptor binding protein 2; MAPK, mitogen-activated protein kinase; p70^{S6K}, p70-S6 kinase; BP, circulating binding protein; S, steroid hormone; AR, androgen receptor; HSP, heat shock protein.

binding proteins remains to be further studied, especially in relationship to adaptations in skeletal muscle consequent to resistance training.

The understanding of GH has essentially been achieved through the examination of the 22-kDa immunoreactive polypeptide or through administration of this recombinant isoform. The anabolic effects of growth hormone on skeletal muscle are thought to have both direct and indirect effects. Although not yet completely understood, some of the effects of GH are thought to be mediated by stimulating the cell-released insulin-like growth factors (IGFs) (liver vs. muscle types) via autocrine, paracrine and/or endocrine mechanisms (Florini *et al.* 1996a,b). Some data have shown that GH does bind to skeletal muscle in pigs (Schnoebelen-Combes *et al.* 1996). Exogenous GH administration in children and adults who are GH deficient in addition to healthy adults have been shown to increase muscle mass and decrease body fat (Cuneo *et al.* 1991; Rooyackers & Nair 1997). Such observations have lead to the obvious conclusion that GH plays a significant anabolic role in skeletal

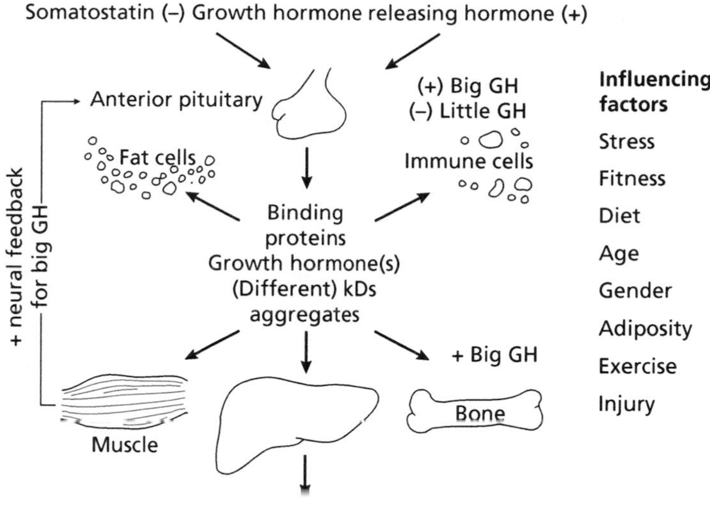

Fig. 5.4 Typical paradigm for growth hormone secretion and its target effects.

muscle growth. Adaptations are likely mediated by growth hormone's positive effects on muscle protein synthesis (i.e. increases) and protein breakdown (i.e. decreases) (Fryburg & Barrett 1995). Also, GH is known to stimulate the release of the availability of amino acids for protein synthesis *in vivo*, as well as the release of other growth factors (e.g. IGF-I) from muscle cells, thereby implicating GH in recovery and tissue repair (Florini *et al.* 1996a). It is the repair and remodelling from resistance exercise stress that mediates the adaptive responses in the contractile unit. Moreover, studies have shown that increases occur in circulating GH concentrations during and/or after heavy-resistance exercise in men (Kraemer *et al.* 1990, 1998b), women (Kraemer *et al.* 1993) and the elderly (Kraemer *et al.* 1998a, 1999) further indicating a potential stimulatory effect on GH secretion and enhanced potential for receptor interactions consequent to heavy-resistance exercise stress directed at improving muscular size, strength and power.

Some important factors related to GH and its various physiological actions include the pulsatile nature of GH release, multiple second messenger mechanisms activated by GH binding with its membrane receptor, the heterogeneity of the hormone's action on different target tissues, heterogeneity of GH aggregates, post-translational processing, heterogeneity of the GH molecular forms and a complex cybernetic regulation of the GH/IGF systems. Furthermore, the complexity of a family of GH polypeptides has started to be accepted by the scientific community. The pulsatile nature of GH secretion is characterized by its diurnal variations, with the highest concentrations of circulating GH observed during sleep. This pattern of GH secretion may be related to mechanisms important for tissue repair consequent to resistance exercise stress, as GH can increase whole-body protein synthesis rates in humans. This implicates GH as a primary anabolic hormonal influence important for strength and power adaptations. Figure 5.4 overviews some of the classic regulatory elements of GH secretion and its targets.

Two GH receptors are expressed in humans. The full-length receptor is one type and the other is a truncated form, which lacks most of the intracellular domain. This specific receptor may inhibit the action of the full-length receptor. Circulating GH binding protein is a proteolytically cleaved product from both of these receptors (Fisker *et al.* 2001). The biological actions of growth hormone are in part mediated by GH binding to its membrane receptor (cytokine receptor superfamily) on target tissues. The GH receptors can be found in moderate to high levels in many human tissues (liver, muscle, kidney, heart, epidermis, fat, thymus and gonadal tissues), but interestingly in very low levels in skeletal muscle (Florini *et al.* 1996a). Also, a second GH binding protein, which appears to be formed by post-translational processing of the GH receptor, has also been identified in many human tissues, as well as in the circulation. Briefly, GH binding to its membrane receptor induces receptor dimerization and the recruitment of a tyrosine kinase enzyme, janus kinase 2 (JAK2). The JAK2 is activated and forms a complex with the GH receptor (Argetsinger & Carter-Su 1996). Activation of the GH receptor/JAK2 complex causes phosphorylation (activation) of other tyrosines within both the GH receptor and JAK2. These activated tyrosines then act as binding sites for several signalling molecules including STATs 1, 3 and 5, ERKs 1 and 2, and IRS proteins; which are important for signal transduction and activation of transcription (STAT), cellular growth and differentiation via Ras and mitogen activator kinases (ERK 1 and 2), and cellular metabolic (enzyme) processes (IRS proteins), respectively (Argetsinger & Carter-Su 1996). These different second messenger pathways related to GH receptor signalling (i.e. diacyl-glycerol, calcium, nitric oxide) identify the variety of mechanisms by which growth hormone may mediate its different physiological actions includ-ing its effects on body growth, metabolism and protein synthesis. Whether all of these second messenger pathways are equally activated with every binding event, if separate pathways are activated only in specific tissues, or if binding by different GH isoforms (molecular variants or aggregates) results in differential activation of pathways has not been elucidated. It appears that separate regions of the GH receptor (SH2 domains vs. COOH-terminal half of GH receptor) may mediate the activation of these pathways differently, thus influencing GH's regulation of metabolism and growth (Argetsinger & Carter-Su 1996).

Another very important concept related to the different physiological actions of human growth hormone is the presence of different GH isoforms and the possible variability in their biological activities (Baumann 1991a; Strasburger & Dattani 1997). It is believed that for optimal biological activity, two adjacent growth hormone receptors must be available in order to bind one GH molecule (Ilondo *et al.* 1994). Therefore only those GH isoforms that have two intact binding sites are capable of initiating signal transduction in target cells (Strasburger *et al.* 1996). Whether GH molecules actually possess the two necessary receptor binding sites required for receptor dimerization is thus thought by some investigators to be of crucial importance for assessing the biological activity of growth hormone. However, how other GH isoforms, binding proteins and GH, and GH aggregates mediate their influence on the GH receptor domains may also be of importance with distinct differences from the classic receptor dimerization mechanisms.

The heterogeneity of the family of human growth hormone molecules includes the 22-kDa monomer, the 20-kDa mRNA splice variant, disulphide-linked homodimers and heterodimers of these monomers, glycosylated GH, high molecular weight oligomers, receptor-bound forms of GH, the 5- and 17-kDa GHs and hormone fragments resulting from proteolysis (Baumann 1991a). The distribution of 22-kDa and non-22-kDa isoforms varies in human blood and is thought to be due to differential metabolic clearance, circulating binding proteins and the formation of GH fragments in peripheral tissues (Baumann 1991b). Because of the complex nature of the family of human growth hormone molecules and its numerous physiological actions, it is possible that some of the effect(s) of the hormone on lipid, carbohydrate and protein metabolism, longitudinal bone growth, and skeletal muscle protein turnover may be controlled by different GH isoforms (Rowlinson *et al.* 1996; Hymer *et al.* 2001).

Hymer *et al.* (2001) recently examined the effects of acute heavy-resistance exercise on biologically active circulating growth hormone in young women via immunoassay vs. bioassay techniques. The results from this study indicated that acute resistance exercise significantly increased the lower molecular weight GH isoforms (30–60 kDa and < 30 kDa) when measured by the immunofunctional assay (Strasburger *et al.* 1996), but not in the classic rat tibial line bioassay. However, acute circulatory increases have been seen in men for bioactive GH using the tibial line bioassay (McCall *et al.* 2000). Such data show that our understanding of the dynamics of pituitary function in response to exercise is starting to become more complex and requires careful study before general conclusions can be drawn as to the impact of exercise training on GH. GH isoforms, aggregates and binding proteins could be important hormonal factors for mediating adaptations in muscle consequent on resistance exercise and training. How such isoforms respond to different types of resistance training remains to be studied. One brief report shows that increases in tibial line GH does occur with long-term resistance training in women suggesting that higher molecular weight molecules are adaptive in nature (Rubin *et al.* 2000). Thus, the exact mechanisms by which different GH molecules interact with their receptors to elicit their growth-promoting actions remain unclear, but their complexity continues to be unravelled with each subsequent study.

An important, yet unanswered question regarding the actions of GH is related to whether the 22-kDa GH acts directly on skeletal muscle to stimulate its growth. Some data exist which may indicate a direct effect of GH on skeletal muscle, in that tyrosine phosphorylation of JAK2 and STAT5 increased following intravenous GH administration in rats (Chow *et al.* 1996). However, these data still do not eliminate any mediating influences of the IGFs. With regard to the indirect effects of growth hormone on muscle growth, numerous interactions between GH and the insulin-like growth factors (IGFs) have been reviewed in detail (Florini *et al.* 1996a), and it seems probable that many of the effects of GH can be mediated in part by the actions of IGFs, yet the direct influences of GH on skeletal muscle cannot be ruled out due to the heterogeneity of the GH family of polypeptides.

INSULIN-LIKE GROWTH FACTORS

The insulin-like growth factors (IGFs) are structurally related to insulin (49% and 47% sequence identity for IGF-I and -II, respectively) and thus are members of the insulin/IGF peptide hormone family. The IGFs are small polypeptide hormones (70 and 67 amino acid residues for IGF-I and -II, respectively) that are secreted as they are produced, and therefore they are not stored in large quantities in any organ or tissue. Similar to insulin, as well as other peptide hormones, the IGFs are synthesized as a larger precursor peptide that is post-translationally processed into the final IGF-I or -II molecule. The primary structural difference between the IGFs and insulin, however, is that the IGFs are single-chain polypeptides since the linking C-peptide between the A- and B-chains of the molecule is not removed as it is in the processing of proinsulin into insulin (DeMeyts *et al.* 1994). Because of their structural similarities, the IGFs can bind the insulin receptor (IR), and vice versa. Two IGF receptor types have been identified and they include the type 1 and type 2 IGF receptors. The binding affinities among these molecules and their receptors are as follows: IGF-I binds type 1 >> type 2 >> IR; IGF-II binds type 2 >> type 1 >> IR; and insulin binds IR >> type 1 (Thissen *et al.* 1994). The type 1 IGF receptor binds IGF-II with nearly the same affinity as IGF-I, and the biological actions of both IGF-I and -II appear to be mediated by interactions with the type 1 receptor (DeMeyts *et al.* 1994). Also, the type 2 IGF receptor does not bind insulin, and both IGF-I and -II bind the insulin receptor with only ~ 1% of the affinity of insulin. The fact that insulin can interact with the type 1 IGF receptor partly explains the profound anabolic effects of insulin at high concentrations.

In cell culture studies, IGFs have been shown to stimulate myoblast proliferation and differentiation, inhibit proteolysis, increase glucose and amino acid uptake, and increase protein synthesis in various skeletal muscle cell lines (reviewed by Florini *et al.* 1996a). Several studies have also demonstrated the efficacy of the IGFs to increase protein synthesis in human skeletal muscles (Fryburg 1994, 1996; Russell-Jones *et al.* 1994; Fryburg *et al.* 1995). These mitogenic (proliferation), myogenic (differentiation) and anabolic actions help to qualify the profound growth-potentiating effects of the IGFs on skeletal muscle (Florini *et al.* 1996a; Adams 1998).

The ability of the IGFs to stimulate both the proliferation and differentiation of myoblasts through a single receptor (type 1 IGF receptor) is quite unique because IGFs are one of only a few circulating mitogens known to stimulate differentiation as well as proliferation in skeletal muscle cells (Florini *et al.* 1996b). Recently, a study examining the signalling pathways of the type 1 IGF receptor revealed that two different signalling pathways may mediate these mutually exclusive biological responses (proliferation and differentiation) in skeletal muscle (Coolican *et al.* 1997). Briefly, IGF-I interaction with its type 1 membrane receptor causes autophosphorylation of the receptor and subsequent phosphorylation of an associated tyrosine kinase enzyme. Similar to signalling by the insulin receptor molecule, phosphorylation of tyrosine kinase results in the activation (phosphorylation) of intracellular signalling proteins including the insulin receptor substrate 1 (IRS-1) and SRC homology-containing proteins (Shc). Activation of IRS-1 leads to the activation of the growth factor receptor binding protein 2 (Grb2) pathway which is associated with Ras and Raf-1/mitogen-activated protein (MAP) kinase activation (Florini *et al.* 1996b). Phosphorylation of Shc has also been shown to be important for the activation of the Grb2/Ras-associated pathways leading to MAP kinase activation. According to Coolican *et al.* (1997), the activation of MAP kinase is believed to be the primary molecular mechanism by which IGFs stimulate their mitogenic, or proliferative effects. Secondly, the phosphorylation of IRS-1 also leads to interaction with the p85 regulatory subunit of phosphatidyl-inositol-3 kinase enzyme (PI3-kinase) (Florini *et al.* 1996b). Activation of PI3-kinase results in the phosphorylation of a serine/threonine kinase named p70-S6 kinase, and subsequently the activation of ribosomal S6 components which stimulate the translation of mRNAs. Coolican *et al.* (1997) reported that the activation of PI3-kinase is the primary molecular mechanism responsible for the myogenic, or cell differentiation effects of the IGFs. Such complex signal regulation by the IGF/insulin receptor system identifies diverse mechanisms by which the IGFs, and even insulin, can mediate various processes important for muscle cell growth and development, especially at different stages of growth including muscle adaptations to resistance training in adults.

The role of the IGFs for skeletal muscle growth as a mediator in the GH/IGF system has been well accepted for many years. This system is characterized largely by the fact that circulating 22-kDa GH is an important stimulus for IGF gene expression and release by the liver (Copeland *et al.* 1980). Although the liver is thought to be responsible for the majority of circulating IGFs, they are known to be produced by many other tissues and cells, including muscle. The extent to which circulating IGFs (endocrine) interact with skeletal muscle has been contested largely because most circulating IGFs (> 75%) are bound as a ternary complex with IGF binding protein 3 (IGFBP-3) and an acid-labile subunit (~ 150 kDa when bound) which apparently does not cross the capillary endothelium (Binoux & Hossenlopp 1988). As a result, it has been proposed that circulating IGFs exhibit only a minor effect on skeletal muscle adaptations to mechanical loading (Yarasheski 1994).

Support for the above premise comes from recent resistance training studies which demonstrated no additive effects of doubled serum total IGF-I concentrations on strength performance or on protein synthesis rates following exogenous GH administration with training in elderly subjects (Taaffe *et al.* 1994; Yarasheski *et al.* 1995). Possible shortcomings from these studies, however, may be related to the stimulatory effect that circulating GH is known to have on the secretion of IGFBPs from the liver, in particular IGFBP-3 (Florini *et al.* 1996a). If the exogenous GH treatment resulted in increased IGFBP-3 concentrations (not measured), then the percentage of unbound, biologically active IGF-I may have remained essentially unchanged in these studies (Taaffe *et al.* 1994; Yarasheski *et al.* 1995). Contrary to the argument against a role for circulating IGFs, Borst *et al.* (2001) recently reported a 20% reduction in circulating IGFBP-3 after 25 weeks of multiple-set resistance training (Borst *et al.* 2001). These data suggest that circulating IGFs may become more important for skeletal muscle adaptations with prolonged resistance training, because circulating binding proteins decrease, thereby permitting an increased portion of unbound IGFs to cross the capillary endothelium and thus interact with muscle. This trend for a decrease in IGF binding protein elements has also been recently shown to begin within hours after a heavy-resistance exercise bout. Nindl *et al.* (2001) demonstrated that circulating concentrations of the acid-labile subunits begin to decrease 2 h after a heavy-resistance exercise bout, and are still lower than controls 13 h post exercise (Nindl *et al.* 2001). Furthermore, the study by Borst *et al.* (2001) also reported a 20% increase in circulating IGF-I concentrations following training, and this is not the only study to demonstrate increasing circulating growth factors with long-term training (Kraemer *et al.* 1995). Thus it seems that the IGF system undergoes adaptations with training which in turn improve the ability of the circulating IGFs to interact with skeletal muscle for cell growth and repair. Such adaptations in the endocrine actions of the IGFs on skeletal muscle could theoretically be mediated by, or simply be complementary with, autocrine/paracrine actions of the IGFs.

Support for autocrine/paracrine actions of the IGFs in muscle adaptational processes arises from the results of several studies which have shown significant hypertrophic effects of local IGF infusion directly into rat (Adams & McCue 1998) and human skeletal muscle (Fryburg 1994, 1996; Russell-Jones *et al.* 1994; Fryburg *et al.* 1995). Whether the local production and release of IGFs from skeletal muscle are influenced primarily by circulating GH, or by other factors (e.g. mechanical loading), remains unclear. This 'somatomedin hypothesis' is supported by data showing that GH stimulates IGF-I gene expression in skeletal muscle of rats and pigs (Turner *et al.* 1988; Loughna *et al.* 1992; Lewis *et al.* 2000). However, this relationship is questionable because such a stimulatory influence of GH on muscle IGF has yet to be conclusively demonstrated in humans. GH-independent local IGF-I gene expression has also been demonstrated in skeletal muscle from several animal models including dwarf chickens, cattle, sheep and pigs (Florini *et al.* 1996a). Thus the primary actions of the local IGFs on skeletal muscle do not appear to be influenced greatly by GH, and it seems that other factors (e.g. mechanical loading, stretch, etc.) may be more important for local IGF production and release (Adams 1998).

Recent reports have begun to describe the importance of a specific IGF-I isoform (also known as mechanogrowth factor) that is expressed by skeletal muscle in response to stretch and/or loading (Perrone *et al.* 1995; Yang *et al.* 1996; Goldspink 1998; Bamman *et al.* 2001). In 1996 Yang *et al.* identified an IGF isoform in avian skeletal muscle that was sensitive only to stretch. Stretch has also been shown to cause differentiated avian skeletal muscle cells in tissue culture to secrete IGFBPs in conjunction with IGFs, possibly for enhanced regulatory control of the actions of the IGF system on local muscle growth (Perrone *et al.* 1995). Mechanical loading of human muscle (i.e. resistance exercise) has recently been shown to result in increased muscle, but not serum IGF-I (Bamman *et al.* 2001). The results from this study also showed that the expression of skeletal muscle IGF-I mRNA in humans was greater following an eccentric as compared to a concentric bout of heavy-squat exercise (Bamman *et al.* 2001). Thus it appears that the stretching component of resistance exercise (eccentric) is a potent stimulus for the production and release of local growth factors in skeletal muscle.

Together, these data appear to emphasize the importance of mechanical loading-induced IGF isoforms for mediating muscle mass adaptations to resistance training; however, more studies examining these responses are needed, in particular, obvious difference(s) between more traditional speed concentric and eccentric training movements vs. explosive strength and power movements (e.g. power cleans). The potential role of supramaximal eccentric exercise training (and the concomitant local IGF gene expression) to optimize maximal strength and power training is being investigated. Perhaps such eccentric load-induced growth factors play a less significant role in explosive or maximal concentric strength and power development. This may help explain why many body building type resistance training programmes which emphasize higher volume (sets and repetitions) and slower, more controlled exercise movements (especially eccentric) are used more often for producing gains in muscle size, but not necessarily for strength and power performance (Fleck & Kraemer 1997).

As mentioned above, nearly all IGFs in the circulation, and some IGFs in tissues (muscle), are bound to IGF binding proteins. These IGFBPs regulate IGF availability by prolonging their half-lives in circulation (~ 12–15 h), controlling their transport out of circulation, and localizing IGFs to tissues (Collett-Solberg & Cohen 1996). Also, IGFBPs diminish the hypoglycaemic potential of IGFs by limiting the concentrations of free IGF molecules in circulation (DeMeyts *et al.* 1994). There are currently seven IGF binding proteins (IGFBP-1 to -7) that have been identified, but IGFBP-3 is the most common in the circulation with its primary role in the transport and bioactivity of the circulating IGFs (Zapf 1997). Together with IGF molecules, IGFBPs are produced and secreted by the liver as well as by most other cells including skeletal muscle. In various cell cultures, skeletal muscle cells have been shown to secrete most of the IGFBPs including IGFBP-1, -2, -4, -5 and -6 (Florini *et al.* 1996a; Frost & Lang 1999). Insulin-like growth factor binding protein 4 has a very high affinity for IGF-I, and has been shown to inhibit IGF-I's myogenic (i.e. differentiation) effects on skeletal muscle (Damon *et al.* 1998). Not surprisingly, it appears that resistance exercise results in decreased human skeletal muscle IGFBP-4 mRNA, while muscle IGF-I mRNA is increased (Bamman *et al.* 2001). Such results indicate that free IGF-I concentrations are increased in skeletal muscle following mechanical loading, probably related to an increased need for processes related to tissue growth and repair. Together with the results from Borst *et al.* (2001) who demonstrated that long-term resistance training results in decreased circulating IGFBP-3 concentrations and increased circulating IGF-I concentrations, these studies suggest potential important roles for both acute, local and chronic systemic growth factor-mediated actions on skeletal muscle for strength and power adaptations.

Lastly, differential effects of the IGFBPs are very characteristic, where many BPs can modulate the actions of the IGFs by either inhibiting or further stimulating IGF actions and production (Florini *et al.* 1996a). Insulin-like growth factor binding protein 5 has been shown to stimulate or inhibit the myogenic actions of IGF-I on skeletal muscle cells (Florini *et al.* 1996b; James *et al.* 1996). Frost and Lang (1999) demonstrated that differential regulation can also be mediated directly by the binding protein molecule itself, demonstrating that IGFBP-1 inhibited IGF-I-stimulated protein synthesis, but also inhibited protein degradation by acting independently of IGF-I in cultured human skeletal muscle cells (Frost & Lang 1999). Whether IGFBPs are inhibitory or stimulatory appears to depend upon different post-translational alterations which in turn change the affinity of the binding protein for the IGF molecules. Phosphorylation, dephosphorylation, proteolysis or polymerization of a binding protein can alter the biological effects of the IGFs, including their effects on skeletal muscle protein metabolism (Jones & Clemmons 1995; Sakai *et al.* 2001). Thus it is evident that the production and release of binding proteins by muscle cells, as well as different post-translational modifications of BPs, magnify the complexity of the regulation of skeletal muscle growth by the IGF system.

INSULIN

With its primary function in blood glucose regulation, pancreatic insulin secretion is pulsatile, and this pulsatility is directly influenced by food content as well as by the frequency and quantity of food consumption. Circulating insulin concentrations are also influenced by the sensitivity of peripheral tissues to insulin binding (e.g. skeletal muscles); a factor that is altered by physical activity level and exercise. Consequently, a person who consumes a healthy diet (e.g. three or four balanced meals per day with a lower glycaemic index) and exercises regularly, will generally exhibit less extreme fluctuations of circulating insulin concentrations and better insulin sensitivity than individuals who eat higher glycaemic index foods, miss meals and do not exercise.

The ability of insulin to stimulate an increase in protein mass has been recognized since the 1940s when individuals with type 1 diabetes (i.e. insulin dependent) first began using insulin therapy to help regulate their blood glucose. Unfortunately, it remains unclear whether this increased protein mass in humans is due to increased protein synthesis, decreased protein degradation, or a combination of both (Rooyackers & Nair 1997; Wolfe 2000). Results from most cell culture and animal model studies have demonstrated that insulin increases protein synthesis and decreases protein degradation (Rooyackers & Nair 1997). Results from other *in vitro* studies using human skeletal muscle cells have demonstrated that insulin increases protein synthesis, but protein degradation does not change (Rooyackers & Nair 1997). Even more confusing, results from *in vivo* studies in humans show mixed results, and appear to depend on the scientific methodology used to examine insulin's effects on protein metabolism. When tracer methodology is used to differentiate the balance between the arterial and venous concentrations of an essential amino acid such as phenylalanine (i.e. neither produced nor metabolized by skeletal muscle), the results from most studies have supported a decrease in protein degradation, but no change in protein synthesis (Rooyackers & Nair 1997). It is believed that insulin-induced hypoaminoacidaemia may help to explain the lack of an effect of insulin on protein synthesis rates, suggesting that insulin would increase protein synthesis if intracellular amino acid concentrations were maintained or enhanced. Studies which used amino acid infusion have in fact demonstrated a stimulatory effect of insulin on muscle protein synthesis (Castellino *et al.* 1987; Tessari *et al.* 1987). Also, Wolfe (2000) has argued that studies using tracer methodologies do not account for intracellular amino acids that originate from protein degradation, as well as amino acids that were originally released by protein degradation, but were reincorporated back into muscle protein before reaching the circulation. By accounting for such ongoing intracellular amino acid turnover processes (protein metabolism), more accurate measures of total protein synthesis and degradation appear to be possible (Biolo *et al.* 1995).

Although unclear, physiological concentrations of insulin appear to increase protein synthesis as long as intracellular amino acid availability is maintained. The mechanisms by which insulin stimulates skeletal muscle protein synthesis include increases in the activation of enzymes, translation of mRNA and gene transcription (Wolfe 2000). It appears, however, that changes in translational processes occur first, then transcriptional processes may be activated later. As mentioned earlier, insulin can bind IGF receptors, and thus at higher concentrations, such as after a large carbohydrate meal, may also contribute to IGF type 1 receptor-mediated increases in protein synthesis.

The influence of insulin on protein degradation is implicated in its effects on two different protein degradation pathways, the ATP-dependent ubiquitin proteolytic system and lysosomal protein degradation (Wolfe 2000). It has been proposed that the ATP-dependent ubiquitin proteolytic system is suppressed by normal resting concentrations of insulin, but that this low-level suppression may not be altered by acute elevations in insulin concentrations (after meals) (Wolfe 2000). This type of ongoing regulation by insulin of the proteolytic breakdown system would thus help explain why, in the absence of insulin such as that observed with untreated insulin-dependent diabetes mellitus, muscle protein degradation is increased and muscle mass decreases over time. Conversely, processes related to lysosomal protein degradation naturally increase following exercise (Kesperek *et al.* 1992), and this may help to explain why a post-exercise meal can reduce muscle protein degradation, since the meal would cause the pancreas to increase insulin secretion causing a transient physiological hyperinsulinaemia (Biolo *et al.* 1995). Thus in normal daily life, resting insulin concentrations induce a low-level suppressive effect on protein degradation via reduced ATP-dependent ubiquitin proteolysis, but with acute exercise that typically results in lower circulating insulin, the inhibitory effects of insulin on lysosomal protein degradation are reduced, and protein degradation increases transiently. At what concentrations insulin has the most dramatic effects on protein synthesis remains unclear but it may only be during times of very low or very high levels of protein synthesis (Szanberg *et al.* 1997; Farrell *et al.* 2000). Thus the role of insulin in resistance training adaptations in humans remains speculative as to the timing of its most important contribution to the protein accretion phenomenon.

Testosterone

Testosterone is an anabolic steroid hormone that is synthesized in the gonadal organs by a series of enzymatic conversions of cholesterol into testosterone. In females the adrenal cortex also contributes an important source of adrenal androgens. In specific tissues, testosterone can also be converted by 5α-reductase or aromatase into other active metabolites including dihydrotestosterone or oestradiol, respectively. While dihydrotestosterone is important for the development of external gen-italia, prostate and seminal vesicles and second-ary hair growth in men, it is believed that very little 5α-reductase enzyme is found in skeletal muscle, and thus testosterone is considered the primary hormone which interacts with skeletal muscles for cell growth (Wu 1997). Oestradiol, on the other hand, is important since it has been demonstrated that testosterone indirectly stimulates GH and IGF-I secretion by way of its conversion to oestradiol (Mauras *et al.* 1987; Hobbs *et al.* 1993; Weissberger & Ho 1993).

Another anabolic mechanism of action for testosterone is believed to occur independently of androgen receptors. In this regard, testosterone may act as an anticatabolic hormone by inhibiting cortisol's stimulatory effect on protein degradation. Thus, testosterone is a potent anabolic hormone that can exert its actions on skeletal muscle growth and repair by directly binding to cytoplasmic receptors in muscle to increase protein synthesis, by mediating the responses of other hormones which increase protein synthesis and decrease protein degradation (GH, IGF-I), or by acting as an antiglucocorticoid to suppress protein degradation (Wu 1997).

Many factors of steroid physiology influence the mechanisms by which testosterone stimulates and maintains muscle mass and these include a unique cytoplasmic binding mechanism, and the ability to alter transcription, their need for binding proteins to enable regulated transport to target tissues and their pulsatile secretion. Because it is a steroid hormone, testosterone is lipid soluble and thus can freely diffuse through the cell membrane and interact with cytoplasmic (or possibly nuclear) receptors. An activated cytoplasmic receptor–ligand complex diffuses into the nucleus and binds hormone response elements on DNA. By doing this, testosterone increases RNA transcription, leading to increased translation of specific proteins necessary for tissue growth and repair. Another factor unique to steroid and other lipophilic hormones is the need for high-affinity binding proteins. Since steroid hormones have the capacity for passive diffusion, their entry into and interaction with target cells must be regulated. As a result, most testosterone in the circulation is bound to sex hormone binding globulin (SHBG) (~ 60%) or other binding proteins (e.g. ~ 38% bound to albumin) thereby prolonging the half-life of testosterone and regulating its biological activity. Lastly, the pulsatile secretion of testosterone is characterized by a diurnal pattern where circulating testosterone is elevated during the morning hours and slowly decreases throughout the day with the lowest values occurring in the evening. Such diurnal variation does not appear to be altered by acute resistance exercise performed at different times of the day, despite the known effects of such activities on anabolic hormonal responses (Kraemer *et al.* 2001). Therefore, it may be that the diurnal variation of testosterone secretion, especially the higher concentrations in the morning, is an overriding stimulus because of accelerated morning metabolic rates. With accelerated metabolism, protein turnover is increased, and such higher concentrations of testosterone are important for maintaining a homeostatic nitrogen balance.

The direct effects of testosterone on skeletal muscle growth may not be as dramatic as other growth factors. This theory is based on cell culture studies which show greater protein synthesis after exposure to insulin or IGFs than after testosterone (Florini 1987). Also, it has been argued that supraphysiological doses of anabolic steroids in eugonadal men ultimately cause a plateau of biological responses (e.g. skeletal muscle growth) due to saturation of androgen receptors (Wu 1997), and this has been demonstrated *in vitro* (Bartsch *et al.* 1983). If testosterone is a less potent anabolic hormone, then perhaps it is because of differential effects on amino acid uptake into muscle cells as compared with other hormones.

Ferrando *et al.* (1998) recently demonstrated that testosterone injection in healthy young men increased protein synthesis but did not affect amino acid transport, suggesting that testosterone promotes the reutilization of intracellular amino acids for increased protein synthesis and accretion. These findings are in contrast to the proposed stimulation of inward amino acid transport by insulin, IGF-I and GH (Biolo *et al.* 1992). In fact, the ability of insulin and IGFs to stimulate protein synthesis has been proposed to be limited by the availability of amino acids (Wolfe 2000). It may be that testosterone stimulates protein synthesis (i.e. directly and/or indirectly) up to a stimulus (i.e. physical activity) and genetic sensitive threshold, and any further increase in muscle size due to testosterone would be a result of other indirect effects of testosterone (e.g. stimulation of increased GH and/or IGF-I secretion).

Testosterone is known to increase growth hormone secretion in children during puberty (Mauras *et al.* 1987) and in healthy adult men (Weissberger & Ho 1993). This effect of testosterone on circulating GH is at least in part mediated by the aromatization of testosterone to oestradiol in tissues (Weissberger & Ho 1993); however, a direct effect of testosterone on anterior pituitary somatotrophs cannot be ruled out. Because of increased circulating GH concentrations, liver IGF production and secretion increases, and such activation of the GH/IGF system has been demonstrated following testosterone administration in healthy men (Hobbs *et al.* 1993; Weissberger & Ho 1993). In fact, in elderly men not involved in a regular resistance exercise programme, 4 weeks of testosterone injections sufficient to produce concentrations similar to those of younger men resulted in increases in muscle IGF-I mRNA and decreased muscle IGFBP-4 mRNA (Urban *et al.* 1995). Together these data give support to the hypothesis that testosterone's anabolic effects on skeletal muscle may in part be mediated by changes in circulating factors of the GH/IGF system. In addition, changes in local cell-released growth factors may also be important.

Testosterone is also believed to exert anabolic action(s) in muscle via an androgen receptor-independent mechanism, where circulating testosterone may act as an antiglucocorticoid (Wu 1997). For this mechanism, it is theorized that testosterone may block or displace glucocorticoids such as cortisol from interacting with glucocorticoid receptors which help regulate protein degradation in muscle. Increased protein mass due to a decreased rate of protein degradation in skeletal muscle following testosterone administration has been demonstrated (Mayer & Rosen 1977), although such inhibitory effects on protein breakdown may be limited to supraphysiological doses of testosterone (Hickson *et al.* 1990). Furthermore, supraphysiological doses of testosterone, such as with steroid administration, are thought to be associated with extensive down-regulation of the glucocorticoid receptor (~ 90%), and therefore testosterone may also exert anticatabolic effects via reductions in the cortisol receptors (Hickson & Marone 1993). Most studies have reported that testosterone increases muscle mass primarily by increasing protein synthesis with no effect on rates of protein degradation; thus whether physiological concentrations of testosterone can decrease protein degradation remains unclear (Griggs *et al.* 1989; Urban *et al.* 1995; Ferrando *et al.* 1998).

Nevertheless, profound anabolic actions of testosterone, independent of any additive effects of resistance exercise, have been recently demonstrated in skeletal muscle of men. Replacement doses of testosterone for 12–24 weeks in hypogonadal men have been shown to increase fat-free mass and muscle size (Bhasin *et al.* 1997) by increasing protein synthesis and accretion (Griggs *et al.* 1989; Brodsky *et al.* 1996). Furthermore, replacement doses of testosterone in older men (> 60 years) (Urban *et al.* 1995) and supraphysiological doses of testosterone in normal men have been shown to increase muscle strength, despite the fact that no resistance exercise was performed (Bhasin *et al.* 1996). It is evident from such data, and from the pronounced differences in muscle mass between the genders, that testosterone is a potent anabolic factor for muscle cell growth. For athletes, this is especially important because circulating testosterone concentrations are known to increase during and immediately following heavy-resistance exercise in men (Kraemer 1988; Kraemer *et al.* 1990) and women (Kraemer *et al.* 1993), and these acute responses over time, as with long-term resistance training, appear to help mediate changes in muscle size, and strength and power adaptations.

Other anabolic factors

Although a considerable amount of research remains to be undertaken in this area of study, it is becoming increasingly evident that other factors also potentiate skeletal muscle growth. Other hormones (e.g. angiotensin II, tibial peptide) and nerve factors (e.g. glial growth factor 2) have been implicated in skeletal muscle anabolic processes in animal and cell culture models. Angiotensin II is thought to be important for overload-induced cardiac and skeletal muscle hypertrophy. Gordon *et al.* (2001) recently demonstrated that angiotensin-converting enzyme (ACE) inhibition in overloaded rat soleus muscle resulted in decreased hypertrophy (96%), while angiotensin II perfusion restored 71% of the hypertrophic response. The exact mechanism by which angiotensin II influences muscle hypertrophy has yet to be clearly elucidated, but concomitant changes in other factors (e.g. angiotensin II type 1 receptor density) also appear to be important. Ultimately, angiotensin II may very well be yet another important factor involved in the complex hormonal pathways associated with the intracellular signalling needed for tissue growth and repair following heavy-resistance exercise.

Another much less understood hormone, called 'tibial line peptide', was recently identified in human plasma and human post-mortem pituitary tissue (Hymer *et al.* 2000). This peptide is proposed to be stored in a secretion granule associated with a specific subpopulation of growth hormone cells, and it contains an amino acid residue sequence not found in human growth hormone. Interestingly, this small peptide (~ 5 kDa) demonstrated bioactivity in the tibial line bioassay, but not in the growth hormone immunoassay. Thus, this peptide appears to be a biologically active hormone that is neither another GH isoform nor a fragment of growth hormone polypeptide family and may have growth-promoting activity.

The importance of the nervous system to skeletal muscle function has been studied in detail, and it has generally been accepted that the type of motor unit innervating a skeletal muscle fibre (i.e. fast or slow) largely dictates the resultant fibre cell type (i.e. Type I or Type II muscle fibres), and its capacity for force production. Recently, evidence supporting myotrophic nerve factors that elicit growth and differentiation actions on muscle without direct physical contact has been mounting. The neuregulin family of neurotrophic proteins is characterized by glycosylated, transmembrane proteins including heregulin, neu differentiation factor and glial growth factors (Florini *et al.* 1996). Glial growth factor 2, unlike its fellow family members, is not a transmembrane protein and thus it may function as a cell-released nerve factor. Florini *et al.* (1996b) demonstrated that glial growth factor 2 is a potent myotrophic factor (i.e. stimulates growth and differentiation) in cultured myoblasts, exhibiting slower, prolonged stimulation over 6 days (Florini *et al.* 1996). Thus, at least in embryonic muscle cells, glial growth factor 2 may be important for the long-term regulation or maintenance of muscle protein accretion. Such long-term myotrophic effects are thought to be different from the well-accepted role that nerve impulses play in influencing muscle fibre type, therefore suggesting an autocrine/paracrine mechanism of action by glial growth factor 2.

Catabolic hormones

Adrenocortical steroid hormones such as cortisol were originally given the name glucocorticoids because of their effects on intermediary metabolism. This is because in the fasted state, cortisol helps to maintain blood glucose by stimulating gluconeogenesis and peripheral release of substrates, both of which are catabolic processes. In peripheral tissues, cortisol stimulates lipolysis in adipose cells, and increased protein degradation and decreased protein synthesis in muscle cells, resulting in greater release of lipids and amino acids into circulation, respectively (Hickson & Marone 1993). Also an important action of the glucocorticoids is local and systemic inflammatory mechanisms related to cytokine-mediated cortisol secretion via the hypothalamic–pituitary–adrenal axis (reviewed by Smith 2000). Perhaps the most notable function of the glucocorticoids, however, is their various roles in the body's responses to stressful stimuli (i.e. injury, surgery, physical activity, etc.). Although evidence supporting other related concepts is mounting, Hans Selye's original general adaptation syndrome (i.e. stress-induced secretion of glucocorticoids enhances and mediates stress responses) remains a heavily researched topic (Selye 1936; Pacak *et al.* 1998; Sapolsky *et al.* 2000). Overall, the importance of the glucocorticoids to strength and power adaptations is related to their catabolic effects on skeletal muscle.

Although the specific mechanisms of catabolism are not completely understood yet, the numerous catabolic actions of the glucocorticoids are regulated by a complex integration of permissive, suppressive, stimulatory and preparative actions which theoretically work together in order to help maintain (or re-establish) a homeostatic cellular environment and ultimately to help prevent any lasting deleterious effects of an acute stress on the body (Sapolsky *et al.* 2000). In this regard, resistance exercise can be thought of as an adaptive microtrauma which can lead to local acute inflammation, chronic inflammation and systemic inflammation, and ultimately to activation of the hypothalamic–pituitary–adrenal axis and the subsequent rapid increase in circulating cortisol concentrations for tissue repair and remodelling (Smith 2000).

Cortisol secretion responds quite rapidly to various stresses (e.g. exercise, hypoglycaemia, surgery, etc.), typically within minutes. While most inflammatory and blood glucose regulatory actions of glucocorticoids may be directly associated with these rapid responses, changes in muscle protein turnover are mostly controlled by the classic steroid hormone binding mechanism. Like testosterone, cortisol binds a cytoplasmic receptor and activates a receptor complex so that it can enter the nucleus, bind specific hormone response elements on DNA, and act directly at the level of the gene. By doing this, cortisol alters transcription and the subsequent translation of specific proteins, but these processes take many hours to days.

Similar to other hormones, the biological activity of the glucocorticoids is regulated by the percentage of freely circulating hormone. About 10% of circulating cortisol is free, while ~ 15% is bound to albumin and 75% is bound to corticosteroid binding globulin. The primary pathway for cortisol secretion begins with the stimulation of the hypothalamus by the central nervous system, which can occur as a result of hypoglycaemia, flight/fight response or exercise. Cytokine-mediated cortisol release is implicated in high-volume and high-intensity exercise (especially eccentric muscle actions), and occurs as a result of adaptive microtrauma injury to the muscle tissue which causes the infiltration of neutrophils and monocytes into the tissues (Smith 2000). The monocytes can then be activated in circulation, or in the tissues where they remain and become macrophages. Whether by circulating monocytes or tissue macrophages, these activated immune cells are capable of secreting hundreds of different cytokines which mediate local and systemic inflammatory processes. Interleukin 1 (IL-1) and IL-6 are pro-inflammatory cytokines secreted by activated monocytes (or macrophages) that are known to activate the hypothalamic–pituitary–adrenal axis (Kalra *et al.* 1990; Path *et al.* 1997). These cytokines interact with receptors on the hypothalamus and cause the sequential secretion of corticotrophin-releasing hormone (CRH), adrenocorticotrophic hormone (ACTH) and cortisol from the hypothalamus, anterior pituitary and adrenal cortex, respectively (Smith 2000). At each level of interaction (i.e. neutrophils to monocytes to cytokines to other cytokines to hypothalamus, etc.), all of these responses can be amplified dramatically, but the magnitude(s) will ultimately depend upon the severity of the initial adaptive microtrauma (e.g. intensity of exercise). Severe inflammatory responses appear to occur only after severe injury, trauma, infection, very high intensity resistance exercise or very high volume endurance training and thus are implicated in the overtraining syndrome (Stone *et al.* 1991; Fry & Kraemer 1997; Smith 2000). However, daily exercise training is also associated with local and systemic cytokine responses at different levels, depending on the intensity of the exercise (Moldoveanu *et al.* 2001).

Many studies have utilized various ratios comparing cortisol and testosterone concentrations in the blood to estimate the anabolic status of the body during prolonged resistance training or with overtraining (Häkkinen *et al.* 1985; Stone *et al.* 1991; Fry & Kraemer 1997). However, this is probably an oversimplification of anabolic status in muscle since many other factors contribute to protein and nitrogen balance. As with any hormone, tissue receptor content as well as circulating binding protein concentrations can change in response to differential circulating concentrations of a hormone, thereby altering bioactivity (Hickson & Marone 1993). Also, ligand uptake and metabolism, nutritional status and responses of other hormonal factors will ultimately influence the resultant anabolic/catabolic hormonal milieu. Nonetheless, chronic hypersecretion of glucocorticoids, such as in disease states like Cushing's syndrome, are known to be associated with decreased muscle size and strength. Furthermore, the delicate balance between catabolic and anabolic factors remains crucial to protein turnover rates, and the glucocorticoids represent the primary catabolic influence on muscle. We have seen that after 7 weeks of resistance training in rats, testosterone can be secreted in normal fashion from the testis despite the high concentrations of corticosterone. Normal binding activities can also occur. This appears to be due to a 'disinhibition' of the testosterone receptor with exercise training mediated via the nitric oxide/β-endorphin and fluid flow mechanisms. Thus, the incidence of high concentrations of cortisol may not necessarily mean that catabolic processes dominate at all the cellular levels. With cortisol the important role of preserving the use of glucose by inhibiting those processes which primarily utilize glucose to function (e.g. immune cell metabolism) may be part of the overall distress syndrome addressed by Selye, and with training these acute effects may be overridden biologically.

Cytokines

Although more *in vivo* research is still needed, it is becoming increasingly evident that different cytokines may elicit catabolic effects which can either directly or indirectly (i.e. through interactions with other growth factors) influence muscle growth and differentiation. Cytokines are soluble glycoprotein substances produced and secreted by nearly all immune and non-immune cells. Hundreds of different cytokines have been identified and many are involved in either anti- or proinflammatory functions. Perhaps the most notable cytokine that is known to affect muscle mass is tumour necrosis factor α (TNF-α). This proinflammatory cytokine is known to be elevated in various muscle wasting pathologies such as acquired immune deficiency syndrome (AIDS) and can either directly or indirectly inhibit muscle protein synthesis. It has recently been demonstrated that TNF-α decreases circulating [illegible] of IGF-I and these decreases are related to the reduced rate of muscle protein synthesis in septic animals (Lang *et al.* 1996). More recently, TNF-α has been shown to directly inhibit protein synthesis in a dose-dependent manner in cultured human myoblast and myotube cells (Frost *et al.* 1997). Thus hypersecretion of TNF-α, such as during infection, trauma or intense damaging exercise, can negatively influence muscle protein turnover directly or by suppressing the IGF system.

Other cytokines also indirectly inhibit muscle cell proliferation via their suppressive effects on the IGF system. McCusker and Clemmons (1994) suggest that some cytokines function to regulate the circulating concentrations of IGF–IGFBP complexes in extracellular fluids by inhibiting IGFBP secretion. Specifically, secretion of IGFBP-4, which is thought to inhibit the proliferative and differentiation effects of IGFs on muscle cells, and IGFBP-5 (which can be either stimulatory or inhibitory) is decreased by transforming growth factor β_1 (TGF-β_1) in cultured rat and mouse muscle cell lines (McCusker & Clemmons 1994). In this manner, cytokines such as TGF-β_1 are proposed to limit the circulating IGF–IGFBP complexes from exceeding a threshold concentration at which muscle cell growth and differentiation are optimal for survival. Another member of the transforming growth factor β superfamily, myostatin, is also a potent inhibitory regulator of skeletal muscle growth. *In vitro*, myostatin decreases cell proliferation and protein synthesis in mouse skeletal muscle cells, while circulating concentrations of myostatin protein in humans have been found to be significantly higher in patients with AIDS and severe muscle loss than in healthy men (Gonzalez-Cadavid *et al.* 1998; Taylor *et al.* 2001). Whether significant inhibitory effects from such cytokines on muscle growth can be observed in healthy adult men and women (*in vivo*) in response to exercise, sleeplessness or other trauma has yet to be conclusively demonstrated, and thus such novel regulators of muscle growth must be studied further in athletic and non-athletic exercising populations in order to better understand the role(s), if any, that cyto- [illegible] size and strength.

Summary

Ultimately, the mechanisms related to the anabolic and catabolic hormones' interactions with skeletal muscle consequent to resistance exercise are just starting to be understood from basic research findings. There are many potential strategies at the molecular and cellular levels that can translate to increased protein synthesis and accretion and altered structural form of muscle. Now the challenge will be to describe and elucidate those mechanisms that are operational consequent to various 'specific' types of resistance training programmes that can be performed in the weight room. In this process, our understanding of the plasticity of the neuroendocrine system and the complex concept of hypertrophy will be revealed. Ultimately these factors will affect the ability of a specific resistance training programme to produce improvements in strength and power performances. The paramount biological 'principle of specificity' for both the exercise stimulus and the series of biological mechanisms it initiates will no doubt be of dramatic importance when trying to unravel the many possible sequences of strategies that can be used to mediate adaptations in muscle to produce enhanced muscle strength and power.

References

Adams, G. (1998) Role of insulin-like growth factor-I in the regulation of skeletal muscle adaptation to increased loading. *Exercise and Sport Sciences Reviews* **26**, 31–60.

Adams, G. & McCue, S. (1998) Localized infusion of IGF-I results in skeletal muscle hypertrophy in rats. *Journal of Applied Physiology* **84**, 1716–1722.

Argetsinger, L.S. & Carter-Su, C. (1996) Mechanisms of signaling by growth hormone receptor. *Physiological Reviews* **76**, 1089–1107.

Bamman, M.M., Shipp, J.R., Jiang, J. *et al.* (2001) Mechanical load increases muscle IGF-I and androgen receptor mRNA concentrations in humans. *American Journal of Physiology* **280**, E383–E390.

Bartsch, W., Krieg, M. & Voigt, K.D. (1983) Regulation and compartmentalization of androgens in the rat prostate and muscle. *Journal of Steroid Biochemistry* **19**, 929–937.

Baumann, G. (1991a) Growth hormone heterogeneity: genes, isohormones, variants, and binding proteins. *Endocrine Reviews* **12**, 424–443.

Baumann, G. (1991b) Metabolism of growth hormone (GH) and different molecular forms of GH in biological fluids. *Hormone Research Supplement* **36**, 5–10.

Bhasin, S., Storer, T., Berman, N. *et al.* (1996) The effects of supraphysiological doses of testosterone on the muscle size and strength in normal men. *New England Journal of Medicine* **335**, 1–7.

Bhasin, S., Storer, T.W., Berman, N. *et al.* (1997) Testosterone replacement increases fat-free mass and muscle size in hypogonadal men. *Journal of Clinical Endocrinology and Metabolism* **82**, 407–413.

Binoux, M. & Hossenlopp, P. (1988) Insulin-like growth factor (IGF) and IGF-binding proteins: comparison of human serum and lymph. *Journal of Clinical Endocrinology and Metabolism* **67**, 509–514.

Biolo, G., Chinkes, D., Zhang, X. & Wolfe, R.R. (1992) A new model to determine in vivo the relationship between amino acid transmembrane transport and protein kinetics in muscle. *Journal of Parenteral and Enteral Nutrition* **16**, 305–315.

Biolo, G., Fleming, R.Y.D. & Wolfe, R.R. (1995) Physiologic hyperinsulinemia stimulates protein synthesis and enhances transport of selected amino acids in human skeletal muscle. *Journal of Clinical Investigation* **95**, 811–819.

Borst, S.E., DeHoyos, D.V., Garzarella, L. *et al.* (2001) Effects of resistance training on insulin-like growth factor-1 and IGF binding proteins. *Medicine and Science in Sports and Exercise* **33**, 648–653.

Brodsky, I.G., Balagopal, P. & Nair, K.S. (1996) Effects of testosterone replacement on muscle mass and muscle protein synthesis in hypogonadal men—a clinical research center study. *Journal of Clinical Endocrinology and Metabolism* **81**, 3469–3475.

Castellino, P., Luzi, L., Simonson, D.C., Haymond, M. & DeFronzo, R.A. (1987) Effect of insulin and plasma amino acid concentrations on leucine metabolism in man. Role of substrate availability on estimates of whole body protein synthesis. *Journal of Clinical Investigation* **80**, 1784–1793.

Chow, J.C., Ling, P.R., Qu, Z. *et al.* (1996) Growth hormone stimulates tyrosine phosphorylation of JAK2 and STAT5, but not IRS-1 or SHC proteins in liver and skeletal muscle of normal rats in vivo. *Endocrinology* **137**, 2880–2886.

Collett-Solberg, P.F. & Cohen, P. (1996) The role of the insulin-like growth factor binding proteins and the IGFBP proteases in modulating IGF action. *Endocrinology and Metabolism Clinics of North America* **25**, 591–614.

Coolican, S.A., Samuel, D.S., Ewton, D.Z., McWade, F.J. & Florini, J.R. (1997) The mitogenic and myogenic actions of insulin-like growth factors utilize distinct signaling pathways. *Journal of Biological Chemistry* **272**, 6653–6662.

Copeland, K.C., Underwood, L.E. & Van Wyk, J.J. (1980) Induction of immunoreactive somatomedin-C in human serum by growth hormone: dose–response relationships and effect on chromatographic profiles. *Journal of Clinical Endocrinology and Metabolism* **50**, 690–697.

Cuneo, R.C., Salomon, F., Wiles, C.M., Hesp, R. & Sonksen, P.H. (1991) Growth hormone treatment in growth hormone-deficient adults. I. Effects on muscle mass and strength. *Journal of Applied Physiology* **70**, 688–694.

Damon, S.E., Haugk, K.L., Birnbaum, R.S. & Quinn, L.S. (1998) Retrovirally mediated overexpression of insulin-like growth factor binding protein 4: evidence that insulin-like growth factor is required for skeletal muscle differentiation. *Journal of Cell Physiology* **175**, 109–120.

DeMeyts, P., Wallach, B., Christoffersen, C.T. *et al.* (1994) The insulin-like growth factor-I receptor. *Hormone Research* **42**, 152–169.

Deschenes, M.R., Maresh, C.M., Armstrong, L.E., Covault, J., Kraemer, W.J. & Crivello, J.F. (1994) Endurance and resistance exercise induce muscle fiber type specific responses in androgen binding capacity. *Journal of Steroid Biochemistry and Molecular Biology* **50**, 175–179.

Farrell, P.A., Hernandez, J.M., Fedele, M.J., Vary, T.C., Kimball, S.R. & Jefferson, L.S. (2000) Eukaryotic initiation factors and protein synthesis after resistance exercise in rats. *Journal of Applied Physiology* **88**, 1036–1042.

Ferrando, A.A., Tipton, K.D., Doyle, D., Phillips, S.M., Cortiella, J. & Wolfe, R.R. (1998) Testosterone injection stimulates net protein synthesis but not tissue amino acid transport. *American Journal of Physiology* **275**, E864–E871.

Fisker, S., Kristensen, K., Rosenfalck, A.M. *et al.* (2001) Gene expression of a truncated and the full-length growth hormone (GH) receptor in subcutaneous fat and skeletal muscle in GH-deficient adults: impact of GH treatment. *Journal of Clinical Endocrinology and Metabolism* **86**(2), 792–796.

Fleck, S.J. & Kraemer, W.J. (1997) *Designing Resistance Training Programs*, 2nd edn. Human Kinetics, Champaign, Illinois.

Florini, J.R. (1987) Hormonal control of muscle growth. *Muscle and Nerve* **10**, 577–598.

Florini, J.R., Ewton, D.Z. & Coolican, S.A. (1996a) Growth hormone and the insulin-like growth factor system in myogenesis. *Endocrine Reviews* **17**, 481–517.

Florini, J.R., Samuel, D.S., Ewton, D.Z., Kirk, C. & Sklar, R.M. (1996b) Stimulation of myogenic differentiation by a neuregulin, glial growth factor 2: are neuregulins the long-sought muscle trophic factors secreted by nerves. *Journal of Biological Chemistry* **271**, 12699–12702.

Frost, R.A. & Lang, C.H. (1999) Differential effects of insulin-like growth factor I (IGF-I) and IGF-binding protein-1 on protein metabolism in human skeletal muscle cells. *Endocrinology* **140**, 3962–3970.

Frost, R.A., Lang, C.H. & Gelato, M.C. (1997) Transient exposure of human myoblasts to tumor necrosis factor-α inhibits serum and insulin-like growth factor-I stimulated protein synthesis. *Endocrinology* **138**, 4153–4159.

Fry, A.C. & Kraemer, W.J. (1997) Resistance exercise overtraining and overreaching. *Sports Medicine* **23**, 106–129.

Fryburg, D.A. (1994) Insulin-like growth factor I exerts growth hormone- and insulin-like actions on human muscle protein metabolism. *American Journal of Physiology* **267**, E331–E336.

Fryburg, D.A. (1996) NG-monomethyl-L-arginine inhibits the blood flow but not the insulin-like response of forearm muscle to IGF-I: possible role of nitric oxide in muscle protein synthesis. *Journal of Clinical Investigation* **97**, 1319–1328.

Fryburg, D.A. & Barrett, E.J. (1995) Insulin, growth hormone and IGF-I regulation of protein metabolism. *Diabetes Reviews* **3**, 93–112.

Fryburg, D.A., Jahn, L.A., Hill, S.A., Oliveras, D.M. & Barrett, E.J. (1995) Insulin and insulin-like growth factor-I enhance human skeletal muscle protein anabolism during hyperaminoacidemia by different mechanisms. *Journal of Clinical Investigation* **96**, 1722–1729.

Goldspink, G. (1998) Cellular and molecular aspects of muscle growth, adaptation and aging. *Gerodontology* **15**, 35–43.

Gonzalez-Cadavid, N., Taylor, W.E., Yarasheski, K.E. *et al.* (1998) Organization of the human myostatin gene and expression in healthy men and HIV-infected men with muscle wasting. *Proceedings of the National Academy of Sciences of the United States of America* **95**, 14938–14943.

Gordon, S.E., Davis, B.S., Carlson, C.J. & Booth, F.W. (2001) ANG II is required for optimal overload-induced skeletal muscle hypertrophy. *American Journal of Physiology* **280**, E150–E159.

Griggs, R.C., Kingston, W., Jozefowicz, R.F., Herr, B.E., Forbes, G. & Halliday, D. (1989) Effect of testosterone on muscle mass and muscle protein synthesis. *Journal of Applied Physiology* **66**, 498–503.

Häkkinen, K., Pakarinen, A., Alén, M. & Komi, P.V. (1985) Serum hormones during prolonged training of neuromuscular performance. *European Journal of Applied Physiology* **53**, 287–293.

Hickson, R.C. & Marone, J.R. (1993) Exercise and inhibition of glucocorticoid-induced muscle atrophy. *Exercise and Sport Sciences Reviews* **21**, 135–167.

Hickson, R.C., Czerwinski, S.M., Falduto, M.T. & Young, M.R. (1990) Glucocorticoid antagonism by exercise and androgenic-anabolic steroids. *Medicine and Science in Sports and Exercise* **22**, 331–340.

Hobbs, C.J., Plymate, S.R., Rosen, C.J. & Adler, R.A. (1993) Testosterone administration increases insulin-like growth factor-I levels in normal men. *Journal of Clinical Endocrinology and Metabolism* **77**, 776–779.

Hymer, W.C., Kirshnan, K., Kraemer, W.J., Welsch, J. & Lanham, W. (2000) Mammalian pituitary growth hormone: applications of free flow electrophoresis. *Electrophoresis* **21**, 311–317.

Hymer, W.C., Kraemer, W.J., Nindl, B.C. *et al.* (2001) Characteristics of circulating growth hormone in women following acute heavy resistance exercise. *American Journal of Physiology* **281**, E878–E888.

Ilondo, M.M., Damholdt, A.B., Cunningham, B.A., Wells, J.A., De Meyts, P. & Shymko, R.M. (1994) Receptor dimerization determines the effects of growth hormone in primary rat adipocytes and cultured IM-9 lymphocytes. *Endocrinology* **134**, 2397–2403.

James, P.L., Stewart, C.E. & Rotwein, P. (1996) Insulin-like growth factor binding protein-5 modulates muscle differentiation through an insulin-like growth factor-dependent mechanism. *Journal of Cell Biology* **133**, 683–693.

Jones, J.I. & Clemmons, D.R. (1995) Insulin-like growth factors and the binding proteins: biological actions. *Endocrine Reviews* **16**, 3–34.

Kalra, P.S., Sahu, A. & Kalra, S.P. (1990) Interleukin-1 inhibits the ovarian steroid-induced luteinizing hormone surge and release of hypothalamic luteinizing hormone-releasing hormone in rats. *Endocrinology* **126**, 2145–2152.

Kesperek, S.J., Conway, G.R., Krayeski, D.S. & Lohne, J.J. (1992) A reexamination of the effect of exercise on rate of muscle protein degradation. *American Journal of Physiology* **263**, E1144–E1150.

Kraemer, W.J. (1988) Endocrine responses to resistance exercise. *Medicine and Science in Sports and Exercise* **20** (Suppl.), S152–S157.

Kraemer, W.J., Marchitelli, L.J., Gordon, S.E. *et al.* (1990) Hormonal and growth factor responses to heavy resistance exercise protocols. *Journal of Applied Physiology* **69**, 1442–1450.

Kraemer, W.J., Fleck, S.J., Dziados, J.E. *et al.* (1993) Changes in hormonal concentrations after different heavy-resistance exercise protocols in women. *Journal of Applied Physiology* **75**, 594–604.

Kraemer, W.J., Patton, J., Gordon, S.E. *et al.* (1995) Compatibility of high-intensity strength and endurance training on hormonal and skeletal muscle adaptations. *Journal of Applied Physiology* **78**, 976–989.

Kraemer, W.J., Häkkinen, K., Newton, R.U. *et al.* (1998a) Acute hormonal responses to heavy resistance exercise in younger and older men. *European Journal of Applied Physiology* **77**, 206–211.

Kraemer, W.J., Volek, J.S., Bush, J.A., Putukian, M. & Sebastianelli, W.J. (1998b) Hormonal responses to consecutive days of heavy-resistance exercise with or without nutritional supplementation. *Journal of Applied Physiology* **85**, 1544–1555.

Kraemer, W.J., Häkkinen, K., Newton, R.U. *et al.* (1999) Effects of heavy-resistance training on hormonal response patterns in younger vs. older men. *Journal of Applied Physiology* **87**, 982–992.

Kraemer, W.J., Loebel, C.C., Volek, J.S. *et al.* (2001) The effect of heavy resistance exercise on the circadian rhythm of salivary testosterone in men. *European Journal of Applied Physiology* **84**(1–2), 13–18.

Lang, C.H., Fan, J., Cooney, R. & Vary, T. (1996) IL-1 receptor antagonist attenuates sepsis-induced alterations in the IGF system and protein synthesis. *American Journal of Physiology* **270**, E430–E437.

Lewis, A.J., Wester, T.J., Burrin, D.G. & Dauncey, M.J. (2000) Exogenous growth hormone induces somatotrophic gene expression in neonatal liver and skeletal muscle. *American Journal of Physiology* **278**, R838–R844.

Loughna, P.T., Mason, P. & Bates, P.C. (1992) Regulation of insulin-like growth factor I gene expression in skeletal muscle. *Symposium of the Society for Experimental Biology* **46**, 319–330.

McCall, G.E., Grindeland, R.E., Roy, R.R. & Edgerton, V.R. (2000) Muscle afferent activity modulates bioassayable growth hormone in human plasma. *Journal of Applied Physiology* **89**, 1137–1141.

McCusker, R.H. & Clemmons, D.R. (1994) Effects of cytokines on insulin-like growth factor binding protein secretion by muscle cells in vitro. *Endocrinology* **134**, 2095–2201.

Mauras, N.M., Blizzard, R.M., Link, K., Johnson, M.L., Rogol, A.D. & Veldhuis, J.D. (1987) Augmentation of growth hormone secretion during puberty: evidence for a pulse amplitude-modulated phenomenon. *Journal of Clinical Endocrinology and Metabolism* **64**, 596–601.

Mayer, M. & Rosen, F. (1977) Interaction of glucocorticoids and androgens with skeletal muscle. *Metabolism* **26**, 937–962.

Moldoveanu, A.I., Shephard, R.J. & Shek, P.N. (2001) The cytokine response to physical activity and training. *Sports Medicine* **31**, 115–144.

Nindl, B.C., Kraemer, W.J., Marx, J.O. *et al.* (2001) Overnight responses of the circulating IGF-I system after acute, heavy-resistance exercise. *Journal of Applied Physiology* **90**, 1319–1326.

Pacak, K., Palkovits, M., Yadid, G., Kvetnansky, R., Kopin, I.J. & Goldstein, D.S. (1998) Heterogeneous neurochemical responses to different stressors: a test of Selye's doctrine of nonspecificity. *American Journal of Physiology* **275**, R1247–R1255.

Path, G., Bornstein, S.R., Ehrhart-Bornstein, M. & Scherbaum, W.A. (1997) Interleukin-6 and the interleukin-6 receptor in the human adrenal gland: expression and effects on steroidogenesis. *Journal of Clinical Endocrinology and Metabolism* **82**, 2343–2349.

Perrone, C.E., Fenwick-Smith, D. & Vandenburgh, H.H. (1995) Collagen and stretch modulate autocrine secretion of insulin-like growth factor-1 and insulin-like growth factor binding proteins from differentiated skeletal muscle cells. *Journal of Biological Chemistry* **270**, 2099–2106.

Razandi, M., Pedram, A., Greene, G.L. & Levin, E.R. (1999) Cell membrane and nuclear estrogen receptors (Ers) originate from a single transcript: studies of ER alpha and ER beta expressed in Chinese hamster ovary cells. *Molecular Endocrinology* **13**, 307–319.

Rooyackers, O.E. & Nair, K.S. (1997) Hormonal regulation of human muscle protein metabolism. *Annual Review of Nutrition* **17**, 457–485.

Rowlinson, S.W., Waters, M.J., Lewis, U.J. & Barnard, R. (1996) Human growth hormone fragments 1–43 and 44–191: in vitro somatogenic activity and receptor binding characteristics in human and nonprimate systems. *Endocrinology* **137**, 90–95.

Rubin, M.R., Kraemer, W.J., Nindl, B.C. *et al.* (2000) Periodized resistance training potentiates in vivo bioactivity of human growth hormone. *Medicine and Science in Sports and Exercise* **32**, S186 (Abstract).

Russell-Jones, D.L., Umpleby, A., Hennessey, T. *et al.* (1994) Use of leucine clamp to demonstrate that IGF-I actively stimulates protein synthesis in normal humans. *American Journal of Physiology* **267**, E591–E598.

Sakai, K., Busby,W.H., Jr, Clarke, J.B. & Clemmons, D.R. (2001) Tissue transglutaminase facilitates the polymerization of insulin-like growth factor-binding protein-1 (IGFBP-1) and leads to loss of IGFBP-1's ability to inhibit insulin-like growth factor-I stimulated protein synthesis. *Journal of Biological Chemistry* **276**, 8740–8745.

Sapolsky, R.M., Romero, L.M. & Munck, A.U. (2000) How do glucocorticoids influence stress responses? Integrating permissive, suppressive, stimulatory, and preparative actions. *Endocrine Reviews* **21**, 55–89.

Schnoebelen-Combes, S., Louveau, I., Postel-Vinay, M.C. & Bonneau, M. (1996) Ontogeny of GH receptor and GH-binding protein in the pig. *Journal of Endocrinology* **148**(2), 249–255.

Selye, H. (1936) A syndrome produced by diverse nocuous agents. *Nature* **138**, 32.

Smith, L.L. (2000) Cytokine hypothesis of overtraining: a physiological adaptation to excessive stress? *Medicine and Science in Sports and Exercise* **32**, 317–331.

Stone, M.H., Keith, R.E., Kearney, J.T., Fleck, S.J., Wilson, G.D. & Triplett, N.T. (1991) Overtraining: a review of the signs, symptoms, and possible causes. *Journal of Applied Sports Science Research* **5**, 35–50.

Strasburger, C.J. & Dattani, M.T. (1997) New growth hormone assays: potential benefits. *Acta Paediatrica Supplement* **423**, 5–11.

Strasburger, C.J., Wu, Z., Pfaulm, C. & Dressendorfer, R.A. (1996) Immunofunctional assay of human growth hormone (hGH) in serum: a possible consensus of quantitative hGH measurement. *Journal of Clinical Endocrinology and Metabolism* **81**, 2613–2620.

Szanberg, E., Jefferson, L.S., Lundholm, K. & Kimball, S.R. (1997) Postprandial stimulation of muscle protein synthesis is independent of changes in insulin. *American Journal of Physiology* **272**, E841–E847.

Taaffe, D.R., Pruitt, L., Reim, J. *et al.* (1994) Effect of recombinant human growth hormone on the muscle strength response to resistance exercise in elderly men. *Journal of Clinical Endocrinology and Metabolism* **79**, 1361–1366.

Taylor, W.E., Bhasin, S., Artaza, J. *et al.* (2001) Myostatin inhibits cell proliferation and protein synthesis in C_2C_{12} muscle cells. *American Journal of Physiology* **280**, E221–E228.

Tessari, P., Inchiostro, S., Biolo, G. *et al.* (1987) Differential effects of hyperinsulinemia and hyperaminoacidemia on leucine-carbon metabolism in vivo. Evidence for distinct mechanisms in regulation of net amino acid deposition. *Journal of Clinical Investigation* **79**, 1062–1069.

Thissen, J.P., Ketelslegers, J.M. & Underwood, L.E. (1994) Nutritional regulation of the insulin-like growth factors. *Endocrine Reviews* **15**, 80–101.

Turner, J.D., Rotwein, P., Novakofski, J. & Bechtel, P.J. (1988) Induction of messenger RNA for IGF-I and -II during growth hormone-stimulated muscle hypertrophy. *American Journal of Physiology* **255**, E513–E517.

Urban, R.J., Bodenburg, Y.H., Gilkison, C. *et al.* (1995) Testosterone administration to elderly men increases skeletal muscle strength and protein synthesis. *American Journal of Physiology* **269**, E820–E826.

Wallace, J.D., Cuneo, R.C., Bidlingmaier, M. *et al.* (2001) The response of molecular isoforms of growth hormone to acute exercise in trained adult males. *Journal of Clinical Endocrinology and Metabolism* **86**(1), 200–206.

Weissberger, A.J. & Ho, K.K. (1993) Activation of the somatotropic axis by testosterone in adult males: evidence for the role of aromatization. *Journal of Clinical Endocrinology and Metabolism* **76**, 1407–1412.

Wolfe, R.R. (2000) Effects of insulin on muscle tissue. *Current Opinion in Clinical Nutrition and Metabolic Care* **3**, 67–71.

Wu, F.C.W. (1997) Endocrine aspects of anabolic steroids. *Clinical Chemistry* **43**, 1289–1292.

Yang, S., Alnaqeeb, M., Simpson, H. & Goldspink, G. (1996) Cloning and characterization of an IGF-1 isoform expressed in skeletal muscle subjected to stretch. *Journal of Muscle Research and Cell Motility* **17**, 487–495.

Yarasheski, K.E. (1994) Growth hormone effects on metabolism, body composition, muscle mass, and strength. *Exercise and Sport Science Review* **22**, 285–312.

Yarasheski, K.E., Zachwieja, J.J., Campbell, J.A. & Bier, D.M. (1995) Effect of growth hormone and resistance exercise on muscle growth and strength in older men. *American Journal of Physiology* **268**, E268–E276.

Zapf, J. (1997) Total and free IGF serum levels. *European Journal of Endocrinology* **136**, 146–147.

Chapter 6

Exercise-Related Adaptations in Connective Tissue

RONALD F. ZERNICKE AND BARBARA LOITZ-RAMAGE

Fibrous and bony connective tissues provide the essential infrastructure that allows the human body to strive for the Olympic ideal—*citius, altius, fortius* (faster, higher, stronger). During movements, strong but pliant tendons transmit the forces generated by muscles to bones serving as effective levers, while ligaments and menisci maintain the intricate articulations of the skeletal levers. The adaptive ability of fibrous and bony connective tissues in response to training and exercise is discussed in this chapter. The dynamic responses of a bone to its functional demands have been recognized for more than a century, but the responsiveness of fibrous connective tissues to exercise and conditioning has been appreciated only more recently. It is becoming more and more apparent that all fibrous and bony connective tissues are sensitive to mechanical loads. The quality and quantity of the loading to the tissue, however, can determine whether the outcome is positive or injurious.

There is a plethora of significant information about connective tissues, much more than could be covered in this chapter. Thus, we limit our discussion to major load-transmitting connective tissues (bone, tendon, ligament and meniscus) and emphasize the adaptive and maladaptive changes that occur in these tissues as a consequence of exercise and conditioning after providing an overview of the structure of each tissue.

Bone

The dynamic nature of bone has long been recognized, as Wolff in 1892 stated that: 'every change in the function of bone is followed by certain definite changes in internal architecture and external configuration in accordance with mathematical laws' (Carter 1984, p. S19). To date, however, the mechanisms underlying bone's ability to translate loading events into cellular responses remain largely unexplained. Cowin *et al.* (1984) listed several questions about bone remodelling dynamics that remain to be answered, including: (i) How do mechanically derived stimuli compete with systemic stimuli? (ii) What is the nature of the mechanical stimuli that influence bone remodelling? (iii) What are the structural objectives of bone remodelling?

Structure

Bone matrix comprises three elements: organic, mineral and fluid. Organic components account for 39% of bone's total volume, containing 95% type I collagen and 5% proteoglycans. Minerals include primarily calcium hydroxyapatite crystals and contribute 49% to bone's total volume. Fluid-filled vascular channels and cellular spaces constitute the remaining volume (Frost 1987). Mineral components give bone its stiffness, while the organic matrix contributes to bone strength. Resistance to deformation under load may be the most important physical property of bone (Albright & Skinner 1987), and thus bone must be of adequate stiffness and strength not to break under dynamic or static loading (Currey 1984). Bone mechanical characteristics reflect a balance between mineral and organic phases.

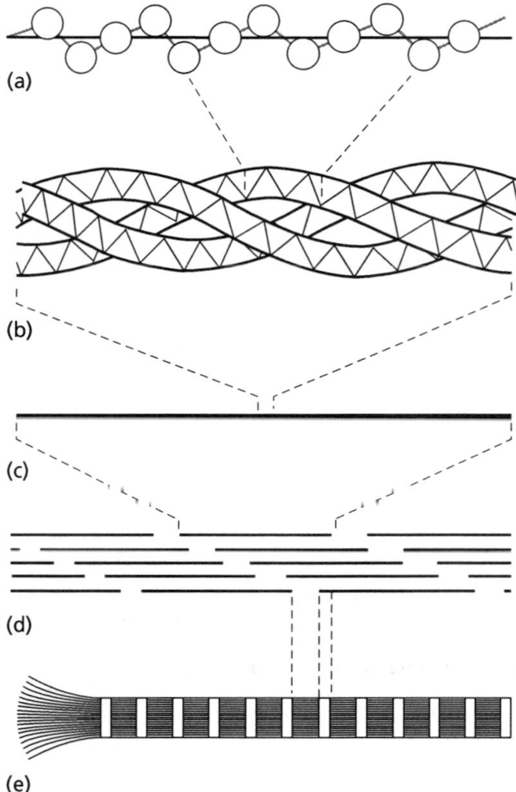

Fig. 6.1 Schematic diagram of a collagen fibril: (a) amino acids join to form an α chain; (b) three α chains coil to form the triple helix procollagen molecule; (c) procollagen bundles link to form tropocollagen, which packs in a staggered orientation (d) that gives the collagen fibril (e) a striated appearance. (From Prockop & Guzman 1977; Nordin & Frankel 1989.)

Collagen, the most abundant mammalian protein (Buckwalter & Cooper 1987), provides a major structural support for connective tissues. Collagen constitutes perhaps one-third of the total protein in the body and therefore about 6% of body weight (White *et al.* 1964). Collagen tensile strength results from polypeptides arranged in α chains (Fig. 6.1). Each α chain consists of amino acids, with glycine, lysine and proline being particularly important. Glycine, the smallest of the three, occupies every third position in the α chain and, in so doing, allows the chain to assume a helical shape. Hydroxyl groups attach to lysine and proline molecules in a completed α chain, and hydroxylation plays a critical role in determining collagen's stiffness. After hydroxylation and attachment of carbohydrates, the α chains coil around each other to form a triple helix called procollagen. Osteoblasts secrete procollagen into the surrounding matrix where cleavage of terminal peptides allows procollagen bundles to link together, forming tropocollagen molecules, the most fundamental molecular structure of collagenous tissues (White *et al.* 1964; Ham 1974). Strong cross-links between procollagen's hydroxylysine molecules give tropocollagen its strength. Intramolecular cross-links join tropocollagen molecules to form collagen fibrils. The extent of hydroxylysine cross-linking changes with age and between types of connective tissues; more cross-links produce a stiffer tissue (Butler *et al.* 1978).

Mineral content distinguishes bone from other connective tissues and gives bone its unique stiffness and a role in maintaining mineral homeostasis in the body. Skinner (1987) suggested that bone mineralization relies on a specific link between type I collagen and hydroxyapatite crystals in bone.

Although different in shape and size, all bones share certain structural features. Bone has two basic forms, woven and lamellar. Woven bone forms quickly and assumes an irregular pattern of collagen fibres and osteocytes. A sporadic mineral distribution also limits woven bone's ability to withstand mechanical loads (Albright & Skinner 1987). Fracture callus, active endochondral ossification sites and some pathological sites contain woven bone, but it is not typically found in the healthy, adult human skeleton. During skeletal maturation, lamellar bone systemically replaces woven bone, providing the adult skeleton with its functional stiffness (Frost 1987).

Lamellar bone plays an important role in transmitting loads. Compact lamellar bone (Fig. 6.2) always surrounds cancellous lamellar bone, covering all external bony surfaces. Its relative thickness varies, from thin vertebral bodies to thick long bone diaphyses. Cancellous lamellar bone assumes a three-dimensional latticework continuous with the endosteal surface of cortical

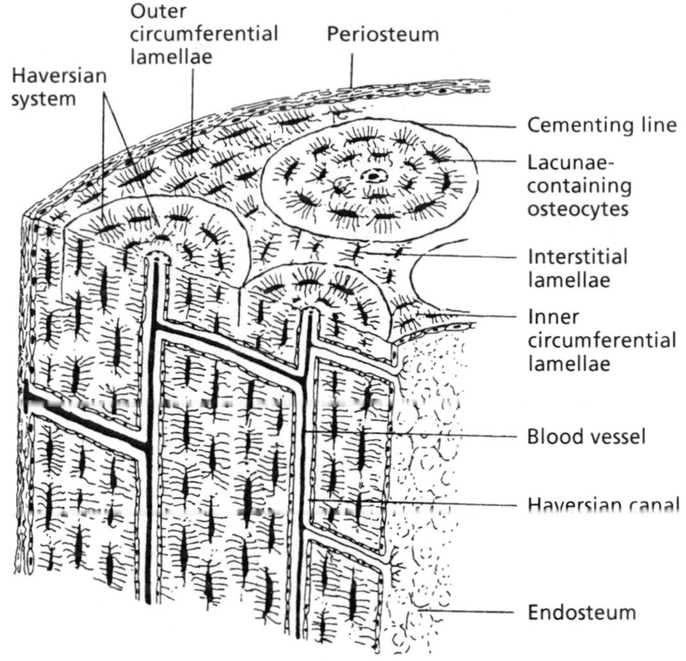

Fig. 6.2 Compact lamellar bone, with the transverse plane showing osteocytes arranged in Haversian systems and circumferential and interstitial lamellae. Vascular channels course longitudinally and transversely throughout the bone. (From Ham 1974.)

bone. Individual columns or plates of bone (trabeculae) orientate parallel to the principal strain axes, providing maximal strength with minimal material (Clark *et al.* 1975).

Remodelling

Electrical phenomena may alter remodelling and fracture repair, and electrical effects are a likely means of information transfer between mechanical deformation and cellular response. While the mechanisms producing electrical potentials remain to be fully explained, Currey (1984) cites two possible sources of electrical phenomena: piezoelectricity and streaming potentials. Crystals having a lattice structure and no central symmetry develop a net separation of charge between anions and cations when deformation occurs. Charge separation causes a potential difference, the piezoelectric potential, to develop between opposite ends of the crystals. Wet collagen stiffened by minerals may react like a lattice crystal when deformed and may provide the piezoelectric potentials generated by bone strain (Eriksson 1976). Piezoelectricity is highly directional, a noteworthy feature that may help to explain bone's differing sensitivity to compressive and tensile strains.

When a solid surface carrying a surface charge contacts a polar liquid, oppositely charged ions from the fluid migrate toward the surface. If the fluid flows, weakly connected ions move, creating a current such that a potential difference (streaming potential) develops between upstream and downstream sites. When bone deforms, polarized extracellular fluid tends to move. The resulting streaming potentials may provide information concerning the strain stimulus.

Lanyon and Hartman (1977) demonstrated that during bending, the tensile surface of a wet bone sample developed a positive charge, the compressive side became negatively charged, and the peak difference depended on both the strain rate and magnitude. When bone experienced a static load, the potential decayed to zero within approximately 2 s (Cochran *et al.* 1968). Eriksson (1976) postulated that such strain-induced polarization resulted from streaming potentials generated by unidirectional flow of positively charged extracellular fluid in transversely orientated channels. Bending forced channel diameters to decrease on the concave surface and increase on the convex surface, moving fluid toward the convexity, thereby creating a strain-induced voltage. This theory supports bone's insensitivity to static load (Hert *et al.* 1971; Lanyon & Rubin 1984) and sensitivity to variations in strain rate and magnitude (Rubin & Lanyon 1985). When static loading is superimposed upon normal activity, however, new periosteal bone apposition results (Meade *et al.* 1984). Not unexpectedly, when intermittent bending loads are applied in physiological ranges, Liskova and Hert (1971) report that periosteal and endosteal bone is deposited. O'Connor *et al.* (1982) suggest that a principal determinant of new bone deposition in a weightbearing bone is the rate of change of strain that closely approximates that developed during normal locomotion. Several investigators (Carter *et al.* 1981; Churches & Howlett 1981) have reported a differential response to bending loads, indicating that more bone deposition occurs in areas of increased compressive strains as opposed to areas of tensile strains.

Skerry *et al.* (1988, 1990) proposed that loading-related reorientation of proteoglycans may be a link between mechanical loading and remodelling. They measured collagen and proteoglycan reorientation following load applications, and collagen orientation showed no difference between loaded and control bones. Proteoglycans, however, showed a significant 36% difference in orientation between control and loaded bones. Forty-eight hours after the cessation of loading, no difference was found in control and loaded bones. Skerry *et al.* concluded that dynamic loading affected the proteoglycan orientation in a manner related to the load's magnitude and distribution, similar to previous descriptions relating strain and bone remodelling. Proteoglycan reorientation may therefore provide a strain-induced stimulus to the osteocyte that signals the bone's recent dynamic strain history.

Studies measuring prostaglandin (PG) concentrations in cultured osteoblasts led Yeh and Rodan (1984) and Binderman *et al.* (1984) to conclude that PGE_2 may act as a transducer between mechanical strain and osteoblasts. Yeh and Rodan compared PG synthesis between bone cells cultured on collagen ribbons left undisturbed and cells cultured on ribbons stretched eight times over a 2-h period. Stretching increased PG synthesis 3.5-fold compared to the non-stretched ribbons, supporting PG's role in the translation of mechanical stimuli to cellular activity. Binderman *et al.* concluded, similarly, that the osteoblast's membrane may have a specific mechanoreceptor system capable of being stimulated by straining to increase PGE_2 synthesis.

Remodelling occurs when existing bone undergoes degradation and new bone forms in its place. This sequence has been referred to as ARF—activation, resorption and formation (Martin & Burr 1989). Therefore, the first step in remodelling is activation of osteoclasts to resorb existing bone. A line of osteoclasts, the osteoclastic front, cuts a longitudinal cone through the bone by secreting acid phosphatase, collagenase and other proteolytic enzymes (Buckwalter & Cooper 1987). The cutting cone resorbs approximately three times its volume and, when completed, leaves a resorptive channel 1000–10 000 mm deep (Albright & Skinner 1987).

Osteoblasts follow the resorptive front, first laying mineralized matrix around the walls of the resorptive channel, forming a cement line. Cement lines contain 10–15% less mineral than surrounding bone, rendering the lines less stiff and providing paths for crack propagation. Osteoblasts then produce new matrix that fills the volume eroded by the osteoclasts. Refilling the cone requires three times longer than resorption, in spite of osteoblasts outnumbering osteoclasts by more than 200 to one (Jaworski 1984). The distance between the osteoclasts and osteoblasts represents the time needed to reverse the resorptive process into one of formation. Generally, this latent period is about 1 week (Albright & Skinner 1987). Osteoblasts then become osteocytes as they trap themselves within the new matrix, changing their role from bone formation to bone maintenance.

Examination of a long bone cross-section reveals that remodelling occurs in three separate areas or envelopes. Though the sequence of osteoclast and osteoblast activity applies to all three envelopes, each surface exhibits unique behaviour to given stimuli and therefore needs to be considered independently when describing remodelling. The inner and outer bony surfaces are the endosteal and periosteal envelopes, and the cortical bone in between forms the intracortical envelope. Measurement of changes in periosteal and endosteal diameters and cortical density is therefore important in studying skeletal diseases and effects of disuse or exercise on bone.

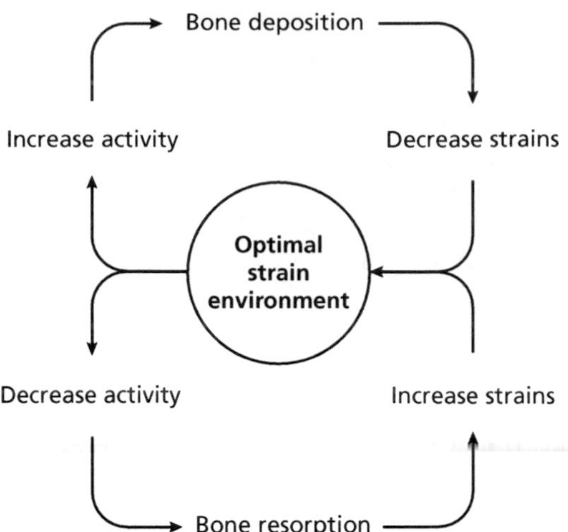

Fig. 6.3 Hypothesized relations among activity level, bone strain and remodelling response. The bone resorption and deposition balance appears to maintain an optimal strain environment. (From Rubin & Lanyon 1987.)

Functional adaptation and exercise-related changes

Judex *et al.* (1999) described the mechanical measures used to quantify bone's mechanical environment as '. . . forces, stresses (forces normalized to unit area), strains (normalized deformations), strain frequency (number of strain cycles per unit time), strain rate (change in strain per unit time), and strain gradients (change in strain per unit length) in various directions within the bone.' (Judex *et al.* 1999, p. 235). In terms of exercise-related adaptation, identifying potent stimuli is critical to optimize the exercise effects. If strain rate, for example, is the strongest stimulus for remodelling, an exercise that applies loads rapidly should be undertaken. Identifying the potent stimuli during exercise is difficult, however, because exercise-induced adaptation may also be influenced by physiological events such as alterations in blood flow or release of systemic factors such as cytokines.

Lanyon (1987) described remodelling as an 'interpretation and purposeful reaction' to a bone's strain state, allowing for adaptation to both increased and decreased strains. 'Functional strains are both the objective and the stimulus for the processes of adaptive modelling and remodelling' (Lanyon 1987, p. 1084). Similarly, Rubin and Lanyon (1985) hypothesized that if functional strains were too high, the incidence of damage and probability of failure increased. If strains were too low, the bone was unnecessarily active, and energy was wasted in the synthesis and maintenance of its matrix. Thus, functional strain appears to be the most relevant parameter to control (Fig. 6.3). As noted by Judex *et al.* (1999), however, the *specific* characteristic of strain (e.g., rate, gradient or magnitude) that is most osteogenic remains unclear.

During the past 30 years, experimental data have emerged to describe, quantitatively, the relation between bone structure and function. Numerous studies have been conducted to correlate known loading events with changes in bone geometry and strength. Among the approaches that have been used are functional overload, artificial loading and *in vivo* strains.

FUNCTIONAL OVERLOAD

Skeletal adaptation to overload has been documented in dogs (Chamay & Tschantz 1972; Carter *et al.* 1980; Meade *et al.* 1984), sheep (Radin *et al.* 1982), swine (Goodship *et al.* 1979; Woo *et al.*

1981), rats (Smith 1977; Gordon *et al.* 1989), mice (Saville & Whyte 1969; Kiiskinen & Heinninen 1973; Kiiskinen 1977) and humans (Jones *et al.* 1977; Krolner *et al.* 1983; Smith *et al.* 1984; Simkin *et al.* 1987). Chamay and Tschantz (1972) performed unilateral radial excisions on dogs, placing the entire forelimb loadbearing responsibility on the ulna. Within 9 months, ulnar cortical thickness increased twofold. Following ulnar excisions in swine, Goodship *et al.* (1979) reported rapid bone deposition, and after 3 months the area of the remodelled radius equalled that of the contralateral radius and ulna together. Surface strains were approximately equal in the radius before ulnar removal and after remodelling, despite dramatic changes in bone geometry. These overload studies support a hypothesis that mechanical loads stimulate bone remodelling and that remodelling continues until strains achieve a predetermined, site-specific level.

ARTIFICIAL LOADING

Artificial load application through cortical pins facilitates precise measurement of loads experienced by bone and allows correlations between loads and remodelling changes. Applied loads may produce strains less than, equal to, or greater than those applied during normal activities. In this way, effects can be quantified of both diminished and excessive loads. Rubin and Lanyon (1985) deprived turkey ulnae of normal loads by performing metaphyseal osteotomies, then applied known loads through diaphyseal pins. A dose : response relationship ($r = 0.83$) was found, with loads producing strain less than 1000 microstrain (μstrain) resulting in bone loss, strains between 1000 and 2000 μstrain maintaining bone mass, and strains exceeding 2000 μstrain stimulating osteogenesis. Using a similar experimental design, Lanyon and Rubin (1984) also reported the remodelling effects of dynamic vs. static loads. Ulnae deprived of all loads and those that experienced static loads displayed increased endosteal diameters and intracortical porosity, resulting in a 13% decreased cortical cross-section. Ulnae exposed to cyclical loading of 1 Hz for 100 s day^{-1} showed a 24% increased cortical cross-section, with new bone deposited primarily on the periosteal surface. Rubin (1984) reported maintained bone mass in rooster ulnae with only four bending cycles per day. Strain magnitudes generated by loads in each of these experiments did not exceed strains measured during wing flapping. From their numerous studies, Lanyon and Rubin concluded that bone appears to be sensitive to magnitude and distribution of dynamic strains and that the insensitivity to static experimental strains reflects the skeleton's natural insensitivity to adapt to static loading situations. Lanyon (1996) also reported bone's sensitivity to strain distribution. If bone is loaded such that strain magnitude remains the same but the strain distribution changes within the section, new bone formation occurs.

IN VIVO STRAINS

Evans (1953) reported the first use of a single-element strain gauge to measure bone strains of a dog's tibia during walking, although the data were of somewhat limited value because the strains were only measured along the axis of the strain gauge. Lanyon (1973) improved this early technique when he placed rosette (three-element) gauges on sheep calcanei and calculated compressive, tensile and shear strains during walking. Gradients of longitudinal normal strain have also been found to correlate well with specific sites of periosteal bone formation (Gross *et al.* 1997). Although such data improved our understanding of the link between bone's mechanical environment and adaptive response, the complex interactions among strain-related mechanical variables elude identification of a specific mechanical stimulus responsible for initiating bone remodelling.

EXERCISE EFFECTS

Disuse-related changes in bone resulting from immobilization (e.g. Uhthoff & Jaworski 1978), spaceflight (e.g. Morey & Baylink 1978; Jee *et al.* 1983; Shaw *et al.* 1988) and hindlimb suspension

(Shaw *et al.* 1987) support a hypothesis that bone requires loadbearing strains to maintain its mass. Similarly, studies quantifying exercise-related changes in bone reiterate bone's dynamic nature by increased cortical thickness (Jones *et al.* 1977; Woo *et al.* 1981), bone mineral content (Krolner *et al.* 1983) and bone mass (Wittich *et al.* 1998) following exercise regimes. Variations among exercise protocols and measurement techniques, however, limit the generalizability of many results and conclusions about the precise effects of exercise on bone. Additionally, studying bone adaptation exclusively among professional or elite athletes violates assumptions of random sampling of the general population.Woo *et al.* (1981) studied the effects of long-term exercise on cortical bones. Five immature swine ran approximately 40 km·week^{-1} at 65–80% maximum heart rate for 12 months. After the animals were killed, 4-mm wide strips of cortical bone taken from the anterior, posterior, medial and lateral femoral diaphyses were loaded in four-point bending tests to failure. Biochemical components of cortical samples were also measured. The authors reported exercise-related increases in bone strength resulting from changes in bone geometry, with exercised animals developing a 17% increased cortical thickness and 23% increased cortical cross-sectional area. Analyses of bone composition showed similar biochemical constituents and bone density between exercise and control animals. Woo *et al.* concluded that exercise-induced internal stresses stimulated remodelling changes without altering bone's composition. No attempt was made, however, to differentiate between growth- and exercise-related influences. Matsuda *et al.* (1986) studied exercise effects on growing chicks and found that moderately strenuous exercise increased cortical cross-sectional area but decreased the bone's strength. From the findings of Matsuda *et al.* it is conceivable that the bones may have initially laid down poorly mineralized matrix in response to the early exercise-related stresses. Given the duration of the Woo *et al.* exercise protocol, remodelling may have improved the quality of the immature bone so that after a year the resulting bone would be no different from that of the control bones. A relationship that appeared to exist between remodelling and duration of an exercise protocol may have accounted for the disparity between data from these studies.

Judex and Zernicke (2000a) exercised growing roosters on a treadmill for short bouts (5 min), three times daily for 8 weeks. *In vivo* strains measured during running revealed an 19% increase in the peak strain magnitude, a 136% increase in peak strain rate, and an 18% increase in peak strain gradients. Despite this stimulus, after the 8-week training protocol, mid-diaphyseal areal or mechanical properties and normalized ash weight did not differ between the runners and sedentary controls. The data suggested that the detrimental effects noted by Matsuda *et al.* may have been mitigated by reducing the number of loading cycles. Additionally, the authors suggested that for exercise to induce significant adaptation, the exercise-related mechanical environment must differ markedly from the habitual environment.

Defining exactly how 'exercise or conditioning' affects the skeletal system is a profoundly complex problem. Exercise intensity, skeletal maturity, type of bones (trabecular or cortical) and anatomical location (axial or extremity bones) all can influence the specific response of a bone to exercise. Regular, prolonged exercise can increase the skeletal mass of adults and athletes (Dalen & Olsson 1974; Pirnay *et al.* 1987), but particularly strenuous training, in the immature skeleton, can delay collagen cross-link maturation in joint connective tissues (Pedrini-Mille *et al.* 1988), slow the rate of long bone growth (Kiiskinen & Heikkinen 1973; Kiiskinen 1977; Matsuda *et al.* 1986) or deleteriously affect bone mechanical characteristics (Matsuda *et al.* 1986). Rapidly growing bone appears to be more affected by mechanical loading environment than mature bone (Steinberg & Trueta 1981; Carter 1984), and trabecular bone, with its rapid turnover (Bhasin *et al.* 1988), may even be more sensitive to remodelling stimuli than is cortical bone (Rambaut & Johnson 1979). McDonald *et al.* (1986) reported age-related differences in rat bone mineralization patterns after exercise, with axial bones being less mineralized than weight-bearing bones. In response to a programme of strenuous running, Hou *et al.* (1991) showed the differential effects that strenuous exercise may have on the mechanical properties of immature trabecular bone in the rat femoral neck as opposed to the lumbar vertebrae. In response to 10 weeks of strenuous exercise, the structural and material properties of the weightbearing femoral neck were significantly and adversely affected, but the lumbar vertebrae did not change significantly. It is not clear whether a more moderate training programme would have the same effect on bone and its mechanical properties. Careful and well controlled studies need to be conducted to characterize the dose–response relation of exercise training to bone geometry and mechanical properties. On the plus side, Silbermann *et al.* (1990) examined the effects of long-term, moderate physical exercise on trabecular bone volume and composition. They showed that if the physical activity started at an early age (prior to middle age) and was extended to old age, the exercise positively influenced trabecular bone mass and mineralization. They did not find the same benefits if the training programme was initiated after middle age. Silbermann *et al.* suggested that while young animals (mice) responded favourably to moderate physical exercise, older animals lost some of the ability to adapt.

EXERCISE–GROWTH INTERACTION

Exercise-related changes in growing bones have been examined by Keller and Spengler (1989), Biewener *et al.* (1986), Matsuda *et al.* (1986) and Judex and Zernicke (2000b). Interest in the exercise–growth interaction stems from the lack of quantitative descriptions of whether all growing bones react similarly to exercise and whether such reactions are site specific within the same bone.

Keller and Spengler (1989) implanted *in vivo* strain gauges on femora of six 30-week-old rats. One treatment group walked on a wire mesh wheel for 2 min·day^{-1}, while the other exercised 45 min·day^{-1} at the same rate (0.2 m·s^{-1}) and intensity (25% maximal effort). No statistically significant differences were found for any *in vivo* stress or strain parameters between the activity groups. Compared with sedentary age-matched controls, the exercise animals also showed no significant differences. Keller and Spengler concluded that the loading threshold for positive bone change may have been greater than that elicited by the estimated 25% effort. Biewener *et al.* (1986) performed a similar study with 3-week-old chicks trained to run on a treadmill at 35% maximal speed 15 min·day^{-1}. The exercise regime continued until animals reached 4–17 weeks of age. *In vivo* strain measurements were made on the tibiotarsus of animals 4, 8, 12 and 17 weeks old. Their data closely paralleled those reported by Keller and Spengler, with strain magnitudes, orientations and distributions remaining consistent despite growth- and exercise-related stimuli. Biewener and colleagues postulated a genetically predefined strain environment directing bone remodelling. A conclusion similar to that made by Keller and Spengler relative to exercise intensity, however, must also be considered.

Matsuda *et al.* (1986) addressed the limitations of the previous studies by exercising growing chicks at a moderately strenuous intensity (70–80% of maximum aerobic capacity). Animals ran on a treadmill for 35–45 min·day^{-1}, 5 days a week for 5 or 9 weeks. Muscle fumerase activity of the lateral gastrocnemius demonstrated significantly increased aerobic capacity in the exercised animals. Significant differences were found in the geometry and structural properties of the tarsometatarsus bones between runners and controls. The runners' average flexural rigidity was 40% less than those of controls after 5 weeks of exercise and 52% less than those of controls after 9 weeks of exercise. Runners had greater cortical cross-sectional areas after both 5 and 9 weeks of exercise. The cortical cross-sectional area results supported the hypothesis that exercise stimulates surface bone remodelling in growing animals. Data also suggest, however, that high-intensity exercise produces a decrease in material strength. The authors theorized that

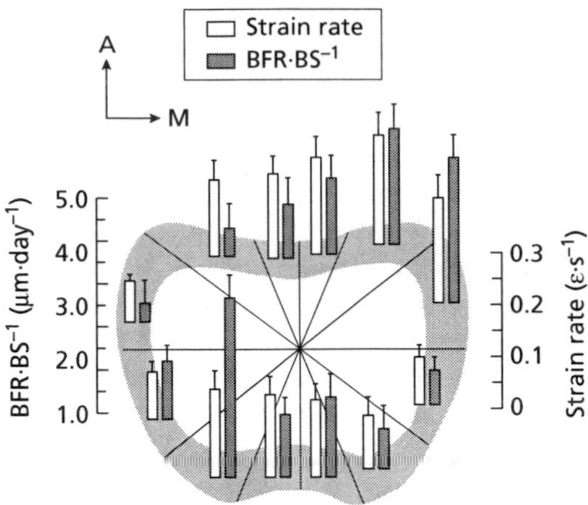

Fig. 6.4 Endocortical distribution of peak strain rates induced by drop jumping and differences in BFR/BS (bone formation rate per bone section) between jumpers and controls superimposed on a mid-diaphyseal tarsometatarsus section (means ± SE). (From Judex & Zernicke 2000b, with permission.)

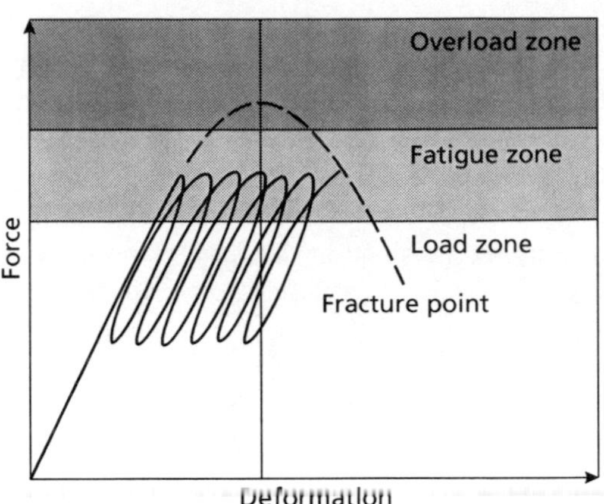

Fig. 6.5 Force–deformation curve illustrating fatigue that may result from repetitive loading (solid line) or fracture from single load application (dashed line). Cyclic forces in the fatigue can lead eventually to fatigue failure. Fracture may result from a single application of load with magnitude within the overload zone. (From Chamay & Tschantz 1972, with permission.)

high-intensity exercise undertaken during rapid growth may have altered calcification of the newly deposited matrix, making the bone less stiff despite an increased cortical area.

Judex and Zernicke (2000b) investigated whether high-impact drop jumps could increase mid-diaphyseal bone formation in the tarsometatarsus of growing roosters. *In vivo* strain measurements revealed a large (+740%) increase in peak strain rate with only a moderate (+30%) increase in strain magnitude and no difference in strain distribution. After an exercise programme of 200 drop jumps a day for 3 weeks, the exercise animals had a significant increase in bone formation rates at the periosteal (+40%) and endocortical (+370%) surfaces. Strain rate correlated significantly with bone formation rate at the endocortical sites (Fig. 6.4) but not at the periosteal surfaces. Their data support a conclusion that growing bone is sensitive to high strain rates.

FATIGUE

'Fatigue in compact bone is the process of gradual mechanical failure caused by repetitive loading at stresses or strains far lower than those required to fracture bone in a single application of force' (Schaffler *et al.* 1989, p. 207) (Fig. 6.5). Multiple loading of a bone may eventually lead to fatigue processes that are intimated in normal and pathological physiology of bone. Fatigue-related microdamage during exercise may stimulate bone remodelling. If the loading is too extensive and the microdamage excessive, however, fatigue fractures may develop (Lafferty & Raju 1979; Carter & Caler 1985). As compact bone fatigues, it progressively loses its stiffness and strength, leading to a fatigue failure (Carter & Caler 1985). The exact characteristics of the multiple loading episodes (e.g. the number, magnitude and strain rate) remain to be quantified. Vigorous exercise undoubtedly generates high strain rates as well as high strain magnitudes. Because bone is viscoelastic (exhibits strain rate dependency) the loading at higher strain rates may increase bone stiffness (Currey 1988; Schaffler & Burr 1988), which may increase the fatigue resistance in compact bone. The fatigue behaviour of compact bone is like that in composite materials that exhibit a progressive loss of stiffness and strength (Hahn & Kim 1980). Nevertheless, the details of how exercise-related strain rates and magnitudes relate to bone fatigue properties remain to be quantified.

Tendons and ligaments

Without tendons and ligaments, normal motion of the human skeleton could not occur. But while important information has already been revealed about the properties of tendons and ligaments (e.g. Booth & Gould 1975; Tipton *et al.* 1975; Butler *et al.* 1978; Akeson *et al.* 1985; Buckwalter *et al.* 1987; Zernicke & Loitz 1990), significant gaps exist in our explanation of the effects of training and conditioning on these important dense fibrous connective tissues. Part of the lack of information about training can be linked to earlier suggestions that tendons and ligaments were virtually inert (Butler *et al.* 1978). In the past two decades, however, it has become clear that these dense fibrous tissues exhibit a viable metabolism and are uniquely adaptable (e.g. Vailas *et al.* 1981).

Structure

The principal fibre in tendons and ligaments is collagen. As described earlier, the tropocollagen molecule (Viidik 1973) provides the fundamental molecular structure in tendons and ligaments. Generally, five parallel tropocollagen molecules are staggered to form a microfibril (Viidik 1973; Kastelic *et al.* 1978). Sequentially, microfibrils are organized into fibrils and into collagen fibres (Viidik 1973) (Fig. 6.6). A primary fibre bundle is a group of fibres enclosed in an endotenon. A group of these primary bundles is called a fascicle (Kastelic *et al.* 1978) and is surrounded by an epitenon sheath. The eventual tendon or ligament is a group of collagen fascicles enclosed within a sheath called a paratenon (Butler *et al.* 1978). The arrangement and organization of the fascicles within a tendon or ligament is thought to relate to the direction of pull in the collagen fibres (Elliott 1965). Tendons are usually thick, white collagenous bands that connect muscle to bone and transmit tensile forces. The collagen content of tendon is roughly 70% of its dry mass (Harkness 1968). The fascicles within a tendon are usually parallel to each other (Viidik 1973), but the insertion of tendon into bone involves a gradual transition from tendon to fibrocartilage, to mineralized fibrocartilage, to lamellar bone (Cooper & Misol 1970). Collagenous Sharpey's fibres connect the tendon to the underlying subchondral bone and blend with the collagenous fibres of the periosteum. At the other end, tendon attaches to the muscle via the myotendinous junction; intracellular myofibrils join to extracellular collagen fibres. Recent studies have revealed the relatively complex multilayered interface that is found at the connection of the actin filament of the terminal sarcomere to the tendon collagen fibres (Trotter *et al.* 1983; Ovalle 1987). The membranous folding in the myotendinous

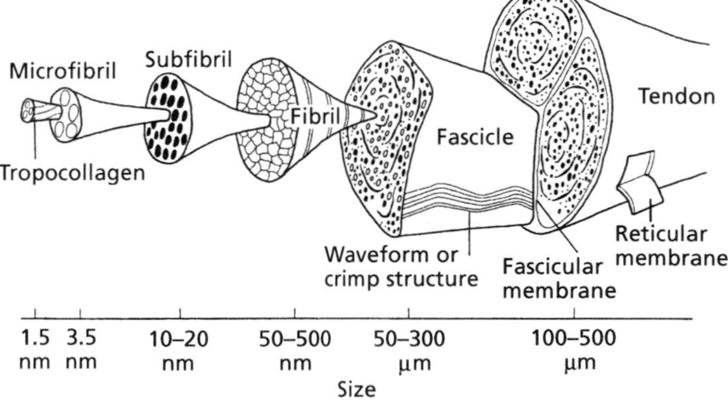

Fig. 6.6 Schematic diagram of tendon structure. Fibrils are bound by endotenons, epitenons bind fibril bundles together to form a fascicle, and these are bundled together by paratenons to form the tendon. (From Kastelic *et al.* 1978, with permission.)

junction enhances the surface area and thus reduces the stress on the junction. Work by Tidball (1983, 1984) revealed that the strength of the adhesive junction between the muscle and the tendon depended both on the properties of the adjoining tissues and on the orientation of the forces that cross the junction. Junctions loaded in shear are stronger than junctions that have a large tensile component which is perpendicular to the membrane.

Under a light microscope, tendon appears crimped and wave-like because of the buckling phenomena created by the intercellular matrix impinging on collagen fibres (Butler *et al.* 1978). In the intercellular matrix, besides collagen, tendon contains small amounts of mucopolysaccharides and elastin (Hooley *et al.* 1980).

Ligaments join together adjacent bones at their ends and may support organs (Butler *et al.* 1978). Ligaments can be internal or external to the joint capsule or they may blend with the capsule. The colour of collagenous ligaments is a dull white due to the greater percentage of elastic and reticular fibres between the collagen fibre bundles.

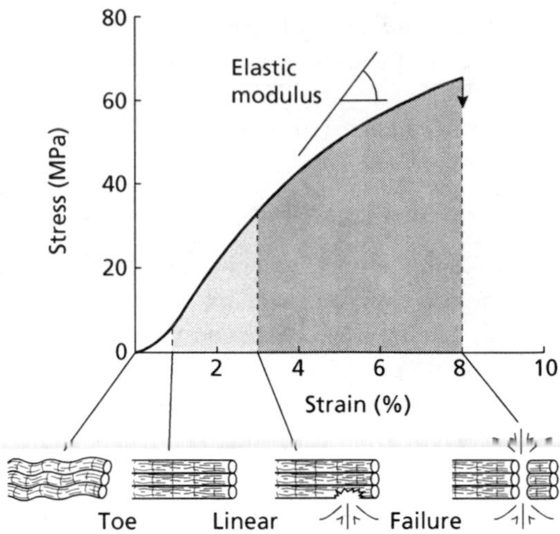

Fig. 6.7 Exemplar stress–strain curve for collagen. Each area of the curve reflects collagen's behaviour during tensile loading. (From Butler *et al.* 1978.)

Mechanical properties

Collagenous tissues, such as tendons and ligaments, provide resistance to tensile loads. During a typical force elongation test, the initial load applied to the tissue results in a concave portion of the curve, termed the 'toe' region (Elliott 1965; Viidik 1973) (Fig. 6.7). The relative elongation of the tissue at the end of this region has been reported to be between 1.5 and 4% (Viidik 1973; Butler *et al.* 1978). Following the toe region is a relatively linear response. The fibres in the tissue become more parallel and lose their wavy appearance (Viidik 1973; Butler *et al.* 1978). If collagen fibres are tested alone, the strain limit of the linear region may be from 2 to 5% (Elliott 1965). Microfailure occurs at the end of the linear loading region; once maximum load is attained, complete failure occurs rapidly, and the load-supporting ability of the ligament is lost (Butler *et al.* 1978). As with bone, fibrous connective tissues are viscoelastic and display a sensitivity to different strain rates (Fung 1967, 1972; Butler *et al.* 1978). Noyes *et al.* (1974a) demonstrated that strain rate has a significant effect on the maximal loads that a ligament can withstand.

The myotendinous junction is also viscoelastic, and its mechanical behaviour depends on the duration, frequency and magnitude of the applied loads (Tidball & Daniel 1986). Tidball and Daniel (1986) suggested that the duration of loading helps establish the degree of myotendinous folding that occurs at the junction. They reported that slow-twitch muscle cells have a greater junctional surface area than fast-twitch muscle cells. Presumably, the greater surface area prevents muscle cell lysis under conditions of prolonged loading because of the reduction in stress at the membrane.

Exercise effects

Dense fibrous tissues are sensitive to both disuse and training (Booth & Gould 1975; Buckwalter *et al.* 1987). The underlying mechanisms responsible for these adaptive changes, however, are not clearly understood. Most of the information about the response of dense fibrous tissues to exercise is related to ligaments. Little quantita-

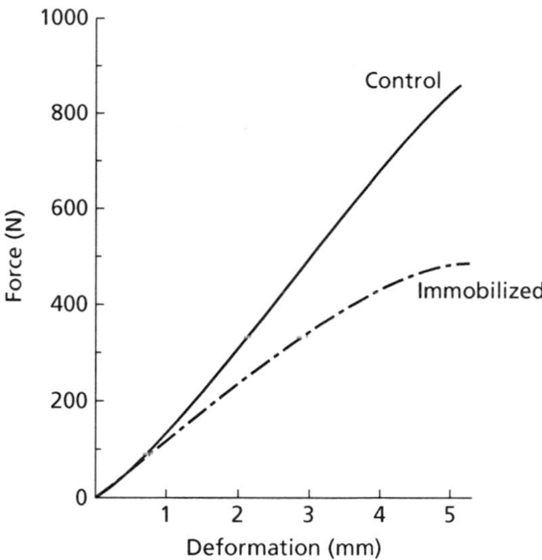

Fig. 6.8 Joint immobilization detrimentally affects the structural properties of the femur–anterior cruciate ligament–tibia unit. Immobilized tissues are less stiff and withstand less load at maximum and failure points. (From Butler *et al.* 1978.)

tive information exists about exercise-related adaptations of tendon (Woo *et al.* 1982; Michna 1984). Tipton *et al.* and Viidik *et al.* provided some of the most systematic and extensive investigations of the influences of training and physical activity on ligaments (Viidik 1973; Tipton *et al.* 1975). Generally, it was shown that with immobilization or significant disuse, noteworthy changes occurred in the substance of ligaments (Akeson *et al.* 1967; Woo *et al.* 1975) (Fig. 6.8). Immobilization decreases the glycosaminoglycan and water content of ligamentous and tendinous tissues, increases the non-uniform orientation of the collagen fibrils, and increases collagen cross-linking. The collagen synthesis and degradation rates increase with immobilization so that the proportion of new to old collagen increases in unloaded ligaments (Amiel *et al.* 1982). Total collagen mass (Amiel *et al.* 1982) and the stiffness of the ligament may also decrease (Noyes *et al.* 1974b; Tipton *et al.* 1974). Tipton *et al.* (1975) concluded that the strength of the junction between the bone and ligament was closely related to the type of exercise regimen and not only to the duration of the exercise. Most researchers investigating exercise effects on ligaments report an increase in the ultimate strength of the maximum load at separation–junction strength (e.g. Adams 1966; Tipton *et al.* 1967, 1970, 1974, 1975; Zuckerman & Stull 1969, 1973; Laros *et al.* 1971). Normal everyday activity (without training) appears to be sufficient to maintain 80–90% of ligament's mechanical potential (Frank 1996). Exercise may increase ligament strength and stiffness by up to an additional 10–20%. Single exercise bouts or sprint training, however, does not appear to result in significant increases in junction strength although the sprint training produced marked increases in ligament mass (Tipton *et al.* 1967, 1974). Tipton and coworkers showed that although tendons and ligaments can be influenced by hormones (Dougherty & Berliner 1968), chronic endurance training can increase the knee ligament junction strengths of thyroidectomized and hypophysectomized rats (Tipton *et al.* 1971; Vailas *et al.* 1978).

Of the studies available that specifically quantify tendon's response to changes in load environment, Michna (1984), Woo *et al.* (1980) and Curwin *et al.* (1988) have provided details of the changes that occur with exercise. Mice that were exercised 1 week on a treadmill showed increased numbers and size of the collagen fibrils and larger cross-sectional areas in digital flexor tendons than did sedentary controls (Michna 1984). After 7 weeks of continued training, the average fibril diameter was less than the control group, and it appeared that fibrils were splitting. By the end of 10 weeks, the flexor tendon cross-sectional areas were comparable for both groups. Woo *et al.* (1980) exercised immature swine for 1 year and examined the adaptations in the extensor tendons. After this period of moderate exercise, there were no differences in the mechanical properties or cross-sectional area between the control and exercised swine. Currently, there is no quantitative information about how weightbearing, mature extensor tendons adapt to exercise, but Curwin *et al.* (1988) have shown marked biochemical changes in immature tendon after a regiment of strenuous exercise. Collagen synthesis increased dramatically, but the Achilles tendon dry weight and collagen concentration did not change, suggesting that synthesis matched degradation.

Using a compensatory overload model, Zamora and Marini (1988) reported marked changes in plantaris tendon morphology. They reported a substantial increase in a number of active fibroblasts in the tendon. The fibroblast cytoplasm contained many vacuoles, indicating active protein synthesis. Zamora and Marini further described the changes in the myotendinous junction after an overload regimen. The adaptive changes to the overloading consisted of enhanced collagen synthesis, with intensive membrane renewal and recycling. Barfred (1973) summarized an extensive set of literature related to human tendons, indicating that physical activity and training apparently maintain tendon strength and integrity and reduce the probability of tendon rupture with age.

Meniscus

Menisci are fibrocartilage structures that bear loads and enhance rotation in synovial joints (Slocum & Larson 1968; Shrive 1974; Krause *et al.* 1976), and the absence of knee menisci can increase joint laxity and propensity for articular cartilage degeneration (Slocum & Larson 1968; Lufti & Sudan 1975). After meniscectomy, articular cartilage has been shown to degenerate morphologically and biochemically (Cox *et al.* 1975; Krause *et al.* 1976).

While menisci must transmit a variety of mechanical loads (Shrive 1974; Walker & Erkman 1975; Krause *et al.* 1976; Uezaki *et al.* 1979; Jaspers *et al.* 1980), little information is available about the adaptability of the important meniscal fibrocartilage in response to exercise. Some *in vitro* experiments involving chondrocytes obtained from fibrocartilage indicate that cyclic compression enhances the synthesis of collagen, proteoglycans and deoxyribonucleic acid (Veldhuijzen *et al.* 1979; De Witt *et al.* 1984). In addition, a study by Vailas *et al.* (1986) suggested the meniscal fibrocartilage also is sensitive to exercise-related loading. After detailing the distinct regional characteristics of the rat knee meniscus composition, morphology and biomechanical properties (Vailas *et al.* 1985; Zernicke *et al.* 1986), Vailas and coworkers trained rats to run on a motor-driven treadmill, 5 days a week for 12 weeks. There was a significant training effect that occurred, as evidenced by the 65% increase in gastrocnemius succinate dehydrogenase. In addition, in the region of the meniscus (posterior lateral horn) that probably received the principal compressive cyclic loading, there was a significant increase in collagen, proteoglycan and calcium concentrations.

Egner (1982) indicated that the longitudinal fibres of collagen ensure tension resistance in the meniscus while the transverse fibre bundles bind the longitudinal fibres to retain the shape of the meniscus. The increase in collagen and proteoglycan concentration in the meniscus as a result of exercise-induced loading should enhance the tissue's ability to accommodate mechanical loading (Mow *et al.* 1984). Although researchers have doubted the capacity of meniscal fibrocartilage for adaptation—because of its low metabolic activity and poor blood supply (Videman *et al.* 1979; Danzig *et al.* 1983; Amiel *et al.* 1985)—data suggested that the amount of nutrient delivery to the tissue is strongly related to the degree of tissue surface exposure to synovial fluid (Amiel *et al.* 1985). During exercise, cyclic loading and unloading may improve delivery to the matrix.

Concluding comments

In the past several decades, significant research has emerged about the responses of connective tissues to exercise and training. It is readily apparent from available data that fibrous and bony connective tissues are adaptive and very sensitive to the type of mechanical loads that are transmitted. Nevertheless, many of the relations among the biochemical, morphological and biomechanical properties of bony and fibrous connective tissues and the quantity and quality of physical activity remain to be established. The search for the underlying mechanisms of remodelling and adaptation in these tissues persists as a prime challenge for continuing research.

References

Adams, A. (1966) Effect of exercise upon ligament strength. *Research Quarterly for Exercise and Sport* **37**, 163–167.

Akeson, W.H., Amiel, D. & LaViolette, D. (1967) The connective-tissue response to immobility. *Clinical Orthopaedics and Related Research* **51**, 183–197.

Akeson, W.H., Frank, C.B., Amiel, D. & Woo, S.L.-Y. (1985) Ligament biology and biomechanics. In: *Symposium on Sports Medicine: The Knee* (ed. G.A.M. Finerman), pp. 111–151. C.V. Mosby, St. Louis.

Albright, J.A. & Skinner, H.C. (1987) Bone. Structural organization and remodeling dynamics. In: *The Scientific Basis of Orthopaedics* (eds J.A. Albright & R.A. Brand), 2nd edn, pp. 161–198. Appleton-Lange, Connecticut.

Amiel, D., Woo, S.L., Harwood, F.L. & Akeson, W.H. (1982) The effect of immobilization on collagen turnover in connective tissue. *Acta Orthopaedica Scandinavica* **53**, 325–332.

Amiel, D., Abel, M.F. & Akeson, W.H. (1985) Nutrient delivery in the diarthrial joint: An analysis of synovial fluid transport in the rabbit knee. *Transactions of the Orthopaedic Research Society* **10**, 196 (Abstract).

Barfred, T. (1973) Achilles tendon rupture: aetiology and pathogenesis of subcutaneous rupture assessed on the basis of the literature and rupture experiments on rats. *Acta Orthopaedica Scandinavica Supplement* **152**.

Bhasin, S., Sortoris, D.J., Felllingham, L., Zlatkin, M.B., Andre, M. & Resnick, D. (1988) Three dimensional quantitative CT of the proximal femur: Relationship to vertebral trabecular bone density in postmenopausal women. *Radiology* **167**, 145–149.

Biewener, A.A., Swartz, S.M. & Bertram, J.E. (1986) Bone modelling during growth: Dynamic strain equilibrium in the chick tibiotarsus. *Calcified Tissue International* **39**, 390–395.

Binderman, I., Shimshone, Z. & Somjen, D. (1984) Biochemical pathways involved in the translation of physical stimulus into biological message. *Calcified Tissue International* **36**, S82–S85.

Booth, F.W. & Gould, E.W. (1975) Effects of training and disuse on connective tissue. *Exercise and Sport Sciences Reviews* **3**, 83–112.

Buckwalter, J.A. & Cooper, R.R. (1987) *The Cells and Matrices of Skeletal Connective Tissue*. In: *The Scientific Basis of Orthopaedics* (eds J.A. Albright & R.A. Brand), 2nd edn, pp. 1–30. Appleton-Lange, Connecticut.

Buckwalter, J.A., Maynard, J.A. & Vailas, A.C. (1987) Skeletal fibrous tissues. Tendon, joint capsule, and ligament. In: *The Scientific Basis of Orthopaedics* (eds J.A. Albright & R.A. Brand), 2nd edn, pp. 387–405. Appleton-Lange, Connecticut.

Butler, D.L., Grood, E.S., Noyes, F.R. & Zernicke, R.F. (1978) Biomechanics of ligaments and tendons. *Exercise and Sport Sciences Reviews* **6**, 125–181.

Carter, D.R. (1984) Mechanical loading histories and cortical bone remodelling. *Calcified Tissue International* **36**, S19–S24.

Carter, D.R. & Caler, W.E. (1985) A cumulative damage model for bone fracture. *Journal of Orthopaedic Research* **3**, 84–90.

Carter, D.R., Smith, D.J., Spengler, D.M., Daly, C.H. & Frankel, V.H. (1980) Measurement and analysis of in vivo bone strains on the canine radius and ulna. *Journal of Biomechanics* **13**, 27–38.

Carter, D.R., Caler, W.E., Spengler, D.M. & Frankel, V.H. (1981) Fatigue behavior of adult cortical bone: The influence of mean strain and strain range. *Acta Orthopaedica Scandinavica* **52**, 481–490.

Chamay, A. & Tschantz, P. (1972) Mechanical influences in bone remodelling. Experimental research on Wolff's law. *Journal of Biomechanics* **5**, 173–180.

Churches, A.E. & Howlett, C.R. (1981) The response of mature cortical bone to controlled time-varying loading. In: *Mechanical Properties of Bone*, Vol. 45 (ed. S.C. Cowin), pp. 69–80. American Society of Mechanical Engineers, New York.

Clark, E.A., Goodship, A.E. & Lanyon, L.E. (1975) Locomotor bone strain as the stimulus for bone's mechanical adaptability. *Journal of Physiology* **245**, 57P.

Cochran, G.V., Pawluk, R.J. & Bassett, C.A. (1968) Electromechanical characteristics of bone under physiologic moisture conditions. *Clinical Orthopaedics and Related Research* **58**, 249–270.

Cooper, R.R. & Misol, S. (1970) Tendon and ligament insertion. *Journal of Bone and Joint Surgery* **52A**, 1–21.

Cowin, S.C., Lanyon, L.E. & Rodan, G. (1984) The Kroc Foundation conference on functional adaptation in bone tissue. *Calcified Tissue International* **36**, S1–S6.

Cox, J.S., Nye, C.E., Schaefer, W.W. & Woodstein, I.J. (1975) The degenerative effects of partial and total resection of the medial meniscus in dogs' knees. *Clinical Orthopaedics and Related Research* **109**, 178–183.

Currey, J.D. (1984) *The Mechanical Adaptations of Bones*. Princeton University Press, New Jersey.

Currey, J.D. (1988) Strain rate and mineral content in fracture models of bone. *Journal of Orthopaedic Research* **6**, 32–38.

Curwin, S.L., Vailas, A.C. & Wood, J. (1988) Immature tendon adaptation to strenuous exercise. *Journal of Applied Physiology* **65**, 2297–2301.

Dalen, N. & Olsson, K.E. (1974) Bone mineral content and physical activity. *Acta Orthopaedica Scandinavica* **45**, 170–174.

Danzig, L., Resnick, D., Gonsalves, M. & Akeson, W.H. (1983) Blood supply to the normal and abnormal menisci of the human knee. *Clinical Orthopaedics and Related Research* **172**, 271–276.

De Witt, M.T., Handley, C.J., Oakes, B.W. & Lowther, D.A. (1984) In vitro response of chondrocytes to mechanical loading. The effect of short-term mechanical tension. *Connective Tissue Research* **12**, 97–109.

Dougherty, T.F. & Berliner, D.L. (1968) The effects of hormones on connective tissue cells. In: *Treatise on Collagen*, Vol. 2. *Biology of Collagen* (ed. B.S. Gould), Part A, pp. 361–394. Academic Press, London.

Egner, E. (1982) Knee joint meniscal degeneration as it relates to tissue fibre structure and mechanical resistance. *Pathology, Research and Practice* **173**, 310–324.

Elliott, D.H. (1965) Structure and function of mammalian tendon. *Biological Reviews* **40**, 392–421.

Eriksson, C. (1976) Electrical properties of bone. In: *The Biochemistry and Physiology of Bone*, Vol. IV. *Calcification and Physiology* (ed. G.H. Bourne), 2nd edn, pp. 329–384. Academic Press, New York.

Evans, F.G. (1953) Methods of studying the biomechanical significance of bone form. *American Journal of Physical Anthropology* **11**, 413–436.

Frank, C.B. (1996) Ligament injuries. Pathophysiology and healing. In: *Athletic Injuries and Rehabilitation* (eds J.E. Zachazewski, D.J. Magee & W.S. Quillen), pp. 9–26. Saunders, Philadelphia.

Frost, H.M. (1987) Mechanical determinants of skeletal architecture. In: *The Scientific Basis of Orthopaedics* (eds J.A. Albright & R.A. Brand), 2nd edn, pp. 241–265. Appleton-Lange, Connecticut.

Fung, Y.C.B. (1967) Elasticity of soft tissues in simple elongation. *American Journal of Physiology* **213**, 1532–1544.

Fung, Y.C.B. (1972) Stress-strain relations of soft tissue in simple elongation. In: *Biomechanics: its Foundations and Objectives* (eds Y.C.B. Fung, N. Perrone & M. Anliker), pp. 181–209. Prentice Hall, Englewood Cliffs.

Goodship, A.E., Lanyon, L.E. & MacFie, H. (1979) Functional adaptation of bone to increased stress. *Journal of Bone and Joint Surgery* **61A**, 539–546.

Gordon, K.R., Perl, M. & Levy, C. (1989) Structural alterations and breaking strength of mouse femora exposed to three activity regimens. *Bone* **10**, 303–312.

Gross, T.S., Edwards, J.L., McLeod, K.J. & Rubin, C.T. (1997) Strain gradients correlate with sites of periosteal bone formation. *Journal of Bone and Mineral Research* **12**, 982–988.

Hahn, H.T. & Kim, R.V. (1980) Fatigue behavior of composite laminates. *Journal of Composite Materials* **10**, 156–180.

Ham, A.W. (1974) *Histology*. J.B. Lippincott, Philadelphia.

Harkness, R.D. (1968) Mechanical properties of collagenous tissues. In: *Treatise on Collagen*, Vol. 2. *Biology of Collagen* (ed. B.S. Gould), Part A, pp. 241–310. Academic Press, London.

Hert, J., Liskova, M. & Landa, J. (1971) Reaction of bone to mechanical stimuli. Part 1. Continuous and intermittent loading of tibia in rabbit. *Folia Morphologica* **19**, 290–300.

Hooley, C.J., McCrum, N. & Cohen, R.E. (1980) The viscoelastic deformation of tendon. *Journal of Biomechanics* **13**, 521–528.

Hou, J.C.-H., Salem, G.J., Zernicke, R.F. & Barnard, R.J. (1991) Structural and mechanical adaptations of immature trabecular bone to strenuous exercise. *Journal of Applied Physiology* **69**, 1309–1314.

Jaspers, P., Lange, A., Huiskes, R. & Van Reus, T.G. (1980) The mechanical function of the meniscus, experiments on cadaveric pig knee joints. *Acta Orthopaedica Belgica* **46**, 663–668.

Jaworski, Z.F.G. (1984) Lamellar bone turnover system and its effector organs. *Calcified Tissue International* **36**, S46–S55.

Jee, W.S., Wronski, E.R., Morey, E.R. & Kimmel, D.B. (1983) Effects of spaceflight on trabecular bone in rats. *American Journal of Physiology* **244**, R310–R314.

Jones, H.H., Prienst, J.B., Hayes, W.C., Tichenor, C.C. & Nagel, A. (1977) Humeral hypertrophy in response to exercise. *Journal of Bone and Joint Surgery* **59A**, 204–208.

Judex, S. & Zernicke, R.F. (2000a) Does the mechanical milieu associated with high-speed running lead to adaptive changes in diaphyseal growing bone? *Bone* **26**, 153–159.

Judex, S. & Zernicke, R.F. (2000b) High-impact exercise and growing bone: Relation between high strain rates and enhanced bone formation. *Journal of Applied Physiology* **88**, 2183–2191.

Judex, S., Whiting, W.C. & Zernicke, R.F. (1999) Exercise-induced bone adaptation: Considerations for designing an osteogenically effective exercise program. *International Journal of Industrial Ergonomics* **24**, 235–238.

Kastelic, J., Galeski, A. & Baer, E. (1978) The multicomposite structure of tendon. *Connective Tissue Research* **6**, 11–23.

Keller, T.S. & Spengler, D.M. (1989) Regulation of bone stress and strain in the immature and mature rat femur. *Journal of Biomechanics* **22**, 1115–1128.

Kiiskinen, A. (1977) Physical training and connective tissue in young mice—physical properties of Achilles tendon and long bone growth. *Growth* **41**, 123–127.

Kiiskinen, A. & Heikkinen, E. (1973) Effects of physical training on development and strength of tendons and bone in growing mice. *Scandinavian Journal of Clinical and Laboratory Investigation* **29** (Suppl. 123), 60.

Krause, W.R., Pope, M.H., Johnson, R.J. & Wilder, D.G. (1976) Mechanical changes in the knee after meniscectomy. *Journal of Bone and Joint Surgery* **58A**, 599–604.

Krolner, B., Toft, B., Nielson, S.P. & Tondevold, E. (1983) Physical exercise as prophylaxis against involutional vertebral bone loss: a controlled trial. *Clinical Science* **64**, 541–546.

Lafferty, J.F. & Raju, P.V.V. (1979) The influence of stress frequency on the fatigue strength of cortical bone. *Journal of Biomechanical Engineering* **101**, 112–113.

Lanyon, L.E. (1973) Analysis of surface bone strain in the calcaneus of sheep during normal locomotion. *Journal of Biomechanics* **6**, 41–49.

Lanyon, L.E. (1987) Functional strain in bone tissue as an objective and controlling stimulus for adaptive bone remodelling. *Journal of Biomechanics* **20**, 1083–1093.

Lanyon, L.E. (1996) Using functional loading to influence bone mass and architecture: objectives, mechanisms, and relationship with estrogen of the mechanically adaptive process in bone. *Bone* **18**, 37S–43S.

Lanyon, L.E. & Hartman, W. (1977) Strain related electrical potentials recorded in vitro and in vivo. *Calcified Tissue Research* **22**, 315–327.

Lanyon, L.E. & Rubin, C.T. (1984) Static vs. dynamic loads as an influence on bone remodelling. *Journal of Biomechanics* **16**, 897–905.

Laros, G.S., Tipton, C.M. & Cooper, R.R. (1971) Influence of physical activity on ligament insertions in the knees of dogs. *Journal of Bone and Joint Surgery* **53A**, 275–286.

Liskova, M. & Hert, J. (1971) Reaction of bone to mechanical stimuli. Part 2: Periosteal and endosteal reaction of tibial diaphyses in rabbit to intermittent loading. *Folia Morphologica* **19**, 301.

Lufti, A.M. & Sudan, K. (1975) Morphological changes in the articular cartilage after meniscectomy: An experimental study in the monkey. *Journal of Bone and Joint Surgery* **57B**, 525–527.

McDonald, R., Hegenauer, J. & Saltman, P. (1986) Age-related differences in the bone mineralization pattern of rats following exercise. *Journal of Gerontology* **41**, 445–452.

Martin, R.B. & Burr, D.B. (1989) *Structure, Function, and Adaptation of Compact Bone*. Raven Press, New York.

Matsuda, J.J., Zernicke, R.F., Vailas, A.C., Pedrini, V.A., Pedrini-Mille, A. & Maynard, J.A. (1986) Structural and mechanical adaptation of immature bone to strenuous exercise. *Journal of Applied Physiology* **60**, 2028–2034.

Meade, J.B., Cowin, S.C., Klatwitter, J.J., Van Buskirk, W.C. & Skinner, H.B. (1984) Bone remodeling to continuously applied loads. *Calcified Tissue International* **36**, S25–S30.

Michna, H. (1984) Morphometric analysis of loading-induced changes in collagen-fibril populations in young tendons. *Cell and Tissue Research* **236**, 465–470.

Morey, E.R. & Baylink, D.J. (1978) Inhibition of bone formation during space flight. *Science* **201**, 1138–1141.

Mow, V.C., Holmes, M.H. & Lai, W.M. (1984) Fluid transport and mechanical properties of articular cartilage: a review. *Journal of Biomechanics* **17**, 377–394.

Nordin, M. & Frankel, V.H. (1989) *Basic Biomechanics of the Musculoskeletal System*, 2nd edn. Lea & Febiger, Philadelphia.

Noyes, F.R., De Lucas, J.L. & Torvik, P.J. (1974a) Biomechanics of anterior cruciate ligament failure: An analysis of strain-rate sensitivity and mechanisms of failure in primates. *Journal of Bone and Joint Surgery* **56A**, 236–253.

Noyes, F.R., Torvik, P.J., Hyde, W.B. & De Lucas, J.L. (1974b) Biomechanics of ligament failure. *Journal of Bone and Joint Surgery* **56A**, 1406–1418.

O'Connor, J.A., Lanyon, L.E. & McFie, H. (1982) The influence of strain rate on adaptive bone remodeling. *Journal of Biomechanics* **15**, 767–781.

Ovalle, W.K. (1987) The human muscle–tendon junction: a morphological study during normal growth and at maturity. *Anatomy and Embryology* **176**, 281–294.

Pedrini-Mille, A., Pedrini, V.A., Maynard, J.A. & Vailas, A.C. (1988) Response of immature chicken meniscus to strenuous exercise: Biochemical studies of proteoglycan and collagen. *Journal of Orthopaedic Research* **6**, 196–204.

Pirnay, F., Bodeux, M., Crielaard, J.M. & Franchimont, P. (1987) Bone mineral content and physical activity. *International Journal of Sports Medicine* **8**, 331–335.

Prockop, D.J. & Guzman, N.A. (1977) Collagen diseases and the biosynthesis of collagen. *Hospital Practice* December, 61–68.

Radin, E.L., Orr, R.B., Kelman, J.L., Paul, I.L. & Rose, M.R. (1982) Effect of prolonged walking on concrete on the knees of sheep. *Journal of Biomechanics* **15**, 487–492.

Rambaut, P.C. & Johnson, R.S. (1979) Prolonged weightlessness and calcium loss in man. *Acta Astronautica* **6**, 1113–1122.

Rubin, C.T. (1984) Skeletal strain and the functional significance of bone architecture. *Calcified Tissue International* **36**, S11–S18.

Rubin, C.T. & Lanyon, L.E. (1985) Regulation of bone mass by mechanical strain magnitude. *Calcified Tissue International* **37**, 411–417.

Rubin, C.T. & Lanyon, L.E. (1987) Osteoregulatory nature of mechanical stimuli: Function as a determinant for adaptive remodeling in bone. *Journal of Orthopaedic Research* **5**, 300–310.

Saville, P.D. & Whyte, M.P. (1969) Muscle and bone hypertrophy: Positive effect of running exercise in the rat. *Clinical Orthopaedics and Related Research* **65**, 81–88.

Schaffler, M.B. & Burr, D.B. (1988) Stiffness of compact bone: The effect of porosity and density. *Journal of Biomechanics* **21**, 13–16.

Schaffler, M.B., Radin, E.L. & Burr, D.B. (1989) Mechanical and morphological effects of strain rate on fatigue on compact bone. *Bone* **10**, 207–214.

Shaw, S.R., Zernicke, R.F., Vailas, A.C., DeLuna, D., Thomason, D.B. & Baldwin, K.B. (1987) Mechanical, morphological and biochemical adaptations of bone and muscle to hindlimb suspension and exercise. *Journal of Biomechanics* **20**, 225–234.

Shaw, S.R., Vailas, A.C., Grindeland, R.E. & Zernicke, R.F. (1988) Effects of one-week space-flight on the morphological and mechanical properties of growing bone. *American Journal of Physiology* **254**, R78–R83.

Shrive, N. (1974) The weight-bearing role of the meniscus of the knee. *Journal of Bone and Joint Surgery* **56B**, 381–387.

Silbermann, M., Bar-Shira-Maymon, B., Coleman, R. *et al.* (1990) Long-term physical exercise retards trabecular bone loss in lumbar vertebrae of aging female mice. *Calcified Tissue International* **46**, 80–93.

Simkin, A., Ayalon, J. & Leichter, I. (1987) Increased trabecular bone density due to bone-loading exercises in postmenopausal women. *Calcified Tissue International* **40**, 59–63.

Skerry, T.M., Bitensky, L., Chayen, J. & Lanyon, L.E. (1988) Loading-related reorientation of bone proteoglycan in vivo. Strain memory in bone tissue? *Journal of Orthopaedic Research* **6**, 547–551.

Skerry, T.M., Suswillo, R., El Haj, A.J., Ali, N.N., Dodds, R.A. & Lanyon, L.E. (1990) Load-induced proteoglycan orientation in bone tissue in vivo and in vitro. *Calcified Tissue International* **46**, 318–326.

Skinner, H.C. (1987) *Bone Mineralization*. In: *The Scientific Basis of Orthopaedics* (eds J.A. Albright & R.A. Brand), 2nd edn, pp. 199–212. Appleton-Lange, Connecticut.

Slocum, D.B. & Larson, R.L. (1968) Rotatory instability of the knee. *Journal of Bone and Joint Surgery* **50A**, 211–225.

Smith, S.D. (1977) Femoral development in chronically centrifuged rats. *Aviation Space and Environmental Medicine* **48**, 828–835.

Smith, E.L., Smith, P.E., Ensign, C.J. & Shea, M.M. (1984) Bone involution decrease in exercising middle-aged women. *Calcified Tissue International* **36**, 5129–5138.

Steinberg, M.E. & Trueta, J. (1981) Effects of activity on bone growth and development in the rat. *Clinical Orthopaedics and Related Research* **156**, 52–60.

Tidball, J.G. (1983) The geometry of actin filament–membrane associations can modify adhesive strength of the myotendinous junction. *Cell Motility* **3**, 439–447.

Tidball, J.G. (1984) Myotendinous junction: Morphological changes and mechanical failure associated with muscle cell atrophy. *Experimental and Molecular Pathology* **40**, 1–12.

Tidball, J.G. & Daniel, T.L. (1986) Myotendinous junctions of tonic muscle cells. Structure and loading. *Cell and Tissue Research* **245**, 315–322.

Tipton, C.M., Schild, R.J. & Tomanek, R.J. (1967) Influence of physical activity on the strength of knee ligaments in rats. *American Journal of Physiology* **212**, 783–787.

Tipton, C.M., James, S.L., Mergner, W. & Tcheng, T.K. (1970) Influence of exercise on strength of medial collateral knee ligaments of dogs. *American Journal of Physiology* **218**, 894–902.

Tipton, C.M., Tcheng, T.K. & Mergner, W. (1971) Influence of immobilization, training, exogenous hormones, and surgical repair on knee ligaments from hypophysectomized rats. *American Journal of Physiology* **221**, 1144–1150.

Tipton, C.M., Matthes, R.D. & Sandage, D.S. (1974) In situ measurements of junction strength and ligament elongation in rats. *Journal of Applied Physiology* **37**, 758–761.

Tipton, C.M., Matthes, R.D., Maynard, J.A. & Carey, R.A. (1975) The influence of physical activity on tendons and ligaments. *Medicine and Science in Sports* **7**, 165–175.

Trotter, J.A., Eberhard, S. & Samora, A. (1983) Structural connections of the muscle–tendon junction. *Cell Motility* **3**, 431–438.

Uezaki, N., Kobayashi, A. & Matushige, K. (1979) The viscoelastic properties of the human semilunar cartilage. *Journal of Biomechanics* **12**, 65–73.

Uhthoff, H.K. & Jaworski, Z.F. (1978) Bone loss in response to long-term immobilization. *Journal of Bone and Joint Surgery* **60B**, 420–429.

Vailas, A.C., Tipton, C.M., Laughlin, H.L., Tcheng, T.K. & Matthes, R.D. (1978) Physical activity and hypophysectomy on the aerobic capacity of ligaments and tendons. *American Journal of Physiology* **44**, 542–546.

Vailas, A.C., Tipton, C.M., Matthes, R.D. & Gart, M. (1981) Physical activity and its influence on the repair process of medial collateral ligaments. *Connective Tissue Research* **9**, 25–31.

Vailas, A.C., Zernicke, R.F., Matsuda, J. & Peller, D. (1985) Regional biochemical and morphological characteristics of rat knee meniscus. *Comparative Biochemistry and Physiology* **82B**, 283–285.

Vailas, A.C., Zernicke, R.F., Matsuda, J., Curwin, S. & Durivage, J. (1986) Adaptation of rat knee meniscus to prolonged exercise. *Journal of Applied Physiology* **60**, 1031–1034.

Veldhuijzen, J.P., Bourret, L.A. & Rodan, G.A. (1979) In vitro studies of the effect of intermittent compressive forces on cartilage cell proliferation. *Journal of Cellular Physiology* **98**, 299–306.

Videman, T., Eronen, I., Friman, C. & Langenskiold, A. (1979) Glycosaminoglycan metabolisms of the medial meniscus, the medial collateral ligaments and the hip joint capsule in experimental osteoarthritis caused by immobilization of the rabbit knee. *Acta Orthopaedica Scandinavica* **50**, 465–470.

Viidik, A. (1973) Functional properties of collagenous tissues. *International Review of Connective Tissue Research* **6**, 127–215.

Walker, P.S. & Erkman, M.J. (1975) The role of menisci in force transmission across the knee. *Clinical Orthopaedics and Related Research* **109**, 184–191.

White, A., Handler, P. & Smith, E.L. (1964) *Principles of Biochemistry*. McGraw-Hill, New York.

Wittich, A., Mautalen, C.A., Oliveri, M.B., Bagur, A., Somoza, F. & Rotemberg, E. (1998) Professional football (soccer) players have a markedly greater skeletal mineral content, density and size than age- and BMI-matched controls. *Calcified Tissue International* **63**, 112–117.

Woo, S.L.-Y., Matthews, J.V., Akeson, W.H., Amiel, D. & Convery, F.R. (1975) Connective tissue response to immobility. Correlative study of biochemical measurements of normal and immobilized rabbit knees. *Arthritis and Rheumatism* **18**, 257–264.

Woo, S.L.-Y., Ritter, M.A., Amiel, D. *et al.* (1980) The biomechanical and biochemical properties of swine tendons—long-term effects of exercise on the digital extensors. *Connective Tissue Research* **7**, 177–183.

Woo, S.L.-Y., Kuei, S.C., Amiel, D. *et al.* (1981) The effect of physical training on the properties of long bone: a study of Wolff's law. *Journal of Bone and Joint Surgery* **63A**, 780–787.

Woo, S.L.-Y., Gomez, M.A., Woo, Y.K. & Akeson, W.H. (1982) Mechanical properties of tendons and ligaments. II. The relationships of immobilization and exercise on tissue remodeling. *Biorheology* **19**, 397–408.

Yeh, C.K. & Rodan, G.A. (1984) Tensile forces enhance prostaglandin E synthesis in osteoblastic cells grown on collagen ribbons. *Calcified Tissue International* **36**, S67–S71.

Zamora, A.J. & Marini, J.F. (1988) Tendon and myotendinous junction in an overloaded skeletal muscle in the rat. *Anatomy and Embryology* **179**, 89–96.

Zernicke, R.F. & Loitz, B.J. (1990) Myotendinous adaptation to conditioning. In: *Sports-Induced Inflammation* (eds J. Buckwalter, S. Gordon & W. Leadbetter), pp. 687–698. American Academy of Orthopaedic Surgeons, Park Ridge, Illinois.

Zernicke, R.F., Vailas, A.C., Shaw, S.R., Bogey, R.S., Hart, T.J. & Matsuda, J. (1986) Heterogeneous mechanical responses of rat knee menisci to thermochemical stress. *American Journal of Physiology* **250**, R65–R70.

Zuckerman, J. & Stull, G.A. (1969) Effects of exercise on knee ligament separation force in rats. *Journal of Applied Physiology* **26**, 716.

Zuckerman, J. & Stull, G.A. (1973) Ligamentous separation force in rats as influenced by training, detraining and cage restriction. *Medicine and Science in Sports* **5**, 41–49.

Chapter 7

Contractile Performance of Skeletal Muscle Fibres

K.A. PAUL EDMAN

Skeletal muscle represents the largest organ in the body. It makes up approximately 40% of the total body weight and it is organized into hundreds of separate entities, or body muscles, each of which has been assigned a specific task to enable the great variety of movements that are essential to normal life. Each muscle is composed of a great number of subunits, muscle fibres, which are arranged in parallel and typically extend from one tendon to another. In order to understand the performance of muscle it is essential to know the mechanical properties of the individual fibres. With the laboratory techniques now available it is possible to study, in considerable detail, the contractile behaviour of intact single fibres that have been isolated from amphibian muscles and kept immersed in a physiological salt solution. Such fibres, if properly treated, are remarkably stable in their contractile behaviour, showing almost identical responses to electrical stimulation over a whole day of experimentation. In addition, the single-fibre preparation offers the possibility of studying the mechanical performance under strict control of sarcomere length. The latter aspect is of particular importance as the sarcomere length reflects the state of overlap between the two sets of interdigitating filaments that constitute the main functional elements of the contractile system. The following account will elucidate some basic contractile properties of the skeletal muscle fibre, and an attempt will be made to relate these properties to the structure of the contractile system.

Structure of the force generating system

The muscle fibre is a cable-like structure that is composed of tightly packed subunits, myofibrils, that fill up most of the fibre volume (Fig. 7.1). The myofibrils are approximately 1 μm wide and run the entire length of the fibre. They contain the contractile apparatus and are therefore the structures within the muscle that are responsible for force generation and active shortening. The myofibrils exhibit a characteristic band pattern of alternating dark and light segments when viewed in an ordinary light microscope. As the dark and light segments coincide in adjacent myofibrils the entire muscle fibre assumes a striped appearance in the microscope. Skeletal muscle is therefore often referred to as 'striated muscle'. As will become apparent from the following, the striated appearance is an expression of the remarkable regularity in which the contractile machinery is organized within the myofibril.

The principal elements in the myofibrillar structure are two sets of filaments of different thickness that show a highly ordered, segmental arrangement that corresponds to the striated appearance of the myofibril. The thicker filaments occupy the dark bands of the fibre (see Fig. 7.1) and are made up of a fibrous protein, myosin (Hanson & Huxley 1953; Hasselbach 1953). It is the specific optical properties of these filaments in their ordered state in the muscle that make the segment appear dark in the microscope when the

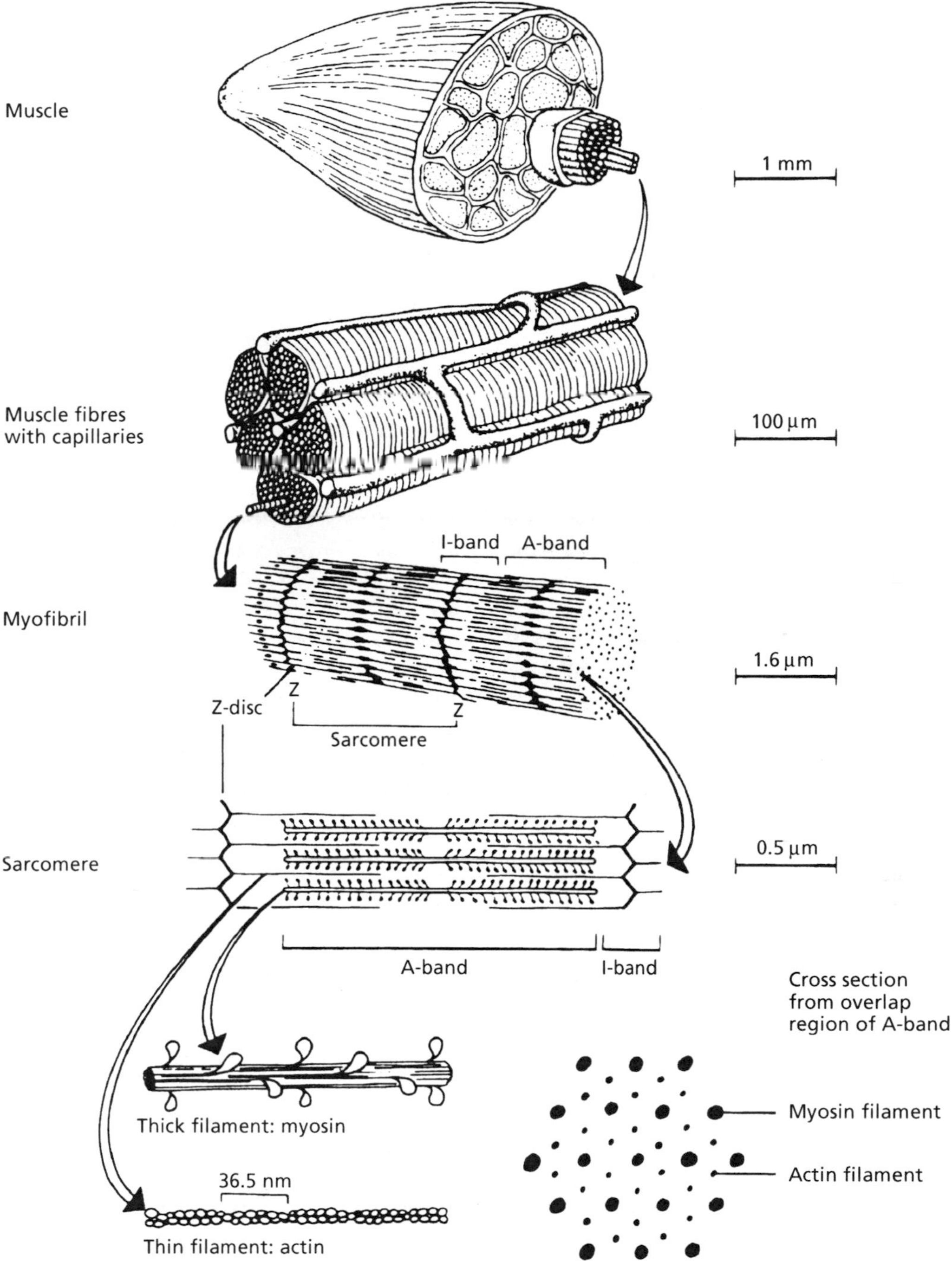

Fig. 7.1 Schematic illustration of muscle structure. For further explanation, see text. (From di Prampero, 1985.)

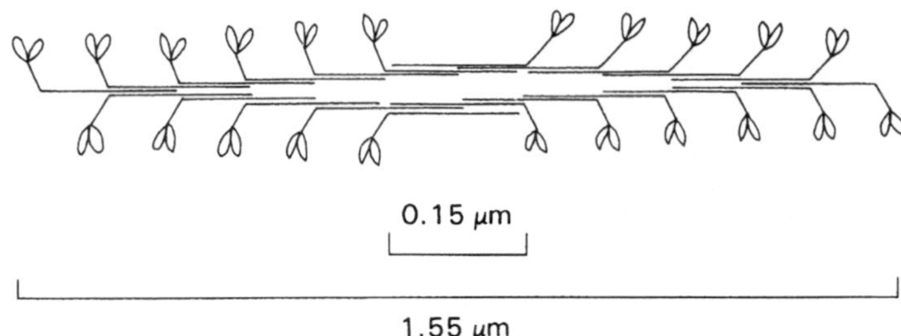

Fig. 7.2 Simplified drawing of the myosin filament (not drawn to scale) illustrating arrangement of myosin molecules. Note that the two halves of the filament are symmetrical and that a central zone, *c.* 0.15 μm wide, is free of myosin extensions (bridges). (After model presented by Huxley 1963.)

fibre is illuminated under standard conditions. Synonymous names of the filaments are: thick filaments, myosin filaments or, referring to their optical (anisotropic) properties, A-filaments.

The second set of filaments is mainly built up of a globular protein, actin. These filaments are anchored in the Z-disc, which is located in the centre of the light band (Fig. 7.1). They extend from either side of the Z-disc and reach into the adjacent A-band where they overlap to some degree with the thick filaments (Hanson & Huxley 1953). These thin (actin) filaments have optical properties (isotropic) that differ from those of the thick filaments, explaining the characteristic appearance of the segment they occupy. The thin filaments are often referred to as I-filaments, and the segments they fill up are generally named I-bands. A cross-sectional view of the myofibril makes clear that the two sets of filaments are arranged in a highly ordered fashion relative to one another (Fig. 7.1). Each A-filament is surrounded by six I-filaments in a hexagonal array. An individual A-filament is thus in a position to interact simultaneously with six adjacent I-filaments, and each I-filament is able to interact with three neighbouring A-filaments. This spatial arrangement of the myofilaments is of great functional significance as it lends stability to the contractile system during activity. The fact that any given filament is able to interact with several adjacent filaments simultaneously ensures that the individual filaments do not coalesce side to side but remain separated from one another during muscle contraction.

Myosin, which is the main constituent of the thick filament, is a large club-like structure composed of a long shaft with two globular heads at one end. The myosin molecules are packed together in such a way (Fig. 7.2) that the shafts form the backbone of the thick filament. However, a substantial portion of the myosin molecule, namely the two heads and a part of the shaft, extends from the rod-like structure to form side-pieces (myosin cross-bridges) at regular intervals along the filament. The cross-bridges are spaced in such a way that every sixth bridge, going from the centre towards the tip of the filament, will face a given thin filament. The two halves of the filament are mirror images of one another (Fig. 7.2), and there is a central region, *c.* 0.15 μm in length, that is free of cross-bridges (the 'inert zone'). The total length of the thick filament is approximately 1.55 μm.

As is shown in Fig. 7.3 the actin monomer is the main building stone of the thin filament. The actin molecules are polymerized to form two helical strands that are wound together. Each actin molecule constitutes a site where an adjacent thick filament may interact to form a cross-bridge connection during muscle activity (see further below). Another important constituent of the thin filament is the protein system that regulates the degree of interaction between the thick and thin filaments. This system is located in the grooves between the two actin strands and is an integral part of the thin filament. It is formed by tropomyosin and troponin, whose functions are now quite well understood (Ebashi & Endo 1968; Ebashi 1980; Gordon *et al.* 2000). The tropomyosin molecules are rod shaped. They are polymerized end to end to form a string that lies in each of the two grooves between the actin

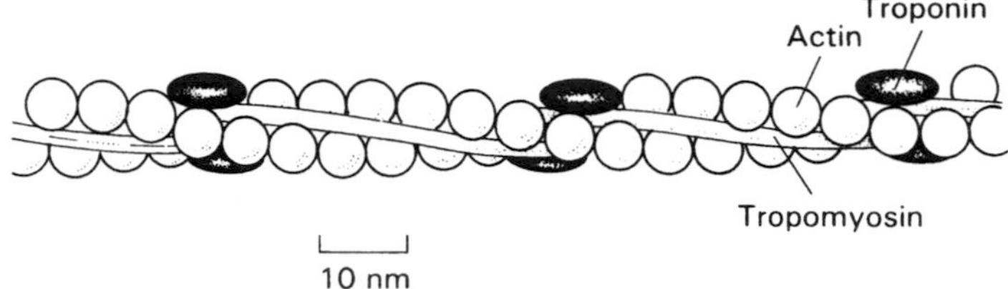

Fig. 7.3 Schematic drawing of a portion of the thin filament showing the two helical strands of actin molecules. The regulatory proteins, troponin and tropomyosin, are positioned in each of the two grooves between the actin strands. (From Ebashi, 1980.)

strands along the entire I-filament. Each tropomyosin molecule has a troponin entity attached to it as is shown in Fig. 7.3. Troponin, in reality a protein complex, has a high affinity for calcium. Binding of calcium to troponin causes a structural change of the troponin–tropomyosin complex that leads to contractile activation as is described subsequently.

In addition to actin, myosin and the regulatory proteins, which make up the thick and thin filaments as described above, there is a fine network of filamentous structures that form a cytoskeleton serving to keep the filaments aligned within the sarcomere and to uphold the lateral register of the sarcomeres across the muscle fibres (see reviews by Waterman-Storer 1991; Wang 1996; Linke 2000). A part of this network of elastic structures is made up by the giant proteins titin and nebulin. Each titin molecule forms a long filament that extends all the way from the Z-disc to the middle of the A-band, attaching at regular sites along the thick (myosin) filaments. The titin filaments in both halves of the sarcomere will, by this arrangement, assist in keeping the myosin filaments aligned and positioned in the centre of the sarcomere. The free portion of the titin filament, i.e. the part extending from the end of the myosin rod to the Z-disc, is compliant and accounts for a major part of the resting elasticity of the muscle fibre. Nebulin, likewise a large protein molecule, forms a long filament that extends from the Z-disc along the entire thin (actin) filament, forming regular connections with actin units. Another part of the cytoskeleton is made up by the proteins desmin, vimentin and synemin which form a filament system that wraps around the Z-disc and interconnects neighbouring Z-discs both transversely across the muscle fibre and longitudinally along each individual myofibril. This supportive filament system is to a great extent responsible for the axial register of the sarcomeres that gives the muscle its striated appearance in a microscope. Damage to these structures by excessive exercise may lead to disorder of the sarcomere pattern and impairment of the contractile function.

For more information about the structure of the contractile system see monographs by Squire (1981, 1997), Woledge *et al.* (1985) and Gordon *et al.* (2000).

Molecular events during contraction

Our knowledge about the structural organization of the contractile system in the form of two distinct sets of filaments, as outlined above, stems from the pioneering work of H.E. Huxley and J. Hanson in the early 1950s (Hanson & Huxley 1953; Huxley 1953; Huxley & Hanson 1954). Their observation that the thick and thin filaments remain constant in length during muscle contraction, while the region of overlap between the two filaments changes with fibre length, led these authors to suggest that muscle contraction is based on a sliding motion of the two sets of interdigitating filaments. A similar conclusion was reached at the same time by A.F. Huxley and Niedergerke (1954). The latter authors were able to demonstrate that the length of the A-bands (occupied by the thick filaments) stays essentially constant as a muscle fibre shortens whereas the I-band spacing varies with the overall length of the fibre. The idea that muscle contraction involves a sliding movement of the thick and thin filaments, with no significant change of their length, has now gained general

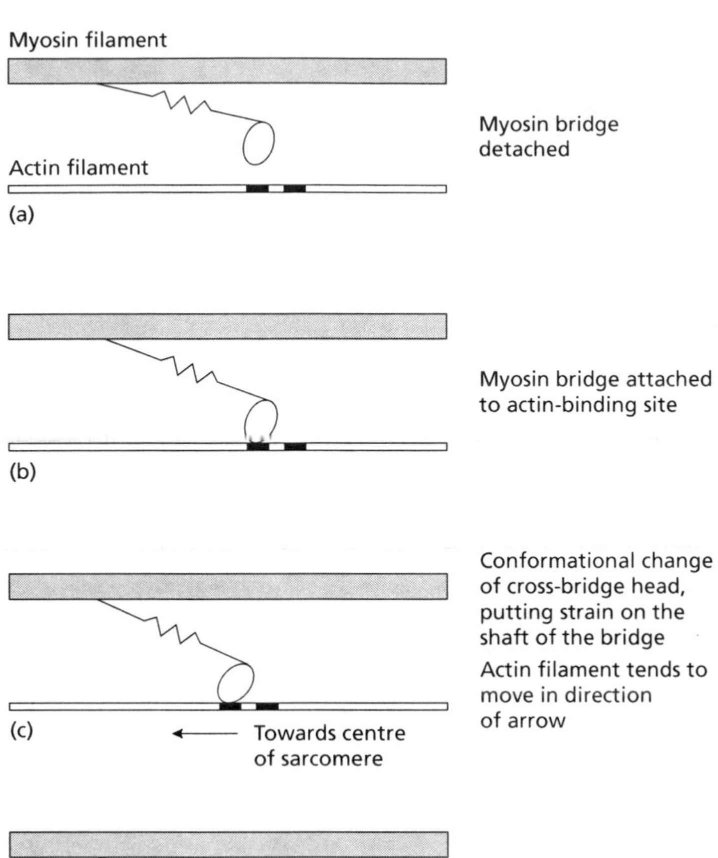

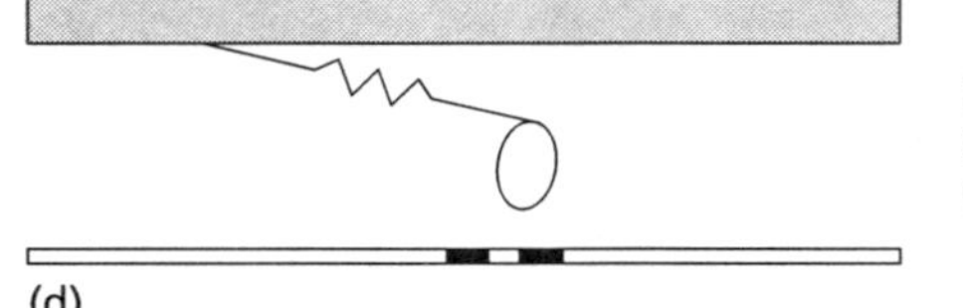

Fig. 7.4 Schematic illustration of the cross-bridge cycle. Two binding sites on the actin filament are marked to illustrate the sliding of the thin filament relative to the cross-bridge from (a) to (d).

acceptance. According to this view the driving force for the sliding motion is generated by the myosin cross-bridges within the region where the thick and thin filaments overlap. The experimental evidence suggests that the myosin bridges make repeated contacts with adjacent thin filaments and that each such contact makes a contribution to the force developed during contraction. However the precise mechanism by which force is generated by the cross-bridge still remains to be established.

Figure 7.4 is a schematic illustration of the cross-bridge cycle according to current views. The process starts as the calcium concentration around the myofibrils is raised above a certain level. This occurs when the fibre is stimulated and calcium is released into the myoplasm from its storage site in the sarcoplasmic reticulum. Binding of calcium to troponin initiates a conformational change of the troponin–tropomyosin complex that leads to retraction of tropomyosin into the groove between the actin strands of the thin filament (Ebashi & Endo 1968; Squire 1981; Gordon *et al.* 2000). In this way, the steric hindrance for interaction between the thick and thin filaments is eliminated, and myosin cross-bridges get the opportunity to attach to actin molecules that are within their reach on neighbouring thin filaments.

The mode of action of the cross-bridge is not known in detail. As already pointed out, each myosin bridge has two heads that conceivably work in an alternating way, i.e. only one head may be in action at a given time. Figure 7.4(a–d) illustrates, schematically, the series of events that are likely to occur during a cross-bridge cycle. A connection is formed between one of the globular heads of the bridge and an actin site (b). This leads to a conformational change within the head region (schematically illustrated as a tilt of the myosin head) that puts strain on the shaft of the bridge (c). The force so produced will tend to move the thin filament further into the array of thick filaments. After the 'power stroke' the cross-bridge head is detached from the thin filament; this occurs as a molecule of adenosine triphosphate (ATP) binds to the myosin head. The bound ATP molecule is rapidly split and the bridge resumes its original ('relaxed') shape. The bridge is thereafter ready to attach again to the actin filament for a new cycle of activity (d). Each complete working cycle of the cross-bridge thus requires the hydrolysis of one molecule of ATP which, accordingly, serves as the immediate source of energy for the contractile process (see further Woledge *et al.* 1985). The ATP consumed is continuously replenished. This is partly achieved by reutilizing the breakdown products, adenosine diphosphate (ADP) and inorganic phosphate (P_i), for formation of ATP. However, accumulation of ADP, P_i and H^+ does occur during excessive exercise and this has an unfavourable effect on the performance of the cross-bridges and is a cause of muscle fatigue (see further below).

According to the cross-bridge hypothesis (Huxley 1957) bridges are thought to act as independent force generators, i.e. the performance of any one bridge is assumed to be uninfluenced by the activity of other bridges. The number of cross-bridges formed is determined by the degree of activation of the contractile system (governed by calcium ions, see above) and by the amount of overlap between the thick and thin filament. Bridges attach to the thin filament in a position where they are able to produce active force, and if the filaments are restrained from sliding (which can be achieved by holding the sarcomere length constant by feedback control) the bridges will remain in a force-producing position as long as they are attached to the thin filament. However, some turnover of bridges does occur even under isometric (constant length) conditions, i.e. bridges dissociate spontaneously and are replaced by new ones, keeping the total number of attached bridges at a given level. This results in there being some energy expenditure even during a purely isometric action when the muscle produces no work.

When the ends of the muscle are free to move, the force produced by the cross-bridges make the thin filaments slide towards the centre of the thick filaments. The sliding movement decreases the probability of cross-bridge formation since the myosin bridges will be exposed to a potential binding site for a shorter time as the filaments slide. Thus, as a muscle is allowed to shorten at progressively higher speeds (which is achieved by decreasing the load on the muscle), the number of attached bridges is steadily reduced. By this mechanism the muscle is able to adjust the number of active cross-bridges (and therefore its energy expenditure) to precisely match the load that is lifted during shortening.

Due to the movement of the filaments some of the attached bridges will come into a braking position and counteract the sliding motion. When the load on the muscle is reduced to zero, the number of braking cross-bridges is just equal to the number of bridges that are in a pulling (force-producing) position. The distribution between pulling and braking cross-bridges will always be such that no net force is created for the sliding movement (Huxley 1957). This ensures that the muscle shortens at a constant velocity. If a net force for the sliding movement were to arise, due to a mismatch between pulling and braking bridges, the muscle would accelerate throughout the shortening phase, a behaviour that would tend to make the body movements jerky and probably less precise.

Contractile performance of striated muscle

The length–tension relationship

It has been known for a long time that a muscle's capacity to produce force depends on the length

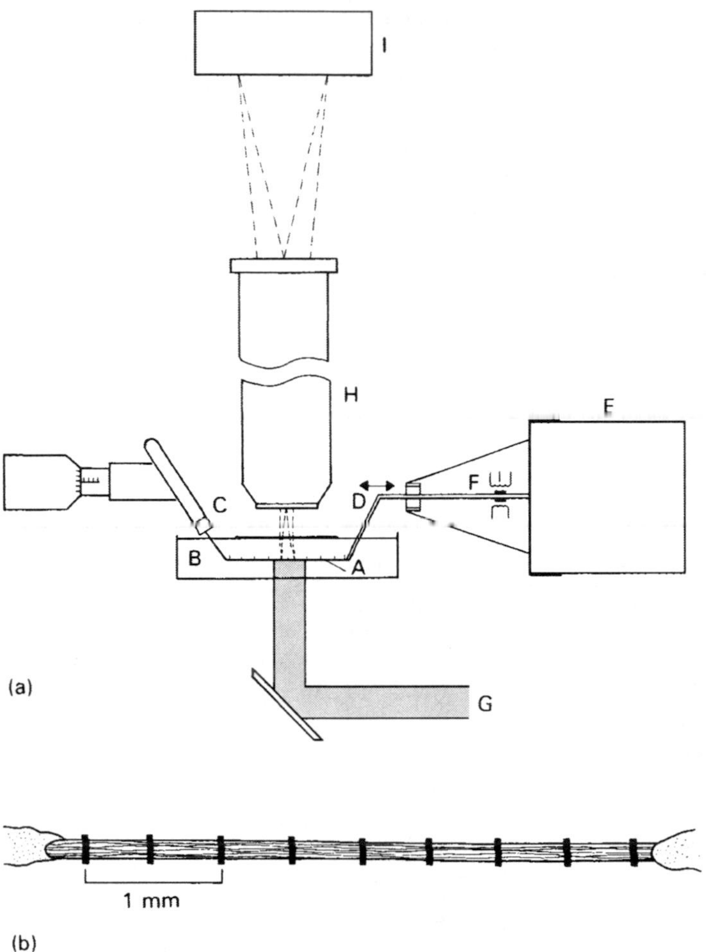

Fig. 7.5 (a) Apparatus for recording force and movement in discrete short segments of intact single muscle fibre. A, single muscle fibre; B, muscle chamber filled with saline; C, force transducer; D, shaft movable in the horizontal plane; E, electromagnetic puller; F, transducer for recording movements of shaft D; G, path for laser beam; H, monocular microscope onto which an image of fibre (and markers) is projected. A photodiode assembly, I, positioned in the plane of the image records the distance between adjacent markers. (b) Drawing of a single muscle fibre with markers attached on the surface.

at which the muscle is held, maximum force being delivered near the length that the muscle normally takes up in the body. This length dependence of the contractile performance has attracted much interest as it has become clear that the relationship between force and sarcomere length provides information of relevance to the elucidation of the sliding filament mechanism of muscle contraction. A study of the sarcomere length–tension relationship, however, is made difficult by the fact that the sarcomere pattern is not precisely uniform within a muscle fibre but varies to some extent from one region to another along the fibre. In order to eliminate this problem, techniques have been developed that enable recording of isometric force from merely a part of the intact fibre. Gordon *et al.* (1966) were first to present such a method. With their 'spot follower' technique these authors were able to length-clamp a 7–10-mm portion of a muscle fibre during tetanus, in this way excluding the end regions of the fibre from force recording. Later experiments (Edman & Reggiani 1984, 1987) have demonstrated, however, that there is a need to length-clamp a considerably smaller fibre segment (*c.* 0.5 mm in length) to eliminate the error in the length–tension measurement that may arise from non-uniform sarcomere behaviour.

Figure 7.5 illustrates the approach used for length-clamping a discrete, short segment of an isolated muscle fibre (for further details, see Edman & Höglund 1981; Edman & Reggiani 1984; Edman & Lou 1990). Illustrated is a single fibre (A) that is mounted horizontally in physiological saline (B) between a force transducer (C) and the shaft (D) of an electromagnetic puller (E). The fibre is stimulated by means of two platinum plate electrodes (not illustrated) that are placed along either side of the fibre in the bath. Discrete segments, approximately 0.5 mm in length, are defined by thin opaque markers that are firmly attached to the upper surface of the fibre. The relative position of any two adjacent markers (outlining one segment) can be measured with a high degree of accuracy by means of a photoelectric recording device (I). For length clamping a given segment the puller (E) is commanded to adjust the overall length of the fibre in such a way that the segment's length is maintained constant throughout the contraction. For this manoeuvre the puller is continuously guided by the signal that is provided by the photoelectric device. It is possible in this way to keep the sarcomere length of a small fibre segment very nearly constant (to within 0.1%) during a tetanus. The clamped segment is thus neither shortening nor lengthening during contraction. The tension recorded from the fibre under these conditions is therefore the true isometric force of the length-clamped segment. Typically, the force so produced remains quite stable during the tetanus period as is illustrated in Fig. 7.6 (record b).

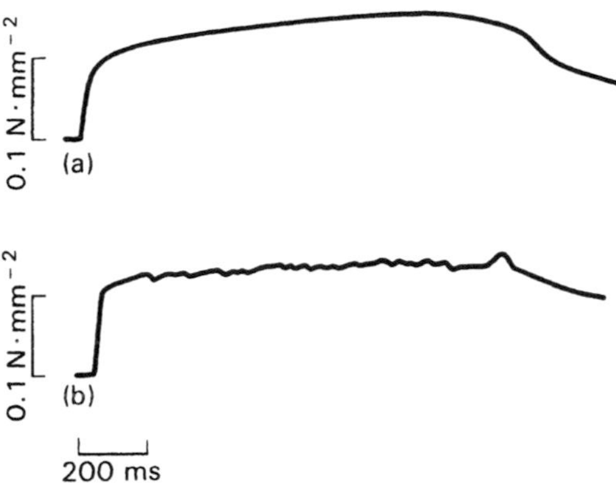

Fig. 7.6 Tetanic force recorded in a single muscle fibre from a frog at 2.95-μm sarcomere length. (a) Conventional recording with the ends of the fibre fixed. Note continuous creep of tension indicating non-uniform behaviour of sarcomeres along the fibre. (b) Recording from a short segment held at constant length during contraction by servo mechanism described in Fig. 7.5. Note constant force production indicating uniform sarcomere behaviour within the short segment.

The relationship between maximum tetanic force and sarcomere length is illustrated in Fig. 7.7. The curve is based on measurements from short length-clamped segments, as described above, and can therefore be supposed to reflect the mechanical performance of a uniform sarcomere population of the fibre. It can be seen that maximum force is attained near a sarcomere length of 2.0 μm and that force is progressively reduced above and below this length. The measured force approaches zero when the sarcomeres are extended to 3.6–3.7 μm.

The sarcomere length–tension relationship described above differs in some respects from the polygonal length–tension curve that was originally described by Gordon *et al.* (1966). The new data show that the length–tension relationship has no distinct plateau between 2.0 and 2.2 μm sarcomere length (see comparison of curves in Fig. 7.8). Furthermore, the length–tension relationship has a smoother shape than postulated earlier.

Assuming that active force is proportional to the degree of overlap between the thick and thin filaments, the length–tension relationship can be used to estimate the average functional length of the A- and I-filaments and the variability of overlap between them. The results of such an analysis (for details, see Edman & Reggiani 1987) suggest that in frog skeletal muscle the thick and thin filaments have a mean length of 1.55 and 1.94 μm, respectively, and that the amount of overlap between the two sets of filaments within a fibre cross-section varies with a standard deviation of 0.21 μm. The filament lengths so derived agree closely with the values of the A- and I-filament lengths (1.55 and 1.92–1.96 μm, respectively) that have been presented by Page (1968) and Huxley (1973) on the basis of electron

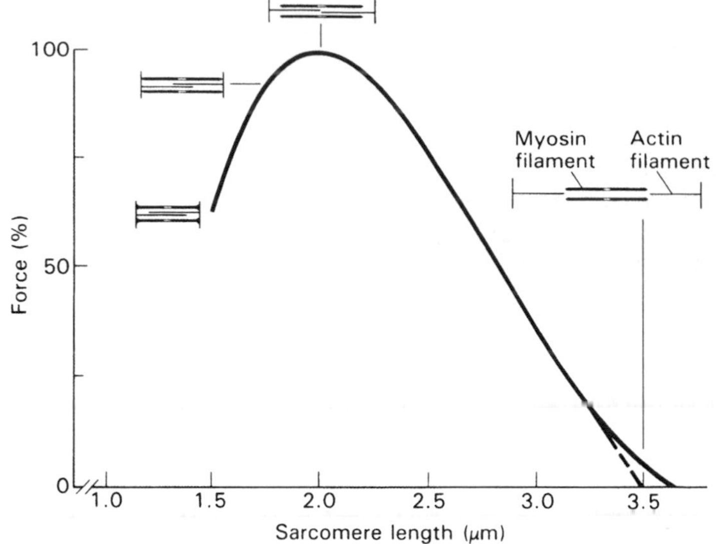

Fig. 7.7 Variation of maximum tetanic force with sarcomere length. Insets show degree of filament overlap at four different sarcomere lengths. The dashed line shows extrapolation to abscissa of the steep portion of the length–tension relation. The intersection of the dashed line with the abscissa shows the sarcomere length at which the majority of the A- and I-filaments are in end-to-end position. For further information, see text (From Edman & Reggiani, 1987.)

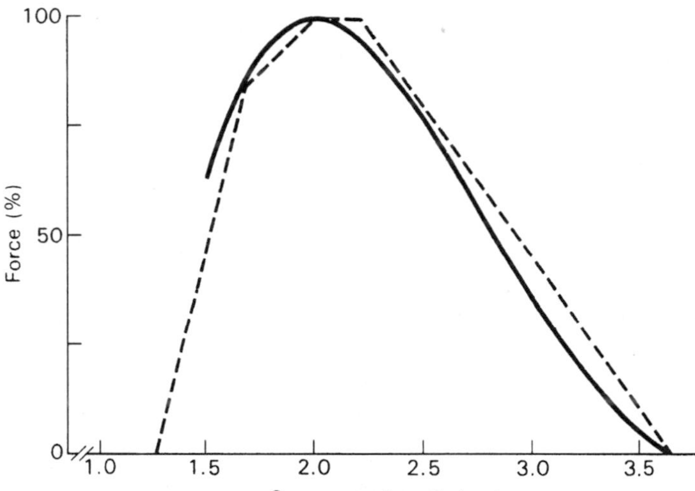

Fig. 7.8 The length–tension relationship shown in Fig. 7.7 (—) compared with the classic polygonal length–tension curve (---) described by Gordon *et al.* (1966).

microscopical measurements. The variation in filament overlap is partly due to imperfect alignment of the filaments and accounts for the smooth shape of the length–tension curve.

It is instructive to consider the relative position of the thick and thin filaments at some representative points along the length–tension curve. As illustrated in Fig. 7.7 (insets), the A- and I-filaments are in end-to-end position at the sarcomere length (approximately 3.5 μm) where active force is close to zero. At 2.0 μm sarcomere length, on the other hand, the ends of the I-filaments are at the centre of the A-filament. This degree of overlap would consequently provide the maximum number of active cross-bridge in line with the finding that maximum force is reached at this point.

The overlap situation becomes more difficult to interpret as the sarcomere length is reduced below 2.0 μm (ascending limb of the length–tension curve). If the sarcomeres are shortened below optimum length, for instance to 1.8 μm, the I-filaments will pass into the opposite half of the sarcomere causing double filament overlap, as is shown in Fig. 7.7. The functional significance of the double overlap cannot be assessed at the present time, but it is reasonable to suppose that the phenomenon is causally related to the decline in active force that occurs at these lengths (for further discussion, see Edman & Reggiani 1987). At sarcomere lengths shorter than 1.7 μm the thick filaments will be compressed when coming up to the Z-discs (Fig. 7.7). This will counteract further sliding and markedly reduce the force produced by the fibre at these lengths.

Incomplete activation of the muscle fibre is yet another possible cause of the decline in tension at very short lengths. As demonstrated by Taylor and Rüdel (1970) the interior of the fibre may not become fully activated at lengths shorter than approximately 1.6 μm due to failure of the inward spread of the action potential under these conditions. However, this complication does not seem to be of any concern within the range of sarcomere lengths considered here. This is indicated by the fact that increasing the release of activator calcium in the fibre (by addition of caffeine) does not affect the length–tension curve depicted in Fig. 7.7 (Edman & Reggiani 1987).

The force–velocity relationship

As already pointed out, muscle has an inherent capacity to adjust its active force to precisely match the load that is experienced during shortening. This remarkable property, which distinguishes muscle from a simple elastic body, is based on the fact that active force continuously adjusts to the speed at which the contractile system moves. Thus, when the load is small, the active force can be made correspondingly small by increasing the speed of shortening appropriately. Conversely, when the load is high, the muscle increases its active force to the same level by reducing the speed of shortening sufficiently. Fenn and Marsh (1935) were first to demonstrate that there exists a given relationship between active force and velocity of shortening. Hill (1938) further characterized the force–velocity relationship and he emphasized the importance of this parameter in the study of muscle function. The force–velocity relationship has attracted much new interest in recent years after it was demonstrated (Huxley 1957) that this relationship is consistent with the cross-bridge mechanism of muscle contraction.

Figure 7.9 shows the classic load– or force–velocity curve that was published by Hill (1938). It shows the inverse relationship between force and velocity of shortening in an isolated *whole* sartorius muscle of the frog. Hill demonstrated that this relationship had a hyperbolic shape and he provided a general formula for its description that has been widely used in muscle physiology. The maximum speed of shortening (V_{max}) can be seen to occur when the load is zero. Maximum force (P_0), on the other hand, is produced when the muscle is stationary, i.e. neither shortening nor lengthening.

Experiments with single muscle fibres (Edman *et al.* 1976; Edman 1988) have demonstrated that the force–velocity relationship has a more complex shape than that observed in whole muscle. As illustrated in Fig. 7.10, the force–velocity relationship contains *two* distinct curvatures, each one with an upward concavity. The two curvatures are located on either side of a breakpoint near 75% of isometric force, P_0.

When the load exceeds P_0 the muscle begins to lengthen (eccentric action) as indicated by the negative velocities in Fig. 7.10. However, the force–velocity curve can be seen to be remarkably flat in the force range around P_0. For instance, as the load is increased from 0.9 to 1.2 P_0, a 30% change in load, the velocity of shortening or elongation is altered by less than 2% of V_{max}. The flat region of the force–velocity relationship around P_0 is of great significance to muscle function in that it promotes stability within the contractile system. For instance, a muscle that is loaded above its own P_0 value (this may occur during jumping or downstairs walking) will nevertheless be able to withstand the load quite well, i.e. the muscle will not yield appreciably. Due to the low speed of lengthening the total length change that the sarcomeres will

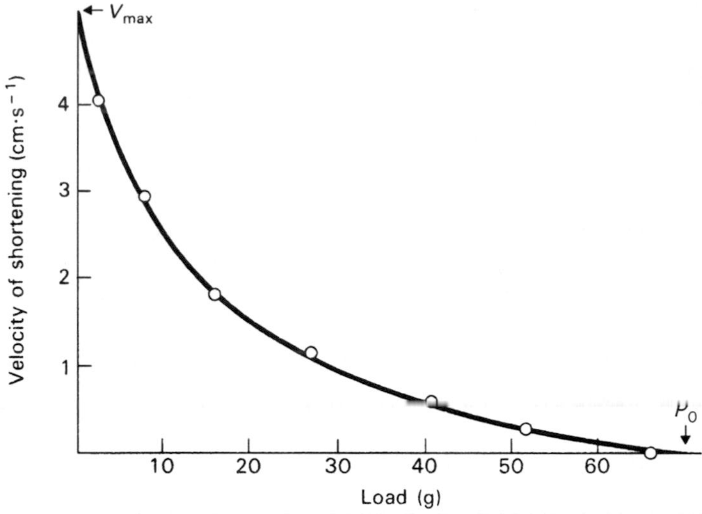

Fig. 7.9 Relationship between force and velocity of shortening measured in a whole sartorius muscle of the frog. The equation for the curve, which is a single hyperbola, is given by Hill (1938). For further information, see text. (From Hill, 1938.)

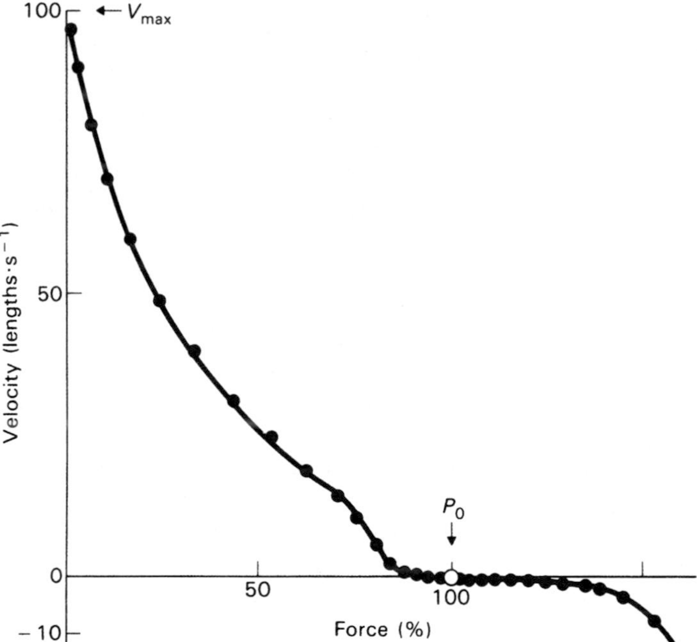

Fig. 7.10 Relationship between force and velocity of shortening recorded in a single muscle fibre of the frog. Note that the force–velocity relation has two distinct curvatures on either side of a break point near 75% of P_0. When the load exceeds the isometric force (P_0), the muscle lengthens, i.e. the velocity assumes a negative value. (From Edman, 1988.)

undergo during the eccentric action will be relatively small. Only when the load is raised by more than 40–50% above P_0 will the muscle elongate at a high speed (see Fig. 7.10). The flat region of the force–velocity relationship may thus be said to represent a highly effective intracellular servo mechanism that helps to keep the sarcomere pattern uniform when the muscle works at a high load and, of great significance, that prevents the muscle from being improperly stretched in situations when the load is suddenly raised above the isometric level.

The force–velocity relationship is likely to reflect the kinetic properties of the cross-bridges

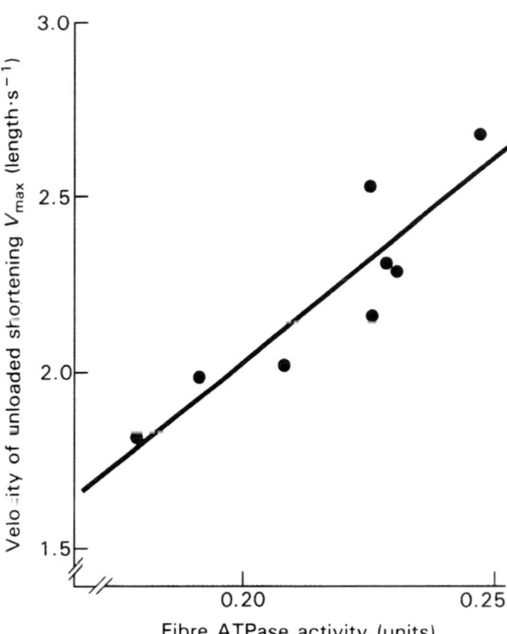

Fig. 7.11 Relationship between myofibrillar ATPase activity and maximum speed of shortening, V_{max}, recorded in single muscle fibres. (From Edman *et al.* 1988.)

and attempts have been made to evaluate the various steps in the cross-bridge cycle using the information provided by the force–velocity curve (e.g. Huxley 1957; Eisenberg & Hill 1978; Edman *et al.* 1997). There is reason to believe that V_{max} expresses the maximum cycling rate of the cross-bridges. In support of this view, V_{max} has been found to correlate well with the maximum rate of splitting of ATP within the contractile system. This was first demonstrated in studies of whole muscles (Bárány 1967) and later, in a more quantitative way (Edman *et al.* 1988), by comparing V_{max} and myofibrillar ATPase activity in isolated single muscle fibres (Fig. 7.11).

If V_{max} represents the maximum speed at which the cross-bridges are able to cycle, V_{max} may be presumed to be independent of the actual number of bridges that interact with the thin filaments. By way of comparison, a light carriage pulled by only one or two horses would reach the same maximum speed as one pulled by many horses. Maximum speed of shortening would thus be expected to remain constant at different degrees of overlap between the thick and thin filaments and also at different states of activation of the contractile system. These predictions have been verified experimentally as illustrated in Fig. 7.12. Here V_{max} is compared with the tetanic force as the sarcomere length is changed from 1.7 to 2.7 μm. It can be seen that whereas the tetanic force varies considerably, the maximum speed of shortening remains constant over this wide range of sarcomere lengths. Thus, in contrast to the fibre's ability to produce force, the maximum speed of shortening does not depend on the number of myosin bridges that are able to interact with thin filaments. Figure 7.13 shows that V_{max} is likewise independent of the degree of activation of the contractile system. These findings thus fully support the sliding filament model and the theory of independent force generators (Huxley 1957).

Various muscles in the body differ considerably with respect to their maximum speed of shortening (see for example Buchthal & Schmalbruch 1980). There is reason to believe that these differences are based on structural heterogeneity of the contractile proteins among the muscles, resulting in different kinetic properties of the myofilament system (for references, see Edman *et al.* 1985; Schiaffino & Reggiani 1995). Individual fibres within a muscle generally exhibit marked differences with respect to their shortening characteristics. This is most pronounced in mammalian and avian muscles in which different types of fibres, fast-twitch and slow-twitch fibres, are regularly found to coexist. Predominance of one particular fibre type determines whether a muscle will acquire fast or slow properties.

Recent studies have demonstrated that the differentiation of the kinetic properties within a muscle extends to *below* fibre level. This is indicated by the finding that both V_{max} and the shape of the force–velocity relationship vary substantially from one part to another along the fibre (Edman *et al.* 1985). Typically, as illustrated in Fig. 7.14, V_{max} varies by 10–45% along the length of a frog muscle fibre. The variation in V_{max} *within* a given fibre may in some cases be as large

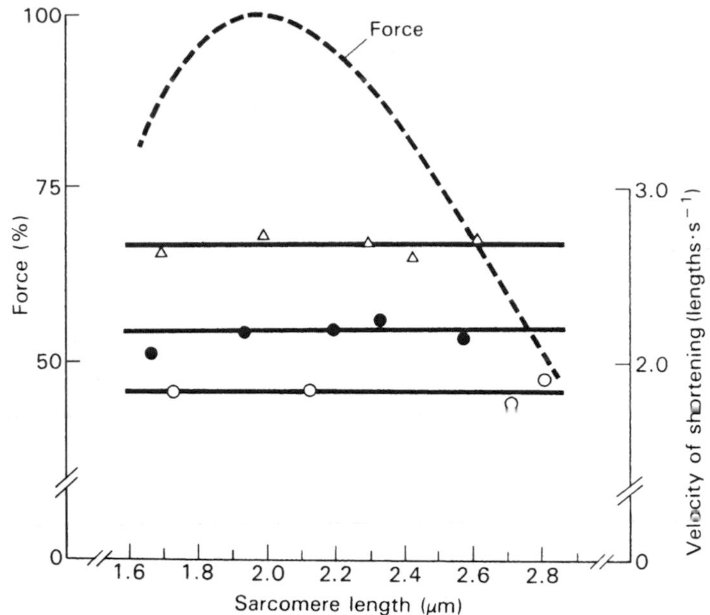

Fig. 7.12 Maximum velocity of shortening, V_{max}, measured at various sarcomere lengths in three different fibres (indicated by different symbols). V_{max} can be seen to remain very nearly constant as sarcomere length is changed. The dashed line shows, for comparison, the variation in isometric force within the range of sarcomere lengths (1.6–2.8 μm) considered. (From Edman, 1979.)

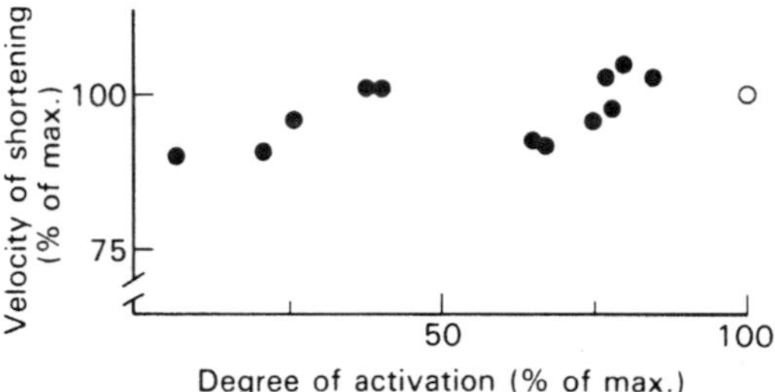

Fig. 7.13 Maximum speed of shortening, V_{max}, recorded at different degrees of activation of single muscle fibres. ○, V_{max} during tetanus, i.e. at full activation. •, measurements of V_{max} during twitch contractions representing various degrees of submaximal activation as indicated on abscissa. Note that V_{max} remains virtually constant as activation is changed. (From Edman, 1979 (Table 1).)

as that recorded *among* different fibres in a muscle. Each fibre has a unique pattern of V_{max} differences. It is of interest to note, however, that there is a clear trend for V_{max} to decrease towards the distal end of the fibre in the body (see Fig. 7.15).

The experimental evidence suggests that the segmental differences in shortening velocity reflect regional differences in myosin isoform composition along the fibre (Edman *et al.* 1988). The rationale behind this heterogeneity in function is unclear, but it may be thought to reflect a subcellular adaptation mechanism. A muscle fibre generally spans the entire length of the muscle and the various parts of the fibre may encounter different working conditions when the muscle operates *in situ* in the body. For instance, the passive resistance to shortening may vary along the fibre due to differences in the amount of connective tissue that holds the fibres together. Furthermore, the distal part of a muscle undergoes a larger translation during shortening than does the proximal part. By adjusting the myosin isoform composition in the various regions appropriately the fibre may be able to compensate for any local differences in the passive resistance to shortening that it may experience *in situ* in the body.

Deactivation by shortening

Skeletal muscle that shortens during activity loses temporarily some of its contractile strength. This depressant effect of shortening has been demonstrated both in muscle *in situ* in the body

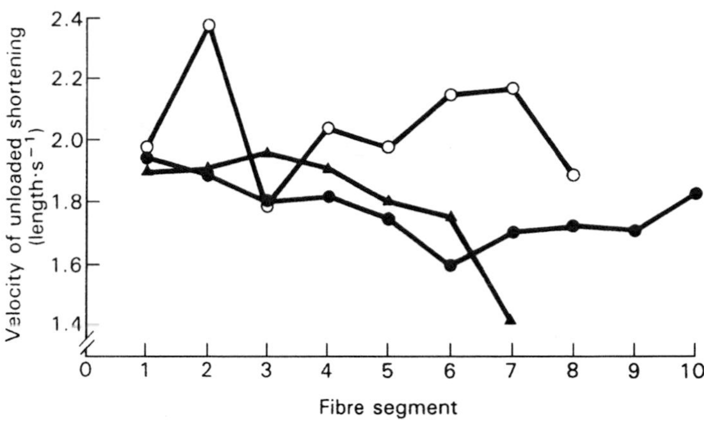

Fig. 7.14 Maximum velocity of shortening, V_{max}, recorded in consecutive segments of three individual muscle fibres (indicated by different symbols). The segments are approximately 0.8 mm in length and are numbered from one tendon insertion to the other in the respective fibre. Note that V_{max} is markedly different along the fibres and that each fibre has a unique velocity pattern. (From Edman *et al.* 1985.)

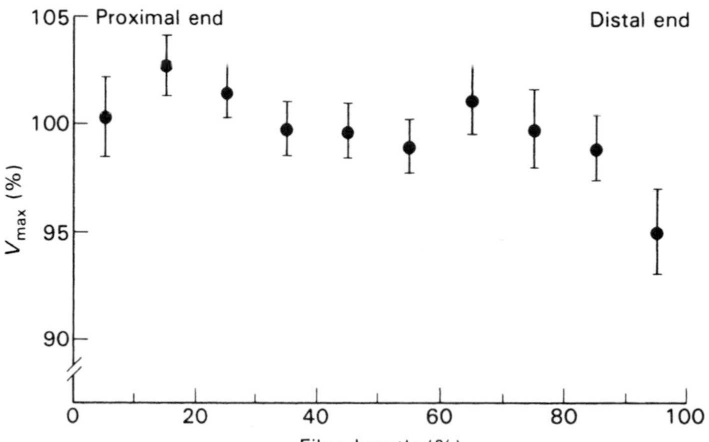

Fig. 7.15 V_{max} of individual fibre segments related to the fibre's orientation in the body. The length of each fibre is normalized to 100%. Data points are mean values (± SE of mean) based on measurements in 14 fibres. Note decline of V_{max} towards the distal fibre end. (From Edman *et al.* 1985.)

(Joyce *et al.* 1969) and in isolated whole muscle (Jewell & Wilkie 1960), and the phenomenon has been explored in considerable detail in isolated single muscle fibres (Edman & Kiessling 1971; Edman 1975, 1980).

Figure 7.16 illustrates the depressant effect of active shortening in an isolated muscle fibre of the frog. The two superimposed myograms, A and B, show the development of force during a partially fused tetanus at a sarcomere length of 2.05 μm, i.e. near optimum length. The responses to the respective stimuli are seen as humps in the records and are referred to as twitches. In myogram A the entire contraction is performed at 2.05 μm sarcomere spacing. In myogram B, on the other hand, the contraction is initiated at a longer sarcomere length, 2.55 μm, and the fibre is allowed to shorten to 2.05 μm during the first twitch period. As can be clearly seen in Fig. 7.16, the active force is greatly depressed after shortening. The peak force of the second twitch in myogram B is thus considerably lower than the force attained in the first twitch of myogram A. This is significant since tension starts from zero level in both cases. The reduced tension in the second twitch of myogram B thus represents a true depression of the fibre's ability to produce force due to preceding shortening. Even the third twitch of myogram B can be seen to be lower than the first twitch in myogram A. It should be noted, however, that the depressant effect of shortening is gradually diminished as contraction goes on; the effect has virtually disappeared by the end of the tetanus period.

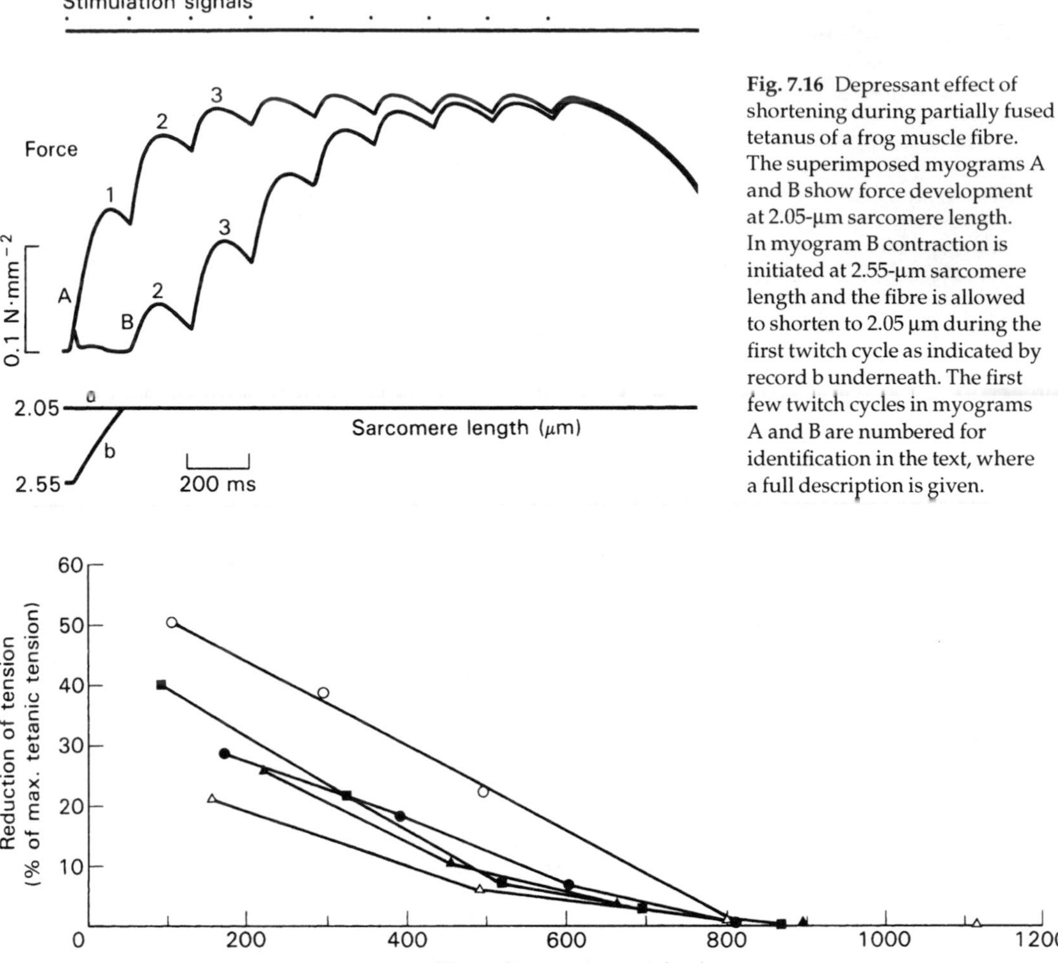

Fig. 7.16 Depressant effect of shortening during partially fused tetanus of a frog muscle fibre. The superimposed myograms A and B show force development at 2.05-μm sarcomere length. In myogram B contraction is initiated at 2.55-μm sarcomere length and the fibre is allowed to shorten to 2.05 μm during the first twitch cycle as indicated by record b underneath. The first few twitch cycles in myograms A and B are numbered for identification in the text, where a full description is given.

Fig. 7.17 Time course of disappearance of the depressant effect of active shortening during incompletely fused tetanus. Results of five experiments (indicated by different symbols) with various degrees of force depression after shortening.

The time needed for the movement effect to disappear is remarkably constant from fibre to fibre as is shown in Fig. 7.17. Although the initial force depression varies in different fibres, depending on the amount of shortening used, a time period of almost 1 s is required for the effect to die away in each case.

The magnitude of force depression depends on the degree of activation of the contractile system when the movement occurs. The movement effect is large during a single twitch or during a *partially* fused tetanus, i.e. under conditions when the contractile system is not fully activated (see Fig. 7.16). On the other hand, the effect is quite small when the movement occurs during a completely fused tetanus (Edman 1980). Since muscle activity *in vivo* is based on partially fused tetani, it is reasonable to suppose that force depression by shortening does play a part in daily life. The effect is also likely to influence the results in certain branches of athletics. In weight-lifting, for instance, the muscles' capacity to lift

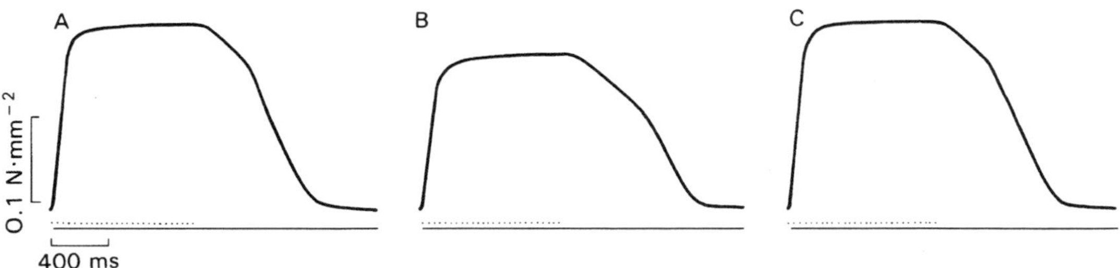

Fig. 7.18 Effects of fatigue on force development during tetanus in a frog muscle fibre. Myogram A shows tetanus during the control period, when intervals between the tetani were 15 min; myogram B shows tetanus after fatiguing stimulation, when intervals between the tetani were 15 s; myogram C shows the return to control stimulation protocol, when intervals between the tetani were 15 min. (From Edman & Mattiazzi, 1981.)

the load can be presumed to decline progressively while the lifting occurs. However, after a brief (1–2-s) pause the muscles will have regained their contractile strength again. The movement effect may serve as a safety mechanism to prevent overuse of the muscles.

It is now possible to conclude that the movement effect is caused by a change within the myofilament system itself. This is indicated by the fact that the depressant effect of shortening also appears in skinned fibres, i.e. preparations in which the cell membrane has been removed, either mechanically or by chemical treatment. In such 'membrane-free' fibres the contractile machinery can be directly controlled by varying the calcium concentration in the surrounding medium. The results of such studies suggest strongly (Ekelund & Edman 1982) that active shortening causes a transitory change of the binding site for calcium on the thin filament. This leads to a decrease in the amount of calcium that is bound to the regulatory proteins, and this in turn reduces the degree of activation of the contractile system. In line with this view it has been possible to demonstrate in intact fibres that calcium is released from its binding sites during shortening (Edman 1996; Vandenboom *et al.* 1998). The decrease in calcium affinity of the binding sites is likely to be a direct consequence of the actin–myosin interaction during shortening as discussed in detail elsewhere (Edman 1975, 1980; Ekelund & Edman 1982). On this basis, then, the depressant effect of shortening may be regarded as an integral part of the sliding filament process.

Cellular mechanism of muscle fatigue

Muscle fatigue may be defined as a reversible decrease in contractile strength that occurs after longlasting or repeated muscular activity. There is reason to believe that human fatigue is a complex phenomenon that includes failure at more than one site along the chain of events that leads to stimulation of the muscle fibres (Edwards 1981; Gandevia *et al.* 1995). It is thus conceivable that human fatigue involves a 'central' component that puts an upper limit on the number of command signals that are sent to the muscles. There is little doubt, however, that muscle fatigue also involves a 'peripheral' component. In fact, part of the muscle's failure to produce force is likely to be caused by a change in the myofilament system itself. This is strongly suggested by the fact that the contractile performance of an isolated muscle fibre is greatly dependent on its preceding mechanical activity. The following account will deal with this 'peripheral' effect of muscle fatigue.

Figure 7.18 shows the characteristic changes in active force that occur when a muscle fibre is fatigued by frequent activation. Myogram A illustrates a control tetanus; before this recording the fibre had been stimulated to produce a 1-s isometric tetanus at 15-min intervals until constant responses were obtained. Myogram B shows, for comparison, an isometric tetanus after development of fatigue; in this case the fibre had been stimulated to produce a tetanus once every 15 s over a time period of several minutes. It can be seen that reducing the resting interval between contractions (from 15 min to 15 s) leads to a decrease in the force output during the tetanus. The total amplitude of the tetanus is thus markedly reduced by fatiguing stimulation. Furthermore, force develops less rapidly in the fatigued state, and the fibre requires a longer time to relax. These changes in the contractile performance are fully reversed after return to the control stimulation protocol (myogram C, Fig. 7.18).

Fatiguing stimulation does not merely affect the muscle's capacity to produce force, it also reduces the speed of shortening of the muscle (Edman & Mattiazzi 1981). The latter effect is illustrated in Fig. 7.19, which shows the simultaneous change in tetanic force and maximum speed of shortening, V_{max}, at different degrees of fatigue in single muscle fibres. It can be seen that as fatigue develops (indicated by the decrease of tetanic force, abscissa), the maximum speed of shortening is also steadily reduced (ordinate). This is a relevant finding as it suggests that muscle fatigue involves a change of the kinetic properties of the cross-bridges.

Further information about the molecular mechanism of fatigue has been obtained by studying muscle stiffness. This measurement provides an index of the number of myosin cross-bridge that are attached to the thin filaments (Ford *et al.* 1977). Muscle stiffness is measured by applying a fast and very small length change to an isolated fibre during activity while recording the corresponding change in force. In principle the approach is the same as that used for testing stiffness of a rubber band; when the stiffness is high there is a large increase in tension as the rubber band is stretched; when the stiffness is small the tension response to the stretch is correspondingly small. For information concerning the techniques used for measuring stiffness throughout the course of a contraction, see Edman and Lou (1990).

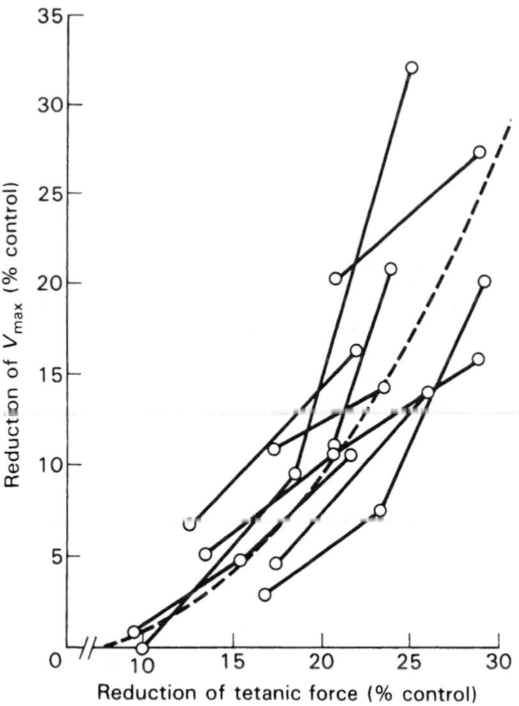

Fig. 7.19 Decrease in maximum speed of shortening (ordinate) in relation to force depression (abscissa) during fatigue of single muscle fibres. Each set of data connected by a solid line is from a single fibre. The dashed line is the calculated mean of all data points. (From Edman & Mattiazzi 1981.)

Muscle stiffness is found to be only slightly changed during moderate fatigue as is demonstrated in Fig. 7.20. For example, a 25% decrease in the muscle's ability to produce force is associated with a mere 9% reduction in muscle fibre stiffness. These findings suggest that the force deficit during fatigue is only partly due to fewer attached cross-bridges. The major portion of the force decline is attributable to reduced force output of the individual bridge.

In summary, the following changes in cross-bridge function are likely to occur during muscle fatigue: (i) a slight decrease in the number of interacting cross-bridges; (ii) reduced force output of the individual cross-bridge; and (iii) reduced speed of cycling of the bridges during muscle shortening. There is reason to believe

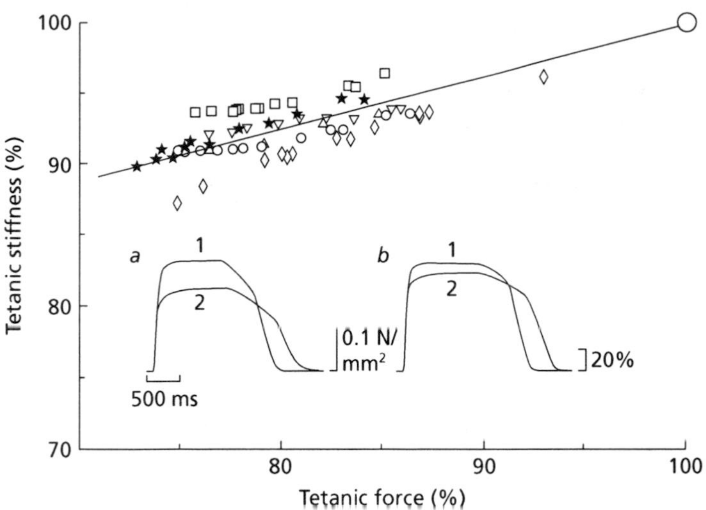

Fig. 7.20 Relationship between force (abscissa) and stiffness (ordinate) recorded during the tetanus plateau as fatigue develops in six single muscle fibres. Data normalized with respect to maximum force and maximum stiffness recorded under resting conditions in respective fibres. The control value (indicated by a large open circle) is the calculated mean for all fibres at rest. Data from a given fibre are denoted by the same symbol. The straight line is the calculated regression of force upon stiffness based on all data points. The insets show example records of tetanic force (*a*) and tetanic stiffness (*b*) under control conditions (traces 1) and, superimposed, after fatiguing stimulation (traces 2). (From Edman & Lou 1990).

that all three changes are ultimately caused by accumulation of breakdown products of ATP hydrolysis within the fibre. Sustained muscular activity leads to increased concentrations of ADP, P_i and H^+ (e.g. Edwards *et al.* 1975; Dawson *et al.* 1978, 1980), and these products affect force production and speed of shortening in a way that is compatible with the changes observed in fatigue (for references and further discussion, see Edman & Lou 1990). Of the three products, increased H^+ concentration would seem to be of particular importance for the development of muscle fatigue. This is suggested by the finding that the contractile changes observed during fatigue (decrease in active force, speed of shortening and power output) can all be simulated remarkably well by lowering the intracellular pH (Edman & Mattiazzi 1981; Curtin & Edman 1989; Edman & Lou 1990). However, the relative role of the various ATP hydrolysis products during development of fatigue may vary in different muscle species (Fitts 1994; Allen *et al.* 1995).

It should be pointed out that the above changes in mechanical performance during fatigue refer to experimental conditions where there is no failure of activation of the contractile system (see further Edman & Lou 1990). Impairment of the excitation–contraction coupling does occur, however, if the isolated muscle is subjected to an extreme fatiguing programme, for example when the contractions are induced at very short (1–2-s) intervals (see, for instance, Eberstein & Sandow 1963; Lännergren & Westerblad 1986). Under such conditions there will be a failure of the inward spread of the action potential along the T-tubules, and the interior of the muscle fibre will therefore be inadequately activated (Gonzalez-Serratos *et al.* 1981; Lou & Edman 1990). The amount of calcium released into the myoplasm from the storage sites of the sarcoplasmic reticulum is reduced under these extreme conditions (Allen *et al.* 1995), resulting in a smaller number of active cross-bridges as indicated by a progressive reduction in fibre stiffness (see further Edman & Lou 1992). It still remains uncertain, however, whether a stimulation programme intense enough to cause such a failure of activation can ever be achieved under *in vivo* conditions in the body before other, more central, fatigue mechanisms put a limit on the stimulation of the muscle (for further reading, see Gandevia *et al.* 1995).

References

Allen, D.G., Westerblad, H. & Lännergren, J. (1995) The role of intracellular acidosis in muscle fatigue. In: *Fatigue, Neural and Muscular Mechanisms. Advances in Experimental Medicine and Biology* (eds S.C. Gandevia, R. M. Enoka, A.J. McComas, D.G. Stuart & C.K. Thomas) **384**, 57–68.

Bárány, M. (1967) ATPase activity of myosin correlated with speed of muscle shortening. *Journal of General Physiology* **50**, 197–218.

Buchthal, F. & Schmalbruch, H. (1980) Motor unit of mammalian muscle. *Physiological Reviews* **60**, 90–142.

Curtin, N.A. & Edman, K.A.P. (1989) Effects of fatigue and reduced intracellular pH on segment dynamics of 'isometric' relaxation of frog muscle fibres. *Journal of Physiology* **413**, 159–174.

Dawson, M.J., Gadian, D.G. & Wilkie, D.R. (1978) Muscular fatigue investigated by phosphorus nuclear magnetic resonance. *Nature* **274**, 861–866.

Dawson, M.J., Gadian, D.G. & Wilkie, D.R. (1980) Mechanical relaxation rate and metabolism studied in fatiguing muscle by phosphorus nuclear magnetic resonance. *Journal of Physiology* **299**, 465–484.

Ebashi, S. (1980) Regulation of muscle contraction. *Proceedings of the Royal Society of London Series B* **207**, 259–286.

Ebashi, S. & Endo, M. (1968) Calcium ion and muscle contraction. *Progress in Biophysics and Molecular Biology* **18**, 125–183.

Eberstein, A. & Sandow, A. (1963) Fatigue mechanism in muscle fibres. In: *The Effect of Use and Disuse on Neuromuscular Functions* (eds E. Gutman & P. Hnik), pp. 515–526. Nakladatelstvi Ceskoslovenske Akademie ved Praha, Prague.

Edman, K.A.P. (1975) Mechanical deactivation induced by active shortening in isolated muscle fibres of the frog. *Journal of Physiology* **246**, 255–275.

Edman, K.A.P. (1979) The velocity of unloaded shortening and its relation to sarcomere length and isometric force in vertebrate muscle fibres. *Journal of Physiology* **291**, 143–159.

Edman, K.A.P. (1980) Depression of mechanical performance by active shortening during twitch and tetanus of vertebrate muscle fibres. *Acta Physiologica Scandinavica* **109**, 15–26.

Edman, K.A.P. (1988) Double-hyperbolic force–velocity relation in frog muscle fibres. *Journal of Physiology* **404**, 301–321.

Edman, K.A.P. (1996) Fatigue vs. shortening-induced deactivation in striated muscle. *Acta Physiologica Scandinavica* **156**, 183–192.

Edman, K.A.P. & Höglund, O. (1981) A technique for measuring length changes of individual segments of an isolated muscle fibre. *Journal of Physiology* **317**, 8–9.

Edman, K.A.P. & Kiessling, A. (1971) The time course of the active state in relation to sarcomere length and movement studied in single skeletal muscle fibres of the frog. *Acta Physiologica Scandinavica* **81**, 182–196.

Edman, K.A.P. & Lou, F. (1990) Changes in force and stiffness induced by fatigue and intracellular acidification in frog muscle fibres. *Journal of Physiology* **424**, 133–149.

Edman, K.A.P. & Lou, F. (1992) Myofibrillar fatigue versus failure of activation during repetitive stimulation of frog muscle fibres. *Journal of Physiology* **457**, 655–673.

Edman, K.A.P. & Mattiazzi, A. (1981) Effects of fatigue and altered pH on isometric force and velocity of shortening at zero load in frog muscle fibres. *Journal of Muscle Research and Cell Motility* **2**, 321–334.

Edman, K.A.P. & Reggiani, C. (1984) Redistribution of sarcomere length during isometric contraction of frog muscle fibres and its relation to tension creep. *Journal of Physiology* **351**, 169–198.

Edman, K.A.P. & Reggiani, C. (1987) The sarcomere length–tension relation determined in short segments of intact muscle fibres of the frog. *Journal of Physiology* **385**, 709–732.

Edman, K.A.P., Mulieri, L.A. & Scubon-Mulieri, B. (1976) Non-hyperbolic force–velocity relationship in single muscle fibres. *Acta Physiologica Scandinavica* **98**, 143–156.

Edman, K.A.P., Reggiani, C. & te Kronnie, G. (1985) Differences in maximum velocity of shortening along single muscle fibres of the frog. *Journal of Physiology* **365**, 147–163.

Edman, K.A.P., Reggiani, C., Schiaffino, S. & te Kronnie, G. (1988) Maximum velocity of shortening related to myosin isoform composition in frog skeletal muscle fibres. *Journal of Physiology* **395**, 679–694.

Edman, K.A.P., Mansson, A. & Caputo, C. (1997) The biphasic force–velocity relationship in frog muscle fibres and its evaluation in terms of cross-bridge mechanism. *Journal of Physiology* **503**, 141–156.

Edwards, R.H.T. (1981) Human muscle and fatigue. In: *Ciba Foundation Symposium 82: Human Muscle Fatigue: Physiological Mechanisms* (eds R. Porter & J. Whelan), pp. 1–18. Pitman Medical, London.

Edwards, R.H.T., Hill, D.K. & Jones, D.A. (1975) Metabolic changes associated with the slowing of relaxation in fatigued mouse muscle. *Journal of Physiology* **251**, 287–301.

Eisenberg, E. & Hill, T.L. (1978) A cross-bridge model of muscle contraction. *Progress in Biophysics and Molecular Biology* **33**, 55–82.

Ekelund, M. & Edman. K.A.P. (1982) Shortening induced deactivation of skinned fibres of frog and mouse striated muscle. *Acta Physiologica Scandinavica* **116**, 189–199.

Fenn, W.O. & Marsh, B.S. (1935) Muscular force at different speed of shortening. *Journal of Physiology* **85**, 277–297.

Fitts, R.H. (1994) Cellular mechanisms of muscle fatigue. *Physiological Reviews* **74**, 49–94.

Ford, L.E., Huxley, A.F. & Simmons, R.M. (1977) Tension responses to sudden length change in stimulated frog muscle fibres near slack length. *Journal of Physiology* **269**, 441–515.

Gandevia, S.C., Enoka, R.M., McComas, A.J., Stuart, D.G. & Thomas, C.K. (eds) (1995) *Fatigue, Neural and Muscular Mechanisms. Advances in Experimental Medicine and Biology* **384**.

Gonzalez-Serratos, H., Garcia, M., Somlyo, A., Somlyo, A.P. & McClellan, G. (1981) Differential shortening of myofibrils during development of fatigue. *Biophysical Journal* **33**, 224a.

Gordon, A.M., Huxley, A.F. & Julian, F.J. (1966) The variation in isometric tension with sarcomere length in vertebrate muscle fibres. *Journal of Physiology* **184**, 170–192.

Gordon, A.M., Homsher, E. & Regnier, M. (2000) Regulation of contraction in striated muscle. *Physiological Review* **80**, 853–924.

Hanson, J. & Huxley, H.E. (1953) The structural basis of the cross-striations in muscle. *Nature* **172**, 530–532.

Hasselbach. W. (1953) Elektronmikroskopische Untersuchungen an Muskelfibrillen bei totaler und partieller Extraktion des L-Myosins. *Zeitschrift für Naturforschung* **8b**, 449–454.

Hill, A.V. (1938) The heat of shortening and the dynamic constants of muscle. *Proceedings of the Royal Society of London Series B* **126**, 136–195.

Huxley, H.E. (1953) Electron-microscope studies of the organization of the filaments in striated muscle. *Biochimica et Biophysica Acta* **12**, 387.

Huxley, A.F. (1957) Muscle structure and theories of contraction. *Progress in Biophysics and Biophysical Chemistry* **7**, 255–318.

Huxley, H.E. (1963) Electron microscope studies on the structure of natural and synthetic protein filaments from striated muscle. *Journal of Molecular Biology* **7**, 281–308.

Huxley, H.E. (1973) Molecular basis of contraction in cross-striated muscle. In: *The Structure and Function of Muscle*, Vol. 1 (ed. G. Bourne), 2nd edn, pp. 301–397. Academic Press, New York.

Huxley, H.E. & Hanson, J. (1954) Changes in the cross-striation of muscle during contraction and stretch and their structural interpretation. *Nature* **173**, 973–977.

Huxley, A.F. & Niedergerke, R. (1954) Structural changes in muscle during contraction: interference microscopy of living muscle fibres. *Nature* **173**, 971–973.

Jewell, B.R. & Wilkie, D.R. (1960) The mechanical properties of relaxing muscle. *Journal of Physiology* **152**, 30–47.

Joyce, G.C., Rack, P.M.H. & Westbury, D.R. (1969) The mechanical properties of cat soleus muscle during controlled lengthening and shortening movements. *Journal of Physiology* **204**, 461–474.

Lännergren, J. & Westerblad, H. (1986) Force and membrane potential during and after fatiguing, continuous high-frequency stimulation of single *Xenopus* muscle fibres. *Acta Physiologica Scandinavica* **128**, 359–368.

Linke, W.A. (2000) Stretching molecular springs: elasticity of titin filaments in vertebrate striated muscle. *Histology and Histopathology* **15**, 799–811.

Lou, F. & Edman, K.A.P. (1990) Effects of fatigue on force, stiffness and velocity of shortening in frog muscle fibres. *Acta Physiologica Scandinavica* **140**, 24A.

Page, S. (1968) Fine structure of tortoise skeletal muscle. *Journal of Physiology* **197**, 709–715.

di Prampero, P.E. (1985) Metabolic and circulatory limitations to $Vo_{2\ max}$ at the whole animal level. *Journal of Experimental Biology* **115**, 319–332.

Schiaffino, S. & Reggiani, C. (1995) Molecular diversity of myofibrillar proteins: gene regulation and functional significance. *Physiological Review* **76**, 371–423.

Squire, J. (1981) *The Structural Basis of Muscular Contraction*. Plenum Press, New York.

Squire, J. (1997) Architecture and function in the muscle sarcomere. *Current Opinion in Structural Biology* **2**, 247–257.

Taylor, S.R. & Rüdel, R. (1970) Striated muscle fibers: inactivation of contraction induced by shortening. *Science* **167**, 882–884.

Vandenboom, R., Claflin, D.R. & Julian, F.J. (1998) Effects of rapid shortening on rate of force regeneration and myoplasmic [Ca^{2+}] in intact frog skeletal muscle. *Journal of Physiology* **511**, 171–180.

Wang, K. (1996) Titin/connectin and nebulin: giant protein rulers of muscle structure and function. *Advances in Biophysics* **33**, 123–134.

Waterman-Storer, C.M. (1991) The cytoskeleton of skeletal muscle: is it affected by exercise? A brief review. *Medicine and Science in Sports and Exercise* **23**, 1240–1249.

Woledge, R.C., Curtin, N.A. & Homsher, E. (1985) *Energetic Aspects of Muscle Contraction*. Academic Press, London.

Chapter 8

Skeletal Muscle and Motor Unit Architecture: Effect on Performance

ROLAND R. ROY, RYAN J. MONTI, ALEX LAI AND V. REGGIE EDGERTON

Introduction

The architectural features of a muscle play an important role in determining the functional properties of individual skeletal muscles. In the previous edition of this book (Roy & Edgerton 1992), we described the basic skeletal muscle structure–function relationships and described the roles of muscle mass, and fibre (fascicle) length and angle of pennation in determining these properties. Several reviews on this topic have been published in the past decade (e.g. Fukunaga *et al.* 1997b; Lieber & Friden 2000). One major advancement in this area has been the determination of these structure–function interrelationships in humans, particularly as this relates to athletic performance and gender differences. These advancements have been possible because of the development of non-invasive imaging techniques, such as ultrasound and magnetic resonance imaging (MRI) (see '*In vivo* strain patterns' below). Abe *et al.* (2000) have reported that elite male sprinters have longer fascicle lengths (vastus lateralis, medial and lateral gastrocnemii) and smaller pennation angles (vastus lateralis, medial gastrocnemius) in selected leg muscles than distance runners. These differences should relate to a 'faster' velocity of contraction in the sprinters than distance runners. Sumo wrestlers have longer fascicle lengths (triceps long head, vastus lateralis and medial gastrocnemius, but not the lateral gastrocnemius) and larger pennation angles (same muscles except for the vastus lateralis) than controls (Kearns *et al.* 2000). These architectural features should translate to an increase in force production capability. It has also been reported that the architectural properties (fascicle length) of skeletal muscles in humans do not contribute to race differences (black and white college football players; triceps long head, vastus lateralis and medial gastrocnemius) or gender differences (college athletes; same muscles) in sprint/jump performance of young, highly trained individuals (Abe *et al.* 1999). Similarly, Ichinose *et al.* (1998) reported a larger mean muscle thickness and fibre pennation angle in the triceps brachii of highly trained male than in female soccer and gymnastic, but not judo, athletes, although these authors point out that the differences in pennation angle were minimal if allowances were made for the differences in muscle size. In a general population of healthy adults, Chow *et al.* (2000) reported that females had longer average muscle fibre bundle lengths and males had thicker muscles and larger angles of pennation in the soleus and gastrocnemius (both heads) muscles. Their interpretation was that these architectural differences help account for the overall greater absolute strength in males than females. Together, these results emphasize the importance of having a clear understanding of the role that architecture can play in defining skeletal muscle function when interpreting human movement or performance. However, much more work is needed in this area before any definitive structure–function interrelationships can be fully substantiated.

In the present review we will focus on two main topics that were introduced in a previous chapter (Roy & Edgerton 1992): (i) the role of architecture in determining the structure–function relationships among motor units and subdivisions of a muscle; and (ii) the role of architecture in determining skeletal muscle stress–strain injuries in humans. The emphasis will be on describing the manner in which the architectural features of the individual fibres, single motor units and whole muscles affect the transmission of force during contractions.

Motor unit structure–function interrelationships

A motor unit includes a motoneurone and all of the muscle fibres that it innervates, and is the basic functional unit of the neuromotor system (Henneman & Olson 1965). Although much is known about the physiological properties of individual motor units and the biochemical characteristics of their constituent fibres (Burke & Edgerton 1975; Burke 1981; Enoka 1995), relatively little data are available concerning the architectural properties of these neuromuscular elements. We have recently published a review describing some of these motor unit and fibre features (Monti *et al.* 2001) and the key points are summarized below.

Motor unit territories

The fibres belonging to a single motor unit are localized within a region of the muscle cross-section. In addition, the extent of the dispersion of the fibres appears to be motor unit type and muscle specific. For example, the motor unit territories within the cat tibialis anterior muscle range from 8 to 24%: slow motor units usually have smaller territories than fast motor units (Bodine *et al.* 1988). In the exclusively slow cat soleus muscle, the territories are somewhat larger, ranging from 41 to 76% of the muscle cross-section. In general, other data on motor unit territory size in mammalian skeletal muscles are consistent with these findings (see Monti *et al.* 2001).

Spatial distribution of motor unit fibres

A common feature of all motor units in control adult animals is that the fibres innervated by a motoneurone are intermingled with fibres innervated by other motoneurones. This arrangement is clearly shown in glycogen-depleted motor units (Fig. 8.1; Bodine *et al.* 1988; Bodine-Fowler *et al.* 1990; Ounjian *et al.* 1991; Bodine-Fowler *et al.* 1993). A number of spatial distribution analyses indicate that: (i) there is little tendency for individual fibres within a motor unit to group or disperse, i.e. the distribution is not different from random; and (ii) motor unit fibres are arranged in small subclusters probably reflecting fibres innervated by a primary branch of the axonal tree. These spatial properties seem to have been established during the innervation process during development (Pfeiffer & Friede 1985; Dahm & Landmesser 1988). Based on electromyographic mapping techniques, the arrangement of motor units in human muscles appears to be similar to that described above (Stalberg 1980; Stalberg & Antoni 1980). However, it is important to note that the spatial distribution of motor units in some species are quite different, e.g. avian flight muscles, and may have unique functional significance (Sokoloff *et al.* 1998; Sokoloff & Goslow 1999).

Motor unit muscle fibre shapes and location within a muscle

The use of maceration techniques to isolate and of glycogen depletion and microinjection of dyes to reconstruct individual fibres within a muscle have provided the following information: (i) there is a wide range of fibre lengths as well as a high percentage of fibres that end intrafascicularly within a muscle (Loeb *et al.* 1987; Chanaud *et al.* 1991; Ounjian *et al.* 1991; Trotter *et al.* 1995; Young *et al.* 2000); and (ii) muscle fibres can have a variety of shapes: e.g. the cross-sectional area of a fibre can be relatively consistent along its entire length or it can taper, i.e. show a decrease in fibre cross-sectional area at one or both ends (Ounjian *et al.* 1991; Trotter 1991; Eldred *et al.* 1993a,b;

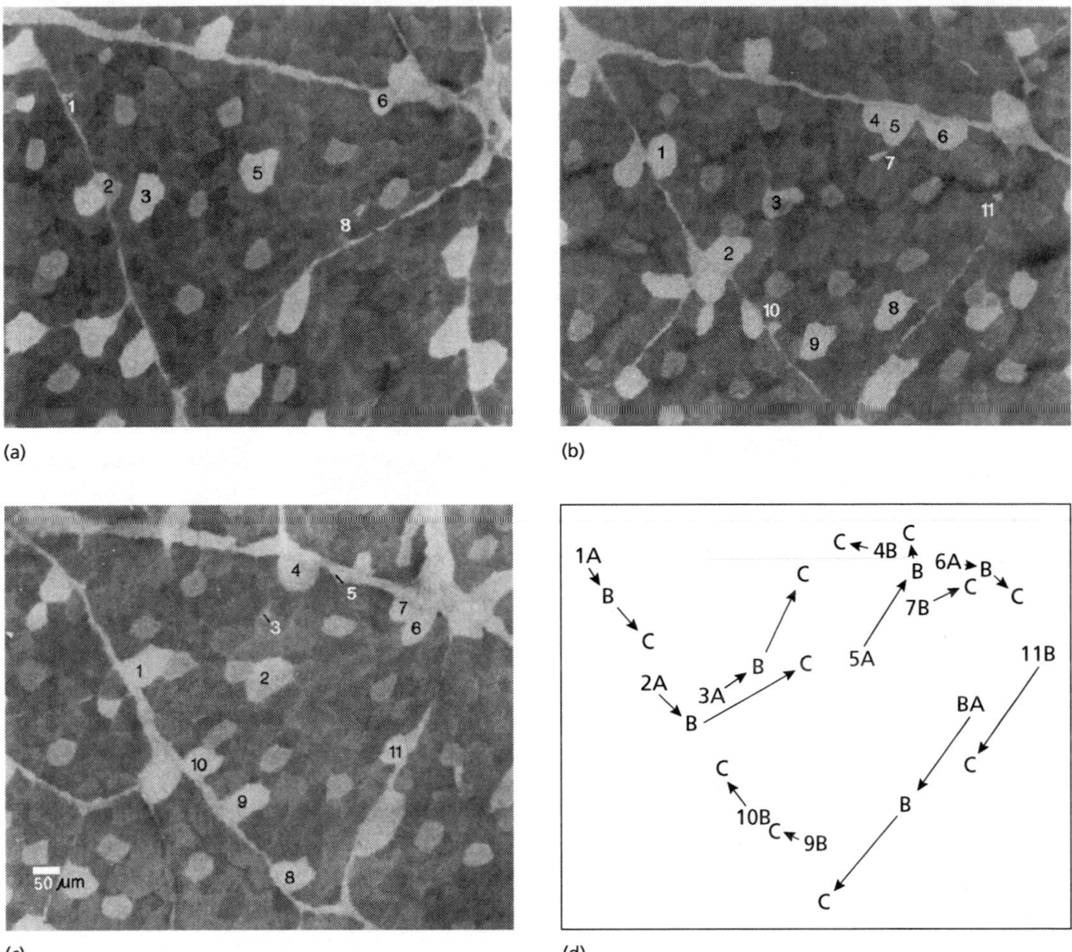

Fig. 8.1 Photomicrographs illustrating the contrast between depleted and surrounding non-depleted fibres of fast, fatigable motor unit at three levels along the muscle, i.e. 17 (a), 28 (b) and 37 (c) mm from the most proximal extent of the motor unit. Plotting of fibre movements was based on analysis of fibre positions observed on 27 selected sections along the length of the fascicle. The histological sections were stained for glycogen by the periodic acid–Schiff reaction and the micrograph taken of the grey-level image on the video terminal of an image-processing system. The bar represents 50 µm. Changes in the relative position of several fibres in the three sections are illustrated in (d). Overlay of the micrographs was approximated by matching the angles described by tangential lines (not shown) drawn along the margins of the fascicle. Numerals identify the particular fibres and the letter indicates the histological section. (Taken from Ounjian *et al.* 1991.)

Trotter *et al.* 1995; Sheard *et al.* 1999; Sheard 2000; Young *et al.* 2000). Although limited data are available, based on glycogen depletion of single motor units and serially sectioning the muscle along its length, the motor unit territory (and thus the fibre shapes and location) along the length of a muscle can be reconstructed (Burke & Tsairis 1973; Burke *et al.* 1974; Kanda & Hashizume 1992; Roy *et al.* 1995). These data show that the territory of a motor unit (i) spans a portion, but not the entire length of the muscle and (ii) is restricted to a portion of the muscle cross-section. This arrangement is shown schematically in Fig. 8.2.

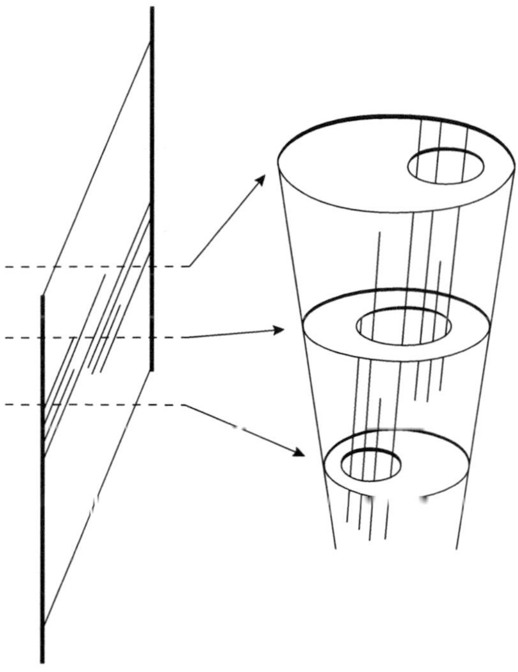

Fig. 8.2 Schematic representation of the territory of a motor unit along the length of a fascicle in a skeletal muscle. Note that the size of the motor unit territory changes along the length of the muscle and, in most cases, may reflect the number of muscle fibres at each muscle level. Muscle fibres can extend the entire fascicle length or end intrafascicularly. Fibres that terminate within the fascicle can have one attachment at either end of the fascicle or end intrafascicularly at both ends. The arrows identify the same muscle level represented by the discs on the right and the dashed lines on the left. Note that the location of the motor unit territory along the muscle length reflects the angle of fibre pennation.

Muscle fibre–connective tissue interface

Skeletal muscle fibres are connected along their length to the extracellular matrix. An extensive system of proteins is responsible for forming a linkage between actin filaments within the cell and the network of fibrillar proteins in the extracellular matrix (Fig. 8.3) (see Monti *et al.* 1999 and Patel & Lieber 1997 for a more detailed review of these proteins and their potential functions). These proteins are organized into a series of bands, called costameres, along the cell membrane (Pardo *et al.* 1983). The spacing of the costameres corresponds closely to that of the Z-line within the underlying sarcomeres, providing anatomical evidence for the role of these proteins in transmitting force across the cell membrane. The costameric proteins can be divided roughly into two groups. In the first group, actin binds to dystrophin, which in turn is linked to laminin-2 (merosin) in the extracellular matrix by a membrane-spanning protein complex. In the second group of costameric proteins, actin binds to talin, which links via vinculin to members of the integrin family of transmembrane proteins that in turn are bound to collagen and laminin-1 in the extracellular matrix. The recent description of clusters of membrane-associated proteins with connections to the extracellular matrix and to adjacent fibres is consistent with a role for these periodic membrane proteins in force transmission (Young *et al.* 2000). In addition, the morphological specializations of the cell membranes of intrafascicularly terminating fibres could function to reduce strains in the membrane relative to the underlying sarcomeres at the sites of force transmission. The discussion of the fibre–connective tissue interface will be continued in the next section.

Skeletal muscle connective tissue and elastic elements

Each muscle cell is enveloped by a basal lamina containing primarily type IV collagen, fibronectin, enactin and laminins. These collagen and laminin molecules provide linkages to transmembrane proteins as discussed above. Consistent with their role in mediating the linkage between muscle cells and the extracellular matrix, congenital deficiencies of members of the laminin family of glycoproteins cause unique types of muscular dystrophy (Wewer & Engvall 1996). The remainder of the extracellular matrix has been divided into three levels of organization based on its relation to the muscle fibres. The endomysium is contiguous with the basal lamina of the muscle cells. The perimysium is the thickened endomysium that circumscribes fascicles

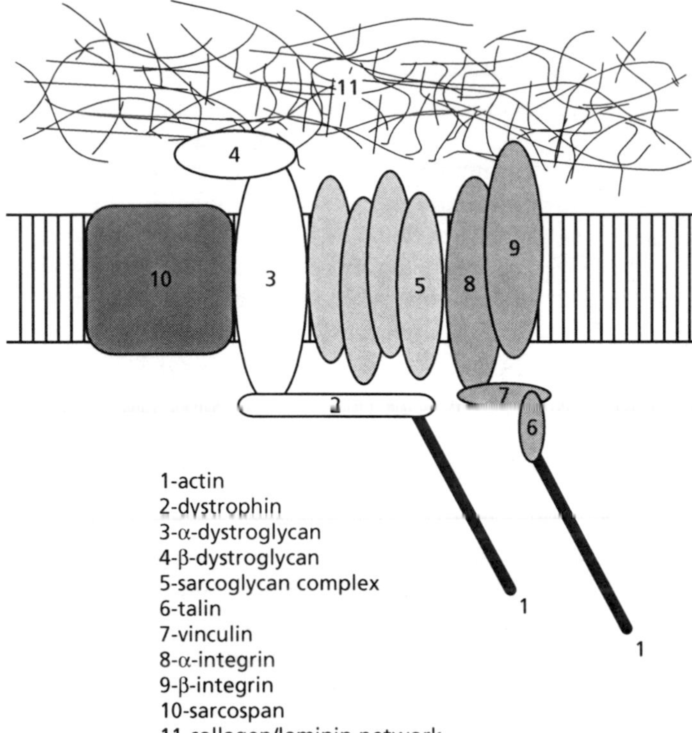

Fig. 8.3 Generalized diagrammatic representation of the protein pathways known or postulated to take part in force transmission to the extracellular matrix. Two chains of proteins have been identified that theoretically could serve this function. In the first, actin binds to dystrophin, which in turn binds to β-dystroglycan. Beta-dystroglycan is then linked to laminin-2 (merosin) in the extracellular matrix by α-dystroglycan. The sarcoglycan complex may function in stabilizing these associations. In a second chain of proteins, actin is bound to talin, which binds to vinculin. Vinculin binds to one of a family of integrins that bind to collagen and laminin-1 in the extracellular matrix. (Taken from Monti *et al.* 1999.)

of muscle fibres. The epimysium surrounds the outer surface of the muscle. These levels of organization are distinguishable primarily by their morphology (Borg & Caulfield 1980), rather than by their composition (Light & Champion 1984). All three are composed primarily of types I and III collagen. The endomysium and perimysium will be referred to collectively in the remainder of this chapter as the intramuscular connective tissue. Although it was originally described as a mesh of randomly orientated collagen fibrils when examined by electron microscopy (Borg & Caulfield 1980; Rowe 1981), more recent analyses have demonstrated that this intramuscular connective tissue is to some degree an ordered array (Purslow & Trotter 1994). At short muscle lengths the arrangement of the collagen is biased toward circumferential, and as muscle length increases the fibrils become increasingly orientated with the long axis of the muscle (Tidball & Daniel 1986; Purslow & Trotter 1994). A dramatic illustration of the three-dimensional structure of the intramuscular connective tissue can be found in Fig. 8.4. If the reader imagines this honeycomb of connective tissue extending to each end of the muscle, it is possible to conceive the muscle as a continuous tendon with muscle fibres embedded within.

What is the series elastic component (SEC)?

In a simple Hill-type model of skeletal muscle, the muscle–tendon unit is represented by a contractile element with elastic elements in parallel and in series (Hill 1938). Because of the potential for an elasticity in series with the contractile element to deform in response to loading and thereby store potential energy, this aspect of muscle modelling has received a great deal of attention. In general, the properties of the series elastic element are assumed to be dominated by those of the free tendon (Zajac 1989). While this is almost certainly the case for distal limb muscles with long tendons, the proximal limb muscula-

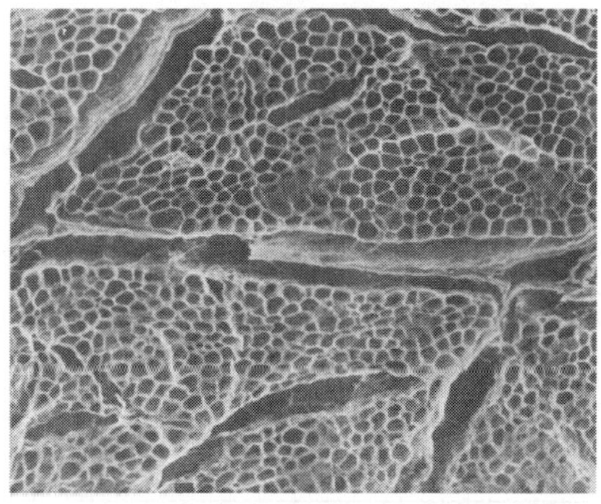

(a)

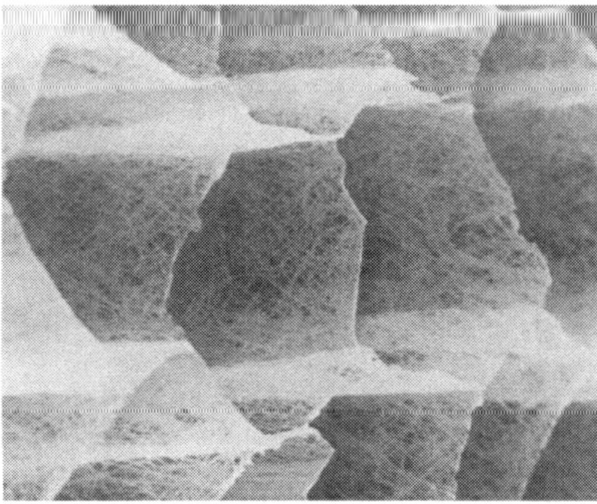

(b)

Fig. 8.4 Scanning electron micrographs of the transversely cut surface of bovine sternomandibularis muscle after sodium hydroxide digestion. (a) Low magnification (× 100) view showing endomysial connective tissue within fascicles separated by perimysial connective tissue. (b) Higher magnification (× 3200) oblique view of cut surface showing the endomysium separating (extracted) individual muscle cells. The planar feltwork of collagen fibrils in the endomysium reticular layer is clearly seen. (Taken from Purslow & Trotter 1994.)

ture frequently contains little or no anatomically identifiable free tendon. The gradation in the length of tendons proximodistally on the limbs indicates that there must be a gradation of their dominance in defining the properties of the SEC relative to the active contractile elements of those muscle fibres arranged in series and indirectly on surrounding fibres arranged in parallel.

What, then, constitutes the series elastic element in the more proximal musculature? Many muscles have a sheet of tendon-like connective tissue called an aponeurosis that serves as an attachment site for muscle fibres at one or both ends of the muscle. A role for the aponeurosis in storing mechanical energy has been suggested by Roberts *et al.* (1997) based on their work in running turkeys. In these animals the tendon of the gastrocnemius muscle is calcified over a portion of its length. Using sonomicrometry techniques they were able to establish that the muscle itself was isometric through much of the stance phase of locomotion. Therefore any work done by length changes in elastic elements would be done primarily by non-tendinous connective tissues like the aponeurosis.

A further potential source of elasticity is the intramuscular connective tissue discussed above. Because muscle fibres are effectively in series with the extracellular matrix through their lateral connections, deformation of this connective tissue may contribute to the series elasticity, perhaps significantly in muscle with no free tendon. Tidball and Daniel (1986) demonstrated that single frog skeletal muscle cells stored more energy during passive, sinusoidal oscillations with the basement membrane intact than with it removed, implying the importance of the transmembrane proteins and extracellular matrix in storing elastic energy.

Tendon and aponeurosis length–force characteristics

The *in vitro* mechanical properties of isolated mammalian tendons have been well characterized. Bennett *et al.* (1986) tested tendons with a variety of functions taken from seven different animals including quadrupeds of different sizes, wallaby and dolphin. They found that all had similar Young's moduli (1.2–1.6 GPa) and failed at similar stresses. In addition, all had a similar capacity to store and return strain energy. This uniformity of tendon mechanical properties across species was confirmed by Pollock and Shadwick (1994), who demonstrated that the elastic modulus of tendons does not scale with body mass, but remains constant at ~ 1.2 GPa for 18 species with body masses ranging from 0.5 to 500 kg. In addition, they found no differences in the mechanical properties of tendons from flexors and extensors of the ankle joint, indicating that mechanical properties of tendinous tissues are not specialized with respect to the function of the attached muscle. One specialized system where this general pattern may not hold true is the human wrist and hand (Loren & Lieber 1995).

The moduli reported above, however, are tangent moduli taken from the linear portion of the stress–strain curves for these tendons. By contrast, the cat soleus (Proske & Morgan 1984; Scott & Loeb 1995) and frog semitendinosus (Lieber *et al.* 1991) remain within the early, non-linear region of their stress–strain curves throughout a range of forces up to the maximum that the muscle can produce. Therefore, the use of a Young's modulus from the linear portion of a stress–strain curve may result in an underestimate of tendon extension during a movement, particularly at low levels of recruitment.

There is no clear consensus on aponeurosis properties, or on the relationship between tendon and aponeurosis properties, in the literature. Rack and Westbury (1984) noted that the total stiffness of the connective tissue of the cat soleus was 3–5 times less than that of the free tendon measured in isolation, indicating that the tendon was much stiffer than other connective tissue elements (i.e. the aponeurosis). Other reports in a variety of species have also indicated differences in the relative mechanical properties of tendon and aponeurosis. In human tibialis anterior, tendon strain is approximately 3 times aponeurosis strain during maximum voluntary contraction (Maganaris & Paul 2000) and in frog semitendinosus is approximately 4 times higher at a passive load equal to maximum tetanic tension (P_0) (Lieber *et al.* 1991). However, some reports have indicated that tendon and aponeurosis have similar mechanical properties. Trestik and Lieber (1993) reported a 2% strain in both tendon and aponeurosis of frog gastrocnemius passively loaded to P_0. Aponeurosis and tendon also have similar stiffness in cat soleus during tetanic contractions (Scott & Loeb 1995). It should be noted that the methods used in studies reporting both similar and different properties for the tendon and aponeurosis include passive and active loads and thus the results cannot be attributed to differences in the method used to load the tissue.

We have studied the rat soleus muscle in an effort to understand the mechanical properties of its aponeurosis and tendon under loads approximating in pattern and magnitude to those encountered *in vivo*. The muscle was contracted by stimulating ventral root filaments, allowing different fractions of the total muscle fibre population to be recruited. Strains were measured by using X-ray videography to visualize small metal particles embedded in the tissues of interest. Figure 8.5 presents the results of these measurements for the free tendon and for the proximal and distal halves of the aponeurosis. The slopes of these lines, while not representing stiffness in its purest sense, represent the load–deformation relationship for the different areas of interest. No significant differences were found in the slopes of these lines across the different regions. Thus, in the rat soleus, the properties of the aponeurosis and tendon are similar.

In some muscles, the stiffness of the aponeurosis also may be non-uniform along its length. During single loading events, strain in the portion of the aponeurosis furthest from the tendon has been reported to be 5 times greater than in the portion closest to the tendon in the rat medial gastrocnemius (Zuurbier *et al.* 1994). The relative strain of the muscular end of the aponeurosis is also 3 times greater than that of the tendinous end in frog semitendinosus (Trestik & Lieber 1993) and human tibialis anterior (Maganaris & Paul 2000). Thus, not only do the properties of tendon and aponeurosis seem to vary relative to one another, but the mechanical properties of the aponeurosis also may vary along its length.

It can be seen again in Fig. 8.5 that the two regions of the aponeurosis exhibit nearly identical

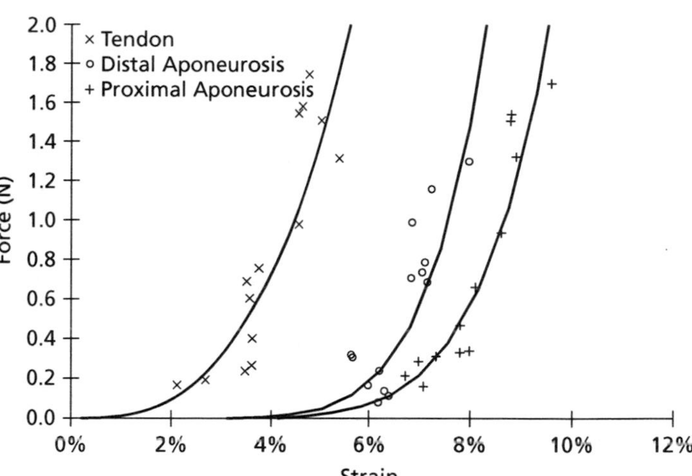

Fig. 8.5 Force–strain plots for the tendon and proximal and distal halves of the aponeurosis of the rat soleus muscle are shown. Strain was measured using X-ray videography during contraction of different subsets of the muscle fibres. The slope of the lines drawn through each set of points is the stiffness of that tissue. The slopes for these three tissues are not different ($P > 0.20$), indicating that all have similar stiffnesses when loaded by muscle stimulation.

stiffness. Thus, within the range of animals discussed here, the mechanical properties of the rat soleus appear highly uniform. This range of properties, from uniform to as much as fivefold variation, across species emphasizes the importance of accurately characterizing individual muscle–tendon units rather than applying average properties derived from a variety of muscles and species. This is especially true when attempting to develop accurate mathematical models of the *in vivo* function of particular muscles.

Skeletal muscle physiology and function

Force transmission

INTEGRATION OF SINGLE-FIBRE AND MOTOR UNIT FORCES

The organization of skeletal muscles into motor units and neuromuscular compartments raises the issue of how these various units interact within the muscle. If a muscle is fully activated, the importance of the mechanical interactions between these units cannot be defined. However, most movements involve the recruitment of muscles at submaximal levels. Thus, a clear understanding of the interaction between these organizational units, whether they are in a passive or an active mode, is important in defining the functional demands placed on the nervous system for controlling skeletal muscle.

One common theme to the interaction of both motor units and neuromuscular compartments is that they interact non-linearly. That is, the sum of the individual forces of two subunits activated separately is frequently different from the force observed when they are activated simultaneously. Both less than linear $[(A + B) < (A) + (B)]$ and more than linear $[(A + B) > (A) + (B)]$ summations of forces among motor units have been observed.

Early observations of less than linear summation during stimulation of whole ventral roots were taken as evidence that some skeletal muscle fibres are innervated by more than one neurone (polyinnervation), thus making them functionally part of more than one motor unit (Hunt & Kuffler 1954). By this explanation, the force deficit during simultaneous stimulation is due to overlap in the populations of muscle fibres innervated by each root. While this remains an accepted mechanism in amphibian muscles, subsequent studies indicated that it is not likely to play a role in adult mammalian skeletal muscles, particularly in the extremities (Brown & Matthews 1960). The principal explanation for non-linearities in mammalian muscles is the interaction of the contractile elements of the muscle fibres with the series elasticity of the muscle, particularly that portion of the SEC shared by most or all of the fibres (i.e. the tendon and aponeurosis). As more muscle fibres contract, the force applied to these elastic elements increases, leading to an increase in the internal shortening of muscle fibres. Thus, for movements starting at optimum length, as is typically done during *in situ* testing, the muscle fibres will shorten onto the ascending limb of their length–tension relationships, reducing their force output. In a recent study, Sandercock (2000) illustrated the role of this mechanism in non-linear summations. He stimulated two bundles of ventral roots, each innervating half of the cat soleus muscle. During contractions at a constant whole muscle length, he observed more or less than linear summation depending on muscle length. He then computed the extension of the SEC expected during the contraction of one half of the muscle, and used a servomotor to counteract the internal shortening of the fibres by lengthening the whole muscle–tendon unit by the computed amount. This movement produced a sharp reduction in the magnitude of the non-linear summation.

Non-linear summation has also been observed at the level of single motor units. Studies have included the cat soleus and medial gastrocnemius (Clamann & Schelhorn 1988), peroneus longus (Emonet-Denand *et al.* 1990), tibialis posterior (Powers & Binder 1991) and lateral rectus muscles (Goldberg *et al.* 1997). Again there is evidence that these non-linearities can be explained by the response of the SEC. Powers and Binder (1991) applied small step length changes to the tibialis posterior during tetanic stimulation of motor unit pairs, and found that steps as small as 50 μm significantly reduced the non-linearity of the interaction. When a single element (i.e. a motor unit or compartment) contracts, it shortens at the expense of the SEC. Contraction of two elements in series will increase the amount of internal shortening. As a result of this additional shortening, the two elements are at a shorter length when contracting together than when contracting alone, placing them on a different region of their force–length relationship. By eliminating the additional shortening, it is possible to reduce or eliminate the non-linearity of the interaction (Powers & Binder 1991; Sandercock 2000).

Until recently, there was no information on how motor unit type might affect the interaction of multiple motor units. Except for the predominantly slow cat soleus, this variable may play a role in all of the muscles mentioned above. Troiani *et al.* (1999) have studied type-identified motor units in the cat peroneus longus. Activation of pairs of slow and/or fast, fatigue-resistant (FR) motor units resulted in a total force in excess of the algebraic sum of the forces of the individual units for 75% of the slow and all of the FR and slow + FR pairs tested. In contrast, activation of different fast, fatigable (FF) motor unit pairs produced more and less than predicted forces in equal proportions. The ratio of measured to predicted force (deviation from linearity) for FF pairs was dependent on stimulation frequency, and was reduced from ± 60% to ± 12% with increased stimulation frequency (24 Hz vs. 72 Hz). It was also reported that the addition of FF motor units to a background of slow + FR units always resulted in less than a linear addition of force. For the FF pairs, contractions at higher frequencies will produce more force, and the motor units will be operating at a stiffer region of the stress–strain curve of the SEC. For mixed pairs, the difference may be due to differences in the force–length properties of different fibre types causing complex interactions among fibres on very different parts of the force–length curves. Alternatively, it may again be a result simply of differences in force production by the different units. For example, Stephens *et al.* (1975) demonstrated that apparent differences in optimum length between fast and slow motor units were not significant when small fast motor units were pooled with large slow motor units.

The architecture of individual fibres and motor units makes the interpretation of interactions among multiple motor units difficult. During submaximal actions the fibres in many motor units will be in contact with passive fibres from other units (Bodine *et al.* 1988). These inactive fibres, particularly those arranged in series, will function as a component of the elasticity

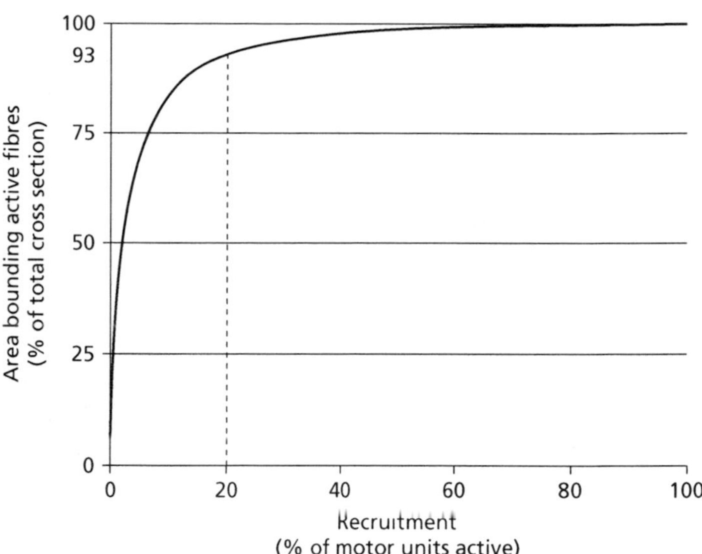

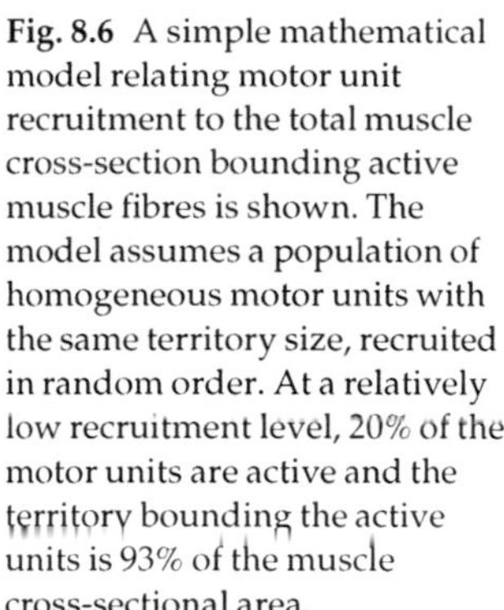

Fig. 8.6 A simple mathematical model relating motor unit recruitment to the total muscle cross-section bounding active muscle fibres is shown. The model assumes a population of homogeneous motor units with the same territory size, recruited in random order. At a relatively low recruitment level, 20% of the motor units are active and the territory bounding the active units is 93% of the muscle cross-sectional area.

experienced by the active motor units. As mentioned earlier, muscle fibres have a system of transmembrane proteins along their lengths connecting them to the extracellular matrix or directly to adjacent muscle fibres. These connections have been implicated in the lateral transmission of forces within muscle. More detailed reviews of this concept of lateral transmission of forces from sarcomeres and the cellular structures involved can be found elsewhere in the literature (Trotter 1993; Patel & Lieber 1997; Monti *et al.* 1999).

Direct evidence supporting the existence of a lateral pathway for force transmission is limited but compelling. Street (1983) demonstrated that both passive and active forces could be transmitted from fibres via linkages between sarcomeres and the cell membrane in bundles of muscle fibres. A few studies have extended her results to the whole-muscle level. Goldberg *et al.* (1997) excised a wedge of the cat lateral rectus muscle extending to a depth of approximately one-third of the muscle width. Despite this large interruption of the muscle fibres, whole-muscle twitch tension fell by only 5%. Thus, although 33% of the fibres of the muscle could not transmit forces along their length, almost no reduction in force production was observed. Huijing *et al.* (1998) have used tenotomy to interrupt the transmission of force from muscle fibres to the tendinous insertion. The rat extensor digitorum longus consists of four neuromuscular compartments, each inserting into a separate distal tendon. After three of the four distal tendons had been cut the force transmitted through the single remaining tendon was more than 80% of that produced by the intact muscle, indicating a well-developed internal mechanism for transmitting force through the intramuscular connective tissue to the remaining tendon.

The functional consequences of the integration of forces within the muscle were clearly illustrated by Proske and Morgan (1984). They split the tendon of the cat soleus muscle longitudinally, attaching each half to a separate force transducer. By stimulating various combinations of motor units they demonstrated that the fraction of the force transmitted to each half of the tendon remained nearly constant when the total muscle force was more than ~ 20% of P_0. For example, if the muscle was stimulated to produce 50% of P_0, both halves of the tendon transmitted 25% of P_0.

The theoretical basis for these observations is illustrated in Fig. 8.6. This figure illustrates the percentage of the muscle cross-section bounding active muscle fibres as a function of recruitment. The model used assumes randomly distributed motor units with a uniform territory size. Motor units were recruited randomly, and the total cross-sectional area of the territory described by the most widely distributed fibres was computed. At 20% recruitment, 93% of the muscle cross-section would be contained within the perimeter described by the most widely distributed muscle fibres. A mixed muscle containing a gradation from slow motor units with small territories to fast motor units with large territories would exhibit an even steeper rise in the percentage of the cross-section containing active fibres. Thus, it is possible that the connective tissue matrix of the muscle filters the mechanical interactions of motor units.

DIRECTION OF FORCE APPLICATION

The variations in fibre and motor unit anatomy raise the possibility that when activated in isolation, motor units may vary in the principal axis along which they produce force. This would, in turn, lead to a variation in the torque applied at a joint by different motor units of the same muscle. Not surprisingly, the degree to which motor units vary in torque direction depends on the morphology of the whole muscle. Sokoloff *et al.* (Sokoloff *et al.* 1997) examined 158 motor units from the cat medial gastrocnemius. They observed some variability in the torque direction of individual motor units when stimulated experimentally. However, when the muscle was activated reflexively in decerebrate animals, the torque direction for the whole muscle did not vary with the level of activation. Thus, when recruitment was accomplished by central nervous system activation, there was no systematic recruitment of motor units with respect to torque. This result indicates that, while some subtle variability may exist among motor unit torques in the cat medial gastrocnemius, this variability is not an important factor in determining the recruitment order of motor units.

In contrast, measurements of the line of action of single motor units in the rabbit masseter showed a wide variation, which was correlated with the physiological properties of the motor units (Turkawski *et al.* 1998). The grouping of motor units by function matched well with the anatomical compartmentalization of the masseter. Thus, the correlation between function and physiology was apparently the result of grouping of fibres of similar types into compartments. However, the observed function of motor units within each compartment agreed with the theoretical function of those compartments during movement of the jaw. Thus, in some muscles (e.g. the cat medial gastrocnemius) the torque applied appears to be constant as activity increases, whereas in others (e.g. rabbit masseter) the nervous system can recruit subpopulations of motor units to produce different movements. The potential functional significance of the force vectors of single motor units, either alone or in combinations, needs to be further addressed in future studies.

Interaction between contractile and elastic elements

FIBRE LENGTH VS. CONNECTIVE TISSUE LENGTH

As mentioned above, tendon lengths vary widely from proximal to distal in the limbs. There are benefits and costs to increasing tendon length, and these trade-offs play a large role in defining the function of a particular muscle *in vivo*. In proximal muscles, the ratio of tendon length to muscle fibre length tends to be relatively small. Thus, any joint displacement controlled by these muscles must be produced primarily by the muscle fibres. In return, the shortening of muscle fibres is reproduced as a movement at the joint. The series elastic element of these muscles is very short, and consequently they have very little capacity for participating in an elastic recovery of mechanical energy. In more distal musculature, tendon length to fibre length ratios tend to increase. These tendons are prime candidates for storing mechanical energy, and have been suggested to play this role in a variety of species

(Alexander 1984; Gregor *et al.* 1988; Griffiths 1989; Biewener & Baudinette 1995; Roberts *et al.* 1997; Biewener 1998). This elasticity could come at the expense of precision in controlling joint position because much of the force generated by muscle fibres will lengthen the tendons at the expense of muscle fibre shortening. The power output of these muscles will be sensitive to their position on their length–tension curves. It has been suggested that the net length of muscle–tendon units with this architecture may remain constant, while the tendon performs much of the mechanical work derived from the energy stored when the active elements shorten (Roberts *et al.* 1997; Biewener 1998). An interesting finding at the wrist joint is that the relationship between muscle fibre architecture and tendon dimensions is highly specialized so that there is a distinction between relatively stiff or compliant muscle–tendon units (Loren & Lieber 1995). This allows stiffer units to actively control joint position, while more compliant units resist perturbations in position by acting in part as shock absorbers.

Relationship between muscle architecture and *in vivo* function

The skeletal muscle structure–function interactions described in the previous section have a number of obvious clinical implications associated with skeletal muscle strain injuries. A fundamental issue is which tissue elements within the muscle–tendon unit architecture are actually 'strained' to the point of injury by exceeding their elastic limits. There have been two main approaches to solving this problem: (i) *in situ* animal studies with passive and active loading of the muscle–tendon unit to failure; and (ii) *in vivo* human and animal studies examining the distribution of strain within the muscle–tendon unit during routine movements.

Location of strain injuries

A major step toward understanding whole-muscle strain injuries has been through the determination of the biomechanical events that comprise a normal human muscle contraction *in vivo*. The fundamental questions are which tissues are strained during normal movement, i.e. muscle contraction; and what is the magnitude of the strain, i.e. their normal range of values? Most work attempting to determine the site of muscle strain injury has been performed using *in situ* animal studies in which the muscle–tendon unit was isolated and stretched to the point of failure: failure being defined as a rupture of the muscle–tendon unit identifiable by gross examination. Using a rabbit model, Garrett and colleagues have reported that the site of injury was found almost always to be within the muscle fibres immediately proximal to the myotendinous junction (MTJ) (see Garrett 1996 for a review). Failure never occurred in the tendon. This was true whether the imposed stretch was passive or active and occurred in muscles having vastly different architectural features, e.g. the tibialis and peroneus longus (fusiform), extensor digitorum longus (unipennate) and rectus femoris (bipennate) muscles (Garrett *et al.* 1988). Tidball *et al.* (1993) strained a whole-muscle preparation of the frog semitendinosus muscle–tendon unit with intact tendon–bone junctions. In both stimulated and non-stimulated muscles the injury occurred at the proximal MTJ, not the distal MTJ. With the aid of electron microscopy, they identified a difference in the site of injury depending on the state of activation of the muscle. When the muscle was not stimulated the site of injury was within the muscle at the proximal MTJ, whereas when the muscle was stimulated the injury was at the lamina lucida of the proximal MTJ.

Garrett and colleagues also have evaluated acute strain injuries in college athletes using computed tomography and/or MRI techniques (Garrett *et al.* 1989; Speer *et al.* 1993). The injuries were localized to the quadriceps, hamstrings, adductors and triceps surae muscle groups, and were associated usually with eccentric actions. In all cases, these imaging studies localized the disruption near the MTJ. As in the *in situ* animal studies, disruption never occurred in the mid-areas of the muscle fibres. Furthermore, the injuries were most prevalent in two-joint muscles (e.g. biceps femoris, rectus femoris and medial gastrocnemius) or in muscles having a complex architecture and function (e.g. adductor longus). Combined, all of these data clearly identify the MTJ junction as the site of the strain injury, and indicate that the susceptibility of a muscle to strain injury increases with the complexity of its architecture.

In vivo strain patterns

SONOMICROMETRY AND TISSUE STRAIN IN ANIMALS

One experimental method that has allowed investigators to begin characterizing the relative strains in skeletal muscle fibres and tendinous structures without relying on *in vitro* estimates of tissue compliance is sonomicrometry. Piezoelectric crystals are implanted into the muscle–tendon unit along the fascicle axis, and the distance between the two crystals is determined using the transit time of an ultrasonic pulse. Griffiths (1991) applied this technique to measure muscle fascicle strain in the cat medial gastrocnemius *in situ* during constant-length contractions, and *in vivo* during walking. He observed as much as 28% shortening with associated lengthening of the passive elements during the *in situ* contractions, but found that during locomotion muscle fibres only shortened by ~ 7%. The lateral gastrocnemius of freely running turkeys shortens less than 6% during the stance phase of a step (Roberts *et al.* 1997). Biewener *et al.* (1998b) studied the strain in plantaris and lateral gastrocnemius muscles of tammar wallabies and found that during normal movement these elements stretch and shorten by approximately 2 and 6%, respectively, which translated to 7 and 34% of the strain experienced by the tendons of each of these muscles. Thus, across a range of animals (including a quadrupedal walking mammal, a bipedal hopping mammal and a bird) tendon strains can be 3–10 times as great as muscle fascicle strains. This would imply that at the ankle joint, where muscles tend to have relatively short fascicle to tendon length ratios, the tendons and associated aponeuroses provide much of the displacement during locomotion.

Not all muscles, however, are designed to utilize tendon strain to generate displacement. During flight, fascicles in the pectoralis muscle of pigeons lengthen to 30–40% beyond resting fascicle length (Biewener *et al.* 1998a). This result fits the expectation for a muscle with very little tendon and long fascicles (see 'Fibre length vs. connective tissue length' above). Biewener and Gillis (1999) also examined the gastrocnemius muscles of mallard ducks and found significant shortening of the fascicles during both swimming (24%) and walking (37%). While these muscles are homologous to those in the cat and turkey discussed above, possessing relatively long free tendons, the morphology of the limb and the cycle rates encountered during swimming and walking may require the muscle fibres to actively shorten to provide displacement.

Taken together, these results indicate that muscle function is correlated with muscle–tendon architecture. As predicted from general architectural relationships, muscle–tendon units with long fascicles and short tendons experience higher strains in the muscle fibres. Muscle–tendon units with long tendons can tolerate higher total strains in their tendons than muscles with shorter tendons.

ULTRASONOGRAPHY AND TISSUE STRAIN IN HUMANS

One inherent limitation of the sonomicrometry technique is that it is invasive: crystals must be implanted in the muscle itself. Thus, to study strain in human muscles, investigators have developed other, less invasive, techniques. Fukunaga and colleagues (Fukashiro *et al.* 1995; Fukunaga *et al.* 1996, 1997a; Ito *et al.* 1998) used ultrasound techniques to study muscle fascicle and aponeurosis movement during an isometric muscle contraction in a single plane. They have reported muscle fascicle shortening of ~ 17% in the tibialis anterior with an associated tendinous stretch of ~ 7%. In the gastrocnemius, both fixed-length contractions and free movement have been studied. Both the tendon and aponeurosis of the gastrocnemius lengthen 5–6% during contractions at a constant joint angle (Muramatsu *et al.* 2001). These investigators have recently extended their results to include fascicle and tendon behaviour during vertical jumping (Kurokawa *et al.* 2001). They observed that fascicles shortened 26%, inducing a 6% lengthening of tendinous structures, during the early part of a jump (350–100 ms before toe-off). During the last 100 ms, the fascicles remained nearly isometric, while the tendon recoiled to its initial length resulting in a 5% shortening of the whole muscle–tendon unit. Thus, during a normal jump from rest, the human medial gastrocnemius muscle fascicles strain about 6%, similar to that seen in the animal studies discussed above.

MRI AND TISSUE STRAIN IN HUMANS

A particular type of MRI using a velocity-encoded cine phase contrast pulse sequence can provide another method of imaging the architectural changes which a muscle–tendon unit experiences *in vivo* and may provide some answers to the issue of the physiological range of strain of tissues in normal movements. In this method the protons within a given volume of tissue are coded for velocity so that their signal intensity (optical density) in the resulting image is a measure of the velocity of that volume of tissue. The displacements, and hence strain, of tissue can be tracked by multiplying a known time constant in between images with the known velocity from the optical density. Successive iterations of these calculations can be performed for each image taken at different phases of a muscle contraction to track the volume of tissue throughout the contraction.

The velocity-encoding technique has several advantages over other imaging techniques: (i) strain measurements can be made in regions that do not have the distinct anatomical features required to measure strains using ultrasound; (ii) tracking of strains at several phases of the isometric action is possible, thus allowing for the determination of different levels of motor unit recruitment; and (iii) imaging in all three anatomical planes, i.e. sagittal, axial and coronal, is provided so that tissue motion in three dimensions can be determined. This technique has proven to be a very effective non-invasive procedure for measuring both *in vivo* muscular and skeletal dynamics. For example, Drace and Pelc (1994) have used velocity-encoded cine phase pulse MRI sequences to track the motion of the muscles of the forearm during flexion and extension of the fingers and of the muscles in the posterior and anterior compartments of the lower extremity during ankle plantarflexion and dorsiflexion in humans. The images identified the most active muscle groups and showed the reciprocal motions of extension and flexion. Using the same techniques, Sheehan *et al.* (1998) determined the velocity profiles of the patella, femur and tibia during leg extensions. Their data indicate that patellar flexion lags behind knee flexion and that the patella tilts laterally and then medially as the knee extends.

Our laboratory is presently using the velocity-encoding technique to investigate the *in vivo* mechanical dynamics of isometric actions of the triceps surae at multiple locations within and among fascicles, aponeuroses and tendons at varying levels of recruitment. The lower extremity of the subject is immobilized in a fibreglass cast to maintain the knee at full extension and the ankle at 90°. The subject is asked to perform a submaximal isometric plantarflexor contraction in synchrony with a flashing metronome at a rate of 49 beats·min^{-1}. The torque generated is measured throughout the contraction via strain gauges attached to the plantar surface of the cast. Before beginning the contractions, a set of morphological fast spin echo images of the lower extremity are taken. These images are reconstructed in three dimensions so that the velocity and strain data from the phase contrast images can be superimposed upon the detailed architecture of the lower extremity. Examples of phase contrast images of the same sagittal section at different phases (Fig. 8.7) and at different sagittal planes (Fig. 8.8) are shown for an isometric contraction. The strain information obtained from

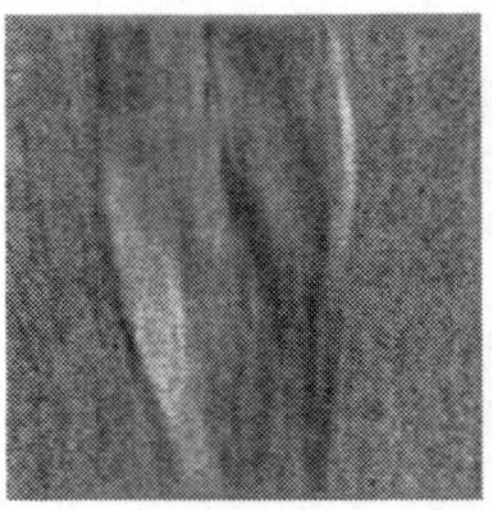
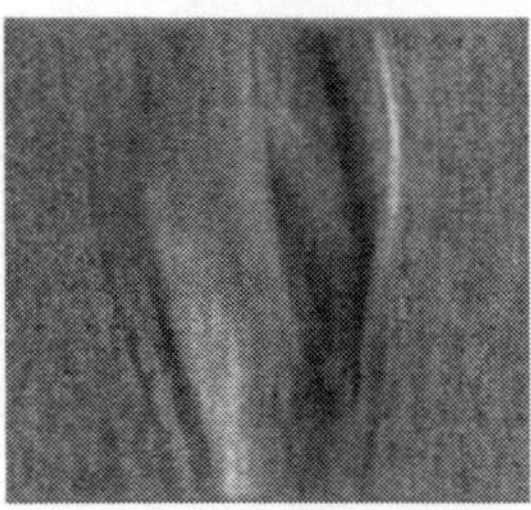
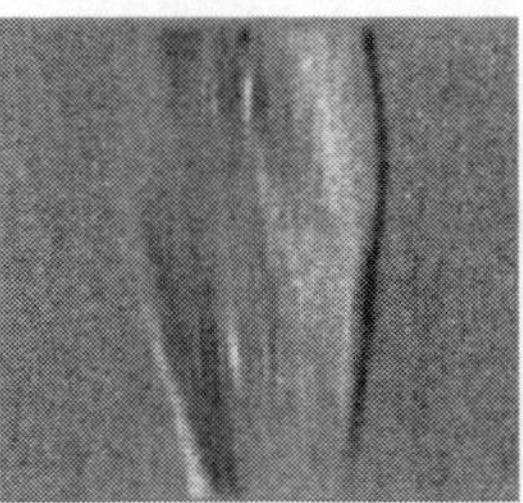
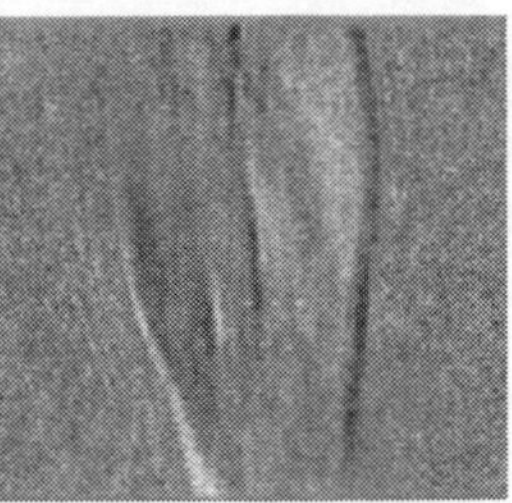

Fig. 8.7 Examples of the cine phase contrast images obtained using the velocity-encoded MRI pulse sequence. The optical density of each pixel is proportional to the velocity of the volume of tissue represented by the pixel. Each image is the same sagittal section of the leg of a normal subject during an isometric plantarflexion action. The left side of the image is anterior and the right side is posterior. The velocities and direction of the movement of a given point are reflected in the optical densities, with the lower scale of optical densities representing movement in one direction and the upper scale of optical densities representing movements in the opposite direction. Note the difference in velocities within and among the muscles of the anterior and posterior compartments. (A. Lai, S. Sinha, J. Hodgson & V.R. Edgerton, unpublished observations.)

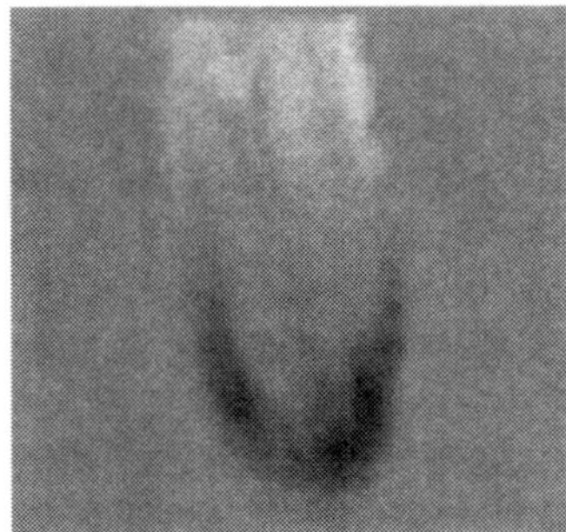
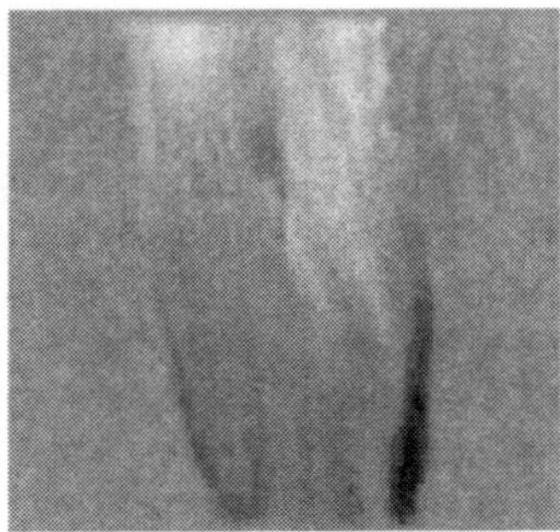
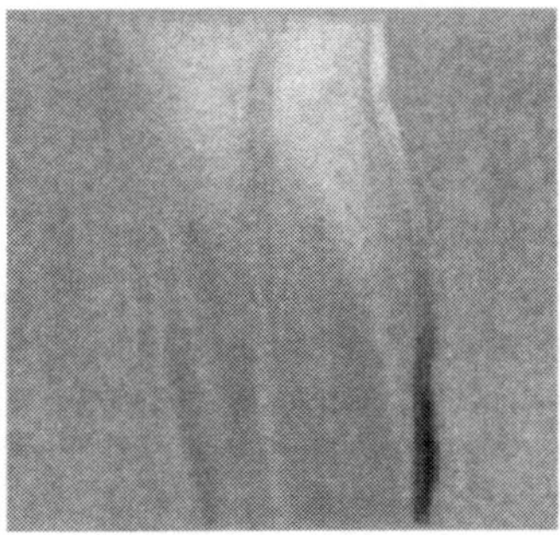

Fig. 8.8 Examples of the cine phase contrast images obtained using the velocity-encoded MRI pulse sequence at different sagittal planes of the leg of a normal subject during an isometric action. Left side of the image is anterior, right side is posterior. (A. Lai, S. Sinha, J. Hodgson & V.R. Edgerton, unpublished observations.)

the phase contrast images in the form of grid markings superimposed on the accompanying anatomical (magnitude) image illustrating the ability to identify areas of high strain during the contraction (indicated by the white arrow) is shown in Fig. 8.9.

Muscle architecture, strain injury and recovery from strain injury

Using velocity-encoding MRI and ultrasound it seems feasible, although very difficult, to begin to understand some of the mechanical interactions of multiple muscles within a group of muscle synergists during normal function. Furthermore, it appears that we will be able to reconstruct the dynamic strain properties of selected structures within and among muscles. For example, one of our initial goals is to define the level and rate of aponeurosis strain for the muscles of the triceps surae during normal contractions.

An understanding of the stress–strain dynamics of shortening and lengthening within a muscle complex during normal movements is a first stage in efforts to understand the aetiology of muscle strain injuries. We think that having the ability to measure strain injury is a prelude to (i) identifying the sites of strain injury; (ii) determining which strain properties of normal movements can lead to a strain injury; and (iii)

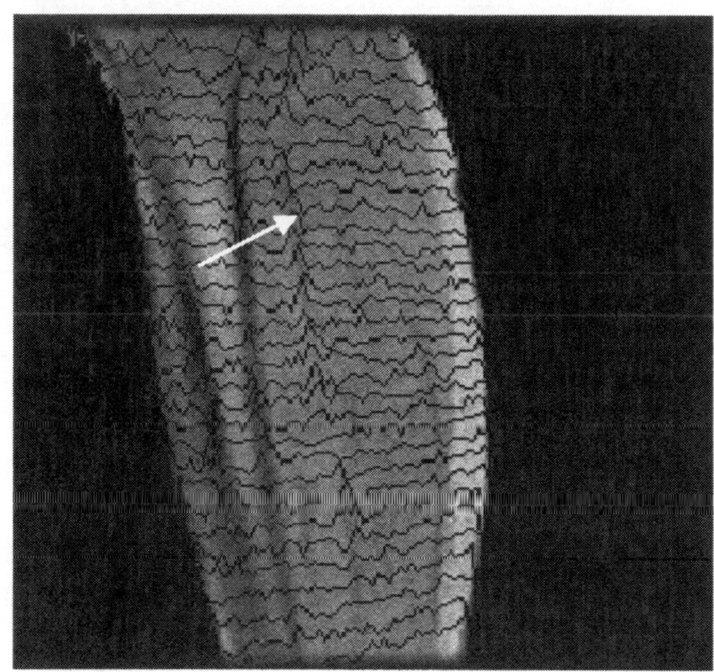

Fig. 8.9 An example of strains at the intersect points of a grid superimposed on a magnitude image taken in the same sagittal plane as the phase contrast image. The magnitude image provides anatomical detail of the leg. The strain grid represents the displacement of each pixel at different time points during the isometric action. The displacement is determined from the phase contrast images by using the velocity information from the phase contrast image and multiplying the known time constant between image acquisitions. Note the high amount of strain in the region of the posterior muscle compartment (indicated by the white arrow) at this point in the isometric contraction. (A. Lai, S. Sinha, J. Hodgson & V.R. Edgerton, unpublished observations.)

developing quantitative methods for following the course of and guiding the type of interventions needed in optimizing the strain properties during the recovery of neuromuscular function.

When strain injury occurs, if the tissues are indeed disrupted as is traditionally believed, then a remodelling process follows and most likely results in changes in the architecture of the muscle–tendon unit (Zarins & Ciullo 1983). The global stimulation of scarring within the muscle following a traumatic injury leads to changes in the properties of connective tissues, in particular the modulus of elasticity of connective tissue structures, within the muscle–tendon unit. Animal models of such injuries demonstrate that these processes alter the distribution and/or mechanical properties of tissues within the muscle–tendon structure (Stauber 1989; Lehto & Jarvinen 1991; Taylor *et al.* 1993; Noonan *et al.* 1994; Stauber *et al.* 1996). Therefore, a more quantitative understanding of the changes in strain of tissues during healing has tremendous clinical significance.

Acknowledgements

The authors thank all of our coworkers who contributed significantly to the work presented in this review. A large portion of this work was supported by NIH Grant NS16333.

References

Abe, T., Brown, J.B. & Brechue, W.F. (1999) Architectural characteristics of muscle in black and white college football players. *Medicine and Science in Sports and Exercise* **31**, 1448–1452.

Abe, T., Kumagai, K. & Brechue, W.F. (2000) Fascicle length of leg muscles is greater in sprinters than distance runners. *Medicine and Science in Sports and Exercise* **32**, 1125–1129.

Alexander, R.M. (1984) Elastic energy stores in running vertebrates. *American Zoologist* **24**, 85–94.

Bennett, M.B., Ker, R.F., Dimery, N.J. & Alexander, R.M. (1986) Mechanical properties of various mammalian tendons. *Journal of Zoology, London (A)* **209**, 537–548.

Biewener, A.A. (1998) Muscle–tendon stresses and elastic energy storage during locomotion in the horse. *Comparative Biochemistry and Physiology*, Part B, *Biochemistry and Molecular Biology* **120**, 73–87.

Biewener, A.A. & Baudinette, R.V. (1995) In vivo muscle force and elastic energy storage during steady-speed hopping of tammar wallabies (*Macropus eugenii*). *Journal of Experimental Biology* **198**, 1829–1841.

Biewener, A.A. & Gillis, G.B. (1999) Dynamics of muscle function during locomotion: accommodating variable conditions. *Journal of Experimental Biology* **202**, 3387–3396.

Biewener, A.A., Corning, W.R. & Tobalske, B.W. (1998a) In vivo pectoralis muscle force–length behavior during level flight in pigeons (*Columba livia*). *Journal of Experimental Biology* **201**, 3293–3307.

Biewener, A.A., Konieczynski, D.D. & Baudinette, R.V. (1998b) In vivo muscle force–length behavior during steady-speed hopping in tammar wallabies. *Journal of Experimental Biology* **201**, 1681–1694.

Bodine, S.C., Garfinkel, A., Roy, R.R. & Edgerton, V.R. (1988) Spatial distribution of motor unit fibers in the cat soleus and tibialis anterior muscles: local interactions. *Journal of Neuroscience* **8**, 2142–2152.

Bodine-Fowler, S., Garfinkel, A., Roy, R.R. & Edgerton, V.R. (1990) Spatial distribution of muscle fibers within the territory of a motor unit. *Muscle and Nerve* **13**, 1133–1145.

Bodine-Fowler, S.C., Unguez, G.A., Roy, R.R., Armstrong, A.N. & Edgerton, V.R. (1993) Innervation patterns in the cat tibialis anterior six months after self-reinnervation. *Muscle and Nerve* **16**, 379–391.

Borg, T.K. & Caulfield, J.B. (1980) Morphology of connective tissue in skeletal muscle. *Tissue and Cell* **12**, 197–207.

Brown, M.C. & Matthews, P.B.C. (1960) An investigation into the possible existence of polyneuronal innervation of individual skeletal muscle fibers in certain hind-limb muscles of the cat. *Journal of Physiology (London)* **151**, 436–457.

Burke, R.E. (1981) Motor units: anatomy, physiology, and functional organization. In: *Handbook of Physiology, Section I, The Nervous System, Volume 2, Motor Control* (ed. V.B. Brooks), pp. 345–422. American Physiological Society, Bethesda, MD.

Burke, R.E. & Edgerton, V.R. (1975) Motor unit properties and selective involvement in movement. *Exercise and Sport Sciences Reviews* **3**, 31–81.

Burke, R.E. & Tsairis, P. (1973) Anatomy and innervation ratios in motor units of cat gastrocnemius. *Journal of Physiology (London)* **234**, 749–765.

Burke, R.E., Levine, D.N., Salcman, M. & Tsairis, P. (1974) Motor units in cat soleus muscle: physiological, histochemical and morphological characteristics. *Journal of Physiology (London)* **238**, 503–514.

Chanaud, C.M., Pratt, C.A. & Loeb, G.E. (1991) Functionally complex muscles of the cat hindlimb. II. Mechanical and architectural heterogeneity within the biceps femoris. *Experimental Brain Research* **85**, 257–270.

Chow, R.S., Medri, M.K., Martin, D.C. & Leekam, R.N. (2000) Sonographic studies of human soleus and gastrocnemius muscle architecture: gender variability. *European Journal of Applied Physiology and Occupational Physiology* **82**, 236–244.

Clamann, H.P. & Schelhorn, T.B. (1988) Nonlinear force addition of newly recruited motor units in the cat hindlimb. *Muscle and Nerve* **11**, 1079–1089.

Dahm, L.M. & Landmesser, L.T. (1988) The regulation of intramuscular nerve branching during normal development and following activity blockade. *Developmental Biology* **130**, 621–644.

Drace, J.E. & Pelc, N.J. (1994) Measurement of skeletal muscle motion in vivo with phase-contrast MR imaging. *Journal of Magnetic Resonance Imaging* **4**, 157–163.

Eldred, E., Garfinkel, A., Hsu, E.S., Ounjian, M., Roy, R.R. & Edgerton, V.R. (1993a) The physiological cross-sectional area of motor units in the cat tibialis anterior. *Anatomical Record* **235**, 381–389.

Eldred, E., Ounjian, M., Roy, R.R. & Edgerton, V.R. (1993b) Tapering of the intrafascicular endings of muscle fibers and its implications to relay of force. *Anatomical Record* **236**, 390–398.

Emonet-Denand, F., Laporte, Y. & Proske, U. (1990) Summation of tension in motor units of the soleus muscle of the cat. *Neuroscience Letters* **116**, 112–117.

Enoka, R.M. (1995) Morphological features and activation patterns of motor units. *Journal of Clinical Physiology* **12**, 538–559.

Fukashiro, S., Ito, M., Ichinose, Y., Kawakami, Y. & Fukunaga, T. (1995) Ultrasonography gives directly but noninvasively elastic characteristic of human tendon in vivo. *European Journal of Applied Physiology and Occupational Physiology* **71**, 555–557.

Fukunaga, T., Ito, M., Ichinose, Y., Kuno, S., Kawakami, Y. & Fukashiro, S. (1996) Tendinous movement of a human muscle during voluntary contractions determined by real-time ultrasonography. *Journal of Applied Physiology* **81**, 1430–1433.

Fukunaga, T., Ichinose, Y., Ito, M., Kawakami, Y. & Fukashiro, S. (1997a) Determination of fascicle length and pennation in a contracting human muscle in vivo. *Journal of Applied Physiology* **82**, 354–358.

Fukunaga, T., Kawakami, Y., Kuno, S., Funato, K. & Fukashiro, S. (1997b) Muscle architecture and function in humans. *Journal of Biomechanics* **30**, 457–463.

Garrett, W.E., Jr (1996) Muscle strain injuries. *American Journal of Sports Medicine* **24**, S2–S8.

Garrett, W.E., Jr, Nikolaou, P.K., Ribbeck, B.M., Glisson, R.R. & Seaber, A.V. (1988) The effect of muscle architecture on the biomechanical failure properties of skeletal muscle under passive extension. *American Journal of Sports Medicine* **16**, 7–12.

Garrett, W.E., Jr, Rich, F.R., Nikolaou, P.K. & Vogler, J.B., 3rd (1989) Computed tomography of hamstring muscle strains. *Medicine and Science in Sports and Exercise* **21**, 506–514.

Goldberg, S.J., Wilson, K.E. & Shall, M.S. (1997) Summation of extraocular motor unit tensions in the lateral rectus muscle of the cat. *Muscle and Nerve* **20**, 1229–1235.

Gregor, R.J., Roy, R.R., Whiting, W.C., Lovely, R.G., Hodgson, J.A. & Edgerton, V.R. (1988) Mechanical output of the cat soleus during treadmill locomotion: in vivo vs in situ characteristics. *Journal of Biomechanics* **21**, 721–732.

Griffiths, R.I. (1989) The mechanics of the medial gastrocnemius muscle in the freely hopping wallaby (*Thylogale billardierii*). *Journal of Experimental Biology* **147**, 439–456.

Griffiths, R.I. (1991) Shortening of muscle fibres during stretch of the active cat medial gastrocnemius muscle: the role of tendon compliance. *Journal of Physiology (London)* **436**, 219–236.

Henneman, E. & Olson, C.B. (1965) Relations between structure and function in the design of skeletal muscle. *Journal of Neurophysiology* **28**, 581–598.

Hill, A.V. (1938) The heat of shortening and the dynamic constants of muscle. *Proceedings of the Royal Society of London Series B: Biological Sciences* **126**, 136–195.

Huijing, P.A., Baan, G.C. & Rebel, G.T. (1998) Non-myotendinous force transmission in rat extensor digitorum longus muscle. *Journal of Experimental Biology* **201**, 683–691.

Hunt, C.C. & Kuffler, S.W. (1954) Motor innervation of skeletal muscle: multiple innervation of individual muscle fibers and motor unit function. *Journal of Physiology (London)* **126**, 293–303.

Ichinose, Y., Kanehisa, H., Ito, M., Kawakami, Y. & Fukunaga, T. (1998) Morphological and functional differences in the elbow extensor muscle between highly trained male and female athletes. *European Journal of Applied Physiology and Occupational Physiology* **78**, 109–114.

Ito, M., Kawakami, Y., Ichinose, Y., Fukashiro, S. & Fukunaga, T. (1998) Nonisometric behavior of fascicles during isometric contractions of a human muscle. *Journal of Applied Physiology* **85**, 1230–1235.

Kanda, K. & Hashizume, K. (1992) Factors causing difference in force output among motor units in the rat medial gastrocnemius muscle. *Journal of Physiology (London)* **448**, 677–695.

Kearns, C.F., Abe, T. & Brechue, W.F. (2000) Muscle enlargement in sumo wrestlers includes increased muscle fascicle length. *European Journal of Applied Physiology and Occupational Physiology* **83**, 289–296.

Kurokawa, S., Fukunaga, T. & Fukashiro, S. (2001) Behavior of fascicles and tendinous structures of human gastrocnemius during vertical jumping. *Journal of Applied Physiology* **90**, 1349–1358.

Lehto, M.U. & Jarvinen, M.J. (1991) Muscle injuries, their healing process and treatment. *Annales Chirurgiae et Gynaecologiae* **80**, 102–108.

Lieber, R.L. & Friden, J. (2000) Functional and clinical significance of skeletal muscle architecture. *Muscle and Nerve* **23**, 1647–1666.

Lieber, R.L., Leonard, M.E., Brown, C.G. & Trestik, C.L. (1991) Frog semitendinosis tendon load-strain and stress-strain properties during passive loading. *American Journal of Physiology—Cell Physiology* **261**, C86–C92.

Light, N. & Champion, A.E. (1984) Characterization of muscle epimysium, perimysium and endomysium collagens. *Biochemical Journal* **219**, 1017–1026.

Loeb, G.E., Pratt, C.A., Chanaud, C.M. & Richmond. F.J. (1987) Distribution and innervation of short, interdigitated muscle fibers in parallel-fibered muscles of the cat hindlimb. *Journal of Morphology* **191**, 1–15.

Loren, G.J. & Lieber, R.L. (1995) Tendon biomechanical properties enhance human wrist muscle specialization. *Journal of Biomechanics* **28**, 791–799.

Maganaris, C.N. & Paul, J.P. (2000) Load–elongation characteristics of in vivo human tendon and aponeurosis. *Journal of Experimental Biology* **203**, 751–756.

Monti, R.J., Roy, R.R., Hodgson, J.A. & Edgerton, V.R. (1999) Transmission of forces within mammalian skeletal muscles. *Journal of Biomechanics* **32**, 371–380.

Monti, R.J., Roy, R.R. & Edgerton, V.R. (2001) Role of motor unit structure in defining function. *Muscle and Nerve* **24**, 848–866.

Muramatsu, T., Muraoka, T., Takeshita, D., Kawakami, Y. & Fukunaga, T. (2001) Mechanical properties of tendon and aponeurosis of human gastrocnemius muscle in vivo. *Journal of Applied Physiology* **90**, 1671–1678.

Noonan, T.J., Best, T.M., Seaber, A.V. & Garrett, W.E., Jr (1994) Identification of a threshold for skeletal muscle injury. *American Journal of Sports Medicine* **22**, 257–261.

Ounjian, M., Roy, R.R., Eldred, E. *et al.* (1991) Physiological and developmental implications of motor unit anatomy. *Journal of Neurobiology* **22**, 547–559.

Pardo, J.V., Siliciano, J.D. & Craig, S.W. (1983) A vinculin-containing cortical lattice in skeletal muscle: transverse lattice elements ('costameres') mark sites of attachment between myofibrils and sarcolemma. *Proceedings of the National Academy of Sciences of the United States of America* **80**, 1008–1012.

Patel, T.J. & Lieber, R.L. (1997) Force transmission in skeletal muscle: from actomyosin to external tendons. *Exercise and Sport Sciences Reviews* **25**, 321–333.

Pfeiffer, G. & Friede, R.L. (1985) The localization of axon branchings in two muscle nerves of the rat. A contribution to motor unit topography. *Anatomy and Embryology* **172**, 177–182.

Pollock, C.M. & Shadwick, R.E. (1994) Relationship between body mass and biomechanical properties of limb tendons in adult mammals. *American Journal of Physiology—Regulatory, Integrative and Comparative Physiology* **266**, R1016–R1021.

Powers, R.K. & Binder, M.D. (1991) Summation of motor unit tensions in the tibialis posterior muscle of the cat under isometric and nonisometric conditions. *Journal of Neurophysiology* **66**, 1838–1846.

Proske, U. & Morgan, D.L. (1984) Stiffness of cat soleus muscle and tendon during activation of part of muscle. *Journal of Neurophysiology* **52**, 459–468.

Purslow, P.P. & Trotter, J.A. (1994) The morphology and mechanical properties of endomysium in series-fibred muscles: variations with muscle length. *Journal of Muscle Research and Cell Motility* **15**, 299–308.

Rack, P.M. & Westbury, D.R. (1984) Elastic properties of the cat soleus tendon and their functional importance. *Journal of Physiology (London)* **347**, 479–495.

Roberts, T.J., Marsh, R.L., Weyand, P.G. & Taylor, C.R. (1997) Muscular force in running turkeys: the economy of minimizing work. *Science* **275**, 1113–1115.

Rowe, R.W. (1981) Morphology of perimysial and endomysial connective tissue in skeletal muscle. *Tissue and Cell* **13**, 681–690.

Roy, R.R. & Edgerton, V.R. (1992) Skeletal muscle architecture and performance. In: *Strength and Power in Sport: Encyclopedia of Sports Medicine* (ed. P.V. Komi), pp. 115–129. Blackwell Scientific Publications, Oxford.

Roy, R.R., Garfinkel, A., Ounjian, M. *et al.* (1995) Three-dimensional structure of cat tibialis anterior motor units. *Muscle and Nerve* **18**, 1187–1195.

Sandercock, T.G. (2000) Nonlinear summation of force in cat soleus muscle results primarily from stretch of the common-elastic elements. *Journal of Applied Physiology* **89**, 2206–2214.

Scott, S.H. & Loeb, G.E. (1995) Mechanical properties of aponeurosis and tendon of the cat soleus muscle during whole-muscle isometric contractions. *Journal of Morphology* **224**, 73–86.

Sheard, P.W. (2000) Tension delivery from short fibers in long muscles. *Exercise and Sport Sciences Reviews* **28**, 51–56.

Sheard, P.W., McHannigan, P. & Duxson, M.J. (1999) Single and paired motor unit performance in skeletal muscles: comparison between simple and series-fibred muscles from the rat and the guinea pig. *Basic and Applied Myology* **9**, 79–87.

Sheehan, F.T., Zajac, F.E. & Drace, J.E. (1998) Using cine contrast magnetic resonance imaging to non-invasively study in vivo knee dynamics. *Journal of Biomechanics* **31**, 21–26.

Sokoloff, A.J. & Goslow, G.E. (1999) Neuromuscular organization of avian flight muscle: architecture of single muscle fibres in muscle units of the pectoralis (pars thoracicus) of pigeon (*Columba livia*). *Philosophical Transactions of the Royal Society of London Series B: Biological Sciences* **354**, 917–925.

Sokoloff, A.J., Cope, T.C., Nichols, T.R. & English, A.W. (1997) Directions of torques produced about the ankle joint by cat medial gastrocnemius motor units. *Motor Control* **1**, 340–353.

Sokoloff, A.J., Ryan, J.M., Valerie, E., Wilson, D.S. & Goslow, G.E. (1998) Neuromuscular organization of avian flight muscle: morphology and contractile properties of motor units in the pectoralis (pars thoracicus) of pigeon (*Columba livia*). *Journal of Morphology* **236**, 179–208.

Speer, K.P., Lohnes, J. & Garrett, W.E., Jr (1993) Radiographic imaging of muscle strain injury. *American Journal of Sports Medicine* **21**, 89–95.

Stalberg, E. (1980) Macro EMG, a new recording technique. *Journal of Neurology, Neurosurgery and Psychiatry* **43**, 475–482.

Stalberg, E. & Antoni, L. (1980) Electrophysiological cross section of the motor unit. *Journal of Neurology, Neurosurgery and Psychiatry* **43**, 469–474.

Stauber, W.T. (1989) Eccentric action of muscles: physiology, injury, and adaptation. *Exercise and Sport Sciences Reviews* **17**, 157–185.

Stauber, W.T., Knack, K.K., Miller, G.R. & Grimmett, J.G. (1996) Fibrosis and intercellular collagen connections from four weeks of muscle strains. *Muscle and Nerve* **19**, 423–430.

Stephens, J.A., Reinking, R.M. & Stuart, D.G. (1975) The motor units of cat medial gastrocnemius: electrical and mechanical properties as a function of muscle length. *Journal of Morphology* **146**, 495–512.

Street, S.F. (1983) Lateral transmission of tension in frog myofibers: a myofibrillar network and transverse cytoskeletal connections are possible transmitters. *Journal of Cellular Physiology* **114**, 346–364.

Taylor, D.C., Dalton, J.D., Jr, Seaber, A.V. & Garrett, W.E., Jr (1993) Experimental muscle strain injury. Early functional and structural deficits and the increased risk for reinjury. *American Journal of Sports Medicine* **21**, 190–194.

Tidball, J.G. & Daniel, T.L. (1986) Elastic energy storage in rigored skeletal muscle cells under physiological loading conditions. *American Journal of Physiology—Regulatory, Integrative and Comparative Physiology* **250**, R56–R64.

Tidball, J.G., Salem, G. & Zernicke, R. (1993) Site and mechanical conditions for failure of skeletal muscle in experimental strain injuries. *Journal of Applied Physiology* **74**, 1280–1286.

Trestik, C.L. & Lieber, R.L. (1993) Relationship between Achilles tendon mechanical properties and gastrocnemius muscle function. *Journal of Biomechanical Engineering* **115**, 225–230.

Troiani, D., Filippi, G.M. & Bassi, F.A. (1999) Nonlinear tension summation of different combinations of motor units in the anesthetized cat peroneus longus muscle. *Journal of Neurophysiology* **81**, 771–780.

Trotter, J.A. (1991) Dynamic shape of tapered skeletal muscle fibers. *Journal of Morphology* **207**, 211–223.

Trotter, J.A. (1993) Functional morphology of force transmission in skeletal muscle. A brief review. *Acta Anatomica* **146**, 205–222.

Trotter, J.A., Richmond, F.J.R. & Purslow, P.P. (1995) Functional morphology and motor control of series-fibered muscles. *Exercise and Sport Sciences Reviews* **23**, 167–213.

Turkawski, S.J., Van Eijden, T.M. & Weijs, W.A. (1998) Force vectors of single motor units in a multipennate muscle. *Journal of Dental Research* **77**, 1823–1831.

Wewer, U.M. & Engvall, E. (1996) Merosin/laminin-2 and muscular dystrophy. *Neuromuscular Disorders* **6**, 409–418.

Young, M., Paul, A., Rodda, J., Duxson, M. & Sheard, P. (2000) Examination of intrafascicular muscle fiber terminations: Implications for tension delivery in series-fibered muscles. *Journal of Morphology* **245**, 130–145.

Zajac, F.E. (1989) Muscle and tendon: properties, models, scaling, and application to biomechanics and motor control. *Critical Reviews in Biomedical Engineering* **17**, 359–411.

Zarins, B. & Ciullo, J.V. (1983) Acute muscle and tendon injuries in athletes. *Clinics in Sports Medicine* **2**, 167–182.

Zuurbier, C.J., Everard, A.J., van der Wees, P. & Huijing, P.A. (1994) Length–force characteristics of the aponeurosis in the passive and active muscle condition and in the isolated condition. *Journal of Biomechanics* **27**, 445–453.

Chapter 9

Mechanical Muscle Models and Their Application to Force and Power Production

WALTER HERZOG AND RACHID AIT-HADDOU

Introduction

This is an interesting time to write a book chapter on force and power production in skeletal muscles and the corresponding mechanical models. Interesting, because the cross-bridge theory of skeletal muscle force production (Huxley 1957; Huxley 1969; Huxley & Simmons 1971) has dominated scientists' thinking on the mechanism of contraction for the past half century. But new techniques for determining the mechanical and biochemical events of single cross-bridge interactions with single actin molecules (Finer *et al.* 1994) have provided experimental results that do not fit the swinging cross-bridge model (Yanagida 1999). Therefore, the question arises, are these new findings incorrect, possibly caused by unresolved problems with a new technique; or are they correct, so that our conceptual thinking of how force is produced in a muscle must change. At the time of writing this chapter, the outcome of this ongoing debate is not clear.

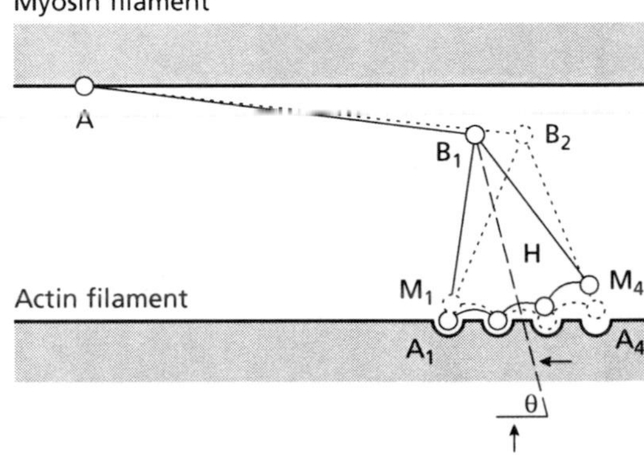

Fig. 9.1 Conceptual swinging cross-bridge model with a series of attachment states, as first proposed by Huxley and Simmons (1971). AB_1 represents the elastic connection of the cross-bridge head to the myosin backbone. A_1......A_4 and M_1.......M_4 are corresponding points of attachment for the actin with the myosin cross-bridge head, respectively. Note how the distance AB_1 is shorter than AB_2, therefore providing a change in the cross-bridge force (the elastic force transmitted by the AB_1/AB_2 element) without a change in the relative position of myosin to actin. Note further how in the 1971 model. rotation of the cross-bridge head occurs about its attachment site, whereas current thinking assumes a rotation about the neck region, with the attachment configuration fixed.

The traditional view of muscle contraction is associated with the swinging cross-bridge theory (Huxley 1969; Huxley & Simmons 1971). According to this theory, side-pieces (cross-bridges) from the thick (myosin) filament attach in a cyclical manner to specific binding sites on the thin (actin) filament. These side-pieces can be in several different attachment states (Fig. 9.1), and contraction (that is, force production and sliding of thin relative to thick filaments) is thought to be produced by a powerstroke of these side-pieces, i.e. a configurational change of the so-called neck region of the cross-bridge (Fig. 9.2). Although there have been competing paradigms of contraction (Iwazumi 1979; Pollack 1995), none of these has gained general acceptance.

With the emergence of optical tweezer methods and the refinement of atomic force microscopy

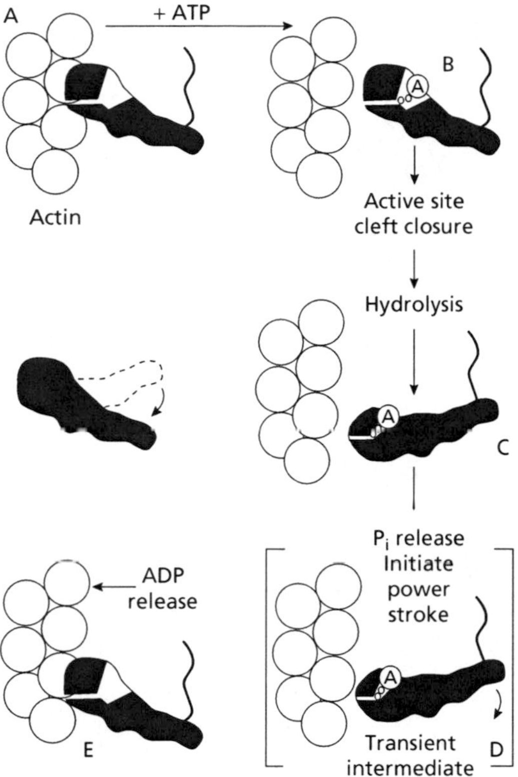

Fig. 9.2 Schematics of the mechanics and biochemistry of a cross-bridge cycle as envisioned by Rayment *et al.* (1993). Note here that the powerstroke is assumed to occur about a point in the neck region of the cross-bridge. Note further how one cross-bridge cycle is associated with one cycle of ATP hydrolysis.

(Finer *et al.* 1994; Kojima *et al.* 1994; Block 1995; Funatsu *et al.* 1995; Molloy *et al.* 1995; Nishizaka *et al.* 1995), it has become possible to study the interactions of single cross-bridges with single actin filaments. With these techniques, experiments can be performed that seemed impossible just a decade ago. The force and step size of a single cross-bridge stroke has been determined using laser tweezers and atomic force microscopy. Based on the traditional, swinging cross-bridge model, and the geometry of the cross-bridge head and its neck region (the part assumed to be responsible for the powerstroke), a skeletal muscle myosin step of about 10 nm is possible. However, step sizes of 11–30 nm have been reported (Yanagida 1999). Furthermore, reducing the neck length in skeletal muscle myosin by mutation did not reduce the step size, as one would expect based on the swinging cross-bridge theory (Yanagida 1999). Similar results in molecular motors other than skeletal muscle gave rise to the idea that contraction may occur, at least in part, through biased Brownian motion, usually referred to as molecular ratchets (Feynman *et al.* 1966).

Molecular ratchets work in a variety of forms; however, they all contain the element that the Brownian motion of molecules becomes directionally biased to cause transport of one molecule relative to another. Such a bias can be produced, for example, by local, asymmetrical potentials in which the molecule becomes trapped (Julicher 1999). The task of describing mechanical models of force/power production is difficult at this time, as the molecular events of force production are not well understood. However, this task is also exciting, as it allows comparison of traditional theories with theories based on new ideas.

With the above comments in mind, this chapter will start with considerations of various models: (i) the Hill-type models, which are based on A.V. Hill's (1938) classic work on the thermodynamics of muscle contraction, and which are still used to a greater extent today than any competing theoretical model in biomechanics; (ii) the cross-bridge models, which are based on the seminal works of A.F. Huxley (1957), Huxley (1969) and Huxley and Simmons (1971); and finally the ratchet-type models which have gained recent notoriety and, if nothing else, provide an actual physical mechanism by which contraction could occur, something that neither Hill nor cross-bridge models do.

Following a conceptual and mathematical description of these models, we will consider how the molecular mechanisms of contraction may translate into whole muscle properties. Finally, we will consider how whole muscle mechanical properties may be used to analyse and optimize athletic performance.

Muscle models

Hill-type models

'It is odd how one's brain fails to work properly when pet theories are involved.' This quotation from Hill (1970) describes his own feelings when scientific evidence suggested that his viscoelastic theory of muscle contraction was wrong. Gasser and Hill (1924) had assumed that the effect of contraction speed on the force exerted by a muscle was caused by an elastic network containing a viscous fluid. A contraction of the muscle with its corresponding change in shape would require the viscous fluid to flow relative to the solid tissue. An increase in the speed of contraction, and therefore an increased rate of change in muscle shape, would cause an increase in the viscous force which in turn would cause a decrease in the force that could be produced externally by the muscle to do mechanical work. Gasser and Hill (1924) believed that this viscous model accounted for most of the force–speed relationship observed in contracting skeletal muscle. If this belief was correct, one would expect that the amount of energy lost as heat during contraction should be proportional to the speed of shortening or lengthening as it represents the change in the viscous force with speed. However, when a muscle is stretched at a slow speed (so that it does not 'slip'), the rate of heat production is less than during an isometric contraction (Hill 1938). Furthermore, the total rate of energy liberation is greatly increased and decreased for concentric and eccentric contractions compared to isometric contractions, respectively. If the biochemical energy liberation during contraction was a 'muscle constant', and viscous fluid flow in an elastic network was to account for the changes in force with speed of contraction (Gasser & Hill 1924), then the above observations could not have been made. Therefore the viscoelastic model proposed by Gasser and Hill (1924) (a viscous fluid in an elastic network) cannot explain the energetic observations made on shortening and lengthening active muscle, and so, must be dismissed as a primary mechanism for the force–velocity relationship. This finding, however, does not imply that muscles do not have viscous or viscoelastic elements and properties.

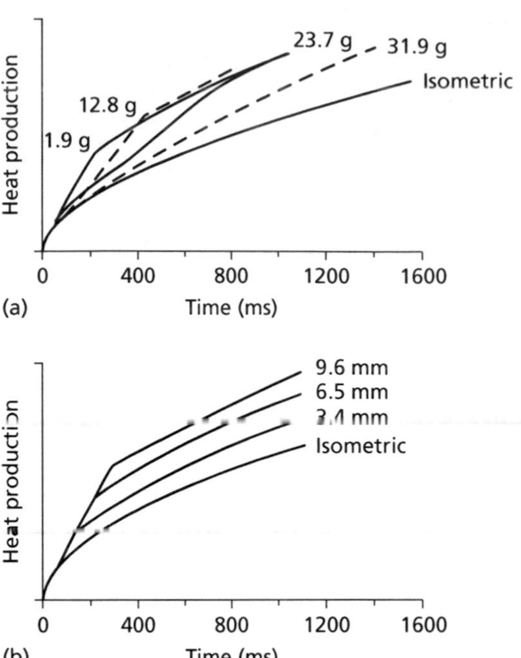

Fig. 9.3 Heat production as a function of time during shortening of tetanized frog skeletal muscle at 0 °C: (a) shortening a constant distance using different loads; (b) shortening different distances against a constant load. Note that the total extra heat produced (i.e. the heat above that observed isometrically) during shortening is approximately proportional to the distance shortened. (Adapted from Hill 1938.)

In his famous experiments on the heat of shortening of skeletal muscle which led to the formulation of the Hill model, Hill (1938) showed that a muscle produced heat during isometric contractions. When the isometrically contracting muscle was suddenly released under a load which allowed for shortening of the muscle, there was an increase in the rate of heat production that was proportional to the speed of shortening and stopped when the muscle stopped shortening (Fig. 9.3a). The total extra heat produced during shortening was proportional to the distance shortened (Fig. 9.3b).

When the size of the muscle is accounted for and the stimulation is constant (typically supramaximal), the shortening heat (H) can be expressed as $H = ax$, where x is the distance shortened during the contraction, and a represents a constant proportionality factor relating the shortening heat and the distance shortened; a takes the units of force.

The value of the constant a depends on the size, or more precisely the physiological cross-sectional area, of the muscle, and further depends on the level of activation. Hill (1938) showed that the value a/P_0 (where P_0 is the maximal isometric force) is reasonably constant (≈ 0.25). This result can be understood by realizing that P_0 (like a) depends on the physiological cross-sectional area and the level of activation (for P_0, the level of activation is maximal, by definition) of the muscle.

During a shortening contraction, a muscle produces extra heat (i.e. heat exceeding that observed during isometric contractions) and mechanical work. Since the extra heat (or shortening heat) is equal to ax, and the work is equal to Px (where P is the force of the muscle), the total energy in excess of that produced during isometric contractions becomes $(P + a)x$. The rate of extra energy liberation becomes $(P + a)dx/dt = (P + a)v$, where v is the speed of shortening.

Hill (1938) showed that the rate of extra energy liberation during shortening was inversely proportional to the load P applied to muscles in afterloaded shortening experiments. By definition, the rate of extra energy liberation is zero during isometric contractions, i.e. when $P = P_0$. Therefore:

$$(P + a)v = b(P_0 - P) \tag{1}$$

where b is a constant (in units of speed) which defines the absolute rate of energy liberation.

Hill (1938) rewrote eqn 1 as:

$$(P + a)(v + b) = (P_0 + a)b = \text{constant} \tag{2}$$

Another way of writing Hill's equation is:

$$P = \frac{P_0 b - av}{b + v} \tag{3}$$

Hill's equation may be verified by measuring the force (P) for different speeds (v) of shortening, or

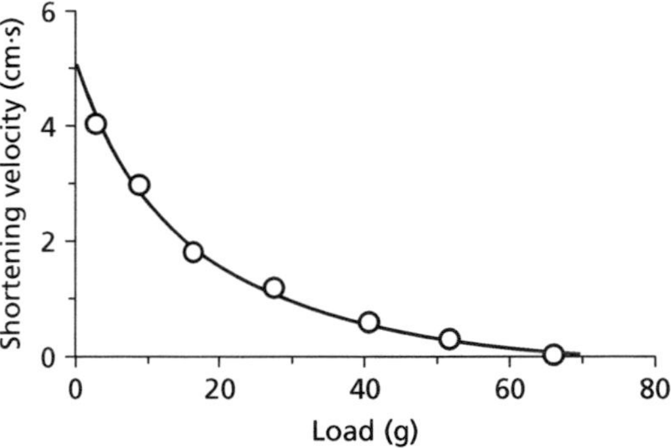

Fig. 9.4 Force–velocity relationship of frog striated muscle at 0 °C. The circles represent the mean of two experimental observations. The line corresponds to the equation $(P + 14.35)(V + 1.03) = 87.6$. Note here that the force–velocity relationship is not a continuous property, but is a discrete relationship of distinct data points. (Adapted from Hill 1938.)

by measuring the shortening speed for different loads exerted on the muscle. Note that this process does not require any heat measurements. Eqns 1–3 describe the loss of force with increasing speeds of shortening for a maximally stimulated muscle at (or near) optimal length. They represent a rectangular hyperbola with asymptotes of $P = -a$ and $v = -b$ (Fig. 9.4).

Based on the experimental work available in 1938, Hill (1938) concluded that skeletal muscle may be seen as a 'two-component system, consisting of an undamped purely elastic element in series with a contractile element governed by the characteristic equation $(P + a)(v + b) = \text{constant}$'. A standard modification of this idea is the introduction of an extra elastic element in parallel with Hill's two-element combination (Fig. 9.5). The contractile element (CE) is a device that introduces the force–velocity relationship 'through the back door', rather than obtaining it as a consequence of the combined behaviour of simpler elements. By the same back-door technique, Hill's CE (originally conceived to operate at the plateau of the force–length relationship) can be generalized to include the full force–length response. Such a generalized CE, to be used in the following model, is governed by an all-or-nothing activation parameter. In the inactive

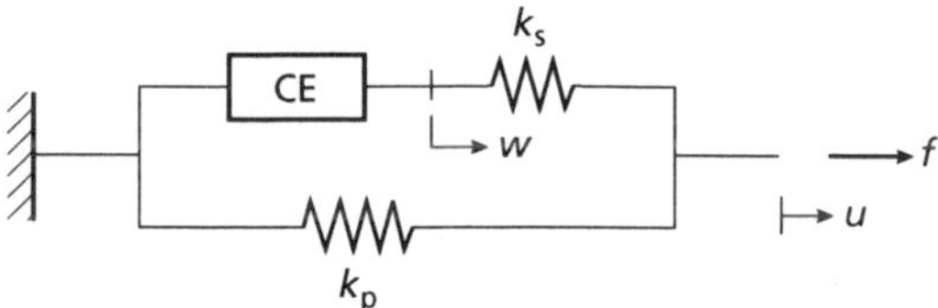

Fig. 9.5 Hill's model, consisting of a contractile element (CE), a series elastic element with stiffness k_s, and a parallel elastic element with stiffness k_p. Note that in Hill's model, the contractile element is endowed (phenomenologically) with the force–velocity (and sometimes even the force–length) properties of the target muscle. Thus, these properties are introduced not based on first principles, but rather through the back door with no explanation of mechanism or origin.

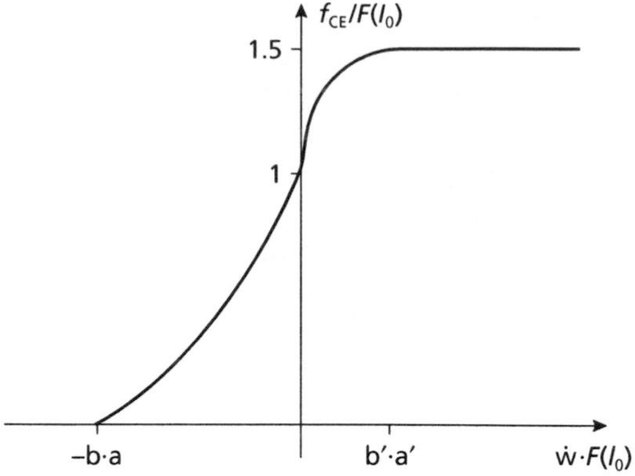

Fig. 9.6 Force–velocity relationship, as described in eqn 8.

state, the CE cannot sustain any force, and its length can be adjusted at will. In the active state, the behaviour of the CE may be described by the equation:

$$f_{CE} = f_{CE}(\dot{w}, l_0) \tag{4}$$

providing the force of the contractile element, f_{CE}, as a function of the speed of contraction $\dot{w}$ and the length l_0 of the CE *at the moment of activation*. This function can be related to empirical data as follows. Let the experimental force–velocity relationship be symbolically expressed as:

$$f_{exp} = f_{exp}(\dot{w}, F_{max}) \tag{5}$$

where F_{max} is the maximal isometric force at the plateau of the force–length relationship. For lengths other than optimal, the formula should be scaled down by the ratio $F(l_0)/F_{max}$, where $F(l_0)$ is the active force–length relationship evaluated at l_0. This scaling can be done in at least two different ways: by requiring either that:

$$f_{CE}(\dot{w}, l_0) = f_{exp}(\dot{w}, F(l_0)) \tag{6}$$

or that:

$$f_{CE} = \frac{F(l_0)}{F_{max}} f_{exp}(\dot{w}, F_{max}) \tag{7}$$

As an example of the former option, one may suggest formulae of the following type:

$$f_{CE} = \begin{cases} 0 & \text{for} \quad \dot{w} \le -F(l_0)\dfrac{b}{a} \\[2ex] \dfrac{F(l_0)b + a\dot{w}}{-\dot{w} + b} & \text{for} \quad -F(l_0)\dfrac{b}{a} < \dot{w} \le 0 \\[2ex] 1.5\,F(l_0) - 0.5\,\dfrac{F(l_0)b' - a'\dot{w}}{\dot{w} + b'} & \\ & \text{for} \quad 0 < \dot{w} \le F(l_0)\dfrac{b'}{a'} \\[2ex] 1.5\,F(l_0) & \text{for} \quad F(l_0)\dfrac{b'}{a'} < \dot{w} \end{cases} \tag{8}$$

where a, b, a', b' are constants. In the shortening range, the equation is a direct rewriting of Hill's law (except that the speed, $\dot{w}$, is considered positive in elongation). The overall appearance of eqn 8 is shown in Fig. 9.6.

To derive the equations governing this three-element model, let us agree to measure displacements, u, from the unique resting state corresponding to the unstretched length, L_p, of the parallel elastic element, and the initial length, l_i, of the inactive contractile element. The unstretched length of the series elastic element is therefore $L_s = L_p - l_i$. Let u_0 be the value of u at the instant in which the activation is applied. At that moment, the elongation of the contractile element must also be u_0, since the force in the series elastic element (and hence its elongation) will be zero up to the instant just before activation. Therefore, the length of the contractile element, at the moment of activation, must be:

$$l_0 = L_p + u_0 - L_s = l_i + u_0 \tag{9}$$

We conclude that the response of the three-element model is governed by the equations:

$$f = k_p u + k_s(u - w) \tag{10}$$

and

$$k_s(u - w) = f_{CE}(\dot{w}, l_0) \tag{11}$$

with l_0 given by eqn 9 and w denoting the elongation of the contractile element with respect to its length at the resting state of the system. Though not necessary, it is possible to eliminate the internal degree of freedom w by reading it off eqn 10, and by introducing the result in eqn 11 to obtain the first-order non-linear differential equation:

$$f - k_p u = f_{CE}\left(\left(1 + \frac{k_p}{k_s}\right)\dot{u} - \frac{\dot{f}}{k_s}, l_0\right) \tag{12}$$

If the applied force $f(t)$ is given, eqn 12 may be used to solve for $u(t)$, and vice versa. Naturally, appropriate initial conditions are to be specified in each case.

CRITIQUE AND POSSIBLE EXTENSIONS OF HILL'S MODEL

There is a subtle point hidden in eqns 10 and 11 that needs further elucidation. For definiteness, we assume that the function f_{CE} is given by eqn 8. Suppose that the muscle is fully activated at an initial length l_0, and is then stretched at a very slow speed (i.e. quasi-statically). According to eqn 11, we obtain (with $\dot{w} = 0$):

$$w = u - \frac{F(l_0)}{k_s} \tag{13}$$

and, by eqn 10:

$$f = k_p u + F(l_0) \tag{14}$$

In other words, the force increases linearly with the displacement, always with a positive stiffness equal to k_p. This is represented schematically in Fig. 9.7. Notice that the positive stiffness remains regardless of whether the initial length is on the ascending or the descending limb of the force–length relationship. This is an important feature of the proposed model, since it means that it is unconditionally stable. This feature stands in sharp contrast to models in which the force is made to depend on the instantaneous length directly, erroneously using the isometric force–length relationship for non-isometric conditions, thereby necessarily leading to instability in the (softening) descending limb. However, softening behaviour of muscle has not been observed experimentally. Quite in contrast to most modelling efforts, it has been shown convincingly that the above-proposed, stable force production on the descending limb of the force–length relationship is much more realistic (Edman *et al.* 1978; Edman *et al.* 1982) than the traditional assumption of instability (Zahalak 1997). In reality, it appears that the instantaneous positive stiffness upon active stretching is not constant, but depends on the initial length of the muscle at activation, l_0 (Edman *et al.* 1982). This feature can be incorporated into the above model by

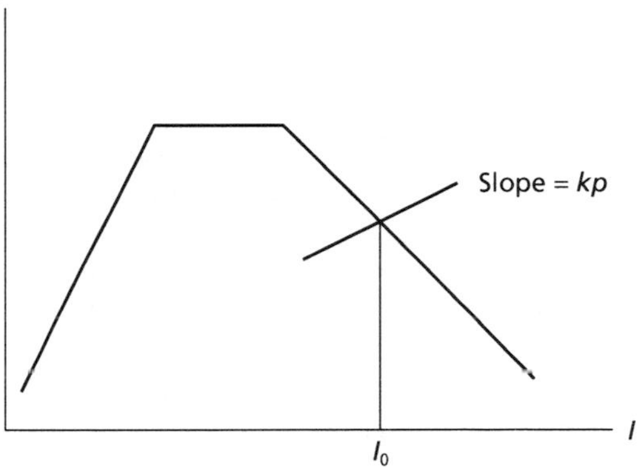

Fig. 9.7 Schematic representation of the force response of a Hill-type muscle model, as described in eqn 8. Note that the force increases linearly with stretching, always with a positive stiffness equal to k_p. This behaviour means that the muscle model is unconditionally stable, an important feature from a theoretical point of view, and likely to be a correct behaviour biologically (Edman *et al.* 1978, 1982).

introducing another parallel elastic element, but one that functions like an elastic rack that is engaged only upon activation (Forcinito *et al.* 1997).

Hill models describe the approximate behaviour of muscles for certain contractile conditions. They do not provide insight into the mechanisms of force production. Despite this limitation, Hill models are more frequently used in biomechanics than any other muscle model. Their success is associated with the mathematical simplicity of the model, and the qualitatively acceptable force predictions. The Hill model is likely to continue to play a major role in whole system musculoskeletal modelling, such as simulation of human locomotion. It has lost its place in research aimed at elucidating the mechanisms of contraction. Similarly, Hill-type models are not tremendously useful in gaining insight into optimal sport performance, as the important features of skeletal muscle contraction are either introduced through 'the back door' (e.g. the force–length and force–velocity relationships) rather than derived from a first principles approach, or are completely ignored (e.g. force enhancement, force depression, potentiation; Herzog 1998).

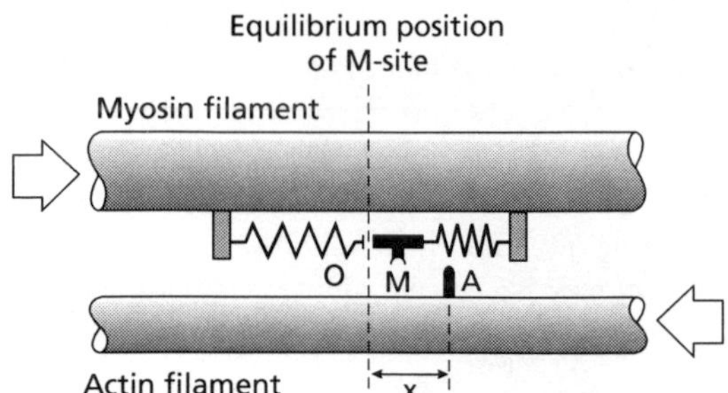

Fig. 9.8 Schematic model of the cross-bridge theory, as first introduced by Huxley (1957). The section shown represents a segment from the right side of a sarcomere with the nearest Z line to the right. The M and A-sites were assumed to combine spontaneously and, because of the loaded springs, the actin filament is thought to be displaced relative to the myosin filament, as indicated by the arrows. The x distance is defined as the distance from the M-site equilibrium position to the nearest actin attachment site, A.

Cross-bridge models

THE 1954 FORMULATION OF THE CROSS-BRIDGE THEORY

Before 1954, most theories of muscular contraction were based on the idea that shortening and force production were the result of some kind of folding or coiling of the myofilaments (particularly the thick filaments) at specialized sites. However, in 1954, H.E. Huxley and Hansen (1954) as well as A.F. Huxley and Niedergerke (1954) demonstrated that muscle shortening was not associated with an appreciable amount of myofilament shortening, and therefore postulated that muscle contraction is likely caused by a sliding of the thin past the thick myofilaments (the sliding filament theory). The mechanism whereby this myofilament sliding is produced was proposed by A.F. Huxley (1957), and is referred to as the cross-bridge theory.

In the cross-bridge theory (Huxley 1957), it was assumed that thick filaments had side-pieces which were connected via elastic springs to the thick filament. The side-piece with its connection point M (Fig. 9.8) was thought to oscillate about its equilibrium position (O) because of thermal agitation. M was assumed to attach to specialized sites (A) on the thin filament, if M came into the vicinity of A. The combination of M-sites with A-sites was thought to occur spontaneously, and was restricted to occur asymmetrically only on one side of O so that a combination of the M- and A-sites would cause a force (because of the tension in the elastic element constraining the side-piece M) and movement which tended to shorten the sarcomere. Attachment and detachment was thought to be governed by rate functions f and g, respectively, and f and g were modelled to be linear functions of the distance of A, the active site on the thin filament, to the equilibrium position, O, of the side-piece (the distance x, Figs 9.8 & 9.9). Since the combination of an M- with an A-site was taken to occur spontaneously, breaking the M–A connection had to be associated with an active, energy-requiring

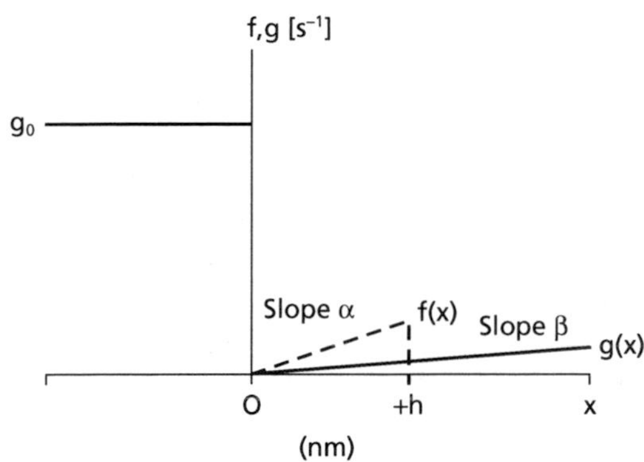

Fig. 9.9 Rate functions of attachment, f, and detachment, g, as proposed first by Huxley (1957) for the two-state cross-bridge model shown in Fig. 9.8. The rate constants were derived by Huxley (1957) in such a way as to fit Hill's (1938) force–velocity curves for frog striated muscle.

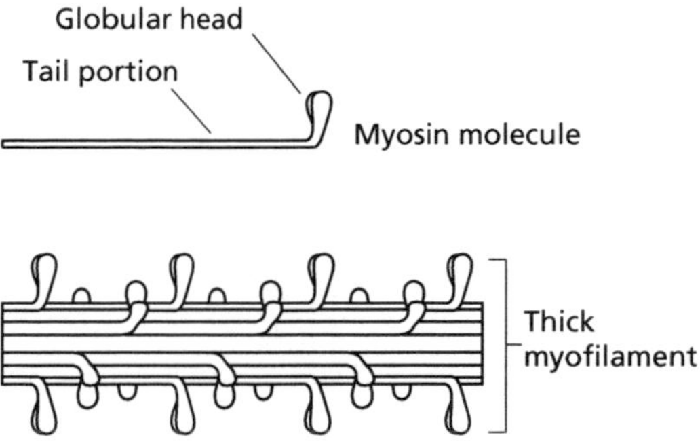

Fig. 9.10 Schematic illustration of the thick myofilament with its myosin molecules. The globular heads, sticking out in pairs, are thought to be the force-generating cross-bridges.

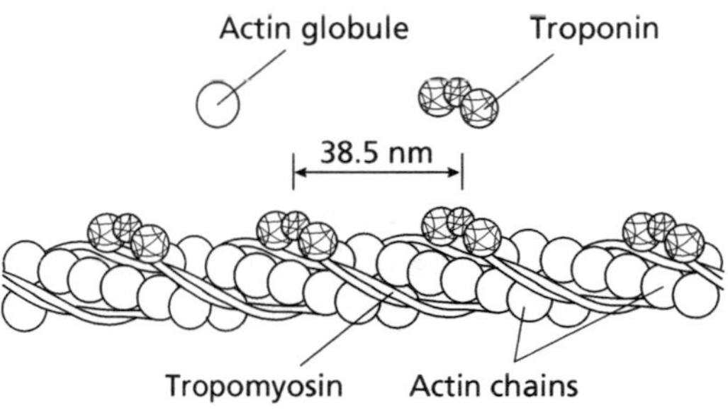

Fig. 9.11 Schematic illustration of the thin myofilament, consisting of two globular strands of actin that are helically interwoven, tropomyosin and troponin. Cross-bridge attachment sites are assumed to be present at intervals of about 38.5 nm.

process. The energy for this process was assumed to come from splitting a high-energy phosphate compound.

For force production to occur smoothly, it was assumed that there was a number of M- and A-sites for possible combination of the thick and thin filaments, which were staggered relative to one another so that different M- and A-sites would come into contact at different relative displacements of the two myofilaments. The M- and A-sites were further assumed to be so far apart that the events at one site would not influence the events at another site.

The cross-bridge theory, and its energetics, are assumed to be associated with defined structures. The M-sites are represented by the S1 subfragment of the myosin protein (the cross-bridge, Fig. 9.10); the A-sites are the attachment sites on the actin near the troponin (Fig. 9.11) and the high-energy phosphate supplying the energy for detachment of the cross-bridges is associated with adenosine triphosphate (ATP). Typically, it is assumed that one ATP is hydrolysed per full cross-bridge cycle.

Since a thick myofilament in mammalian skeletal muscle is about 1600 nm in length and contains cross-bridges along its entire length at intervals of about 14.3 nm (except for about the middle 160 nm where there are no cross-bridges), one-half of the thick filament contains about (720 nm : 14.3 nm) 50 pairs of cross-bridges offset by 180°, and each cross-bridge is thought to contain two heads for possible attachment on the thin filament. Since neighbouring cross-bridge pairs are thought to be offset by 60° (Fig. 9.12), there are about (720 nm : 42.9 nm) 16 side-pieces available on each thick filament for interaction with a given thin filament. Since a given thin filament interacts with three thick filaments (at least in mammalian skeletal muscles), each thin filament can potentially interact with about 48 cross-bridges. Assuming that during a maximal isometric contraction about one-half of all possible cross-bridges are attached at any given

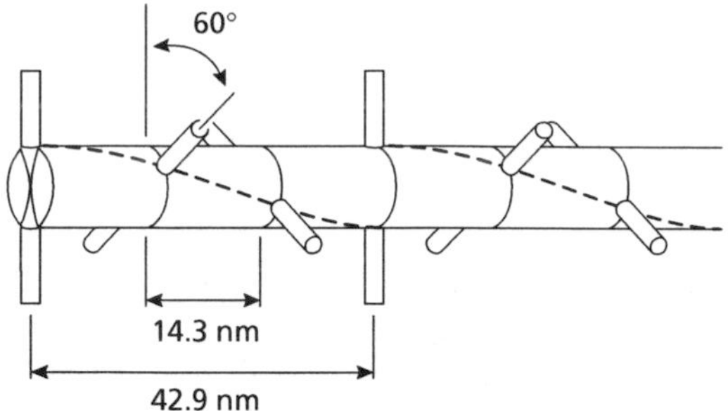

Fig. 9.12 Schematic representation of the geometrical arrangement of cross-bridges on the thick myofilament. Cross-bridges are thought to be offset by a linear distance of about 14.3 nm and a rotational distance of 60°. Since cross-bridges are thought to come in pairs, offset by 180°, two cross-bridges interacting with the same myofilament are separated by a distance of about 42.9 nm (3 × 14.3 nm).

instant (Woledge *et al.* 1985), it appears that a thin filament is never attached to more than about 24 cross-bridges, and typically (for submaximal levels of contraction and dynamic conditions) to much less.

In order to test the cross-bridge model of muscular contraction, Huxley (1957) compared the predictions of his theory (which were formulated in precise mathematical terms) with the experimental force–velocity relationship obtained by Hill (1938) on frog striated muscle during tetanic stimulation at 0 °C. Huxley (1957) found good agreement between the normalized force–velocity relationship of Hill (1938) and his own theoretical predictions. This good agreement was achieved by a careful choice of the rate constants of attachment and detachment (Fig. 9.9). It must be pointed out that these rate constants were not obtained based on any physical or biological reality, but were selected such that Hill's (1938) force–velocity relationship could be represented adequately. Therefore, the structural model of cross-bridge force production breaks down at the level of the description of the rate constants, where it becomes purely phenomenological.

When comparing the predictions of the cross-bridge theory to the properties of active muscle when it is forcibly stretched, several observations were made. Katz (1939) found that the slope of the force–velocity curve for slow lengthening was about 6 times greater than the corresponding slope for slow shortening. Huxley's (1957) theory also predicted this asymmetry in the force–velocity curve about the isometric point with a difference in the slopes of 4.33. Katz (1939) further found that the force produced during rapid lengthening of a stimulated muscle was about 1.8 times the isometric force. Using the rate functions given by Huxley (1957), the force for increasing speeds of lengthening approaches asymptotically a value of 5.33 times the isometric force. This value is much too large, and has proven to be unrealistic for any type of muscle tested to date.

Similarly, Huxley's (1957) theory does not predict well the heat production of a muscle that is stretched. From the theory, it is predicted that the rate of heat liberation increases linearly with the speed of lengthening, a prediction which vastly overestimates the heat production in lengthening muscle (Abbott & Aubert 1952; Abbott & Wilkie 1953). However, Huxley (1957) points out that the discrepancy between experiment and theory could be eliminated quite readily by assuming that during lengthening the cross-bridge connections were broken mechanically rather than released via ATP splitting. This assumption has been implemented in various models to account for experimental observations made during eccentric contractions (e.g. Cooke *et al.* 1994).

THE 1971 FORMULATION OF THE CROSS-BRIDGE THEORY

Another characteristic of muscular contraction which cannot be predicted adequately with the 1957 theory is the force transients following a quick length change. When a muscle is shortened rapidly, the force drops virtually simultaneously with the length change and then recovers quickly (Fig. 9.13). Two force parameters were defined by Huxley and Simmons (1971) for describing these fast force transients: they are referred to as T_1 and T_2. T_1 is defined as the minimum force achieved during the rapid shortening; T_2 is the

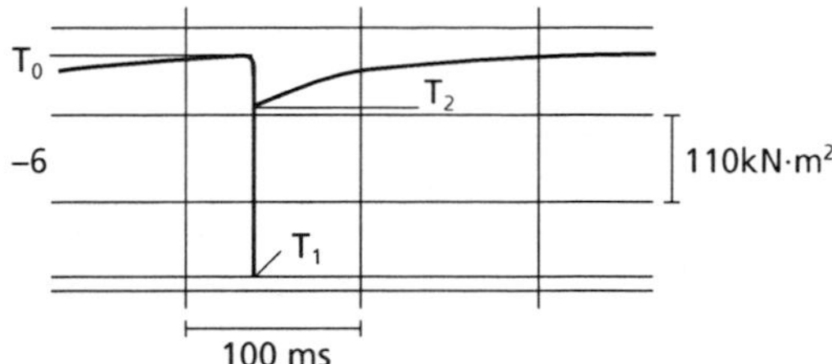

Fig. 9.13 Force-time transient for a sudden decrease in length by 6 nm per half-sarcomere imposed on an isolated frog muscle fibre during contraction at 0 °C. (Adapted from Ford *et al.* 1977.)

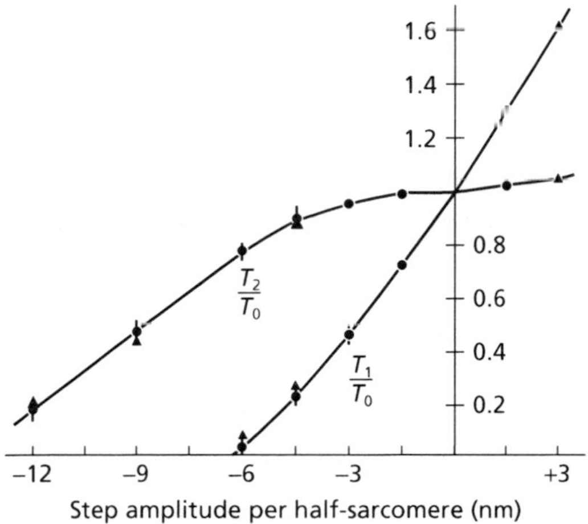

Fig. 9.14 Values of T_1 (the extreme force reached after a sudden length step; see Fig. 9.13), and T_2 (the force reached during the early force recovery following the length step) as a function of the magnitude of the step release. (Adapted from Ford *et al.* 1977.)

force at the end of the quick recovery phase (Fig. 9.13). T_1 becomes progressively smaller with increasing release distances, and was assumed to be linearly related to the release distance (Fig. 9.14). The T_1 vs. length step curve was assumed to represent the undamped elasticity of the contractile machinery. T_2 is always larger than T_1, indicating a force recovery within ms of the length step (Fig. 9.14).

In the 1957 theory, a cross-bridge was either attached or detached. When a fully activated muscle was shortened rapidly, many cross-bridges would detach during the shortening step, and force recovery was dependent on the

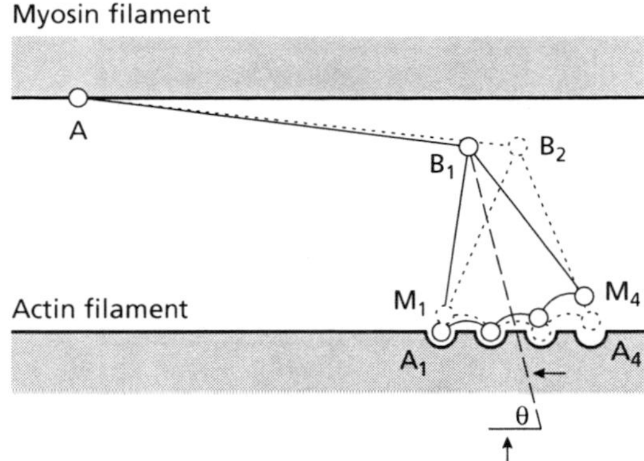

Fig. 9.15 Diagrammatic representation of a multistate cross-bridge model, as first introduced by Huxley and Simmons (1971).

rate of cross-bridge attachment. The rate function for attachment, however, was too slow to account for the quick force recovery. An easy way to remedy this limitation would be to increase the attachment rate of cross-bridges (Podolsky 1960). However, models with substantially increased rate functions for attachment could not predict Hill's (1938) force–velocity relationship as well as the 1957 model, and they could not fit the thermal data observed experimentally during shortening contractions (Woledge *et al.* 1985).

In order to account for the force transients following a stepwise length change and not to lose the good predictive power of the 1957 model, Huxley and Simmons (1971) introduced the concept of different states of attachment for the cross-bridge, thereby allowing the cross-bridge to perform work (while it is attached) in a small number of steps. Going from one stable attachment to the next was associated with a progressively lower potential energy. Furthermore, Huxley and Simmons (1971) assumed that there is an undamped elastic element within each cross-bridge that allows the cross-bridge to go from one stable attachment state to the next without a corresponding relative displacement of the thick and thin filaments. A diagrammatic representation of the 1971 cross-bridge model is shown in Fig. 9.15.

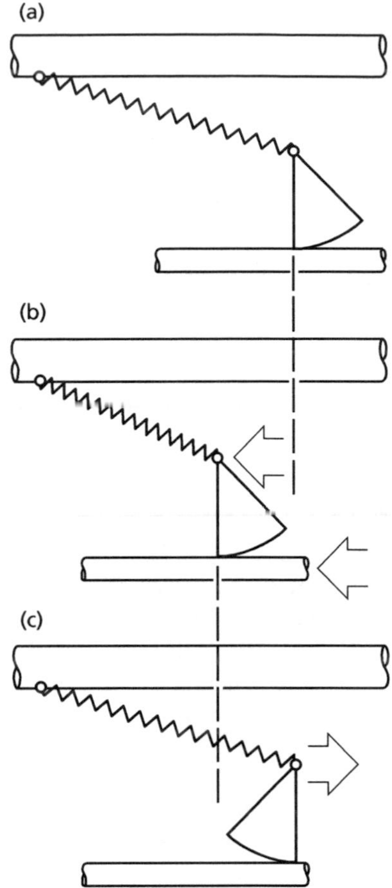

Fig. 9.16 Schematic explanation of the loss of force, and the quick recovery of force, during and following a quick length step (see text for a detailed explanation).

The force transients during a rapid length change are now explained as follows. If a muscle is released infinitely fast, there will be no rotation of the cross-bridge head (Fig. 9.16a,b). Therefore, the drop in force observed during the length step (T_1) corresponds to the force–elongation property of the undamped elastic element within the cross-bridge. Since it had been argued that the relationship between the T_1 value and the distance of the length step was virtually linear (the experimentally observed non-linearity was associated with the beginning of the quick recovery during the large length steps), the cross-bridge elasticity was assumed to be linear as well (2.3×10^{-4} Nm^{-1}; Huxley & Simmons 1971). Once the infinitely fast length step has been completed, the quick recovery of force is possible because of a rotation of the cross-bridge head from a position of high to a position of low potential energy, thereby stretching the elastic link in the cross-bridge, and so increasing the cross-bridge force (Fig. 9.16c). The superiority of the 1971 compared to the 1957 model does not only manifest itself in basic laboratory experiments, but appears to have very practical implications in sports activities. Imagine a sport like alpine skiing where the major working muscle groups of the legs undergo continuous, small length changes because of the vibrations generated by the ground on the skiis. If such vibratory length changes were associated with a continuous release and attachment of cross-bridges (the 1957 model) muscular force would be lost at a great rate. However, if such vibrations could occur without the release of cross-bridges (the 1971 model), forces would tend to fluctuate with the muscular vibrations around a steady value.

Huxley and Simmons (1971) discussed a cross-bridge model with three stable, attached states and derived equations for a system containing two stable states. Many further models with a variety of stable states have been proposed (Eisenberg & Greene 1980; Eisenberg *et al.* 1980) but the basic ideas of these models can all be traced to the 1971 cross-bridge model (Huxley & Simmons 1971).

The cross-bridge model, as discussed here, has dominated our thinking on muscular contraction for the past four decades. It does not account for all observed phenomena; in fact one might argue that it neglects some very basic phenomena, such as the long-lasting, history-dependent force production of muscle following stretch or shortening (Abbott & Aubert 1952; Edman *et al.* 1978; Maréchal & Plaghki 1979; Sugi & Tsuchiya 1988; Granzier & Pollack 1989; Edman *et al.* 1993). Therefore, it could well be that the cross-bridge model may be revised or replaced within the near future. However, at present, it represents the paradigm of choice and it will require strong evidence and convincing theory to replace it.

THEORETICAL FORMULATION

In the original version of the model, Huxley (1957) assumed that the myosin filament is endowed with 'side-pieces which can slide along the main backbone of the filament, the extent of the movement being limited by an elastic connection.' In Fig. 9.8, these moving attachments are denoted by M. We assume that the total spring constant is k. The M-pieces attach to specific sites A fixed along the adjacent thin filaments (Fig. 9.8). These attachments are broken by a chemical reaction requiring ATP. Because of thermal agitation, the unattached sliding element, M, oscillates. Nevertheless, it is assumed that the probability of attachment per unit time is governed by the distance x between the equilibrium (average) position O and the potential attachment site A on the thin filament. This probability distribution for attachment is denoted $f(x)$. Conversely, the probability (per unit time) that a cross-bridge connection will be broken is given by a function denoted $g(x)$ (Fig. 9.9).

If we consider a large number of identical M–A pairs (i.e. pairs having at each instant one and the same value of x), the proportion $n(t)$ of attached pairs will be a function of time alone. We are interested in obtaining a formula for the rate of change of $n(t)$. By definition of $f(x)$ and $g(x)$, we may write:

$$\frac{dn}{dt} = (1 - n)f(x) - ng(x) \tag{15}$$

Eqn 15 is hereafter referred to as Huxley's equation. Note that for a state of dynamic equilibrium, that is, when $dn/dt = 0$, we must have, according to Huxley's equation, the following value for the proportion of attached pairs:

$$n_{eq} = \frac{f(x)}{f(x) + g(x)} \tag{16}$$

as expected on intuitive grounds; the proportion of attached cross-bridges at equilibrium is governed by the probability of attachment.

In order to solve eqn 15 for $n(t)$, we must specify the global relative motion $x = x(t)$, and the initial condition $n_0 = n(0)$. It is sometimes convenient to provide, instead of $x(t)$, the global relative sliding velocity $v = v(t)$, in which case $x(t)$ can be obtained by integration as:

$$x(t) = x(0) + \int_0^t v(T)\, dT \tag{17}$$

where negative v means sarcomere shortening.

So far, we have assumed that all M–A pairs have the same distance $x(t)$. In reality, of course, $x(t)$ would be distributed almost randomly (i.e. uniformly) over the range $[-0.5l_a, 0.5l_a]$, where l_a is the typical distance between actin sites. In that case, we must talk of a distribution function $n(x,t)$ 'per unit length', such that the product $n(x,t)\, dx$ represents, at time t, the proportion of attached cross-bridges whose distance from the (nearest) actin site lies between x and $x + dx$. By the uniformity assumption, the proportion of unattached pairs in the same interval $(x, x + dx)$ is given by:

$$\left[\frac{1}{l_a} - n(x,t)\right] dx \tag{18}$$

Again, we are interested in obtaining the time-rate of change of $n(x,t)$ as seen by an observer fixed at an actin attachment site. It should be noted that this is not the same as the partial derivative $\frac{\partial n(x,t)}{\partial t}$ since, by definition, the partial derivative is calculated while holding x fixed. To take into consideration that the filaments are moving relative to each other, we calculate the *material* time-rate of change by the chain rule of differentiation as:

$$\frac{Dn}{Dt} = \frac{\partial n}{\partial t} + \frac{\partial n}{\partial x} v \tag{19}$$

where v is negative for sarcomere shortening. A careful analysis, in which we assume that the myofilaments are rigid, confirms that the governing differential equation is now:

$$\frac{\partial n}{\partial t} + \frac{\partial n}{\partial x} v = \left(\frac{1}{l_a} - n\right) f(x) - ng(x) \tag{20}$$

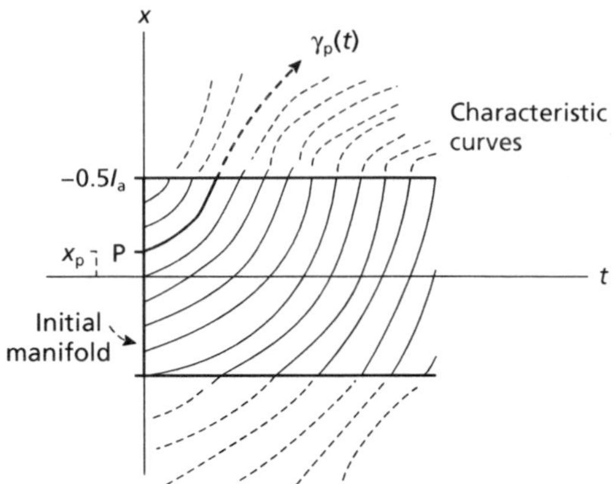

Fig. 9.17 Schematic representation of characteristic curves to solve first-order partial differential equations of the type shown in eqn 20.

The global motion of the relative sliding velocity $v(t)$ is assumed to be given.

To solve an equation of this type (that is, a first-order partial differential equation) one has to specify the values n_0 of the unknown variable n on an initial curve (or initial manifold), most commonly the line $t = 0$. At any given point P of the initial manifold (Fig. 9.17), there passes a unique *characteristic curve*, $x = \gamma_p(t)$, obtained as the solution of the ordinary differential equation:

$$\frac{d\gamma_p(t)}{dt} = v(t) \tag{21}$$

with the initial condition:

$$\gamma_p(0) = x_p \tag{22}$$

Unlike the general case shown in Fig. 9.17, in our case the characteristic curves are all 'parallel' to each other, since at any time t the slope $v(t)$ is independent of x. A careful look at eqn 20 reveals that its left-hand side represents the time derivative of the function $n(\gamma_p(t),t)$, where $\gamma_p(t)$ is the unique characteristic curve passing through the point (x,t). In other words, the integration of the partial differential eqn 20 boils down to the integration of a Huxley-type ordinary differential equation along the characteristic curve through each point P of the initial manifold, namely:

$$\frac{dn_p(t)}{dt} = \left(\frac{1}{l_a} - n_p(t)\right) f(\gamma_p(t)) - n_p(t) g(\gamma_p(t)) \tag{23}$$

with the initial condition:

$$n_p(0) = n_0(P) \tag{24}$$

A similar mathematical treatment also applies to more general partial differential equations of the first order in two independent variables.

ATTACHMENT/DETACHMENT PROBABILITY DISTRIBUTIONS

As pointed out above, the distributions $f(x)$ and $g(x)$ represent the rate constants of the chemical reactions associated with attachment and detachment of M–A pairs, respectively. They are expressed in units of reciprocal time. For the model to give the desired results, it is assumed that $f(x)$ vanishes if A is to the left of M (for the right-hand half of a sarcomere, as shown in Fig. 9.8), whereas, for the same condition, $g(x)$ attains a great constant value. When A is to the right of M, it is assumed that $f(x)$ and $g(x)$ increase linearly, $f(x)$ being truncated at a value $x = h$ (much smaller than $0.5l_a$) representing the range of bonding ability (Fig. 9.9). An explanation for such an odd behaviour of the probability distributions may be found within a more detailed geometric description of the cross-bridges and the molecular structure, which was not available to Huxley in 1957. A possible explanation is given in this chapter under the heading 'Ratchet models' where a physically possible solution is given to the problem of the rate functions. However, it must be pointed out that from a mechanistic point of view, the idea of a ratchet mechanism of contraction is not compatible with the powerstroke idea of the cross-bridge models, although the gross behaviour of muscular force production may appear to be the same in both models. Structurally, and philosophically, ratchet-type and cross-bridge models are not compatible.

MACROSCOPIC QUANTITIES OF THE CROSS-BRIDGE MODEL

From the cross-bridge theory, the total force of a muscle can be calculated. Assuming that half-sarcomeres in series must produce the same force, one must only consider the sum of the contributions of all half-sarcomeres in a physiological cross-section. Let A represent the area of this cross-section, m the number of M-sites per unit volume, and s the instantaneous average sarcomere length. Then, the number of sites contained in all the half-sarcomeres affected by the cross-section is equal to $mAs/2$. The average force per site is obtained by calculating the weighted average of the forces in the individual springs, that is:

$$f_{\mathrm{ave}}(t) = \int_{-\infty}^{\infty} kxn(x,t)\,dx \tag{25}$$

Here the weighting function is the proportion, $n(x,t)$, of attached cross-bridges per unit length. The total force is:

$$F(t) = \frac{mAs}{2}\int_{-\infty}^{\infty} kxn(x,t)\,dx \tag{26}$$

obtained by multiplying the average force per site by the number of sites involved in the cross-section.

Let the muscle be given a constant negative (i.e. shortening) velocity V. This results in a sliding sarcomere velocity:

$$v = \frac{V}{n_{\mathrm{s}}} \tag{27}$$

where n_{s} is the number of half-sarcomeres in one muscle length. Since v, in this case, is a constant, integration of eqn 21 gives the characteristic curves as the straight lines:

$$\gamma_{\mathrm{P}}(t) = x_{\mathrm{P}} + vt,\ (v < 0) \tag{28}$$

A crucial point at this juncture is that, instead of assuming initial conditions at $t = 0$, Huxley effectively moved the initial manifold to the line $x = h$ and specified that $n = 0$ on this line. At first sight, it may seem surprising that the initial conditions could be specified on a line other than $t =$ constant. But the line $x = h$ is a perfectly valid initial manifold, since it satisfies the mathematical restriction of not being anywhere tangent to a characteristic line.

The time of intersection of the characteristic curve through P with the initial manifold is calculated as:

$$t_{\mathrm{P}} = \frac{h - x_{\mathrm{P}}}{v} \tag{29}$$

The solution of eqn 20 must be continuous. Taking into consideration the straight characteristics, the conditions specified at the initial manifold, continuity, and the given probability distributions, the solution of the characteristic differential eqn 23 is obtained by direct integration as (see also Fig. 9.9):

$$n_{\mathrm{P}} = \begin{cases} 0 & \mathit{for}\quad t < \dfrac{h - x_{\mathrm{P}}}{v} \\[2ex] \dfrac{\alpha}{(\alpha+\beta)l_{\alpha}}\left[1 - e^{((\alpha+\beta)/2v)(h^2-(x_{\mathrm{P}}+vt)^2)}\right] & \mathit{for}\quad \dfrac{h - x_{\mathrm{P}}}{v} \le t < -\dfrac{x_{\mathrm{P}}}{v} \\[2ex] \dfrac{\alpha}{(\alpha+\beta)l_{\alpha}}\left[1 - e^{((\alpha+\beta)/2v)h^2}\right]e^{(-g_0/v)(x_{\mathrm{P}}+vt)} & \mathit{for}\quad -\dfrac{x_{\mathrm{P}}}{v} \le t \end{cases} \tag{30}$$

These formulas, although obtained for one characteristic curve, furnish the complete solution $n(x,t)$. Indeed, given a point (x,t), we draw the unique characteristic through it. This line will intersect the vertical axis at $x_{\mathrm{P}} = x - vt$. Substituting this value of x_{P} in the appropriate one of the three formulas (eqn 30), we obtain the value of $n(x,t)$. In this particular case, this procedure is tantamount to substituting x for $x_{\mathrm{P}} + vt$ in the right-hand side of eqn 30. We have used the general procedure to illustrate how the method of characteristics would work even if the specified contractile speed $v(t)$ was not constant in time. In the particular case when the speed is constant, we obtain the same result as Huxley (Huxley 1957), namely:

$$n(x,t) = \begin{cases} 0 & \text{for } x > h \\ \dfrac{\alpha}{(\alpha+\beta)l_\alpha}\left[1 - e^{((\alpha+\beta)/2v(h^2-x^2))}\right] & \text{for } 0 < x \leq h \\ \dfrac{\alpha}{(\alpha+\beta)l_\alpha}\left[1 - e^{((\alpha+\beta)/2v)h^2}\right]e^{-(g_0/v)x} & \text{for } x \leq 0 \end{cases} \tag{31}$$

Let us now use eqns 31 and 26 to calculate the total force F. Note that, since t does not appear explicitly in any of the three formulas in eqn 31, $F(t)$ will turn out to be constant for a given constant speed of contraction, in agreement with the usual interpretation of Hill's experiments. The result of the integration required by eqn 26 is obtained explicitly as:

$$F = \frac{mAsk\alpha}{2(\alpha+\beta)l_\alpha}\left[\frac{1}{2}h^2 + \left(1 - e^{((\alpha+\beta)/2v)h^2}\right)\left(\frac{v}{\alpha+\beta} - \left(\frac{v}{g_0}\right)^2\right)\right] \tag{32}$$

With a judicious choice of constants, this formula may be made to fit Hill's force–velocity law in the shortening range. In fact, by a similar treatment for energy and mechanical power, Huxley was able to match also some of Hill's thermodynamic considerations. Further developments along these lines were proposed by Huxley and Simmons (1971) and by Zahalak and Ma (1990) and Zahalak and Motabarzadeh (1997).

Ratchet models

Hill-type models are purely phenomenological, and the important features, such as the force–velocity and the force–length relationships, are introduced without explanation. Cross-bridge models are more structural than Hill-type models, but they break down, from a mechanistic point of view, at the level of the 'artificially' introduced rate functions that have no biological explanation. Here we present ratchet-type models. The actin–myosin motor is assumed to work by biasing the Brownian motor (myosin) by associating a set of changing and asymmetrical potentials with the motor that cause, on average, directional force and movement. Although ratchet-type models for muscular contraction have not been used or mentioned in the biomechanics literature, it is important to consider them here, because they allow for a physical explanation of muscle contraction which Hill- and cross-bridge-type models cannot.

GENERAL CONSIDERATIONS

In 1993, Magnasco pointed out a simple phenomenon that was inspired by the ratchet and pawl mechanisms discussed by Feynman: a Brownian particle in a sawtooth-shaped potential subjected to external fluctuations, or periodic external forces, is capable of vectorial motion (Magnasco 1993). He also discussed a possible link between this phenomenon and transport and force generation in biological systems, such as muscle contraction and cellular motion. The Brownian particle was referred to as a 'molecular motor' and the system as a 'ratchet model.' Since Magnasco's (1993) seminal work, there have been a great number of contributions aimed at characterizing different systems in which unidirectional motion of a Brownian particle can be induced without a macroscopic gradient force (Astumian & Bier 1996; Julicher *et al.* 1997). Specifically, the ratchet idea has been incorporated into describing the mechanochemical coupling of force generation in muscle contraction (Zhou & Chen 1996; Derenyi & Vicsek 1998) or in the directed walk of kinesin and dynein along microtubules (Derenyi & Vicsek 1996). A common theme in these investigations is that motor proteins may generate force and directed motion by rectifying thermal fluctuations. In such ratchet models, chemical energy is not used directly to produce force. Rather, the molecular motor diffuses along its track by a random walk, and the chemical reaction merely biases the walk so that steps in one direction are more probable than in the other. In the case of muscle contraction, the myosin head is more likely to produce a positive force than a negative one. These theoretical investigations have been supported by results of single myosin–actin interactions (Svoboda *et al.* 1993; Finer *et al.* 1994; Spudich 1994).

In ratchet models, the system consisting of a myosin–actin filament pair is thought of as a small machine operating in a thermal bath, subjected to large fluctuations in conformation and chemical state. In principle, all conformations can be described by a set of conformational variables, $x_1, x_2, \ldots$ which should include all degrees of freedom of the motor molecules (atom positions, bond angles, bond distances, . . .). However, such a detailed description of all conformational variables presents an unrealistic computational challenge, and in most cases is not required in describing the generic features of the system. To proceed further, we assume that the important motions of the system (myosin–actin filament) can be described with just a few conformational variables that are characterized by great relaxation times to the equilibrium compared to the other, neglected, conformational variables. Conformational variables that have quick relaxation times can be ignored because they are considered to be in equilibrium at the time scale of the relaxation of the heat-bath fluctuations. Denote by $x_1, x_2, \ldots, x_n$ the conformational variables with great relaxation times, i.e. a slow dynamics. Since the system is driven by chemical energy, at least one of these conformational variables must reflect the progress of the chemical reactions, and will be called the chemical variable. It will be denoted by x_1. The remaining conformational variables will be called mechanical variables. At least one of these mechanical variables must reflect the position of the myosin relative to the actin filament during muscle contraction. This variable will be denoted by x_2. The remaining mechanical variables all represent a significant conformational change of the myosin motor, such as rotation of the myosin head, tilling of the myosin neck, etc. Each conformation $x_1, x_2, \ldots, x_n$ is associated with a free energy $V(x_1, x_2, \ldots, x_n)$ that has the property that its derivatives with respect to $x_1, x_2, \ldots, x_n$ are the average forces along these variables. In principle, the free energy of each conformation can be calculated using Boltzmann statistical mechanics, provided that the Hamiltonian of the system-bath is known (Mcquarrie 1976; Keller & Bustamante 2000). To simplify the description of the operation of the molecular motor, we consider the case of one chemical variable, x_1, describing the reaction path of the ATP hydrolysis, and one mechanical variable, x_2, describing the position of the centre of mass of the myosin head. In this case the free energy $V(x_1,x_2)$ defines a two-dimensional potential energy surface in which the myosin head moves. At any fixed position x_2, the spatial curve $V(.,x_2)$ will look like a typical reaction free energy diagram, in which the minima represent the stable biochemical states, separated by free energy barriers that represent the activation energy for the progress of the chemical reactions. The rate constants of the chemical reactions can be calculated as the inverse of the mean first passage times of transition among the minima of the free energy potential using a Langevin formalism (Kramers 1940). Note that the rate constants in this description depend on the position of the myosin head, a fact that was recognized by Huxley (1957). Since, after each ATP hydrolysis, the myosin must return to its initial state, and the free energy must have decreased by a fixed amount, the spatial curve $V(.,x_2)$ is a tilted periodic curve with respect to the chemical variable, i.e.

$$V(x_1 + C,x_2) = V(x_1,x_2) + V_0 \tag{33}$$

where V_0 is a constant and C is the period of the chemical reaction.

At any fixed position in the chemical coordinate x_1, the spatial curve, $V(x_1,.)$, represents the change in the free energy associated with the movement of the myosin head along the actin filament. Considering the periodic structure of the actin filament, with a period $d = 38.5$ nm, the overall change in the free energy between any two sites at a distance d in the actin filament has to be zero. Therefore, the spatial curve, $V(x_1,.)$, is periodic with period d, and its minima represent the stable binding sites of the myosin along the actin filament. To implement the ratchet idea, the spatial curve, $V(x_1,.)$, must be asymmetrical over a period for some specific values of the chemical variable x_1. A plausible explanation for this asymmetry would be the structural asymmetry of the actin monomers and the myosin head in certain conformations, such as at the binding of ATP to the myosin head, or at the ATP hydrolysis step. Since force generation in muscle is a result of the movement of the myosin head along the actin filament, we must specify regions on the two-dimensional surface $V(x_1,x_2)$ as force-producing regions. The force generated at any point in these regions can be calculated as the derivative of $V(x_1,x_2)$ with respect to x_2. Note that this force can be negative or positive (a feature that is absent in the Huxley theory immediately upon attachment or in isometric situations) but the ratcheting mechanism gives an overall positive force (where positive is defined as a force that would tend to shorten the sarcomere).

THE STOCHASTIC MOTION OF THE MOLECULAR MOTOR

In the absence of thermal fluctuations, the system would be located in one of the minima of the free energy potential, $V(x_1,x_2)$. However, at a given temperature T, each of the bath variables has energy of the order kT, where k is the Boltzmann constant. The barriers of the free energy potential, $V(x_1,x_2)$, are only a few times greater than the value kT. Therefore, the thermal fluctuations would have a great effect on the motion of the system, and would be responsible for ATP hydrolysis and force generation. A common approach in describing such a system is the Langevin formalism in which a random force (describing the thermal bath) is added to the deterministic equation of motion of the system:

$$\gamma_i \frac{dx_i}{dt} = -\frac{\partial V(x_1,x_2)}{\partial x_i} + F_i(t) + \xi_i(t), i = 1,2 \qquad (34)$$

where γ_i are the damping constants, $F_i(t)$ are the external forces which may include a force opposing the motion of the myosin head, $(F_2(t))$, and a load affecting the temporal progress of the chemical reaction, $(F_1(t))$, and $\xi_i(t)$are Gaussian white noises with short-range correlation, i.e.

$$< \xi_i(t), \xi_i(s) \geq 2\gamma_i kT\delta(t-s), i = 1,2 \qquad (35)$$

where $\delta(x)$ is the Dirac function. The classical inertia force, $m\ddot{x}_i$, has been neglected, assuming that all motions are overdamped. Note that adding a force, $F_1(t)$, to the motion of the chemical coordinate x_1, gives a load-dependent rate constant for the chemical reactions. The random fluctuations of the thermal bath cause the trajectory of the system point $(x_1(t),x_2(t))$ to be random. The choice of a white noise dynamics for the thermal bath destroys all the thermal force correlations after an infinitesimal time. Therefore, the system has no memory and the trajectory $(x_1(t),x_2(t))$ is a Markovian process. However, it is well accepted that skeletal muscle force production has a memory. That is, force depends on the history of the contractile conditions. A ratchet model could account for such history-dependent effects qualitatively, by replacing the white noise by coloured noise that contains specific correlations.

In order to characterize the features of the system, we have to study the statistics of the trajectories $(x_1(t),x_2(t))$. This can be done by defining the probability density for the system, $p(x_1,x_2,t)$, to be in conformation (x_1,x_2) at time t. This probability density follows the Fokker–Planck equations (Chandrasekhar 1943):

$$\frac{\partial p(x_1,x_2,t)}{\partial t} + \frac{\partial J_1(x_1,x_2,t)}{\partial x_1} + \frac{\partial J_2(x_1,x_2,t)}{\partial x_2} = 0 \qquad (36)$$

where $J_i(x_1,x_2,t)$ are the probability current densities defined by

$$J_i(x_1,x_2,t) = -\frac{kT}{\gamma_i}\frac{\partial p(x_1,x_2,t)}{\partial x_i} + \frac{1}{\gamma_i}\left(-\frac{\partial V(x_1,x_2)}{\partial x_i} + F_i(t)\right)p(x_1,x_2,t) \qquad (37)$$

Eqn 37 gives the overall origin of the current density. The first term in eqn 37 is a diffusive current with diffusion constant $D_i = kT/\gamma_i$, according to the Einstein fluctuation–dissipation relationship. The second term is a drift current caused by force acting on the system. Substituting eqn 37 into eqn 36 gives a second-order system of partial differential equations that can be solved for $p(x_1,x_2,t)$ at any given time t, given a known distribution $p_0(x_1,x_2)$ at time $t = 0$. Once p is known, the current probability J (the transport behaviour of the system) can be found using eqn 37.

MULTISTATE RATCHET MODEL

Even with all the simplifications given above (elimination of fast conformational variables, one chemical variable, and one mechanical variable), the general features of eqn 37 are difficult to solve. The available techniques on the theory of stochastic processes in multidimensional space cannot be used to solve such problems. A common approach to solving this type of problem is to convert the two-dimensional dynamics to a one-dimensional dynamics at the expense of a discretization of the chemical coordinate. Using this procedure, the rate constant of the chemical reaction must be given. The myosin head will fluctuate in different potentials that are associated with different states of the chemical reactions. The rate of switching between the potentials is dictated by the rate constants of the chemical reactions. This type of ratchet is referred to as 'flashing ratchet' (Astumian 1997). To derive the stochastic equation of motions, we will use as an example a two-state model, that is equivalent to Huxley's (1957) cross-bridge theory of muscle contraction. A generalization to multistate models is straightforward.

Denote by x the position of the centre of mass of the myosin head. Assume that the chemical variable takes two discrete states: A (attached state) and D (detached state). The chemical reactions produce a switching of the myosin head from the attached to the detached state at a rate $g(x)$, and from the detached to the attached state at a rate $f(x)$. The two rate constants depend on the myosin head position. Contrary to Huxley's theory (Huxley 1957), the rate constants $f(x)$ and $g(x)$ do not need to be asymmetrical to account for the positive force generation in muscle contraction. A common practice is to assume that the rate constant $g(x)$ is localized at a hypothetical binding site on the actin filament. The rate constant $f(x)$ is independent of x since, in the detached state, the myosin head moves freely and far away from the actin filament. Therefore, the chemical reaction would likely be independent of the position of the myosin head. In the detached state (D), the free energy potential $V_D(x)$ of the mechanical variable x can be chosen to be constant, reflecting the fact that the different conformations of the myosin head possess the same free energy and are independent of the position of the myosin head relative to the actin filament. In the attached state (A), the free energy potential $V_A(x)$ is periodic and assumed to be asymmetrical over a period because of the asymmetry of the actin filament. The functioning of the myosin motor can be understood as follows. In the detached state, the myosin head is at a position x and performs a free Brownian motion. The probability distribution of the position of the myosin head follows a Gaussian function that spreads out over time. Once the chemical reaction has advanced the myosin head to the attached state, and because of the asymmetry of the potential in this state, the myosin head is more likely to be located in the region of the potential with a positive slope than the region with negative slope (Fig. 9.18). Therefore, the myosin head is more likely to be in a position to exert positive force (which would tend to shorten the sarcomere) than a position to exert negative force. Denote by $p_D(x,t)$ and $p_A(x,t)$ the probability density of finding the myosin head in state D or state A, respectively, at time t. This probability density satisfies the Fokker–Planck equations:

$$\begin{cases} \dfrac{\partial p_A(x,t)}{\partial t} + \dfrac{\partial J_A(x,t)}{\partial t} = f(x)p_D(x,t) - g(x)p_A(x,t) \\[2ex] \dfrac{\partial p_D(x,t)}{\partial t} + \dfrac{\partial J_D(x,t)}{\partial t} = g(x)p_A(x,t) - f(x)p_D(x,t) \end{cases} \tag{38}$$

where the probability current density is given by:

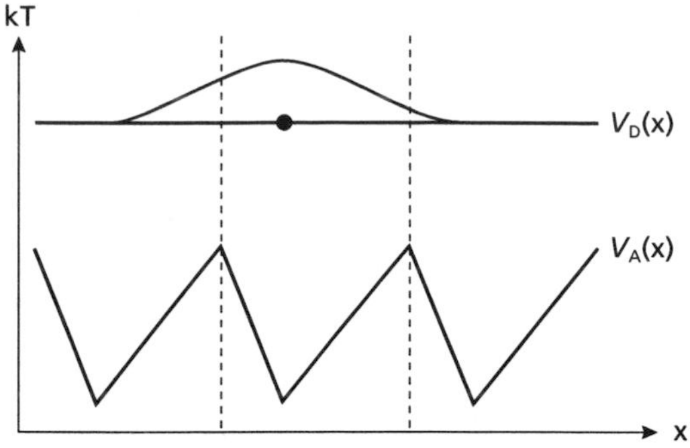

Fig. 9.18 Schematic representation of a particle (myosin head, ●) in a 'flashing' ratchet with a constant potential for the detachment state $V_D(x)$, and an asymmetrical, sawtooth potential for the attached state $V_A(x)$. See text for further explanations.

$$J_i(x,t) = -\frac{kT}{\gamma_i}\frac{\partial p_i(x,t)}{\partial x} + \frac{1}{\gamma_i}\left(-\frac{\partial V_i(x)}{\partial x} + F_{ext}(t)\right)p_i(x,t), i = \mathrm{A,D} \quad (39)$$

$F_{ext}(t)$ is an external load applied to the myosin head. The external load can be understood as a force applied to the actin filament. If this external force is independent of time, it is possible to obtain a stationary solution. In this situation, the velocity of the myosin motor is given by:

$$v_s = \int_0^d J_A(x) + J_D(x)\, dx \quad (40)$$

where d is the periodicity of the actin filament. Eqn 40 gives the load–velocity relationship of the molecular motor. In the experimental setting, the load–velocity relationship has to be understood as follows. For a given load applied to the muscle fibre, eqn 40 gives the steady-state velocity of shortening of the fibre. However, in muscle biomechanics, typically experiments are performed the other way round: i.e. a fibre is shortened at a constant velocity, and the steady-state force is calculated. In order to account for the shortening of the actin relative to the myosin filament, we have to incorporate the x-displacement over time in eqn 38. In this case, the equations become:

$$\begin{cases} \dfrac{dp_A(x(t),t)}{dt} + \dfrac{\partial J_A(x(t),t)}{\partial t} = f(x)p_D(x,t) - g(x)p_A(x,t) \\ \dfrac{dp_D(x(t),t)}{dt} + \dfrac{\partial J_D(x(t),t)}{\partial t} = g(x)p_A(x,t) - f(x)p_D(x,t) \end{cases} \quad (41)$$

By differentiation, this leads to:

$$\begin{cases} \dfrac{\partial p_A(x,t)}{\partial t} - v(t)\dfrac{\partial p_A(x,t)}{\partial x} + \dfrac{\partial J_A(x,t)}{\partial t} \\ = f(x)p_D(x,t) - g(x)p_A(x,t) \\ \dfrac{\partial p_D(x,t)}{\partial t} - v(t)\dfrac{\partial p_D(x,t)}{\partial x} + \dfrac{\partial J_D(x,t)}{\partial t} \\ = g(x)p_A(x,t) - f(x)p_D(x,t) \end{cases} \quad (42)$$

where $v(t)$ is the velocity of shortening (positive) or the velocity of lengthening (negative). The current probabilities have to be changed accordingly, i.e.

$$J_i(x,t) = -\frac{kT}{\gamma_i}\left(\frac{\partial p_i(x,t)}{\partial t} - \frac{1}{\gamma_i}\left(-\frac{\partial V_i(x(t))}{\partial x} + F_{ext}(t)\right)p_i(x,t), i = A,D \quad (43)$$

In order to derive the contractile force of one thin filament in one half sarcomere, we label the myosin heads in sequence by $i = 1,2, \ldots, n$. Each time a myosin head is in the attached state at position x, it transmits a force $F(x) = -\delta V_A(x)/\delta x$. This force is positive or negative, depending on the position x. Denote by $x_i(t)$ the position of the myosin head, labelled i, to the nearest actin binding site; i.e. the distance from the position of the myosin head to the nearest minimum of the potential $V_A(x)$. The force in the filament as a function of time is then given by:

$$F(t) = \sum_{i=1}^{n} -\frac{\partial V_A(x_i(t))}{\partial x} p_A(x_i(t),t) \quad (44)$$

Myosin heads with the same orientation, and therefore interacting with the same actin filament, occur every $a = 42.9$ nm. The repeat distance of the binding site on the actin filament is $d = 38.5$ nm. Therefore, no periodicity occurs as the number of myosin heads from one thick filament to one thin filament is about 16 (in mammalian skeletal muscles). Therefore, the average spacing between adjacent values of x_i can be approximated by a distribution that is uniformly dense over the interval $[-b/2, b/2]$. As a consequence, the expression for the force in eqn 44 can be approximated by an average integral:

$$F(t) = \frac{n}{b} \int_{-b/2}^{b/2} -\frac{\partial V_A(x)}{\partial x} p_A(x,t)\, dx \tag{45}$$

Using eqns 40 and 45, we have formulated the force–velocity and the force production on one thin filament by one thick filament for an actin–myosin motor. From here, force–velocity and force for a single fibre or active muscle could be obtained by appropriate extensions. Also, the force–length relationships would be a basic property of the proposed model (at least for the plateau and descending limb regions), as force is directly proportional to the number of myosin heads attached to the thin (actin) filaments. Therefore, although the above formalism of muscle contraction is somewhat new, and thereby mistrusted, it represents, at the moment, the only physically possible mechanism of force production and movement. The cross-bridge theory fails to explain the asymmetry of the rate constants required to produce force and muscle contraction.

From molecular mechanism to muscle force and power production

Skeletal muscle contraction has been studied on a large range of structural levels: from voluntary, *in vivo* muscle contraction, to the interaction of a single cross-bridge head with an actin filament. Naturally, the question arises, how do properties observed on one structural level (e.g. the molecular level) transfer across to other levels (e.g. the *in vivo* human muscle)? Probably, properties on the molecular level cannot be recognized in the whole muscle and, vice versa, whole muscle properties are not likely to further our understanding of the molecular mechanisms underlying force production and contraction.

However, the cross-bridge model and the ratchet-type models introduced above are molecular-based models, and the Hill model was derived from an isolated, amphibian muscle preparation. Therefore, application of these models to *in vivo* human muscle properties must be done with extreme caution. Here, one can give dozens of examples illustrating the difficulty of using these models for applications in whole body human biomechanics. However, for the sake of brevity, selected examples are given. These relate to the well known force–length and force–velocity properties of skeletal muscle.

The force–length relationship

The force–length relationship of a muscle is typically defined by the maximal, isometric, steady-state force a muscle can exert as a function of its length. Experimentally, a point on the force–length relationship is obtained by setting the muscle to the target length, and then measuring the steady-state force obtained at that length during supramaximal activation. In order to obtain the next data point on the force–length relationship, the muscle is deactivated, set to the new length, and surpramaximally activated again, etc. Therefore, the force–length relationship is a static, discrete relationship, and should not be represented, or thought of, as a continuous property, as is typically done.

According to Huxley (1957), the force–length relationship of a single cross-bridge and an actin filament is a straight line with increasing force for increasing cross-bridge length (extension) (Fig. 9.8). This result comes from the assumption that cross-bridge force is proportional to its extension, and that the extension force comes from a linear spring with the force–length property $F_{ce} = kx$, where F_{ce} is the cross-bridge force, k is the spring stiffness, and x is the extension (or length) of the cross-bridge, defined as the distance from the cross-bridge equilibrium length to the nearest actin attachment site (Huxley 1957).

The exact force–length relationship of a sarcomere is unknown, as sarcomeres cannot be isolated for mechanical testing. However, Gordon *et al.* (1966) took a single-fibre preparation and used a sarcomere clamp method to keep a small segment near the middle of the fibre at a constant (isometric) length. The segment was selected in a region in which sarcomeres were nearly uniform before contraction. It was argued by Gordon *et al.* (1966) that, by keeping the target segment at a constant length and by having chosen a segment of uniform sarcomere length, the forces observed at the end of the fibre reflected the isometric force of those 'clamped' sarcomeres in the target segment. Note that in order to achieve a constant segment length, fibre length could not be kept isometric, but had to be adjusted during contraction to keep the target segment isometric. The 'sarcomere' force–length relationship obtained in this way is shown in Fig. 9.19. The 'fibre' force–length relationship obtained by Ramsey and Street (1940) differs distinctly from the sarcomere force–length relationship (Fig. 9.20). Most notably, the 'fibre' force–length relationship has an extended plateau region and a greater range of the descending limb than the 'sarcomere' relationship.

Finally, force–length relationships of entire muscle are still different from those of single fibres and 'clamped' sarcomeres. Often, muscle force–length relationships are found to be broader than the corresponding fibre properties, presumably because of the range of fibre lengths and the non-uniform average sarcomere lengths across fibres assumed to occur in whole muscle. Also, passive force in whole muscles starts to come into play at different muscle lengths (Fig. 9.21). In some muscles, passive force has a major influence at lengths as short as the plateau region, in others, substantial passive force only occurs in the middle or end range of the descending limb of the force–length relationship.

Last, and possibly most importantly, force–length properties of *in situ* muscles are constrained by the musculoskeletal geometry, and

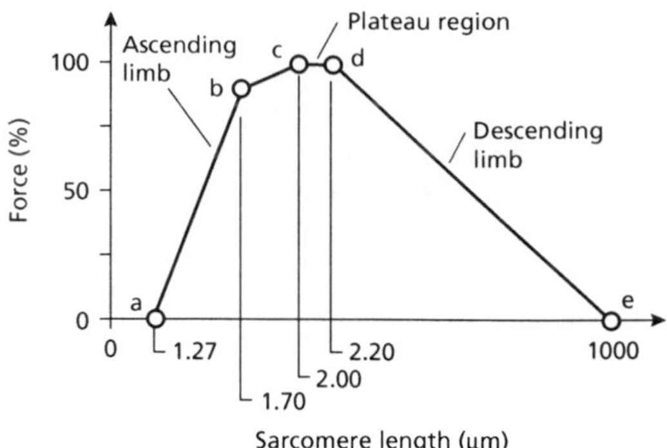

Fig. 9.19 'Sarcomere' force–length relationship as first obtained by Gordon *et al.* (1966) for single intact muscle fibres from frog. Note the straight line of the descending limb that was directly associated with the loss of myofilament overlap with increasing sarcomere length.

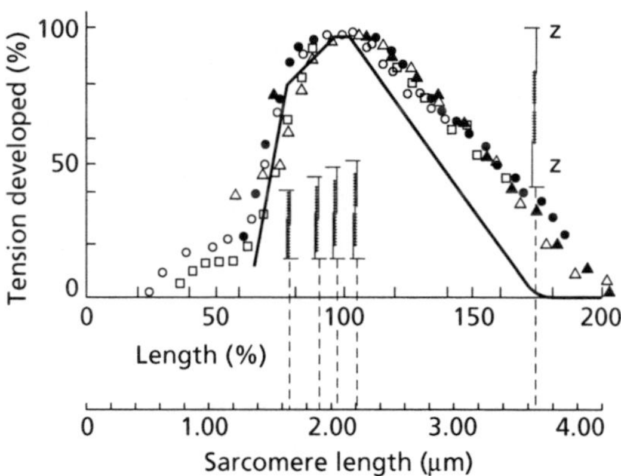

Fig. 9.20 Force–length relationship as obtained by Ramsey and Street (1940)—data points, and by Ford *et al.* (1977).

often the whole range of the force–length relationship is not represented. For example, in human and cat triceps surae, the force–length relationship that is used for normal everyday activities is on the ascending limb and the plateau region of the force–length relationship (Herzog *et al.* 1991b, 1992). Other muscles, such as the frog semimembranosus, work predominantly on the plateau (Lutz & Rome 1993), while still others seem to occupy the descending limb of the force–length relationship, as for example, the frog semitendinosus (Mai & Lieber 1990).

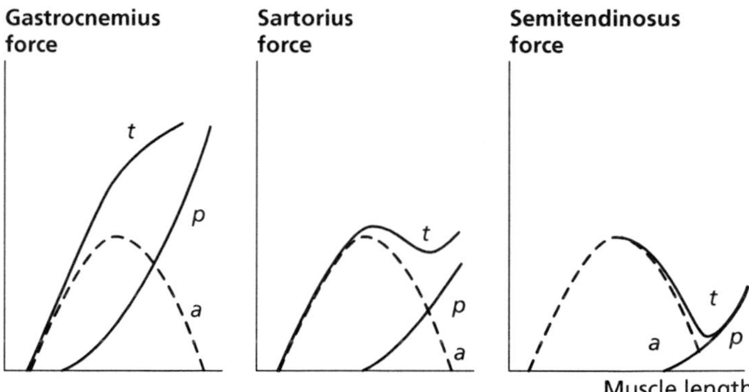

Fig. 9.21 Active (a), passive (p) and total (t) force–length relationship of three frog muscles in which the passive force comes into play at distinctly different regions of the active force–length relationship.

The force–length relationship is an important property of skeletal muscle. For sports activities, the force–length relationship of muscle may severely affect performance. It appears that force–length relationships in athletes competing in different sports requiring distinctly different muscular function may adapt to the functional requirements. In a study on elite-level runners and bicyclists, we found that the rectus femoris in these two athlete populations showed vastly different force–length characteristics (Herzog *et al.* 1991a). Moreover, these different characteristics were suited to the functional requirements of runners and bicyclists, respectively (Fig. 9.22). Therefore, it was concluded that force–length properties of human skeletal muscle can, and will, adapt to chronic functional requirements, as they do in elite-level athletes.

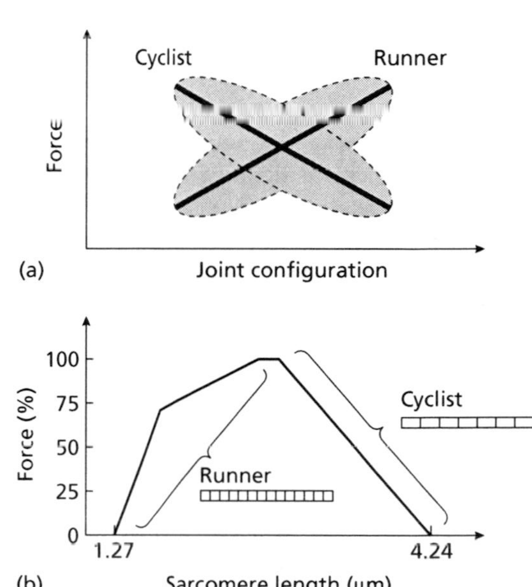

Fig. 9.22 Schematic summary of the force–length results determined for the rectus femoris of elite runners and elite cyclists. The runners appeared to use the rectus femoris on the ascending limb, and the cyclists on the descending limb of the force–length relationship (top graph). This result could be explained if the number of sarcomeres in series in the rectus femoris fibres was greater in the runners compared to the cyclists (bottom graph). This would cause a shift of the force–length relationship of the runners to the left of that for the cyclists. Interestingly, force–length relationships of rectus femoris from non-athletes appear to be in between those shown in this figure.

The force–velocity relationship

As for the force–length relationship discussed above, one could describe and explain force–velocity properties of skeletal muscle across a great range of structural levels. However, there are no force–velocity properties for single cross-bridge interactions with actin. Moreover, force–velocity properties of single fibres are in good agreement, it appears, with those of whole muscle. However, there is one major difference between force–velocity properties of isolated fibres or muscle preparations and those of voluntary human muscle contraction. For the sake of brevity, we will focus on this specific difference.

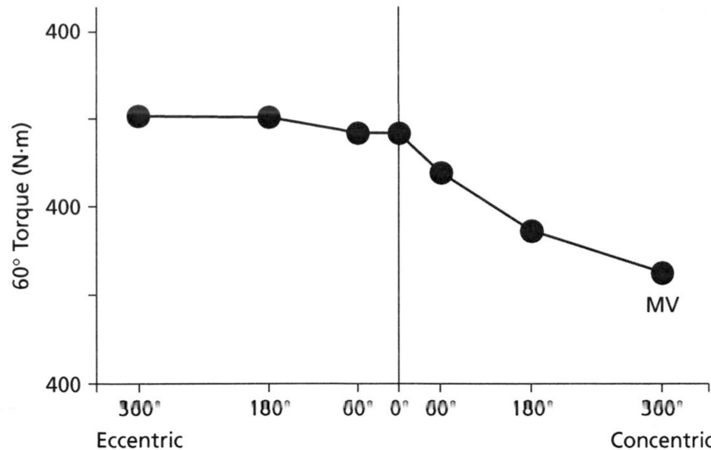

Fig. 9.23 Torque–angular velocity relationship of human knee extensor muscles at maximal voluntary effort, as observed by Westing *et al.* (1990). Note that the force for the eccentric contractions does not increase much beyond the maximal isometric force. This result, for voluntary contractions, is in stark contrast to the force–velocity properties typically observed using artificial electrical stimulation, and used for theoretical modelling (see e.g. Fig. 9.6).

The force–velocity relationship defines the maximal force of a muscle, at a given length (typically optimal length), as a function of the speed of contraction. Typically, a data point on the force–velocity curve is obtained by activating a muscle maximally, releasing the muscle at a constant speed of shortening (or stretch), and measuring the force for the given speed of shortening (stretch) at a defined length. Therefore, as for the force–length relationship, the force–velocity relationship is a discrete and not a continuous property.

The force–velocity property, as described by Hill (1938), approximates a rectangular hyperbola for shortening (Fig. 9.4). For stretching, force increases more rapidly with speed, then it decreases with speed of shortening (Fig. 9.6). Also, at some (relatively low) speed of stretching, muscles reach a constant force of about 1.5–2.0 the value of the isometric force (e.g. Katz 1939). This force–velocity relationship forms the basis of most muscle models. It is based on constant, electrical stimulation of the muscle (or fibre) preparation.

However, for voluntary contractions, the force–velocity property appears to differ distinctly from that of electrically stimulated muscle. The shortening region is similar in both cases; however, for stretching, the increase in force with increasing speeds is virtually absent during voluntary contractions (Westing *et al.* 1990). Eccentric forces reach maximally 1.1–1.2 times the isometric force, rather than 1.5–2.0 times (Fig. 9.23). It is thought, and this has been supported using the superimposed twitch technique and artificial stimulation of *in vivo* human muscle, that the depression of the eccentric force during voluntary contractions is caused by inhibition of α motoneurone drive. Therefore, for voluntary contractions in human muscles, the force–velocity property might be better approximated by Fig. 9.23 than by relationships obtained using electrical stimulation.

Applications

When attempting to apply general knowledge of the properties of skeletal muscle force production to human movement or optimization of sport performance, tremendous difficulties arise. For example, the force–length relationship is well described for tetanically contracting single fibres of frog. However, to the author's knowledge, there is no direct measurement of a force–length relationship of an *in vivo* human muscle. The difficulties are in measuring the dynamically varying and non-uniform fibre length during an isometric (fixed muscle attachment sites) contraction. Other problems involve the definition of a maximal voluntary contraction, muscle inhibition as a function of joint angle (Suter & Herzog 1997), and the non-linearly varying shape of the force–length relationship for submaximal activa-

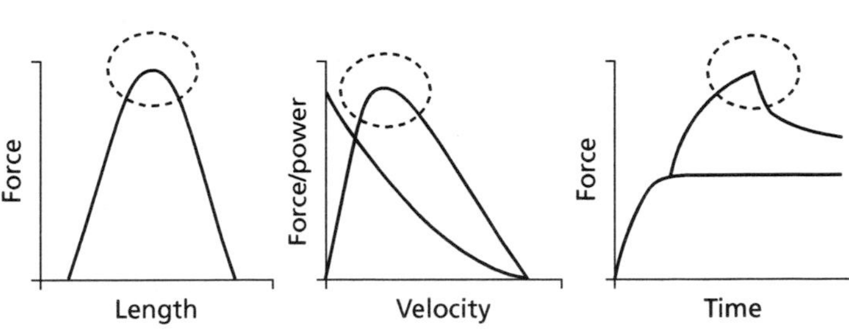

Fig. 9.24 Schematic illustration of how one might obtain maximal force and power output during muscular contraction. (a) Work in the vicinity of the plateau region of the force–length relationship. (b) Work at a constant velocity of shortening that maximizes power output (i.e. about 31% of the maximal speed of shortening). (c) Use a stretch before the shortening contraction to enhance force and power output.

tion (Rack & Westbury 1969) during fatigue and following dynamic contractions. Nevertheless, and for the sake of argument, let us assume that the required muscle properties are known in the following, fully realizing that they are not.

For many sports activities, power output of specific muscles is of utmost importance for athletic success. From throwing a shot, discus or javelin, to sprint running, bicycling or skating, success in all these events depends on muscle power output. How is power output of a muscle, or group of muscles, maximized?

In a study on frog jumping (frogs are extremely good jumpers, definitely much better than humans), Lutz and Rome (1993) argued that, aside from coordination and maximal activation, power output in the frog semimembranosus (an important muscle for jumping) was maximized by working on the plateau region of the force–length relationship and by shortening the muscle at a speed that allows for maximal power output (Fig. 9.24). Maximal power output for a shortening muscle can be directly calculated based on Hill's model introduced earlier in this chapter.

Muscular power (P) is defined as the product of force and velocity ($F \cdot v$). Therefore, for a given force–velocity relation of a muscle, its instantaneous power as a function of velocity of action, $P(v)$, may be determined throughout the range of shortening speeds (Fig. 9.24). For many practical applications, it is of interest to calculate at what speed of shortening, absolute maximal power, P_0, is reached.

By definition:

$$P(v) = F(v)v \tag{46}$$

where:

$$\frac{dP(v)}{dv} = \frac{dF}{dv}v + F(v) \tag{47}$$

and using Hill's equation (eqn 3):

$$\frac{dP(v)}{dv} = \frac{(F_0 + a)b^2 - a(v + b)^2}{(v + b)^2} \tag{48}$$

Realizing that $dP(v)/dv$ needs to be zero for $P(v)$ to become maximal (i.e. P_0), one has:

$$0 = \frac{(F_0 + a)b^2 - a(v + b)^2}{(v + b)^2} \tag{49}$$

Solving eqn 49 for the velocity, v_m, at which P_0 occurs gives:

$$v_m = b\left(\sqrt{(F_0/a) + 1} - 1\right) \tag{50}$$

Assuming that Hill's thermodynamic constants are well approximated for a range of temperatures by $a = 0.25\ F_0$, and $b = 0.25\ V_0$, we can substitute a and b in eqn 50 and obtain:

$$v_m = \frac{v_0}{4}\left(\sqrt{4 + 1} - 1\right) \tag{51}$$

or:

$$v_m \approx 0.31 v_0 \tag{52}$$

which means that the speed of shortening at which maximal muscular power may be produced is about 31% of the maximal speed of shortening.

Therefore, if one wants to maximize power production of a shortening muscle, the muscle should be at optimal length and shorten at a speed of approximately 31% of its maximal speed of shortening. From direct measurements, Lutz and Rome (1993) argued that frog semimembranosus did just that, and therefore was an optimal power producer during frog jumping. Lutz and Rome (1993) further argued that the other frog jumping muscles would also have to produce maximal power output, like the semimembranosus, in order to explain the tremendous jumping ability of frogs.

As far-fetched as it may appear, the above example may be translated into human sports activities. Here, we chose sprint bicycling as an example. Imagine that the goal of the activity is to bicycle 200 m in the shortest time possible with a flying start. This is precisely the event used to qualify and seed athletes in the track bicycle sprinting event. The best riders in the world cover the 200 m distance in about 10 s for men and 11 s for women.

The rules in sprint bicycling demand that the athlete has only a single, fixed gear for the 200-m time trial. Therefore, depending on the gear ratio chosen, the athlete has to perform a precisely known number of pedal revolutions to complete the 200-m race. For example, most riders choose a gear ratio that gives them about 8 m of translation per pedal revolution; therefore 25 full pedal revolutions are required to complete the 200-m race. If the competitor wants to do this in 10 s (a world-class time), 2.5 pedal revolutions per second (or 150 revolutions per minute) are required.

For a fixed gear ratio and a given bicycle design, and assuming the rider sits while performing the sprint (which they normally do), the length range over which the propulsive leg muscles work, and the corresponding speed of contraction can be determined. In order to optimize muscle length for the sprint bicycling task, the geometry of the bike (seat height, pedal length, etc.) may be adjusted, and to optimize the speed of contraction for maximal power output, the gear ratio may be modified. From a theoretical point of view, there is an optimal bicycle design, an optimal posture of the rider, and an optimal choice for the gear ratio to produce maximal muscle power output (Yoshihuku & Herzog 1990). However, such a theoretical analysis is not without difficulties in application. For example, the optimal posture for maximal power output (using bicycle designs that are permitted by the rules of the International Cycling Federation, e.g. reclined bicycles are not permitted) is not ideal in terms of air resistance (Yoshihuku & Herzog 1990). Also, the force–length properties of specific lower limb muscles in well-trained cyclists seem to differ from those of 'normal' (non-cyclist) people (Herzog *et al.* 1991a), a fact that must be considered when specifying an athlete's posture during competition. Furthermore, the gear ratio, and therefore the speed of muscle shortening, will depend on the specific fibre type distribution of the athlete. Everything else being equal, an athlete with a lot of fast-twitch fibres in the major cycling muscles would reach maximal power output at a greater absolute speed of muscle shortening than an athlete with predominantly slow-twitch fibre muscles; therefore the gear ratio should be smaller for the former, so that pedal rate at a maximal power output is greater in the fast-twitch compared to the slow-twitch fibre athlete.

Final comments

There is a variety of muscle models that have been used in biomechanics to predict force and power output of muscles during movement and sports activities. By far the most common of these is the Hill model, typically an adaptation of Hill's (1938) classic work on the force–velocity relationship of tetanically contracting muscle. However, Huxley-type or cross-bridge models have also been used, although typically just as so-called two-stage models, models in which cross-bridges are either attached or detached (Huxley 1957). Different attachment states, as introduced by Huxley and Simmons (1971), have typically not been considered for musculoskeletal modelling, as they are perceived to be too complex mathematically (although with the capacity of today's computers, mathematical complexity does not need to be a concern any more). We did not consider any muscle models based on the actual morphology of muscle, and its three-dimensional deformation during contraction, as such models are typically not used in the analysis of human motion, but serve a more basic need, such as identification of fibre shortening during muscle contraction. Neither were EMG-driven muscle models considered, as these are typically based on a Hill muscle model (discussed above), and a tentative relationship between EMG, contractile conditions and force. Unfortunately, the relationship between EMG and force in dynamically contracting muscle has not been modelled successfully to date, except when using large-scale numerical approaches, such as adaptive filtering or artificial neural network approaches (Savelberg & Herzog 1997; Liu *et al.* 1999).

When attempting to apply muscle models to human movement, at least two basic problems are encountered.

1 Most of the muscle properties are only known for specific experimental conditions. For example, the force–length relationship for an isolated muscle is easily derived through a succession of maximal isometric actions at different lengths. However, we do not know how this relationship changes for submaximal contractions, during fatigue, after potentiation, for dynamic actions, etc.

2 Typically, individual muscle properties are known for isolated and artificially stimulated muscle preparations. The actual, *in vivo* properties might considerably differ from those determined artificially. For example the eccentric part of the force–velocity relationship has a steep rise around the isometric part (i.e. at slow stretch velocities), and reaches a peak force of about 1.5–2.0 times the maximal isometric force. However, *in vivo*, such a steep eccentric force increase is missing, and values of 1.5–2.0 times the isometric force have not been observed *in vivo*. Rather, the eccentric force–velocity relationship appears to be flat, and reaches values close to the isometric forces (Westing *et al.* 1990).

However, aside from all these problems, one could argue that muscle models and individual muscle properties are not as important for athletic performance prediction and training advice as are the overall, *in vivo* properties of entire groups of muscles. Strength curves describe the relationship of forces or moments as a function of joint angles. Strength curves are known for most of the large joints in the human body (Kulig *et al.* 1984). They are easily obtained and describe the combined force–length, activation-length and moment-arm–length relationship of groups of muscles, and so might represent much better the requirements of *in vivo* muscle function than any relationship obtained using artificial stimulation in isolated muscle preparations.

However, despite all the difficulties associated with relating muscle mechanics and models of muscular contraction to sport, there is an inexcusable lack of muscular considerations in the enhancement of sports performance or the training of athletes. Traditionally, muscular considerations have been centred around acquiring strength, i.e. sport-specific strength training. From our point of view, the following muscular considerations have been (virtually) ignored, and they deserve attention.

WHAT IS THE FUNCTIONAL ROLE OF MUSCLES IN GIVEN SPORTS ACTIVITIES?

For example: in most sports, we do not know the most basic aspects of muscle functioning. When is a muscle stretched or shortened in relation to its activation, force production and timing relative to the task at hand? Although such questions might be addressed easily for one-joint muscles, the situation is somewhat more complex for multijoint muscles. Once the relationship between muscle shortening/stretching, activation, force production and timing relative to the task is known, it will be a challenge to relate this information to the contractile element (fibre) level, as it is well known, particularly for pennate, multijoint muscles, that stretch/shortening of the muscle does not reflect well the amount and timing of stretch/shortening on the contractile element level (Hoffer *et al.* 1989; Griffiths 1991). And, after all, it is (presumably) the contractile element length and speed of contraction that determines force production (and regulatory feedback control via muscle spindle pathways).

HOW DO MUSCLE PROPERTIES ADAPT WITH CHRONIC TRAINING?

Although there are a variety of studies on strength adaptation, these are ignored here, as there are entire textbooks on the topic. However, changes associated with adaptations of functional properties of muscles as a function of chronic training have not been systematically studied in elite athletes. More by accident than by design, we discovered a few years ago that the force–length properties of the rectus femoris in runners and bicyclists had exactly opposite characteristics. In runners, the force–length relationship had a positive slope (ascending limb of the force–length relationship), whereas in cyclists it had a negative slope (descending limb). The reason for this adaptation was associated with two specific functional differences. In running, the rectus femoris undergoes an active stretch–shortening cycle and great forces are required at long muscle lengths. In bicycling, the rectus femoris only shortens actively and great forces are required at short muscle lengths. There are a variety of reasons how these differences in the force–length properties can be explained. The most obvious reason (although that does not mean it is the correct one) is that there is an adaptation in the number of sarcomeres that are arranged in series. In our example, runners would be expected to have more sarcomeres in series in the rectus femoris than bicyclists (Fig. 9.22). Therefore, for a given muscle and fibre length, average sarcomere length for the runners would be smaller than for the cyclists. If the difference in sarcomere number is great enough, it could well be, as we observed, that a runner's rectus femoris works predominantly on the ascending, and a bicyclist's rectus femoris works predominantly on the descending limb of the force–length relationship. Interestingly, the force–length relationship of normal (not chronically trained) people lies in between the two extremes seen for the runners and cyclists; i.e. it is centred around the plateau region (Herzog & ter Keurs 1988).

This result has two important messages for top-level athletes: (i) a triathlete (who runs and cycles) can never run (or cycle) as fast as an equally talented athlete who trains the same amount as the triathlete but focuses just on running (or cycling), because the triathlete's muscles will not be able to adapt as effectively to the single task as those of the specialist; (ii) cross-training for top athletes might be great for a variety of reasons (prevention of injury, rehabilitation, overall conditioning, mental break, etc.); however, it is likely not good for optimal muscle adaptation to a single task.

WHAT IS THE FORCE SHARING BETWEEN SYNERGISTIC MUSCLES?

Research in experimental animals has demonstrated that force sharing between synergistic muscles is not always as one might suspect intuitively. For example, the size principle of motor unit recruitment might hold for single muscles, as initially demonstrated by Henneman *et al.* (1965). However, the size principle does not hold across synergistic muscles. For example, in the cat hindlimb, the soleus produces force during quiet stance, whereas, simultaneously, the medial gastrocnemius might be silent (Hodgson 1983). For paw shaking, the reverse is correct: the medial gastrocnemius produces great forces, whereas the soleus is silent (Smith *et al.* 1980; Abraham & Loeb 1985). This represents a complete reversal of force production in these two muscles, and contradicts the idea of motor unit recruitment according to the size principle across muscles. Also, from a functional point of view, the cat soleus does not produce work during locomotion, whereas the medial gastrocnemius does (Herzog & Leonard 2001). Thus, the question arises, what do these two muscles do? How do they share functional requirements? And how might they be trained effectively?

Translated to the human athlete, these results from the cat experiments imply that during maximal effort, high-speed activity, some muscles might not be recruited maximally, and they might not contribute much to the task at hand. For example, during human sprint running, it is likely that not all leg muscles contribute maximally. Therefore, it might be useless to focus training on the non-maximally recruited muscles. Running at 80% of the sprinting speed might do much good for a sprinter's stamina and overall conditioning, but might do little to improve the 100-m time. However, training at high speeds, near, at or even above race speed, can only be done for very short periods of time and limits the total amount of running that can be done. So, one of the questions of a sprint coach might be: 'How can I get at the relevant sprint muscles, and how can I recruit the fastest motor units in these muscles with relatively little effort, so that these muscles and motor units might be subjected to great work loads?' It has been hinted that fast movements with little resistance might do precisely that job. Also, eccentric muscle action has been implicated to recruit large and very fast motor units at relatively low intensities of work. Therefore, eccentric training might be a way to provide great work loads to the motor units and muscles that might otherwise only be recruited at extreme efforts or speeds of (concentric) contraction. However, hard scientific evidence, demonstrating such recruitment patterns unmistakably, is not available.

One safe way to recruit large motor units of the fast-twitch type is by electrical stimulation of the corresponding muscle nerve. It is well known that large motor units have nerve axons of greater diameter than slow-twitch (small) motor units. The greater axon diameter of the fast-twitch motor units compared to the slow twitch motor units causes a decrease in electrical resistance. Therefore, when a muscle nerve is electrically stimulated, large motor axons belonging to large and fast-twitch motor units tend to be recruited preferentially at low stimulation current. Therefore, electrical muscle stimulation may be an easy way to 'train' fast-twitch motor units without great overall muscular effort.

Summarizing, there are a great number of possibilities for applying muscle research, muscular properties and muscular adaptation to sport performance and training. However, little systematic research has been done in this area. It almost appears that muscle research and sport science are divorced from each other, and any reconciliation seems hard. It is not clear why sport science has evolved without much consideration of muscle mechanics. There is a vast array of research possibilities connecting sport science with basic muscle research, and it is hoped that some of the possibilities mentioned here will be explored systematically in the future.

References

Abbott, B.C. & Aubert, X.M. (1952) The force exerted by active striated muscle during and after change of length. *Journal of Physiology* **117**, 77–86.

Abbott, B.C. & Wilkie, D.R. (1953) The relation between velocity of shortening and the tension–length curve of skeletal muscle. *Journal of Physiology* **120**, 214–223.

Abraham, L.D. & Loeb, G.E. (1985) The distal hindlimb musculature of the cat. *Experimental Brain Research* **58**, 580–593.

Astumian, R.D. (1997) Thermodynamics and kinetics of a Brownian motor. *Science* **276**, 917–922.

Astumian, R.D. & Bier, M. (1996) Mechanochemical coupling of the motion of molecular motors to ATP hydrolysis. *Biophysical Journal* **70**, 637–653.

Block, S.M. (1995) One small step for myosin. *Nature* **378**, 132–133.

Chandrasekhar, S. (1943) Stochastic problems in physics and astronomy. *Reviews of Modern Physics* **15**, 1–89.

Cooke, R., White, H. & Pate, E. (1994) A model of the release of myosin heads from actin in rapidly contracting muscle fibers. *Biophysical Journal* **66**, 778–788.

Derenyi, I. & Vicsek, T. (1996) The kinesin walk: a dynamic model with elastically coupled heads. *Proceedings of the National Academy of Sciences of the United States of America* **93**, 6775–6779.

Derenyi, I. & Vicsek, T. (1998) Realistic models of biological motion. *Physica A* **249**, 397–406.

Edman, K.A.P., Elzinga, G. & Noble, M.I.M. (1978) Enhancement of mechanical performance by stretch during tetanic contractions of vertebrate skeletal muscle fibres. *Journal of Physiology* **281**, 139–155.

Edman, K.A.P., Elzinga, G. & Noble, M.I.M. (1982) Residual force enhancement after stretch of contracting frog single muscle fibers. *Journal of General Physiology* **80**, 769–784.

Edman, K.A.P., Caputo, C. & Lou, F. (1993) Depression of tetanic force induced by loaded shortening of frog muscle fibres. *Journal of Physiology* **466**, 535–552.

Eisenberg, E. & Greene, L.E. (1980) The relation of muscle biochemistry to muscle physiology. *Annual Review of Physiology* **42**, 293–309.

Eisenberg, E., Hill, T.L. & Chen, Y.D. (1980) Cross-bridge model of muscle biochemistry to muscle contraction: quantitative analysis. *Biophysical Journal* **29**, 195–227.

Feynman, R.P., Leis, A.A. & Sands, M. (1966) *The Feynman Lectures in Physics*. Addison-Wesley, Reading, MA.

Finer, J.T., Simmons, R.M. & Spudich, J.A. (1994) Single myosin molecule mechanics: piconewton forces and nanometre steps. *Nature* **368**, 113–119.

Forcinito, M., Epstein, M. & Herzog, W. (1997) Theoretical considerations on myofibril stiffness. *Biophysical Journal* **72**, 1278–1286.

Ford, L.E., Huxley, A.F. & Simmons, R.M. (1977) Tension responses to sudden length change in stimulated frog muscle fibers near slack length. *Journal of Physiology* **269**, 441–515.

Funatsu, T., Harada, Y., Tokunaga, M., Saito, K. & Yanagida, T. (1995) Imaging of single fluorescent molecules and individual ATP turnovers by single myosin molecules in aqueous solution. *Nature* **374**, 555–559.

Gasser, H.S. & Hill, A.V. (1924) The dynamics of muscular contraction. *Proceedings of the Royal Society of London Series B* **96**, 398–437.

Gordon, A.M., Huxley, A.F. & Julian, F.J. (1966) The variation in isometric tension with sarcomere length in vertebrate muscle fibres. *Journal of Physiology* **184**, 170–192.

Granzier, H.L.M. & Pollack, G.H. (1989) Effect of active pre-shortening on isometric and isotonic performance of single frog muscle fibres. *Journal of Physiology* **415**, 299–327.

Griffiths, R.I. (1991) Shortening of muscle fibres during stretch of the active cat medial gastrocnemius muscle: the role of tendon compliance. *Journal of Physiology* **436**, 219–236.

Henneman, E., Somjen, G. & Carpenter, D.O. (1965) Functional significance of cell size in spinal motoneurons. *Journal of Neurophysiology* **28**, 560–580.

Herzog, W. (1998) History dependence of force production in skeletal muscle: a proposal for mechanisms. *Journal of Electromyography and Kinesiology* **8**, 111–117.

Herzog, W. & ter Keurs, H.E.D.J. (1988) Force–length relation of in-vivo human rectus femoris muscles. *Pflügers Archiv, European Journal of Physiology* **411**, 642–647.

Herzog, W. & Leonard, T.R. (2001) A new mechanism for force enhancement following stretch for skeletal muscle. *Proceedings of the Society for Experimental Biology Annual Meeting 33*, University of Canterbury, Kent.

Herzog, W., Guimaraes, A.C.S., Anton, M.G. & Carter-Erdman, K.A. (1991a) Moment–length relations of rectus femoris muscles of speed skaters/cyclists and runners. *Medicine and Science in Sports and Exercise* **23**, 1289–1296.

Herzog, W., Read, L.J. & ter Keurs, H.E.D.J. (1991b) Experimental determination of force–length relations of intact human gastrocnemius muscles. *Clinical Biomechanics* **6**, 230–238.

Herzog, W., Leonard, T.R., Renaud, J.M., Wallace, J., Chaki, G. & Bornemisza, S. (1992) Force–length properties and functional demands of cat gastrocnemius, soleus and plantaris muscles. *Journal of Biomechanics* **25**, 1329–1335.

Hill, A.V. (1938) The heat of shortening and the dynamic constants of muscle. *Proceedings of the Royal Society of London* **126**, 136–195.

Hill, A.V. (1970) *First and Last Experiments in Muscle Mechanics*. Cambridge University Press, Cambridge.

Hodgson, J.A. (1983) The relationship between soleus and gastrocnemius muscle activity in conscious cats —a model for motor unit recruitment? *Journal of Physiology* **337**, 553–562.

Hoffer, J.A., Caputi, A.A., Pose, I.E. & Griffiths, R.I. (1989) Roles of muscle activity and load on the relationship between muscle spindle length and whole muscle length in the freely walking cat. In: *Progress in Brain Research* (eds J.H.H. Allum & M. Hulliger), pp. 75–85. Elsevier Science Publishers B.V., Amsterdam.

Huxley, A.F. (1957) Muscle structure and theories of contraction. *Progress in Biophysics and Biophysical Chemistry* **7**, 255–318.

Huxley, H.E. (1969) The mechanism of muscular contraction. *Science* **164**, 1356–1366.

Huxley, H.E. & Hansen, J. (1954) Changes in cross-striations of muscle during contraction and stretch and their structural implications. *Nature* **173**, 973–976.

Huxley, A.F. & Niedergerke, R. (1954) Structural changes in muscle during contraction. Interference microscopy of living muscle fibres. *Nature* **173**, 971–973.

Huxley, A.F. & Simmons, R.M. (1971) Proposed mechanism of force generation in striated muscle. *Nature* **233**, 533–538.

Iwazumi, T. (1979) A new field theory of muscle contraction. In: *Crossbridge Mechanism in Muscle Contraction* (eds H. Sugi & G.H. Pollack), pp. 611–632. University of Tokyo Press, Tokyo.

Julicher, F. (1999) Force and motion generation of molecular motors: a generic description. In: *Transport and Structure in Biophysical and Chemical Phenomena. Lecture Notes in Physics* (eds S.C. Müller, J. Parisi

& W. Zimmermann), pp. 46–74. Springer-Verlag, Berlin.

Julicher, F., Ajdari, A. & Prost, J. (1997) Modeling molecular motors. *Reviews of Modern Physics* **69**, 1269–1281.

Katz, B. (1939) The relation between force and speed in muscular contraction. *Journal of Physiology* **96**, 45–64.

Keller, D. & Bustamante, C. (2000) The mechanochemistry of molecular motors. *Biophysical Journal* **78**, 541–556.

Kojima, H., Ishijima, A. & Yanagida, T. (1994) Direct measurement of stiffness of single actin filaments with and without tropomyosin by in vitro nanomanipulation. *Proceedings of the National Academy of Sciences of the United States of America* **91**, 12962–12966.

Kramers, H.A. (1940) Brownian motion in a field of force and the diffusion theory of chemical reactions. *Physica* 7, 284–304.

Kulig, K., Andrews, J.G. & Hay, J.G. (1984) Human strength curves. In: *Exercise and Sport Sciences Reviews*, Vol. 12 (ed. R.L. Terjung), pp. 417–466. The Collamore Press, Lexington, MA.

Liu, M.M., Herzog, W. & Savelberg, H.C.M. (1999) Dynamic muscle force predictions from EMG: an artificial neural network approach. *Journal of Electromyography and Kinesiology* **9**, 391–400.

Lutz, G.J. & Rome, L.C. (1993) Built for jumping: The design of the frog muscular system. *Science* **263**, 370–372.

Magnasco, M.O. (1993) Forced thermal ratchets. *Physical Review Letters* **71**, 1477–1480.

Mai, M.T. & Lieber, R.L. (1990) A model of semitendinosus muscle sarcomere length, knee and hip joint interaction in the frog hindlimb. *Journal of Biomechanics* **23**, 271–279.

Maréchal, G. & Plaghki, L. (1979) The deficit of the isometric tetanic tension redeveloped after a release of frog muscle at a constant velocity. *Journal of General Physiology* **73**, 453–467.

Mcquarrie, D.A. (1976) *Statistical Mechanics*. Harper & Row, New York.

Molloy, J.E., Burns, J.E., Kendrick-Jones, J., Tregear, R.T. & White, D.C.S. (1995) Movement and force produced by a single myosin head. *Nature* **378**, 209–212.

Nishizaka, T., Miyata, H., Yoshikawa, H., Ishiwata, S. & Kinosita, K.J. (1995) Unbinding force of a single motor molecule of muscle measured using optical tweezers. *Nature* **377**, 251–254.

Podolsky, R.J. (1960) Kinetics of muscular contraction: the approach to the steady state. *Nature* **188**, 666–668.

Pollack, G.H. (1995) Muscle contraction mechanism: are alternative engines gathering steam. *Cardiovascular Research* **29**, 737–746.

Rack, P.M.H. & Westbury, D.R. (1969) The effects of length and stimulus rate on tension in the isometric cat soleus muscle. *Journal of Physiology* **204**, 443–460.

Ramsey, R.W. & Street, S.F. (1940) The isometric length–tension diagram of isolated skeletal muscle fibers of the frog. *Journal of Cellular Composition* **15**, 11–34.

Rayment, I., Holden, H.M., Whittaker, M. *et al.* (1993) Structure of the actin–myosin complex and its implications for muscle contraction. *Science* **261**, 58–65.

Savelberg, H.C.M. & Herzog, W. (1997) Prediction of dynamic tendon forces from electromyographic signals: an artificial neural network approach. *Journal of Neuroscience Methods* **78**, 65–74.

Smith, J.L., Betts, B., Edgerton, V.R. & Zernicke, R.F. (1980) Rapid ankle extension during paw shakes: selective recruitment of fast ankle extensors. *Journal of Neurophysiology* **43**, 612–620.

Spudich, J.A. (1994) How molecular motors work. *Nature* **372**, 515–518.

Sugi, H. & Tsuchiya, T. (1988) Stiffness changes during enhancement and deficit of isometric force by slow length changes in frog skeletal muscle fibres. *Journal of Physiology* **407**, 215–229.

Suter, E. & Herzog, W. (1997) Extent of muscle inhibition as a function of knee angle. *Journal of Electromyography and Kinesiology* **7**, 123–130.

Svoboda, K., Schmidt, B., Schnapp, B.J. & Block, S.M. (1993) Direct observation of kinesin stepping by optical trapping interferometry. *Nature* **365**, 721–727.

Westing, S.H., Seger, J.Y. & Thorstensson, A. (1990) Effects of electrical stimulation on eccentric and concentric torque–velocity relationships during knee extension in man. *Acta Physiologica Scandinavica* **140**, 17–22.

Woledge, R.C., Curtin, N.A. & Homsher, E. (1985) *Energetic Aspects of Muscle Contraction*. Academic Press, London.

Yanagida, T. (1999) Simultaneous observation of individual ATPase and mechanical events by a single myosin molecule during interaction with actin (ed. W. Herzog). *Canmore Symposium on Skeletal Muscle*, p. 22. Canmore, Alberta.

Yoshihuku, Y. & Herzog, W. (1990) Optimal design parameters of the bicycle-rider system for maximal muscle power output. *Journal of Biomechanics* **23**, 1069–1079.

Zahalak, G.I. (1997) Can muscle fibers be stable on the descending limbs of their sarcomere length–tension relations? *Journal of Biomechanics* **30**, 1179–1182.

Zahalak, G.I. & Ma, S.-P. (1990) Muscle activation and contraction: constitutive relations based directly on cross-bridge kinetics. *Journal of Biomechanical Engineering* **112**, 52–62.

Zahalak, G.I. & Motabarzadeh, I. (1997) A re-examination of calcium activation in the Huxley cross-bridge model. *Journal of Biomechanical Engineering* **119**, 20–28.

Zhou, H. & Chen, Y. (1996) Chemically driven motility of Brownian particles. *Phy Rev Lett* **77**, 194–197.

Chapter 10

Stretch–Shortening Cycle

PAAVO V. KOMI

The nature of the stretch–shortening cycle

In Chapter 1, muscle exercises were classified primarily into static and dynamic types. The classification used in Table 1.1 (p. 5) cannot, however, be used to describe the natural form of muscle function. The true nature of muscle function is difficult to assess from isolated forms of isometric, concentric or eccentric actions. In real life, exercise seldom involves a pure form of these types of isolated muscle actions. The natural variation of muscle function is more often a stretch and shortening cycle and thus this model provides a good basis from which to study both normal and fatigued muscle. Two important aspects of this phenomena are (i) preactivation and (ii) variable activation of the muscles preceding the functional phase of a given movement (e.g. ground contact for the leg extensor muscles during running). Other important concepts that need to be addressed are length changes in muscle vs. tendon during the contact phase, and the role of the stretch reflex in the stretch–shortening cycle.

The stretch–shortening cycle (SSC) of muscle function comes from the observation that body segments are periodically subjected to impact or stretch forces. Running, walking and hopping are typical examples in human locomotion of how external forces (e.g. gravity) lengthen the muscle. In this lengthening phase the muscle is acting eccentrically, then a concentric (shortening) action follows. The true definition of eccentric action indicates that the muscles must be active during stretch. This combination of eccentric and concentric actions forms a natural type of muscle function called the stretch–shortening cycle or SSC (Norman & Komi 1979; Komi 1984, 2000) (Fig. 10.1). This type of sequence in muscle function also involves the important features of preactivation and variable activation. SSC muscle function has a well-recognized purpose: enhancement of performance during the final phase (concentric action) when compared to the isolated concentric action. This can be demonstrated in isolated preparations with constant electrical stimulation (e.g. Cavagna *et al.* 1965, 1968), in animal experiments with natural and variable muscle activation (e.g. Gregor *et al.* 1988) and in maximal effort conditions of human SSC actions (Cavagna *et al.* 1968; Komi 1983). Figure 10.2 shows the force potentiation in SSCs in human knee extension muscles when the coupling between the stretch and shortening is varied. When no delay is allowed for coupling the force is clearly potentiated in the concentric phase. In the conditions of Fig. 10.2 maximal electromyographic (EMG) activation was maintained throughout the actions. Considerable effort has been devoted to explaining the mechanisms for this force and power potentiation during an SSC. Cavagna *et al.* (1965) was one of the first to argue that this enhancement comes primarily from stored elastic energy. Since that time many additional alternative explanations (e.g. Huijing 1992; Komi & Gollhofer 1997; van Ingen-Schenau *et al.* 1997) have been presented. However, no

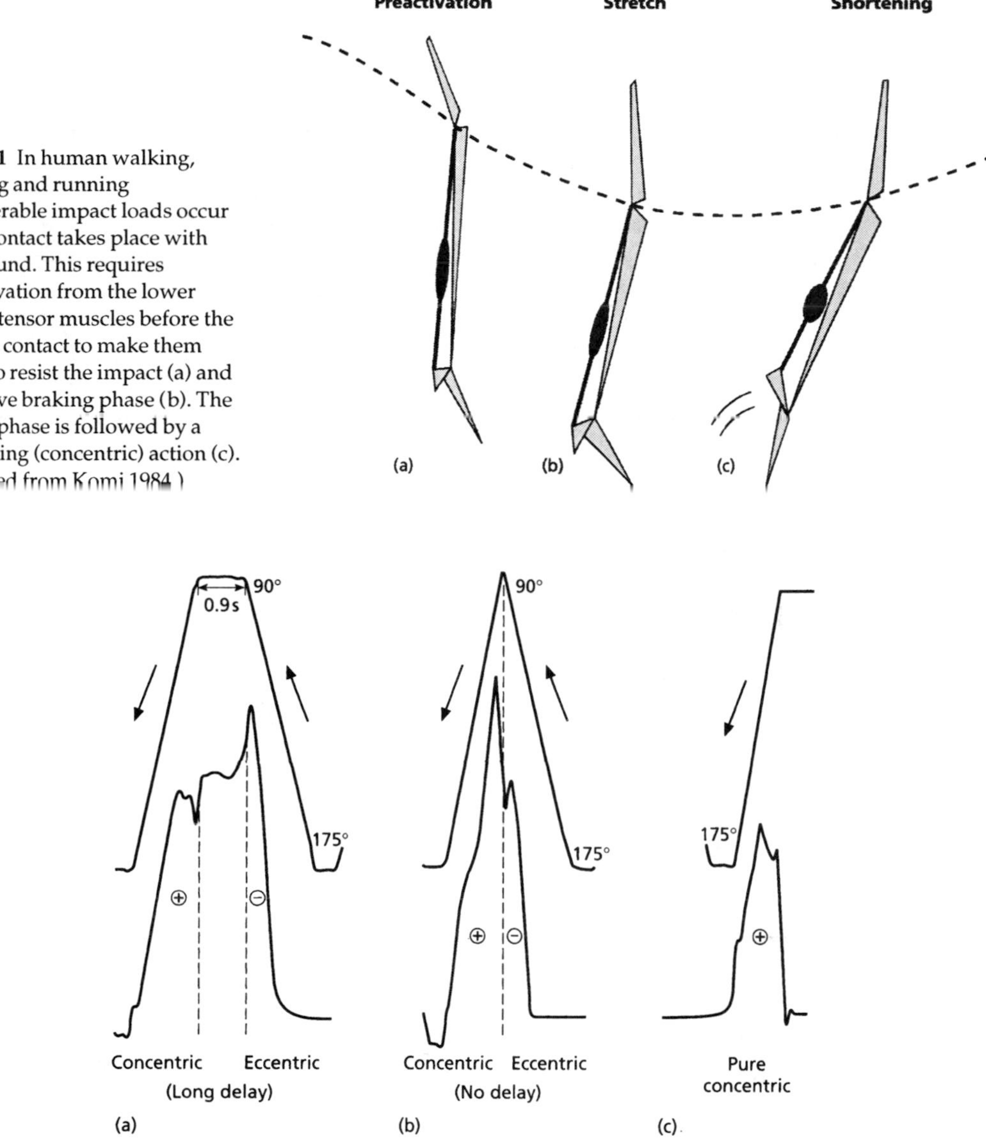

Fig. 10.1 In human walking, hopping and running considerable impact loads occur when contact takes place with the ground. This requires preactivation from the lower limb extensor muscles before the ground contact to make them ready to resist the impact (a) and the active braking phase (b). The stretch phase is followed by a shortening (concentric) action (c). (Adapted from Komi 1984.)

Fig. 10.2 Demonstration of the importance of the short coupling time between eccentric and concentric phases for performance potentiation in the concentric phase of the SSC. Right, pure concentric action of the knee extension from 100° to 175°. Middle, concentric action is preceeded by eccentric (–) action, but no delay is allowed when action type is changed from stretch to shortening. The eccentric (stretch) phase begins in the middle of the movement from the 175° (knee in an extended position) to the 90° position. Note the clear force potentiation in the concentric phase (+) as compared to the condition on the right. Left, a longer delay (0.9 s) was allowed between the eccentric and concentric phases. The potentiation effect on the concentric phase was reduced. Maximal EMG activation was maintained in all conditions. (From Komi 1983.)

convincing evidence has been presented that negates elasticity as an important element in force potentiation during an SSC.

The schematic presentation of Fig. 10.1 takes into consideration the common assumption that in an SSC the contractile and tensile elements are stretched during the eccentric phase. There are, however, arguments in the literature suggesting that the contractile component may maintain a constant length (Hoff *et al.* 1983; Belli & Bosco 1992) or even shorten (Griffiths 1991) during the important early phase of ground contact. However, as will be shown later (Fig. 10.12) the fascicles that primarily represent the contractile tissue can lengthen and shorten, respectively, in the stretching and shortening phases of the SSC.

The present chapter reviews the work of SSC muscle actions performed primarily in human experiments. Admittedly, but perhaps also understandably, much of the work to be referred to comes from our own laboratory. With the limitation of this bias and partly subjective approach, the chapter focuses primarily on demonstrating —with *in vivo* measurement techniques—the recoil nature of the SSC and how the stretch reflexes can play an important role in force potentiation. The material presented is an extension of our previous work on the topic (Komi 1990, 1992, 2000; Komi & Gollhofer 1997; Komi & Nicol 2000).

Use of *in vivo* force measurements to characterize the SSC in human locomotion

Two techniques can be applied to record directly, and *in vivo*, tendon forces in humans: a buckle transducer method and an optic fibre technique.

Buckle transducer method

Of these methods, the buckle technique is the more invasive one and it has been used solely for Achilles tendon (AT) force recordings (e.g. Komi *et al.* 1987b; Komi 1990; Fukashiro *et al.* 1993, 1995). The buckle is surgically implanted around the AT under local anaesthesia, but the subject is able to perform 2–3 h of unrestricted locomotion including walking, running (at different speeds), hopping and jumping. In some cases even maximal long jumps were performed without any discomfort (Kyröläinen *et al.* 1989). Figure 10.3 presents a typical recording obtained during running at a moderate speed. There are several important features to be noted in this figure. First the changes in muscle–tendon length are very small (6–7%) during the stretching phase. This suggests that the conditions favour the potential utilization of short-range elastic stiffness (SRES) (Rack & Westbury 1974) in the muscle. Various length changes are reported in the literature demonstrating that effective range of SRES in *in vitro* preparations is 1–4% (e.g. Huxley & Simmons 1971; Ford *et al.* 1978). In the intact muscle tendon, *in vivo*, this value is increased because series elasticity and fibre geometry must be taken into account. This could then bring the muscle–tendon lengthening to 6–8%. When measurements are made at the muscle fibre level the values could be smaller naturally, as shown by Roberts *et al.* (1997) in turkeys running on level ground.

The second important feature in Fig. 10.3 is that the segmental length changes in these two muscles (gastrocnemius and soleus) take place in phase in both the lengthening and shortening parts of the SSC. This is typical for running and jumping and it has considerable importance because the buckle transducer measures forces of the common tendon for the two muscles. The situation is not so simple in some other activities, such as bicycling (Gregor *et al.* 1991), where the length changes are more out of phase in these two muscles. The third important feature of the example in Fig. 10.3 is that the form of the AT force curve resembles that of a bouncing ball, implying efficient force potentiation.

The buckle technique introduced the basic behaviour of the human AT–triceps surae complex during SSC activities (Komi 1990; Fukashiro *et al.* 1993). Surprisingly, the technique revealed that in bicycling also a small, but meaningful, SSC action could be identified from both gastrocnemius and soleus muscles (Gregor *et al.* 1991).

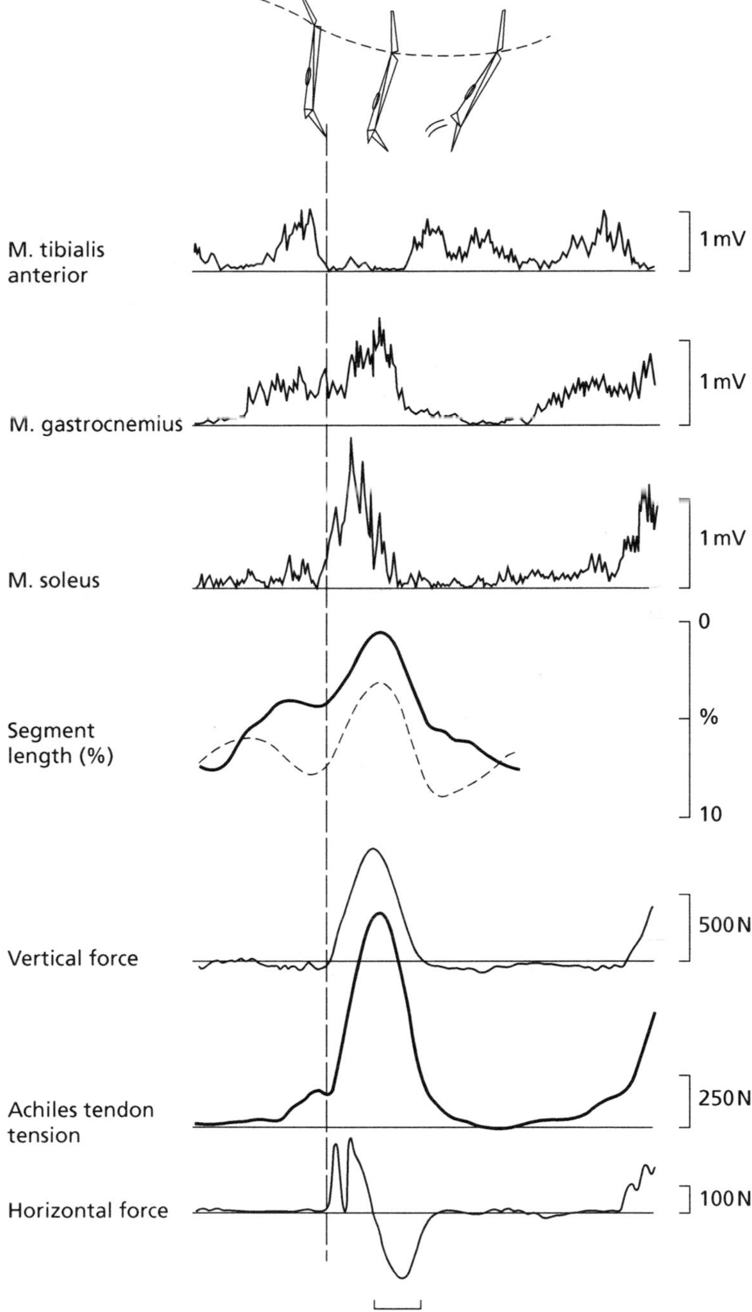

Fig. 10.3 Demonstration of stretch–shortening cycle (SSC) for the triceps surae muscle during the (functional) ground contact phase of human running. Top, schematic position representing the three phases of SSC presented in Fig. 10.1. The rest of the curves represent parameters in the following order (from top to bottom): rectified surface EMG records of the tibialis anterior, gastrocnemius (Ga) and soleus (Sol) muscles; segmental length changes of the two plantar flexor muscles; vertical ground reaction force; directly recorded Achilles tendon force; and the horizontal ground reaction force. The vertical line signifies the beginning of the foot (ball) contact on the force plate. The subject was running at moderate speed. (From Komi 1992.)

The methods also provided the basis of analysing the instantaneous force–velocity curves in both animal (Gregor *et al.* 1988) and human SSC activities (see e.g. Fig. 10.7).

The buckle transducer method is naturally quite invasive, and may receive objections from ethical committees for use in human experiments. An additional disadvantage is a rather long healing time needed before normal locomotion can be resumed after the measurements.

Optic fibre technique

In order to overcome some of the disadvantages of the buckle transducer technique, an alternative method—the optic fibre technique—has recently been developed. As this method is not widely used, but can be applied very well for studying SSC activities, it is appropriate to explain the method in some detail in this chapter.

As was the case for the buckle method, this new optic fibre technique was also first applied to animal tendons (Komi *et al.* 1996). However, it had already earlier been applied with success as a pressure transducer in sensitive skin application (Bocquet & Noel 1987) and for measurement of foot pressure in different phases of cross-country skiing (Candau *et al.* 1993). In fact it was the latter work that resulted in a collaboration with Dr Alain Belli from France in order to develop the method for use as a tendon force transducer (Komi *et al.* 1996). The measurement is based on modulation of light intensity by mechanical modification of the geometric properties of the plastic fibre. The structure of optical fibres used in animal and human experiments (Komi *et al.* 1996; Arndt *et al.* 1998; Finni *et al.* 1998, 2000) consists of two layered cylinders of polymers with small diameters. When the fibre is bent or compressed the light can be reduced linearly with pressure, and the sensitivity depends on the fibre index, fibre stiffness and/or bending radius characteristics. Figure 10.4 characterizes the principle of the light modulation in the two-layer (cladding and core) fibre when the fibre diameter is compressed by external force. The core and cladding will be deformed and a certain amount of light is transferred through the core–cladding interface. In order to avoid the pure effect of bending of the fibre, the fibre when inserted through the tendon (Fig. 10.5) must have a loop large enough to exceed the so-called critical bending radius.

Figure 10.5 demonstrates how the optic fibre is inserted through the tendon. A hollow 19-gauge needle is first passed through the tendon (a). The sterile optic fibre is then passed through the needle; the needle is removed and the fibre remains *in situ* (b). Both ends of the fibre are then attached to the transmitter–receiver unit and the system is ready for measurement. The calibration procedure usually gives a good linear relationship between external force and optic fibre signal. Figure 10.6 gives a representative example of such a relationship for patellar tendon measurements.

Although the optic fibre method may not be more accurate than the buckle transducer method, it has several unique advantages. First of all it is much less invasive and can be reapplied to the same tendon after a few days of rest. In addition, almost any tendon can be studied provided that the critical bending radius is not exceeded. The optic fibre technique can be applied also for measurement of the loading of the various ligaments. In the hands of an experienced surgeon the optic fibre can even be inserted through deeper ligaments such as the anterior talofibular ligament (Alt *et al.* 2002). In such a case, however, special care must be taken

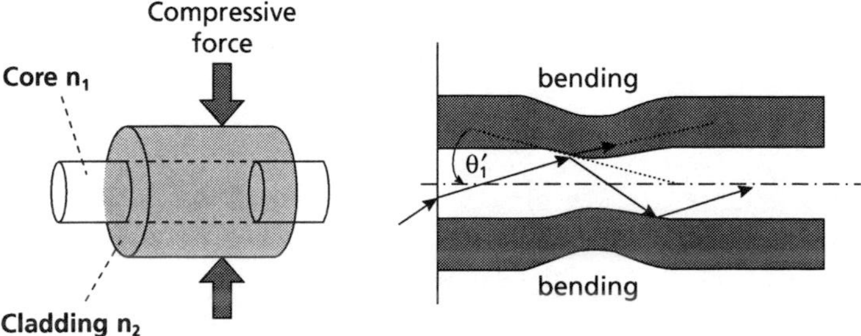

Fig. 10.4 Demonstration of the basic principle behind the compression on the optic fibre (left) causes microbending (right) and less light through the core–cladding interface. (From Alt *et al.* 2002.)

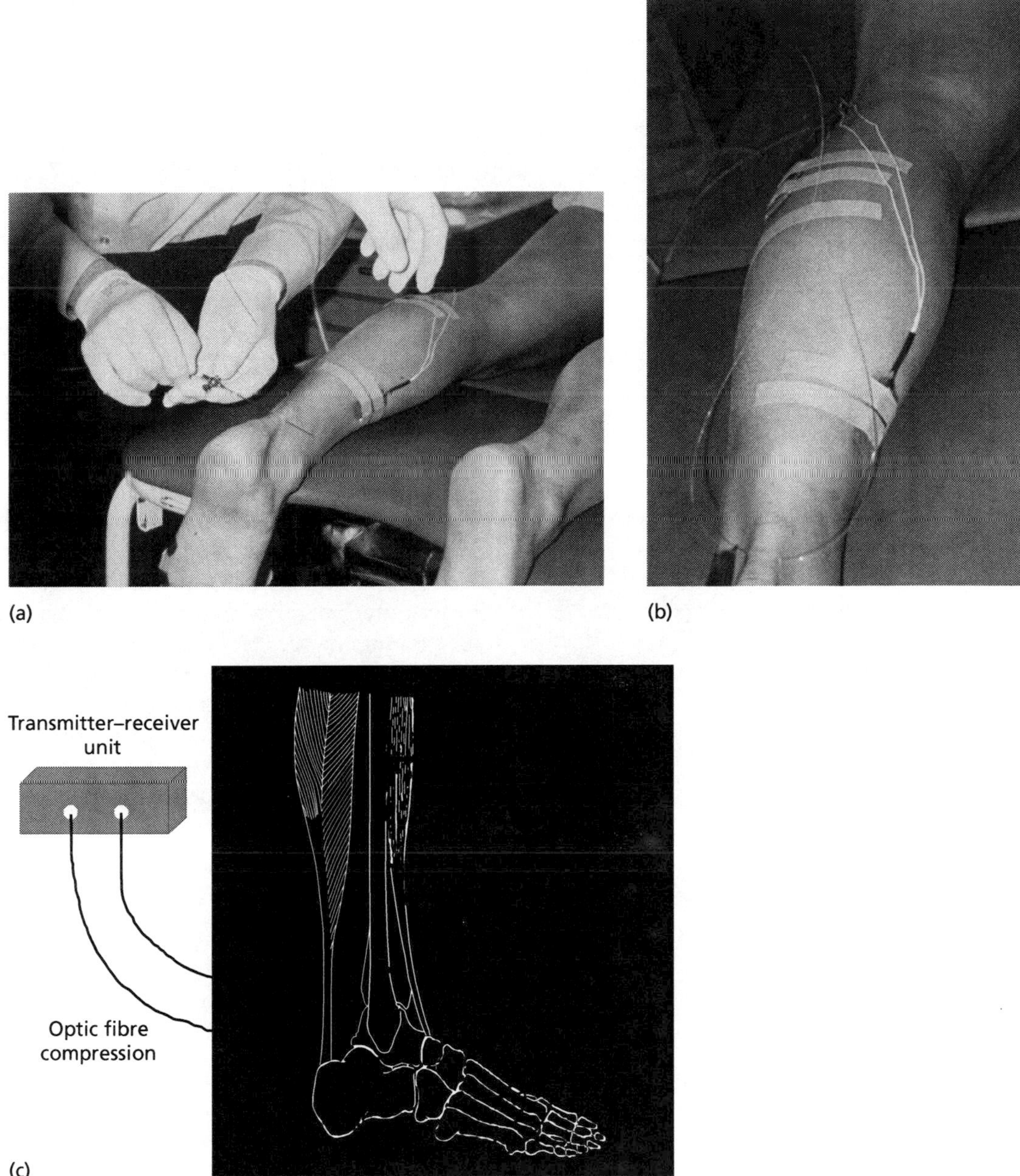

Fig. 10.5 Demonstration of the insertion of the optic fibre into the tendon. a, after the 19-gauge needle has been inserted through the tendon, the 0.5-mm-thick optic fibre is threaded through the needle. The needle is then removed and the optic fibre remains *in situ* inside the tendon (b), and both ends of the fibre are connected to the transmitter–receiver unit. c, in real measurement situations this unit is much smaller and can be fastened onto the skin of the calf muscles.

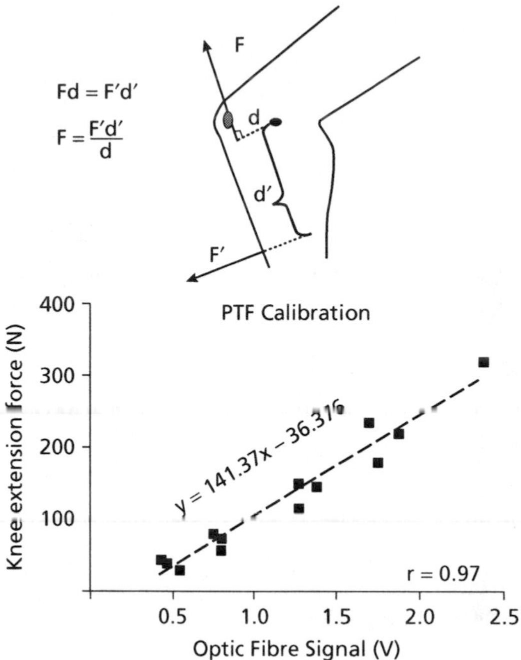

Fig. 10.6 Measured forces and moment arms for the calibration of patellar tendon force (PTF). The optic fibre output was related to the muscle force (F) that had been converted from the external force output (F') using equation $Fd = Fd'$, where d is moment arm of tendon force and d' is moment arm of the foot or leg. (From Finni *et al.* 2000.)

to ensure that the optic fibre is in contact with the ligament only and that it is preserved from interaction with other soft tissue structures by catheters.

Muscle mechanics and performance potentiation in the SSC

The true nature of force potentiation during the SSC can be seen by computing the instantaneous force–length and force–velocity curves from the parameters shown in Fig. 10.3. Figure 10.7 presents the results of such an analysis from fast running, and it covers the functional ground contact phase only. It is important to note from this figure that the force–length curve demonstrates a very sharp increase in force during the stretching phase, which is characterized by a very small change in muscle length. The right-hand side of the figure shows the computed instantaneous force–velocity comparison suggesting high potentiation during the shortening phase (concentric action). Figure 10.8, on the other hand, represents examples of EMG–length and EMG–velocity plots for moderate running. It clearly demonstrates that muscle activation levels are variable and primarily concentrated for the eccentric part

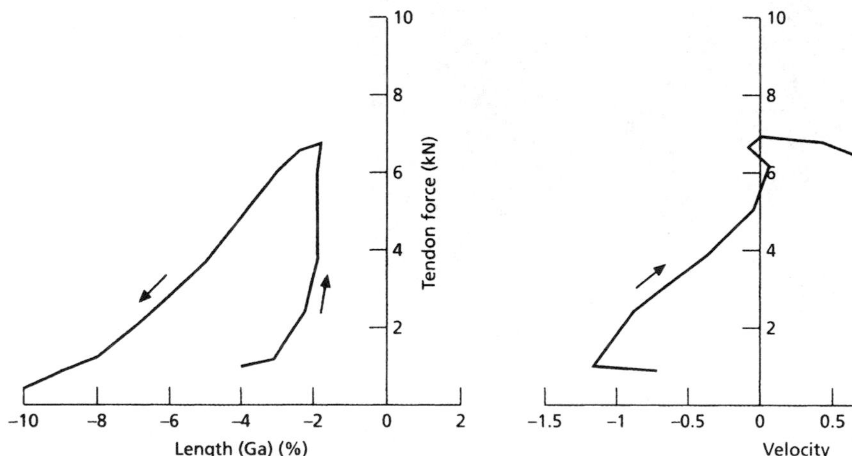

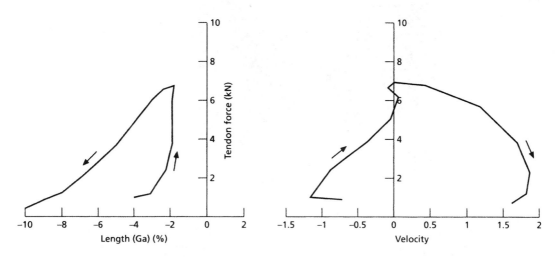

Fig. 10.7 Instantaneous force–length and force–velocity curves of the gastrocnemius muscle for stretch–shortening cycle when the subject ran at a fast speed (9 m·s^{-1}). The upward deflection signifies stretching (eccentric action) and the downward deflection shortening (concentric action) of the muscle during ground contact. The horizontal axes have been derived from segmental length changes according to Grieve *et al.* (1978). (From Komi 1992.)

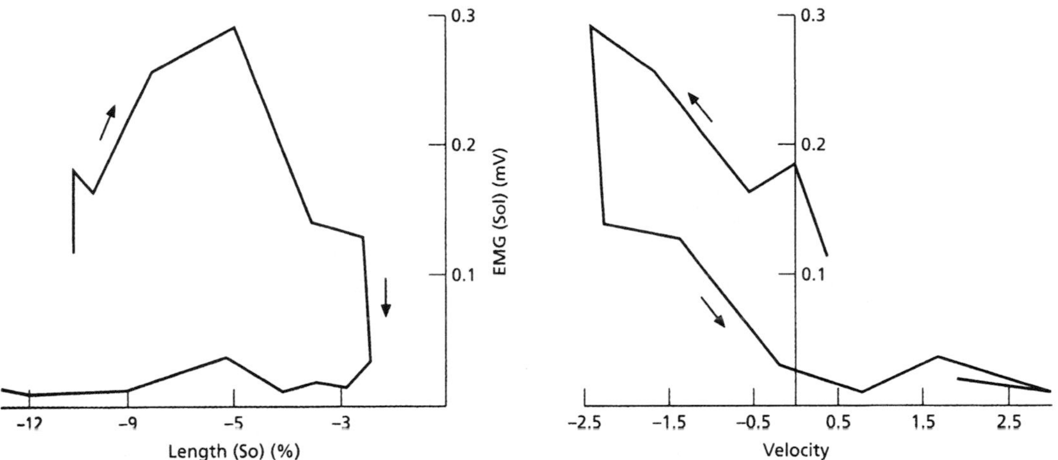

Fig. 10.8 Instantaneous EMG–length and EMG–velocity curves of the soleus muscle for stretch–shortening cycle when the subject ran at moderate speed. The arrows indicate how the events changed from stretching to shortening during the contact phase. Note that the EMG activity is primarily concentrated for the eccentric part of the cycle. Compare these EMG patterns to the rectified EMGs of Fig. 10.3.

of the cycle. This is important to consider when comparing the naturally occurring SSC actions with those obtained with isolated muscle preparations and constant activation levels throughout the cycle.

The classical force–velocity relationship (Hill 1938) describes the fundamental mechanical properties of skeletal muscle (see Chapter 9). Its direct application to natural locomotion, such as SSC, may however, be difficult due to necessity of *in situ* preparations to utilize constant maximal activation. When measured *in vivo* during an SSC the force–velocity curve (Fig. 10.7) is a dramatic demonstration that the curves are very dissimilar to the classical curve obtained for the pure concentric action with isolated muscle preparations (e.g. Hill 1938) or with human forearm flexors (e.g. Wilkie 1950; Komi 1973). Although Fig. 10.7 does not present directly the comparison of the force–velocity curve for the final concentric (push-off) phase with the classical curve, it certainly suggests considerable force potentiation. Unfortunately the human experiment as shown in Fig. 10.7 did not include comparative records obtained in a classical way. However, our recent development of *in vivo* measurements with an optic fibre technique (Komi *et al.* 1995) has now been utilized to obtain these comparisons (Finni *et al.* 1998; Fig. 10.9).

These recent experiments with the optic fibre technique, although not yet performed at high running speeds, suggest similar potentiation. The left side of Fig. 10.9 shows simultaneous plots for both patellar and AT forces during hopping. The records signify that in short-contact hopping the triceps surae muscle behaves with a bouncing ball-type action (see also Fukashiro & Komi 1987, Fukashiro *et al.* 1993). When the hopping intensity is increased or changed to countermovement-type jumps, the patellar tendon force increases and the AT force may decrease (Finni *et al.* 2001a). The classical type of curve obtained with constant maximal activation for an isolated concentric action is also superimposed on the same graph with the AT force (Fig. 10.9a). The shaded area between the two AT curves suggests a remarkable force potentiation for this submaximal effort. It must be emphasized that these performance comparisons have been made between submaximal SSC and maximal isolated concentric action.

The *in vivo* measurement technique for humans has been developed following reports on animal experiments (e.g. Sherif *et al.* 1983).

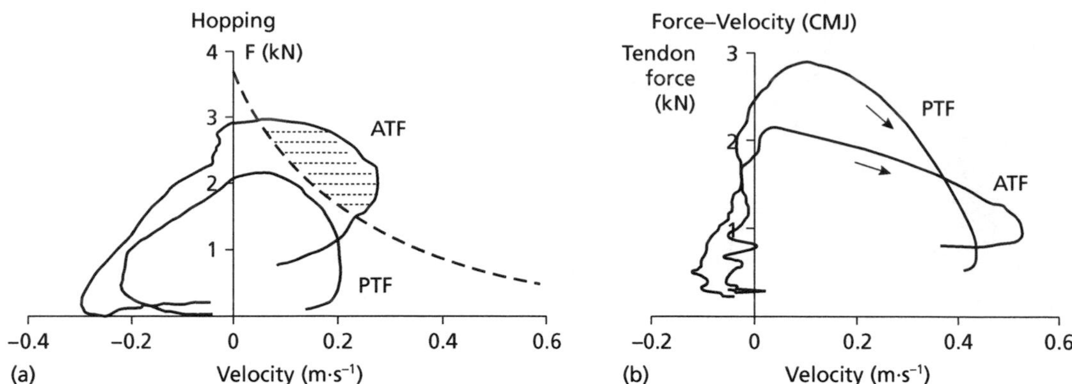

Fig. 10.9 Examples of instantaneous force–velocity curves measured in human hopping and countermovement jumps. a, records (submaximal hopping) present greater loading of the Achilles tendon (ATF) as compared to the patellar tendon (PTF). b, the situation is reversed in case of countermovement jumps. The records signify the functional phases of the ground contact. The left side of both figures represents eccentric action and the right side concentric action. The dashed line signifies the force–velocity curve for plantar flexors measured in the classical way. (From Finni *et al.* 1998 (a) and 2001a (b).)

Many of these animal studies have included similar parameters to those used in our human studies, such as muscle length, force and EMG. The most relevant report for comparison with our human experiments is that by Gregor *et al.* (1988); they measured mechanical outputs of the cat soleus muscle during treadmill locomotion. In that study the results indicated that the force generated at a given shortening velocity during late stance phase was greater, especially at higher speeds of locomotion, than the output generated at the same shortening velocity *in situ*. Thus, both animal and human *in vivo* force experiments seem to give similar results with regard to the force–velocity relationships during an SSC.

The difference between the force–velocity curve and the classical curve in isolated muscle preparations (e.g. Hill 1938) or in human experiments (e.g. Wilkie 1950; Komi 1973) may be partly due to natural differences in muscle activation levels between the two types of activities. While the *in situ* preparations may primarily measure the shortening properties of the contractile elements in the muscle, natural locomotion, primarily utilizing SSC action, involves controlled release of high forces, caused primarily by the eccentric action. This high force favours storage of elastic strain energy in the muscle–tendon complex. A portion of this stored energy can be recovered during the subsequent shortening phase and used for performance potentiation. Both animal and human experiments seem therefore to agree that natural locomotion with primarily SSC muscle action may produce muscle outputs which can be very different to the conditions of isolated preparations, where activation levels are held constant and storage of strain energy is limited. The SSC enables the triceps surae muscle to perform very efficiently in activities such as walking, running and hopping. Recent evidence has demonstrated that the gastrocnemius and soleus muscles also function in bicycling in SSCs, although the active stretching phases are not so apparent as in running or jumping (Gregor *et al.* 1988, 1991).

Important additional features can be seen in Fig. 10.9. The patterns between AT and patellar tendon records differ considerably when the movement is changed from a countermovement jump to a drop-jump. On countermovement jumps—characterized by a smaller eccentric phase—the patellar tendon is much more loaded as compared to the AT which in its turn is more strongly loaded in hopping. Thus the muscle mechanics are not similar in all SSC activities, and generalizations should not be made from one condition and from one specific muscle only. In contrast to hopping, for example, the elastic recoil of the triceps surae muscle plays a much smaller role in countermovement jumps (CMJs) (Fukashiro *et al.* 1993; Finni *et al.* 1998). This is expected because in CMJs the stretch phase is slow and the reflex contribution to SSC potentiation is likely to be much less than in hopping.

One important note of caution must be given when interpreting the muscle mechanics based on the methods shown above. In both animal and human experiments—when the buckles and optic fibres have been applied to the tendons —the measured forces cannot be used to isolate the forces or the movements of the contractile tissue from those of the tendon tissue. The methods can therefore be used to determine the loading characteristics of the entire muscle–tendon complex only. It must be mentioned, however, that as Finni in our laboratory has recently shown (Finni *et al.* 2001b), the fascicle force–velocity curves in isolated forms of maximal eccentric and concentric action resemble quite well the classical force–velocity relationships, and that the instantaneous force–velocity curve in the SSC resembles that of the total muscle-tendon unit, but with a more irregular form.

Fascicle length changes during SSCs

It is evident that although the tendon transducers measure reliably and directly the forces in the tendon, they do not give simultaneous records of the length changes in the muscle–tendon complex. These must be estimated using high-speed video and appropriate anatomical models (e.g. Frigo & Pedotti 1978; Grieve *et al.* 1978). These calculations then need to be synchronized with the tendon force data, as has been done for Figs 10.3, 10.7, 10.8 and 10.9, for example. The obtained results and relationships cannot, however, be used to generate simultaneously information about: (i) the change in length of the muscle fibres; (ii) the change in the fibre orientation with the line of force application; and (iii) the change in length of the tendinous compartment. Successful *in vivo* recordings of changes in muscle fibre length have been made in animal models, such as in cat walking (Griffiths 1991) and turkey running on a treadmill (Roberts *et al.* 1997). The common assumption has been that in SSC activities both the muscle fibre compartment and the tendon would change their lengths in phase. This assumption has recently been challenged, because the muscle fibres may stay at a constant length (Belli & Bosco 1992), or they can even shorten (e.g. Griffiths 1991) while the whole muscle–tendon complex is lengthening.

After the pioneering work of Ikai and Fukunaga (1968) to determine muscle strength per cross-sectional area by means of ultrasonic technique, several decades passed before this technique advanced sufficiently to characterize the muscle architecture *in vivo*. However, the work carried out during the 1990s in Fukunaga's laboratory has produced relevant information regarding the architecture of contracting human muscles (see the review of Kawakami *et al.* 2000). The technique has now been extended to natural locomotion, and the length changes in the fascicles and tendons can be measured *in vivo* (e.g. Fukunaga *et al.* 1996, 1997) Two fundamental problems may arise in these measurements: the behaviour of the entire muscle–tendon complex may not be the same as that of the muscle fibres; and the fascicle velocity may not necessarily be in phase with externally applied isokinetic velocity.

The basic definition of eccentric muscle action (see Chapter 1) refers to lengthening of muscle while it is activated. As this concept has been questioned to apply to the contractile tissue (Griffiths 1991; Belli & Bosco 1992) we decided to examine the fascicle length changes in isolated concentric and eccentric actions as well as in the SSC exercises (Finni *et al.* 2000, 2001c). Figure 10.10 is a typical example of the records obtained for maximal concentric and eccentric actions, and they clearly demonstrate that in knee extension the fascicle of the vastus lateralis (VL) muscle shortens in the concentric mode and lengthens in the eccentric mode (Finni *et al.* 2001c). The magnitude of fascicle shortening in

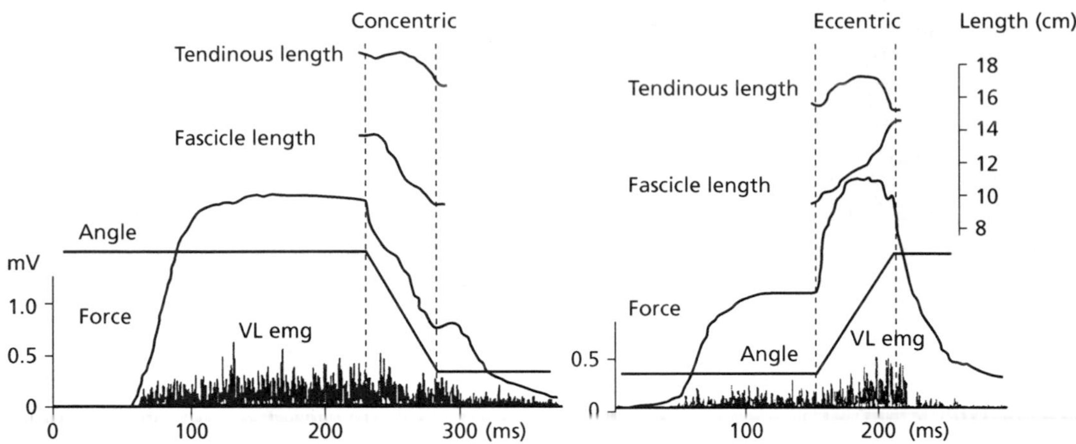

Fig. 10.10 Fascicle and tendon length changes during maximal concentric (left) and eccentric (right) actions. These contractions were produced by maximal preactivation (isometric phase). Note clear shortening of the fascicle in the concentric action as compared to lenthening in the eccentric mode (from Finni *et al.* 2001a).

the concentric mode (2.9 ± 1.4 cm) was smaller than that of lengthening (5.1 ± 1.6 cm) in the eccentric mode. These length changes seemed not to be dependent on the velocity of shortening or lengthening. It must be emphasized in this connection that the lengthening and shortening actions were preceded by isometric preactivation, similar to the method applied in isolated muscle fibre/sarcomeres (see Chapter 9). This provides a good match with the preactivation phase which is so typical in the SSC exercise (e.g. Melvill Jones & Watt 1971; Komi *et al.* 1987a; Horita *et al.* 1999).

In the slow SSC action utilizing CMJs the VL fascicle first demonstrates an increase in length during the eccentric mode followed by shortening in the concentric mode. However, when the CMJ jump was replaced by the faster-type SSC activity, drop-jump, the fascicle demonstrated much smaller length increase in the eccentric phase. Figure 10.11 summarizes the important work of Finni *et al.* (2001b) in these types of muscle functions.

These observations suggest that the muscle lengthening and shortening, respectively, for eccentric and concentric modes of SSC, are naturally occurring events in SSC. The situation is not, however, always this straightforward. In multijoint action especially, there can be conditions where some muscles may demonstrate different patterns from this 'general' rule. For example, if the fascicle of VL is being lengthened in the eccentric phase of CMJ the gastrocnemius muscle can demonstrate either no change in length or shortening of the fascicle.

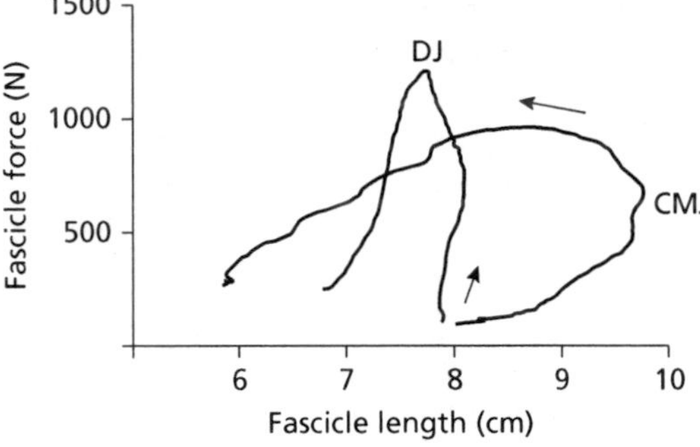

Fig. 10.11 Human skeletal muscle may utilize different portions of the sarcomere force–length curve depending on the type of stretch–shortening cycle action. In this figure of Finni *et al.* (2001b) the fascicle force–length relationships are shown for countermovement jumps (CMJ) and drop-jumps (DJ). Please note the small change in fascicle length in DJ during the entire contact phase on the ground.

Examples of the fascicle behaviour of the vastus lateralis and gastrocnemius muscles during squat-jumps, countermovement jumps and

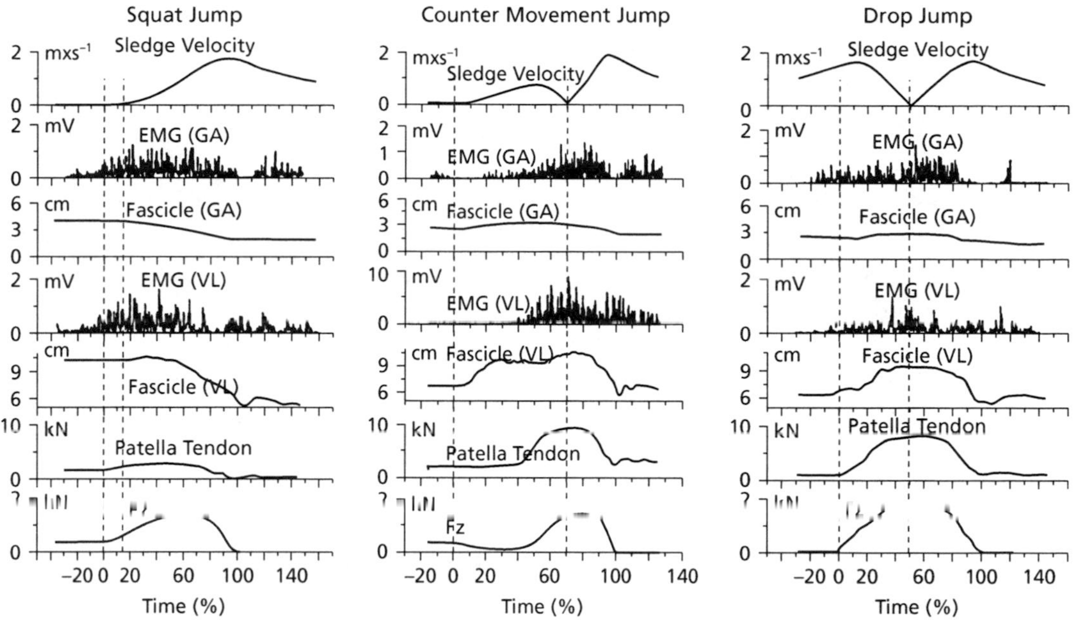

Fig. 10.12 Examples of the fascicle length changes in the vastus lateralis (VL) and gastrocnemius (GA) muscles in squat-jumps (left), countermovement jumps (middle) and drop-jumps (right) on the sledge. The figures also show respective EMG activities as well as the patellar tendon force (optic fibre technique) and the sledge force plate force. The second dashed line refers to the end of the braking phase in the countermovement and drop-jump conditions. (From Ishikawa *et al.* in progress.)

drop-jumps are given in Fig. 10.12. While the data in this figure demonstrate clearly that the fascicle lengthening/shortening parts of the SSC do not occur in phase for the two measured muscles (VL and gastrocnemius) they also suggest that fascicle behaviour is not only effort dependent, as would be expected, but also very much muscle and joint dependent as well as dependent on the type of muscle action or movement. Considering this fact one cannot avoid thinking how difficult it is to model the muscle compartment reliably for different movement tasks.

Importantly, however, isolation of the fascicle and tendon of the muscle–tendon complex can reveal the specific roles the tendon and aponeurosis play in performance potentiation in SSC muscle function. But their potential and individual contribution may be clearly dependent on the type of SSC movement and muscle in question. For example, in contrast to hopping, the elastic recoil of the triceps surae muscle plays a much smaller role in CMJs (Fukashiro *et al.* 1993; Finni *et al.* 1998; see also Fig. 10.9). This is expected because in CMJs the stretch phase is slow and the reflex contribution to SSC potentiation is likely to be much less than in hopping.

Role of stretch reflexes in force enhancement during SSCs

When discussing the possible reflex mechanisms involved in performance potentiation during SSC, the key question is what are the important features of effective SSC function. In our understanding an effective SSC requires three fundamental conditions (Komi & Gollhofer 1997):

1 a well-timed preactivation of the muscle(s) before the eccentric phase;

2 a short and fast eccentric phase; and

3 immediate transition (short delay) between stretch (eccentric) and shortening (concentric) phases.

These conditions are well met in 'normal' activities such as running and hopping, and seem therefore suitable for possible interaction from the stretch reflexes.

Demonstration of short-latency stretch reflexes in SSC

Stiffness regulation is a very important concept in the eccentric part of the SSC, and stretch reflexes play an important role in this task. Hoffer and Andreassen (1981) demonstrated convincingly that when reflexes are intact, muscle stiffness is greater for the same operating force than in an arreflexive muscle. Thus, stretch reflexes may already make a net contribution to muscle stiffness during the eccentric part of the SSC.

In hopping and running, the short-latency stretch reflex component (SLC) can be quite easily observed, especially in the soleus muscle. Figure 10.13 illustrates studies where this component appears clearly in the EMG patterns when averaged over several trials involving two-leg hops with short contact times. Also Voigt *et al.* (1998), in a similar study, measured both the origin to insertion muscle lengthening and the muscle fibre lengthening. Both measurements showed high stretch velocities in the early contact phase, which led the authors to conclude that the conditions were sufficient for muscle spindle afferent activation. The SLC is sensitive to loading conditions as shown in Fig. 10.14, where the stretch loads vary from the preferred submaximal hopping (the records on the top) to drop-jumps. In the highest drop-jump condition (80 cm) the SLC component becomes less clear, suggesting decreased facilitation from the muscle spindles and/or increased inhibitory drive from various sources (e.g. Golgi tendon organ, voluntary protection mechanisms, etc.). In cases where the drop-jumps have been performed from excessive heights, for example from 140 cm (Kyröläinen & Komi 1995), the subjects had to sustain extreme loads during contact. In these situations, the reduced reflex activation

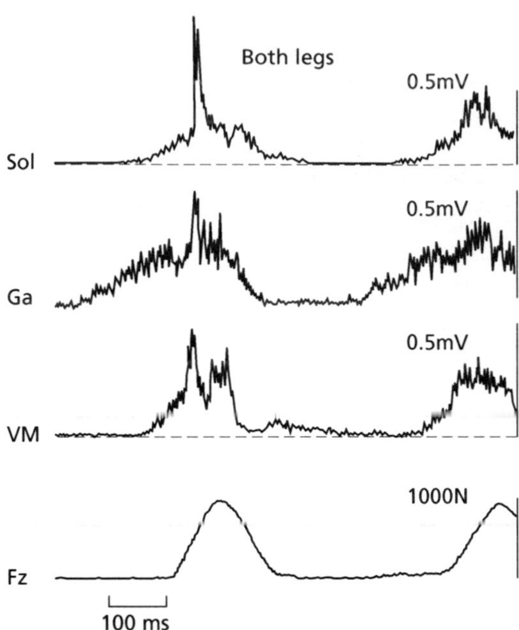

Fig. 10.13 Averaged rectified EMG records of the soleus (SOL), gastocnemius (GA) and vastus medialis (VM) muscles in bilateral hopping. Note the sharp EMG reflex peak in the soleus muscle during early contact phase. (From Komi & Gollhofer 1997, based on Gollhofer *et al.* 1992.)

may functionally serve as a protection strategy to prevent muscle and/or tendon injury.

Magnitude of reflex-induced EMG activity

It has been shown during passive dorsiflexion tests that the SLC and the medium-latency component (MLC) can be dramatically reduced if the measurements are made during ischaemic blockade of the lower limb (e.g. Fellows *et al.* 1993). This method has been applied to conditions of fast running (Dietz *et al.* 1979), in which the control runs made before ischaemia demonstrated that the gastrocnemius EMG had a clear SLC component during contact. The average peak EMG was at least 2 times higher than that measured during a maximal voluntary isometric plantar flexion test (Fig. 10.15). When ischaemic blockade was performed, the gastrocnemius

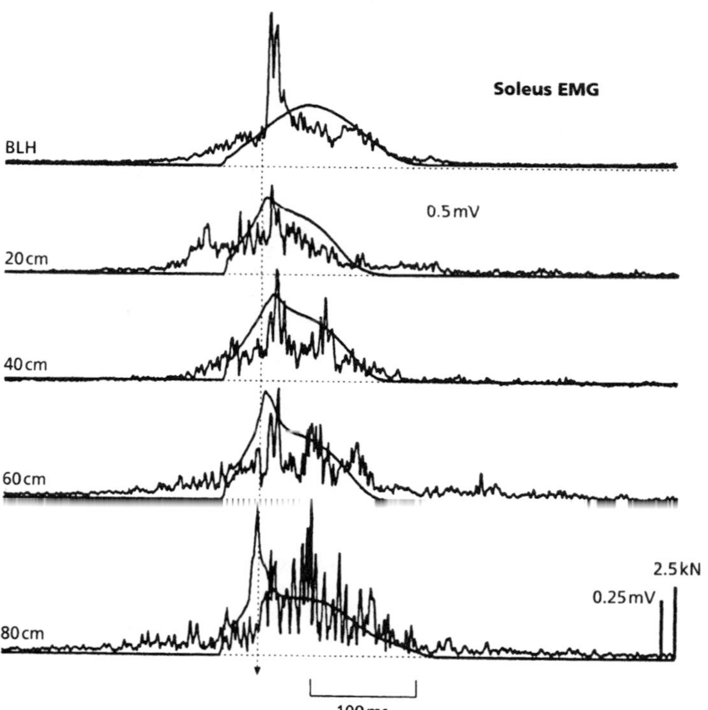

Fig. 10.14 Rectified and averaged EMG pattern of the soleus muscle and vertical ground reaction force in various stretch–shortening cycle drop-jumps with both legs. The figure illustrates the modulation in the pattern and in the force record with increasing stretch load. *From top*: BLH, both-leg hopping in place (see also Fig 10.13 top); 20–80 cm, drop-jumps from 20 to 80 cm height, landing with both legs. The dashed vertical line indicates the initiation of the phasic activation with a latency of 40 ms after ground contact. (From Komi & Gollhofer 1997.)

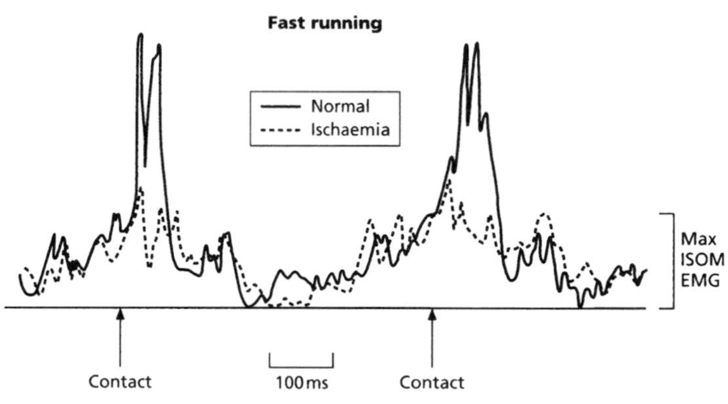

Fig. 10.15 Rectified and averaged EMG activity of the gastrocnemius muscle when the subject was taking many steps during fast running on the spot. The control (normal) before ischaemia shows the typical rapid increase of EMG 40 ms after ground contact. The dashed line indicates the same running after 20 min of ischaemia produced by a tourniquet around the thigh. The stretch-induced EMG activity (SLC component) was reduced to the level of Maximal Isometric EMG (the bar on the right) without reduction in the preactivity before contact. (After Dietz *et al.* 1979.)

EMG during contact was dramatically reduced in the fast running test with the same velocity, but there was no change in preactivation. These results emphasize the potential role of Ia afferent input in SSC-type activities such as running. The ischaemic blockade is used to isolate the Ia afferent information acting on spinal pathways (Fellows *et al.* 1993).

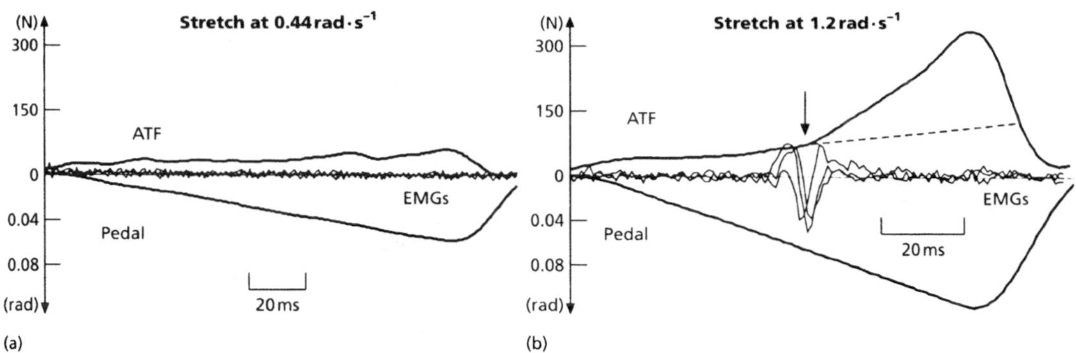

Fig. 10.16 Demonstration of passively induced stretch reflexes on the Achilles tendon force (ATF). Left, passive dorsiflexion at slow stretch caused no reflex EMG response and led to a small and rather linear increase of the ATF (pure passive response). Right, in the case of faster and larger stretches the reflex contribution to ATF corresponds to the additional ATF response above the pure passive influence represented by the dashed line. (From Nicol & Komi 1998.)

Do reflexes have time to be operative during SSC?

As it has been reportedly questioned whether and denied that stretch reflexes can operate and contribute to force and power enhancement during the SSC (van Ingen-Schenau *et al.* 1997), it is important to examine what role the stretch reflexes may play, if any, during the SSC. It is difficult to imagine that proprioceptive reflexes, the existence of which has been known for centuries, would not play any significant role in human locomotion including SSCs. It is true that in normal movements with high EMG activity, the magnitude and net contribution of reflex regulation of muscle force are methodologically difficult to assess. The task becomes much easier when relatively slow (1.2–1.9 rad·s^{-1}) passive dorsiflexions are studied, where the stretch-induced reflex EMG has been reported to enhance AT force by 200–500% over the purely passive stretch without reflex EMG response (Nicol & Komi 1998). Figure 10.16 is an example of these measurements and it shows a typical delay of 12–13 ms between the onset of reflex EMG and onset of force potentiation.

This time delay is similar to electrical stimulation measurements performed together with fibre-optic recordings of the AT force (Komi *et al.* in preparation). Considering the duration of the simple stretch reflex loop of 40 ms, the maximum delay between initial stretch and subsequent force potentiation would be around 50–55 ms. When referred to running, the first contact on the ground would indicate the point of initial stretch. In marathon running the contact phase usually lasts almost 250 ms, implying that this reflex-induced force enhancement would already have functional significance during the eccentric phase of the cycle (Nicol *et al.* 1991). As the contact phase duration (braking and push-off) decreases as a function of the running speed (Luhtanen & Komi 1978) the net reflex contribution will occur at the end of the eccentric phase at faster speeds, and may be extended partly to the push-off phase in maximal sprinting, where the total contact time is only about 90–100 ms (Mero & Komi 1985). These time calculations certainly confirm that stretch reflexes have ample time to operate for force and power enhancement during SSCs, and in most cases during the eccentric part of the cycle. Thus, there are no time restraints for reflexes to be operative in stiffness regulation during SSCs. The large reflex-induced EMG component (see Fig. 10.15) must therefore be regarded as an essential and important contribution to force enhancement in SSCs.

Functional significance of stretch reflexes in SSC activities

Some aspects of the functional importance of stretch reflexes during the SSC have already been referred to above. It is, however, relevant to emphasize that the reflexes contribute to the efficiency of the motor output by making the force output more powerful. In SSCs this can only be accomplished by an immediate and smooth transfer from the preactivated and eccentrically stretched muscle–tendon complex to the concentric push-off, in the cases of running or hopping, for example. The range of high stiffness is, however, limited to that of the 'short-range elastic stiffness' (SRES) (Rack & Westbury 1974; Morgan 1979). In this case the stiffness of the muscle–tendon complex depends not only on the range of motion (Kearney & Hunter 1982), but also on the efficiency of the stretch reflex system (Nichols & Houk 1976; Houk & Rymer 1981). High stretch reflex activity is expected after a powerful stretch of an active muscle (e.g. Dietz *et al.* 1984), and these reflexes are necessary not primarily to enhance SRES, but to linearize the stress strain characteristics (Nichols 1974; Hufschmidt & Schwaller 1987).

It can be assumed that before ground contact in the SSC the initial lengthening of the muscle–tendon complex, shown in Fig. 10.3, occurs in the more or less compliant Achilles tendon. As soon as the 'critical' tension of the fascicles is achieved, which is determined by the amount of activity (preactivation) sent to the muscles prior to contact, the forceful 'yielding' of the cross-links of the actin–myosin complex may take place, with concomitant loss of the potential energy stored in the lengthened cross-bridges (e.g. Flitney & Hirst 1978). From *in vitro* studies it is known that yielding of active cross-bridges can be prevented by intense muscular activation. Such an intense phase-dependent and triggered muscular activation can be provided most effectively by the stretch reflex system, which is highly sensitive to the length and tension changes in the muscle–tendon complex. As discussed earlier, the latencies for the reflex EMG are sufficiently short for it to have functional significance. These latencies (40–45 and 12–14 ms, respectively, for the reflex loop and electromechanical delay) fit well with the occurrence of short- and medium-latency stretch reflex components (e.g. Lee & Tatton 1982). Our recent data on combined stretch and reflex potentiation are well in agreement with the SRES concept, demonstrating that the cross-bridge force resistance to stretch is particularly efficient during the early part of the cross-bridge attachment (Nicol & Komi 1998). Therefore, the reflex-induced cross-link formation appears to play a very rapid and substantial role in force generation during stretch. Furthermore, as demonstrated by Stein (1982) and Nichols (1987), it is the stretch reflex system that provides high linearity in muscular stiffness.

All these aspects may partly contribute to the observation that mechanical efficiency in natural SSCs is higher than that in pure concentric exercise (e.g. Aura & Komi 1986; Kyröläinen *et al.* 1990). The concept of elastic storage favours the existence of reflex activation, and high muscular activation during the eccentric phase of an SSC is a prerequisite for efficient storage of elastic energy, especially in the tendon. Animal studies have shown that an electrically stimulated muscle responds to ramp stretches with linear tension increments, provided the muscle has an intact reflex system (Nichols & Houk 1976; Nichols 1987). This linearity is restricted to small length changes (e.g. Hoffer & Andreassen 1981) and these small changes are indeed relevant to the SSC exercises referred to in the present discussion (see also Figs 10.3 and 10.12).

Overall there seems to be enough evidence to conclude that stretch reflexes play an important role in the SSC and contribute to force generation during touchdown in activities such as running and hopping. Depending on the type of hopping, for example, the amplitude of the SLC peak and its force-increasing or -decreasing potential may vary considerably. However, the combination of the 'prereflex' background activation and the following reflex activation might represent a scenario that supports yield compensation and a fast rate of force development (Voigt *et al.* 1998).

This scenario may be especially effective in a non-fatigued situation, but it can be put under severe stress during increasing stretch loads (see Fig. 10.14) and during progressive SSC fatigue. The clear coupling between reflex activities and mechanical performance reduction during SSC fatigue is a good indication of this scenario. The SSC fatigue will be discussed in detail in Chapter 11.

References

Alt, W., Lohrer, H., Gollhofer, A. & Komi, P.V. (2002) Estimation of ankle ligament load using a fiber optic transducer *in vivo*, submitted for publication.

Arndt, A.N., Komi, P.V., Brüggemann, G.-P. & Lukkariniemi, J. (1998) Individual muscle contributions to the *in vivo* Achilles tendon force. *Clinical Biomechanics* **13**, 532–541.

Aura, O. & Komi, P.V. (1986) The mechanical efficiency of locomotion in men and women with special emphasis on stretch–shortening cycle exercises. *European Journal of Applied Physiology* **55**, 37–43.

Belli, A. & Bosco, C. (1992) Influence of stretch–shortening cycle on mechanical behaviour of triceps surae during hopping. *Acta Physiologica Scandinavica* **144**, 401–408.

Bocquet, J.-C. & Noel, J. (1987) Sensitive skin-pressure and strain sensor with optical fibres. In: *Proceedings of 2nd Congress on Structural Mechanics of Optical Systems*, 13–15 January 1987, Los Angeles, CA.

Candau, R., Belli, A., Chatard, J.C., Carrez, J.-P. & Lacour, J.-R. (1993) Stretch shortening cycle in the skating technique of cross-country skiing. *Science et Motricité* **22**, 252–256.

Cavagna, G.A., Saibene, F.P. & Margaria, R. (1965) Effect of negative work on the amount of positive work performed by an isolated muscle. *Journal of Applied Physiology* **20**, 157–158.

Cavagna, G.A., Dusman, B. & Margaria, R. (1968) Positive work done by a previously stretched muscle. *Journal of Applied Physiology* **24**, 21–32.

Dietz, V., Schmidtbleicher, D. & Noth, J. (1979) Neuronal mechanisms of human locomotion. *Journal of Neurophysiology* **42**, 1212–1222.

Dietz, V., Quintern, J. & Berger, W. (1984) Corrective reactions to stumbling in man. Functional significance of spinal and transcortical reflexes. *Neuroscience Letters* **44**, 131–135.

Fellows, S., Dömges, F., Töpper, R., Thilmann, A. & Noth. J. (1993) Changes in the short and long latency stretch reflex components of the triceps surae muscle during ischaemia in man. *Journal of Physiology* **472**, 737–748.

Finni, T., Komi, P.V. & Lepola, V. (1998) *In vivo* muscle dynamics during jumping. In: *3rd Annual Congress of the European College of Sport Sciences*, 15–18 July 1998, Manchester, UK.

Finni, T., Komi, P.V. & Lepola, V. (2000) *In vivo* triceps surae and quadriceps femoris muscle function in a squat jump and counter movement jump. *European Journal of Applied Physiology* **83**, 416–426.

Finni, T., Komi, P.V. & Lepola, V. (2001a) *In vivo* muscle mechanics during normal locomotion is dependent on movement amplitude and contraction intensity. *European Journal of Applied Physiology* **85**, 170–176.

Finni, T., Ikegawa, S., Lepola, V. & Komi, P.V. (2001b) *In vivo* behavior of vastus lateralis muscle during dynamic performances. *European Journal of Sciences* [on line] 1,1. Human Kinetics and European College of Sport Science. http://www.humankinetics.com/ejss.

Finni, T., Ikegawa, S. & Komi, P.V. (2001c) Concentric force enhancement during human movement. *Acta Physiologica Scandinavica* **173**, 369–377.

Flitney, F.W. & Hirst, D.G. (1978) Cross-bridge detachment and sarcomere 'give' during stretch of active frog's muscle. *Journal of Physiology* **276**, 449–465.

Ford, L.E., Huxley, A.F. & Simmons, R.M. (1978) Tension responses to sudden length change in stimulated frog muscle fibres near slack length. *Journal of Physiology* **269**, 441–515.

Frigo, C. & Pedotti, A. (1978) Determination of muscle length during locomotion. *International Series of Biomechanics* **VI-A**, 355–360.

Fukashiro, S. & Komi, P.V. (1987) Joint moment and mechanical power flow of the lower limb during vertical jump. *International Journal of Sports Medicine* **8**, 15–21.

Fukashiro, S., Komi, P.V., Järvinen, M. & Miyashita, M. (1993) Comparison between the directly measured Achilles tendon force and the tendon force calculated from the ankle joint moment during vertical jumps. *Clinical Biomechanics* **8**, 25–30.

Fukashiro, S., Komi, P.V., Järvinen, M. & Miyashita, M. (1995) *In vivo* Achilles tendon loading during jumping in humans. *European Journal of Applied Physiology* **71**, 453–458.

Fukunaga, T., Ito, M., Ichinose, Y., Kuno, S., Kawakami, Y. & Fukashiro, S. (1996) Tendinous movement of a human muscle during voluntary contractions determined by real-time ultrasonography. *Journal of Applied Physiology* **813**, 1430–1433.

Fukunaga, T., Ichinose, Y., Ito, M., Kawakami, Y. & Fukashiro, S. (1997) Determination of fascicle length and pennation in a contracting human muscle *in vivo*. *Journal of Applied Physiology* **82**, 354–358.

Gregor, R.J., Roy, R.R., Whiting, W.C., Lovely, R.G., Hodgson, J.A. & Edgerton, V.R. (1988) Mechanical output of the cat soleus during treadmill locomotion *in vivo* vs. *in situ* characteristics. *Journal of Biomechanics* **21**(9), 721–732.

Gregor, R.J., Komi, P.V., Browning, R.C. & Järvinen, M. (1991) A comparison of triceps surae and residual muscle moments at the ankle during cycling. *Journal of Biomechanics* **24**, 287–297.

Grieve, D.W., Pheasant, S.Q. & Cavanagh, P.R. (1978) Prediction of gastrocnemius length from knee and ankle joint posture. In: *Biomechanics VI-A* (eds E. Asmissen & K. Jörgensen), pp. 405–412. University Park Press, Baltimore.

Griffiths, R.I. (1991) Shortening of muscle fibres during stretch of the active cat medial gastrocnemius muscle: The role of tendon compliance. *Journal of Physiology* **436**, 219–236.

Hill, A.V. (1938) The heat and shortening of the dynamic constant of muscle. *Proceedings of the Royal Society of London Series B* **126**, 136–195.

Hoff, A.L., Geelen, B.A. & van den Berg, J. (1983) Calf muscle moment, work and efficiency in level walking: Role of series elasticity. *Journal of Biomechanics* **16**, 523–537.

Hoffer, J.A. & Andreassen, S. (1981) Regulation of soleus muscle stiffness in premamillary cats. Intrinsic and reflex components. *Journal of Neurophysiology* **45**, 267–285.

Horita, T., Komi, P.V., Nicol. C. & Kyröläinen, H. (1999) Effect of exhausting stretch–shortening cycle exercise on the time course of mechanical behaviour in the drop jump: possible role of muscle damage. *European Journal of Applied Physiology* **79**, 160–167.

Houk, J.C. & Rymer, W.Z. (1981) Neural control of muscle length and tension. In: *Handbook of Physiology. The Nervous System* II, (ed. V.B. Brooks), pp. 257–323. Waverly Press, Baltimore.

Hufschmidt, A. & Schwaller, I. (1987) Short-range elasticity and resting tension of relaxed human lower leg muscles. *Journal of Physiology* **393**, 451–465.

Huijing, P.A. (1992) Elastic potential of muscle. In: *Strength and Power in Sport* (ed. P.V. Komi), pp. 151–168. Blackwell Scientific Publications, Oxford.

Huxley, A.F. & Simmons, R.M. (1971) Proposed mechanism of force generation in striated muscle. *Nature* **233**, 533–538.

Ikai, M. & Fukunaga, T. (1968) Calculation of muscle strength per unit cross-sectional area of human muscle by means of ultrasonic measurement. *Internationale Zeitschrift fur Angewandte Physiologie Einschliesslich Arbeitsphysiologie* **26**, 26–32.

van Ingen-Schenau, G.J., Bobbert, M.F. & de Haan, A. (1997) Does elastic energy enhance work and efficiency in the stretch–shortening cycle? *Journal of Applied Biomechanics* **13**, 386–415.

Kawakami, Y., Ichinose, M., Kubo, K., Ito, M., Imai, M. & Fukunaga, T. (2000) Architecture of contracting human muscles and its functional significance. *Journal of Applied Biomechanics* **16**, 88–98.

Kearney, R.E. & Hunter, I.W. (1982) Dynamics of human ankle stiffness. Variation with displacement amplitude. *Journal of Biomechanics* **15**, 753–756.

Komi, P.V. (1973) Measurement of the force–velocity relationship in human muscle under concentric and eccentric contraction. In: *Medicine and Sport, Biomechanics III*, Vol. 8 (ed. E. Jokl), pp. 224–229. Karger, Basel.

Komi, P.V. (1983) Elastic potentiation of muscles and its influence on sport performance. In: *Biomechanik und Sportliche Leistung* (ed. W. Baumann), pp. 59–70. Verlag Karl Hofmann, Schorndorf.

Komi, P.V. (1984) Physiological and biomechanical correlates of muscle function: Effects of muscle structure and stretch–shortening cycle on force and speed. *Exercise and Sport Sciences Reviews/American College of Sports Medicine* **12**, 81–121.

Komi, P.V. (1990) Relevance of *in vivo* force measurements to human biomechanics. *Journal of Biomechanics* **23** (Suppl. 1), 23–34.

Komi, P.V. (1992) Stretch–shortening cycle. In: *Strength and Power in Sport* (ed. P.V. Komi), pp. 169–179. Blackwell Scientific Publications, Oxford.

Komi, P.V. (2000) Stretch–shortening cycle: a powerful model to study normal and fatigued muscle. *Journal of Biomechanics* **33**, 1197–1206.

Komi, P.V. & Gollhofer, A. (1997) Stretch reflex can have an important role in force enhancement during SSC-exercise. *Journal of Applied Biomechanics* **13**, 451–460.

Komi, P.V. & Nicol, C. (2000) Stretch–shortening cycle of muscle function. In: *Biomechanics in Sport* (ed. V. Zatsiorsky), pp. 87–102. Blackwell Science, Oxford.

Komi, P.V., Gollhofer, A., Schmidtbleicher, D. & Frick, U. (1987a) Interaction between man and shoe in running: Considerations for more comprehensive measurement approach. *International Journal of Sports Medicine* **8**(3), 196–202.

Komi, P.V., Salonen, M., Järvinen, M. & Kokko, O. (1987b) *In vivo* registration of Achilles tendon forces in man. I. Methodological development. *International Journal of Sports Medicine* **8**, 3–8.

Komi, P.V., Belli, A., Huttunen, V. & Partio, E. (1995) Optic fiber as a transducer for direct *in-vivo* measurements of human tendomuscular forces. In: *Proceedings of the XVth ISB* (eds K. Häkkinen, K.L. Keskinen, P.V. Komi & A. Mero), pp. 494–495. Jyväskylä, Finland.

Komi, P.V., Belli, A., Huttunen, V., Bonnejoy, R., Geyssant, A. & Lacour, J.R. (1996) Optic fiber as a transducer of tendomuscular forces. *European Journal of Applied Physiology* **72**, 278–280.

Kyröläinen, H. & Komi, P.V. (1995) Differences in mechanical efficiency in athletes during jumping. *European Journal of Applied Physiology* **70**, 36–44.

Kyröläinen, H., Avela, J. & Komi, P.V. (1989) Regulation of muscle and stiffness during long jump take-off. In: *Biomechanics* XII (eds R.J. Gregor, R.F. Zernicke & W.C. Whiting), pp. 364–365. UCLA, Los Angeles.

Kyröläinen, H., Komi, P.V., Oksanen, P., Häkkinen, K., Cheng, S. & Kim, D.H. (1990) Mechanical efficiency of locomotion in females during different kinds of muscle actions. *European Journal of Applied Physiology* **61**, 446–452.

Lee, R.G. & Tatton, W.G. (1982) Long latency reflexes to imposed displacements of the human wrist. Dependence on duration of movement. *Experimental Brain Research* **45**, 207–216.

Luhtanen, P. & Komi, P.V. (1978) Segmental contribution to forces in vertical jump. *European Journal of Applied Physiology* **38**, 181–188.

Melvill Jones, G. & Watt, D.G.D. (1971) Observations on the control of stepping and hopping movements in man. *Journal of Physiology* **219**, 709–727.

Mero, A. & Komi, P.V. (1985) Effects of supramaximal velocity on biomechanical variables in sprinting. *International Journal of Sport Biomechanics* **1**(3), 240–252.

Morgan, D.L. (1979) Separation of active and passive components of short-range stiffness of muscle. *American Journal of Physical Medicine* **232**, 45–49.

Nicol, C. & Komi, P.V. (1998) Significance of passively induced stretch reflexes on Achilles tendon force enhancement. *Muscle and Nerve* **21**, 1546–1548.

Nicol, C., Komi, P.V. & Marconnet, P. (1991) Effects of marathon fatigue on running kinematics and economy. *Scandinavian Journal of Medicine and Science in Sports* **1**, 18–24.

Nichols, T.R. (1974) *Soleus muscle stiffness and its reflex control*. PhD dissertation, Harvard University, Cambridge, MA.

Nichols, T.R. (1987) The regulation of muscle stiffness. *Medicine and Science in Sports and Exercise* **26**, 36–47.

Nichols, T.R. & Houk, J.C. (1976) Improvement in linearity and regulation of stiffness that results from actions of stretch reflex. *Journal of Neurophysiology* **39**, 119–142.

Norman, R.W. & Komi, P.V. (1979) Electromechanical delay in skeletal muscle under normal movement conditions. *Acta Physiologica Scandinavica* **106**, 241–248.

Rack, P.M.H. & Westbury, D.R. (1974) The short range stiffness of active mammalian muscle and its effect on mechanical properties. *Journal of Physiology* **240**, 331–350.

Roberts, T.J., Marsch, R.L., Weyand, P.G. & Taylor, C.R. (1997) Muscular force in running turkeys: The economy of minimizing work. *Science* **275**, 1113–1115.

Sherif, M.H., Gregor, R.J., Liu, M., Roy, R.R. & Hager, C.L. (1983) Correlation of myoelectric activity and muscle force during selected cat treadmill locomotion. *Journal of Biomechanics* **16**, 691–701.

Stein, R.B. (1982) What muscle variable(s) does the nervous system control in limb movements? *Behavioral Brain Science* **5**, 535–577.

Voigt, M., Dyhre-Poulsen, P. & Simonsen, E.B. (1998) Modulation of short latency stretch reflexes during human hopping. *Acta Physiologica Scandinavica* **163**, 181–194.

Wilkie, D.R. (1950) The relation between force and velocity in human muscle. *Journal of Physiology* **110**, 249.

Chapter 11

Stretch–Shortening Cycle Fatigue and its Influence on Force and Power Production

CAROLINE NICOL AND PAAVO V. KOMI

In the preceding chapter it was demonstrated that the natural SSC-type locomotion loads the neuromuscular system in a more complex way than any isolated forms of muscle actions. All the major components of performance 'sources' (mechanical, neural and metabolic) are loaded in the SSC so that the induced fatigue differs from that observed e.g. after pure eccentric fatiguing exercise. Thus, SSC exercise has many possibilities of adjustments to the progressive development of the contractile failure. On the other hand, the deterioration of SSC efficacy with fatigue leads to a necessary increase of the concentric work that results in large acute difficulties in maintenance of the required performance level. In addition, SSC-induced fatigue is clearly delayed in nature. The immediate postexercise changes are naturally related primarily to metabolic disturbances, whereas the delayed recovery must be associated with the well-known inflammatory processes related to muscle damage (Faulkner *et al.* 1993).

The present chapter makes an attempt to characterize what is currently understood as SSC fatigue, with its considerable bimodal influences on muscle mechanics and activation that result in major consequences on joint and muscle stiffness regulation, especially in SSC-type performances. As SSC muscle function is very important in most sports activities, it is therefore important to examine this form of fatiguing exercise and to describe how it affects force and power production. The chapter is a follow-up and updated version of our earlier reviews on the topic (Komi & Nicol 2000a,b) with special emphasis on the neural adjustments which depend on the level of the contractile failure as well as on the imposed task.

SSC loading and testing models

The presented material is based on several studies performed in humans during the last 10 years, and which cover a large range of fatiguing SSC exercises. In the experiments to be reviewed in the following paragraphs, the impact loads in the SSC exercises were carefully controlled, but varied in terms of intensity and duration. In most of these studies, kinematic and kinetic techniques were combined with surface electromyograph (EMG) recordings to examine the changes during the course of the exercise as well as during the subsequent days of recovery.

Short- and long-term SSC fatiguing exercise

Short-term SSC exercises consist of intensive and exhaustive series of rebounds performed on a specific sledge apparatus (Horita *et al.* 1996, 1999; Nicol *et al.* 1996a,b). By adjusting the subject's position on the gliding sledge, fatigue can be induced selectively in the upper- (Fig. 11.1a) or the lower-limb (Fig. 11.1b) muscles. The upper-limb protocol (Gollhofer *et al.* 1987a) included 100 submaximal SSCs with both arms. In the basic fatiguing protocol of the leg extensor muscles, the exercise is performed in a sitting position by rebounding as long as possible to a given submaximal rising height (70–80% of the maximal rebound height). Exhaustion is usually

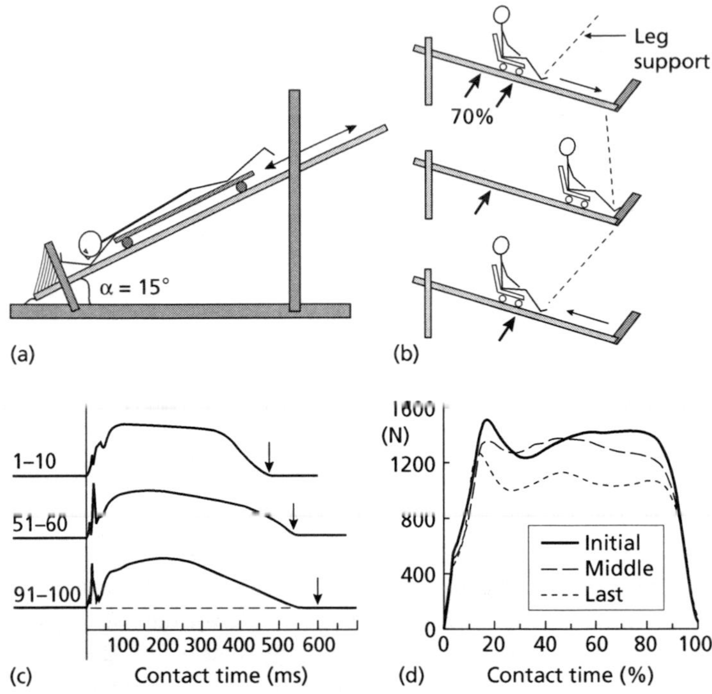

Fig. 11.1 Schematic presentation of the SSC fatigue protocol for either arm (a) or leg (b) exercise. The subjects performed repetitive rebound jumps on the sledge to a submaximal rising height. Both fatiguing exercises demonstrated progressive changes in the reaction force record during the contact phase on the force plate. The records (c,d) have been averaged for 10 successive force–time curves at the beginning, in the middle and at the end of the exercise. Note in the arm exercise the clear increase in the impact peak. In both protocols, the impact is followed by a greater drop in force when fatigue progresses. All figures modified from the originals (a & c: Gollhofer *et al.* 1987a; b: Nicol *et al.* 1996a; d: Horita 2000).

reached after 100–400 repetitions (Horita *et al.* 1996, 1999; Nicol *et al.* 1996a,b), corresponding to 2–5 min of intensive exercise.

Prolonged SSC exercises include different duration–intensity combinations of endurance running and skiing exercises such as a 10-km run by non-endurance runners (Nicol *et al.* submitted), experimental marathon races (Komi *et al.* 1986; Nicol *et al.* 1991a,b,c; Pullinen *et al.* 1997; Avela & Komi 1998a; Avela *et al.* 1999; Kyröläinen *et al.* 2000), a 85-km cross-country skiing race (Viitasalo *et al.* 1982) and a leisure week of alpine skiing (Strojnik *et al.* 2001a,b). These longlasting models serve the purpose of characterizing more specifically the effects of a great number of repeated eccentric muscle actions on various aspects of the neuromuscular function.

Testing protocols

In most studies, the fatigue response is examined during the course of the exercise as well as in static and dynamic strength tests performed immediately before and after the SSC exercise, and repeated several times during the recovery period (after 2 h and 2 days as well as 4–5 and 7–10 days later).

In order to isolate the various components of the SSC-induced fatigue, comparison will be made with the kinetic, kinematic and surface EMG changes in maximal and submaximal SSCs as well as in more isolated types of both active and passive test conditions. Serum levels of creatine kinase (CK) activity, skeletal myoglobin (Mb), troponin I (TnI) and carbonic anhydrase (CAIII) have been used as indirect indicators of exercise-induced muscle damage. Blood lactate concentration is used as an indicator of metabolic fatigue.

Changes during the fatiguing exercise

The progressive development of fatigue during the course of the prolonged SSC exercises is clearly individual and exercise dependent, in both its timing and amplitude. The results of the 10-km (Ftaiti *et al.* 2000) and marathon running

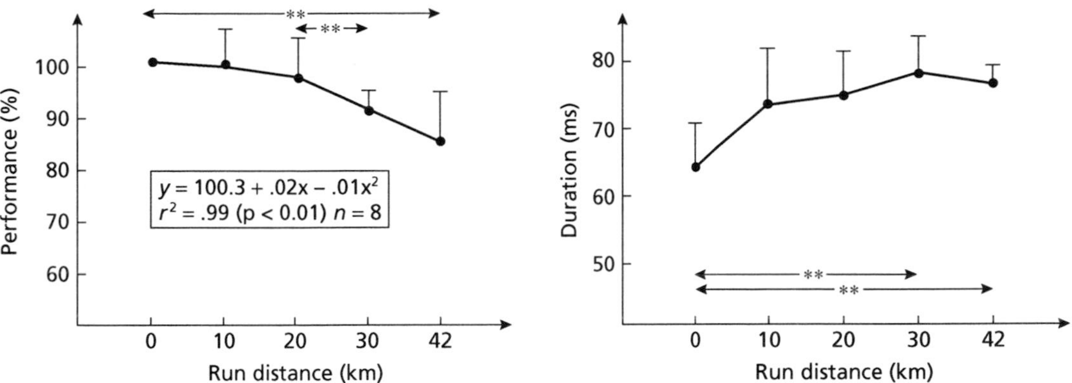

Fig. 11.2 (a) Relative change of the maximal sprint velocity performed every 10 km during the course of a marathon (100% = before marathon value). (b) Duration (mean + SD) of the push-off phase of the sprint runs along the marathon. Adapted by permission, from C. Nicol *et al.* (1991a).

studies (Nicol *et al.* 1991c; Kyröläinen *et al.* 2000) demonstrate that submaximal running kinematics and running economy are not interrelated when fatigue progresses. This suggests that the changes in the running pattern reflect adjustments to fatigue rather than any real failure to compensate for it. However, tests of higher loading level (drop-jump and sprint run) can reveal more homogeneous deterioration of the muscle function (Nicol *et al.* 1991a). This is reflected by a parabolic decrease of the sprinting velocity after the first 20 km (Fig. 11.2a), with associated decrement in the resistance to the impact load and subsequent increased work during the push-off phase (Fig. 11.2b). These results further emphasize that instead of using conventional submaximal running tests, high-intensity loading/velocity tests should be used to reveal the true weakening of the neuromuscular function while performing longlasting SSC exercises. The marathon study of Avela and Komi (1998b) confirms this observation.

Shorter, but more intensive SSC rebound exercises usually lead to an almost 30% increase in contact time as observed both in arm (Gollhofer *et al.* 1987a) and leg (Horita 2000) exercises (Fig. 11.1c,d). Similar to what is observed in prolonged SSC exercises, this is associated with a clear drop in the resistance to stretch. As shown in Fig. 11.1(c), many subjects present a clear and progressive increase in the impact peak (Gollhofer *et al.* 1987a). This implies that the developing contractile failure due to the repeated stretch loads and combined metabolic fatigue eventually becomes so fatiguing that the neuromuscular system needs to change the musculotendon 'stiffness' regulation by increasing the level of preactivation. The resulting increase of the impact peak is then expected to lead to a vicious circle through a reduced tolerance to stretch resulting in a loss of elastic recoil and subsequent need for increased work during the push-off phase. Horita's (2000) finding of a clear turning point in the adjustments to fatigue after the middle stage of an exhaustive leg rebound exercise is in line with this thought. The first two-thirds of the exercise presents rather limited kinetic and kinematic changes during the contact phase (Fig. 11.3b,c), but large kinematic alterations during the flight phase (Fig. 11.3a) accompanied by clear EMG adjustments during the respective preactivation (Fig. 11.4a) and braking (Fig. 11.4b) phases. After an initial trend of learning effect during the first third of the rebound exercise, the activation of the knee extensor muscles shows a linear increase in the braking phase (Fig. 11.4b). The associated stable values of knee joint range of motion (ROM) and contact time demonstrate the effectiveness of this adaptation to counteract the loss of force of the knee

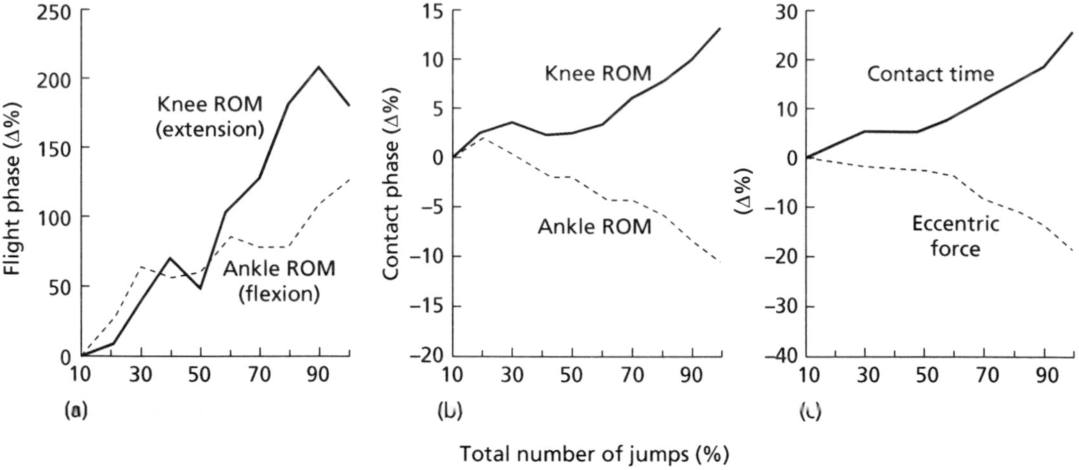

Fig. 11.3 Relative changes in kinematics (a,b) and kinetics (c) during the time course of the SSC exercise. ROM, range of motion. (Ref. 0 = first 10% of the exercise.) (Data from Horita 2000.)

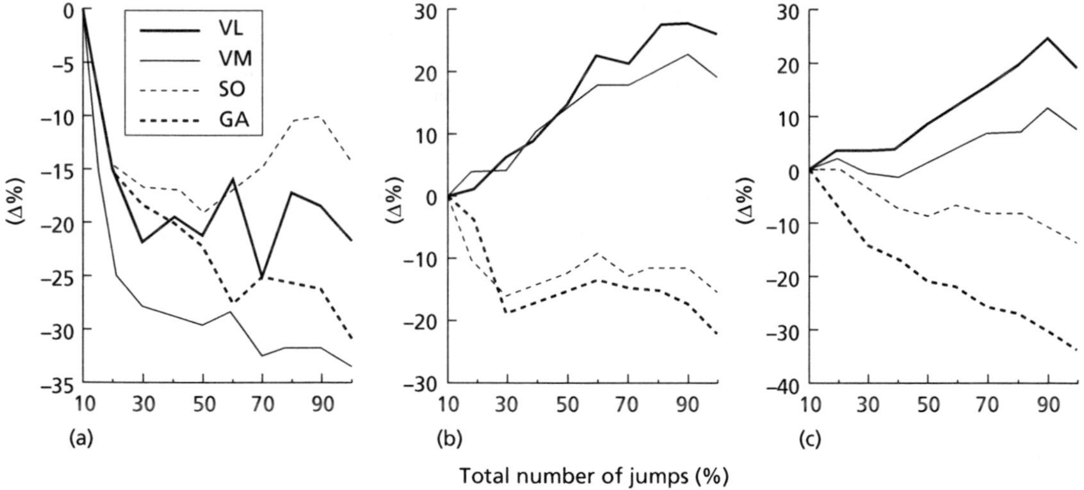

Fig. 11.4 Relative changes in EMG activities of the vastus lateralis (VL), vastus medialis (VM), gastrocnemius (GA) and soleus (SO) muscles during the preactivity, braking and push-off phases along the SSC exercise. The changes are expressed as a percentage of the initial EMG levels recorded during the first 10% of the exercise. (Data from Horita 2000.)

extensors (Fig. 11.3b,c). Thus, the eccentric part of the SSC cycle seems to operate effectively until the middle stage of the exercise. In the second half of the rebound series, however, the pre-landing joint kinematics change dramatically (Fig. 11.3a) and influence significantly the subsequent postlanding stiffness regulation (Fig. 11.3b) and contact time (Fig. 11.3c). In the sledge exercise performed at a submaximal rebound height, the increased contact time then compensates effectively for the reduced force output, thus contributing to the maintained external work output. The opposite trends of knee and ankle ROM changes suggest attempts of compensation among the different segments that may not remain sufficient, however, as indicated by the dramatic increase of the contact time towards the end of the exercise.

These overall results demonstrate that the neuromuscular adaptation process can be clearly modified during exhausting SSC exercise. It is suggested that in the non-fatigued state the muscles are able to damp the impact in SSC by a smooth force increase and smooth joint motion. During the progressive development of fatigue, the time-varying stiffness approach demonstrates a significant interaction between the prelanding kinematics and postlanding stiffness regulation. These results emphasize further the plasticity as well as the efficacy of the neuromuscular adjustments to the increasing fatigue during submaximal SSC exercises. These effective adjustments during the early parts of the fatiguing exercise may explain why in some studies utilizing very moderate SSC exercises, the fatigue effects have been minimal or in some cases even performance enhancing (see e.g. Hortobágyi *et al.* 1991).

Acute and delayed changes

Intensive and/or unaccustomed SSC exercises cause impairment of neuromuscular function that can be both acute and delayed in nature (Komi & Nicol 2000a,b; Komi 2000). Remarkable similarities can be found again in the results of both short- and long-term SSC fatigue studies as well as in the plasticity of the neuromuscular adjustments which depend on the intensity of fatiguing SSC exercise as well as on the demands of the testing task. In the following paragraphs, these respective changes will be referred to as 'fatigue-dependent' and 'task-dependent' effects. In addition, special emphasis will be given to the potential reflex changes as they play an important role in SSC exercises where stretch loads are high and muscle stiffness must be well regulated to meet the external loads.

Influence on maximal neural activation and static force production

Maximal activation and maximal isometric force decline dramatically following SSC exercises.

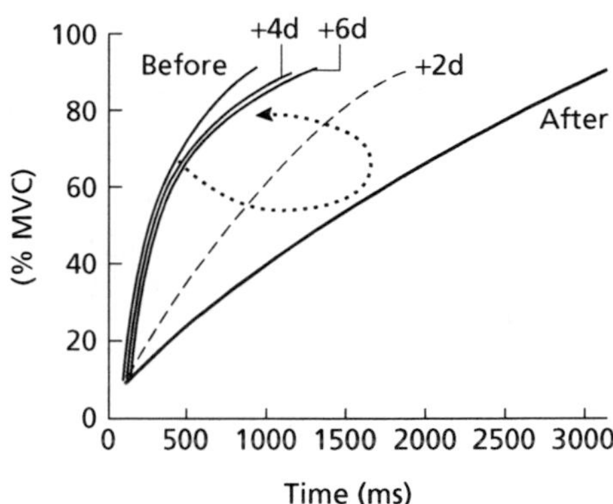

Fig. 11.5 Isometric force–time curves of the maximal knee extension measured immediately before and after a marathon run as well as 2, 4 and 6 days later. Note the large and immediate decrease in the rate of force development and its slow recovery towards the 4th day post marathon. (Data from Pullinen *et al.* 1997.)

Maximal isometric knee extension reportedly decreases by 20–30% after prolonged cross-country skiing (Viitasalo *et al.* 1982) and marathon running (Nicol *et al.* 1991b; Pullinen *et al.* 1997; Avela *et al.* 1999). The rate of force development is also dramatically reduced and accompanied by a slow recovery (Pullinen *et al.* 1997) (Fig. 11.5). In accordance with the concept of 'fatigue-dependent' effect, recovery of both maximal EMG and force may remain incomplete until the 6th day after an intensive SSC exercise (Pullinen *et al.* 1997) (Fig. 11.5), whereas in a less intensive SSC fatigue situation, such as a leisure alpine skiing week, an improved maximal voluntary contraction (MVC) may be already observable during the latter half of the week.

A few attempts have been performed to differentiate the respective role of central and peripheral fatigue. Supporting the hypothesis of a contractile failure, the drop in MVC after a marathon run is associated with a clear decline in the capacity to maintain a 60% isometric force level despite an increased neural activation (Nicol *et al.* 1991b). On the other hand, Strojnik *et al.* (2000) examined the effect of a leisure alpine skiing week on maximal voluntary contraction performed without (MVC) and with additional electrostimulation (MVCES). As shown in Fig.

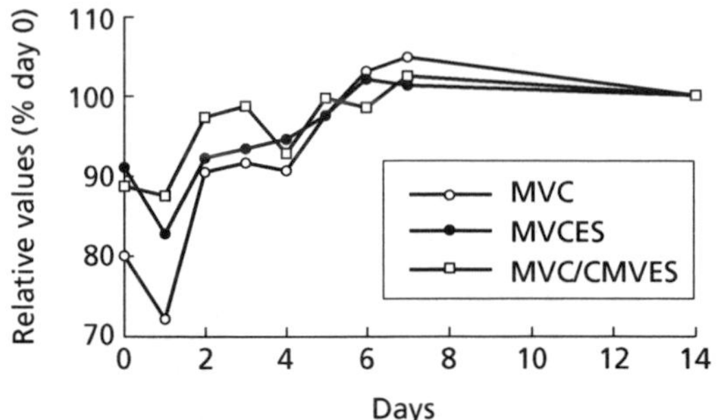

Fig. 11.6 Relative values of maximal voluntary contractions performed without (MVC) and with additional electrostimulation (MVCES), before and during a leisure week of alpine skiing and repeated 7 days later (day 14). (Modified from Strojnik *et al.* 2001a.)

11.6, both MVC and MVCES forces decline after the first skiing day, but on the 4th day only MVC/MVCES is significantly reduced, thus suggesting a central adjustment to the contractile fatigue. This latter change is followed on the subsequent day (day 5) by a significant self-reduction by the skiers of their freely chosen skiing distance.

Influence on dynamic-type performances

Comparison of the fatigue-induced changes in various dynamic testing conditions reveals a continuum of adjustments to the contractile failure. Independently of the type of SSC exercise used to induce fatigue, a clear 'testing task-dependent effect' is observed that emphasizes the plasticity of the neural adjustments. Similar to what is reported in the static testing condition (Nicol *et al.* 1991b), clear trends are observed of either facilitation in tasks with submaximal effort level or inhibition in more stressful maximal testing conditions. In SSC-type performances, both central and reflex adjustments are therefore operative, but they vary during the recovery period as well as depending on the testing task.

TESTS OF SUBMAXIMAL EFFORT LEVEL

Similar to the efficient compensatory adjustments that may take place during the course of the fatiguing SSC exercise itself, maintained submaximal performances are reported after marathon running (Komi *et al.* 1986; Nicol *et al.* 1991c) as well as after prolonged arm rebound exercise (Gollhofer *et al.* 1987a). Fatigue leads to a reproducible series of kinematic and kinetic changes: more extended limb at the impact, subsequent faster and longer limb flexion movement with a clear drop in the vertical ground reaction force after the impact peak. This deterioration of the SSC efficacy during the braking phase is associated with clear increases of the extensor muscle EMG activity and EMG/force ratio during the push-off phase. This increased work during the push-off phase allows the same running or jumping performances to be maintained. Furthermore, an easy SSC testing task that consists of hopping at a preferred frequency is usually characterized by an absence of significant changes in either EMG activity or force production.

The 'task-dependent effect' concept is also substantiated by the specific analysis of the EMG reflex responses. As shown by Fig. 11.7, the short-, medium- and long-latency components of the stretch reflex EMG response vary from facilitation to inhibition with increase of the loading condition (Gollhofer *et al.* 1987b; Komi & Gollhofer 1987). Thus, in the submaximal testing conditions, the stretch reflex contribution during fatigue implies attempts of the nervous system to compensate by an increased activation for the loss of the contractile force to resist repeated impact loads.

TESTS OF MAXIMAL EFFORT LEVEL

Maximal dynamic strength tests can be used to characterize the bimodal recovery of the performance. The bimodal trend refers to a dramatic functional decline immediately after exhaustive SSC exercise, followed by a short-lasting recovery (during the next few hours post exercise) and a subsequent secondary drop around the 2nd or 3rd day post exercise (Horita *et al.* 1999, Horita 2000). Independently of the nature of the fatiguing SSC exercise, parallel acute and delayed reductions affect the preactivity, pre- and postlanding joint stiffness and SSC performance (Avela &

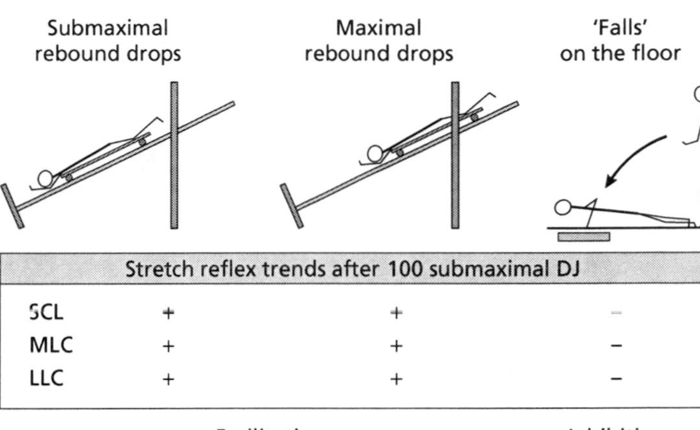

Fig. 11.7 Fatigue effects of 100 repeated rebound 'jumps' performed with the arms on the stretch reflex responses isolated from the global surface EMG records in three testing conditions of increasing intensity (SCL, MLC and LLC, respectively, for short-, medium- and long-latency EMG components of the stretch reflex responses). (Adapted by permission, from P.V. Komi & A. Gollhofer (1987).)

Komi 1998a,b; Horita *et al.* 1999). Supporting the 'task-dependent effect' concept, varying compensatory strategies of both acute and delayed contractile failure can be seen in tests that are less demanding for the subjects. A marathon run may cause no acute changes in maximal countermovement jump (CMJ), but clear declines in isometric as well as in more stressful SSC-type performances (maximal drop-jump, five-jump and sprint running tests) (Nicol *et al.* 1991a,b). An exhaustive rebound exercise may lead to a 2-day delayed decline in SSC (drop-jump) performance with no associated decrement in pure concentric (squat-jump) performance (Horita 2000).

When dealing with the observed EMG changes, there is enough evidence to suggest that coupling exists between the modulation of the neural input to the muscles and the respective changes in the stretch–reflex response. Figure 11.8 demonstrates the parallelism of the bimodal decreases of the active stretch–reflex EMG responses (Fig. 11.8a,b) and landing stiffness regulation (Fig. 11.8a–c), the latter parameter reflecting a clear loss of tolerance to impact (Avela *et al.* 1999). The delayed fatigue-induced changes are well in phase with the delayed increase in CK activity that is expected to result from the occurrence of muscle damage and subsequent inflammatory process. These overall observations confirm earlier findings (Horita *et al.* 1996; Avela & Komi 1998a,b).

Specific reflex responses

As it is not always easy to isolate the stretch–reflex EMG response from the global EMG recordings, the potential effect of SSC fatigue on the EMG reflex response can also be examined indirectly in passive reflex testing conditions (Fig. 11.9). In this case, a powerful engine is used to induce passive stretches of the shank muscles at slow and intermediate angular velocities (60–180°·s^{-1}). To detect potential changes in the spinal excitability level, the Hoffmann reflex test (H-reflex) of the soleus muscle is also recorded. Intensive SSC rebound exercises are found to result in a bimodal trend of decline in peak-to-peak EMG reflex response to passive stretches after a marathon run (Avela *et al.* 1999) as well as after a very intensive rebound exercise on the sledge (Nicol *et al.* 1996a). In the latter case, this was associated with a bimodal decrease of the H-reflex response, a trend that has also been observed after each of three successive exhaustive rebound exercises on the sledge (Nicol *et al.* 1996b) as well as after 75 min of electrical stimulation combined with repeated passive stretches (Ogiso *et al.* in progress). In marathon running, however, Avela *et al.* (1999) did observe an acute reduction in the H/M-wave ratio, but with no secondary decline.

Figure 11.10 combines the findings of two recent studies (Nicol *et al.* submitted; Kuitunen

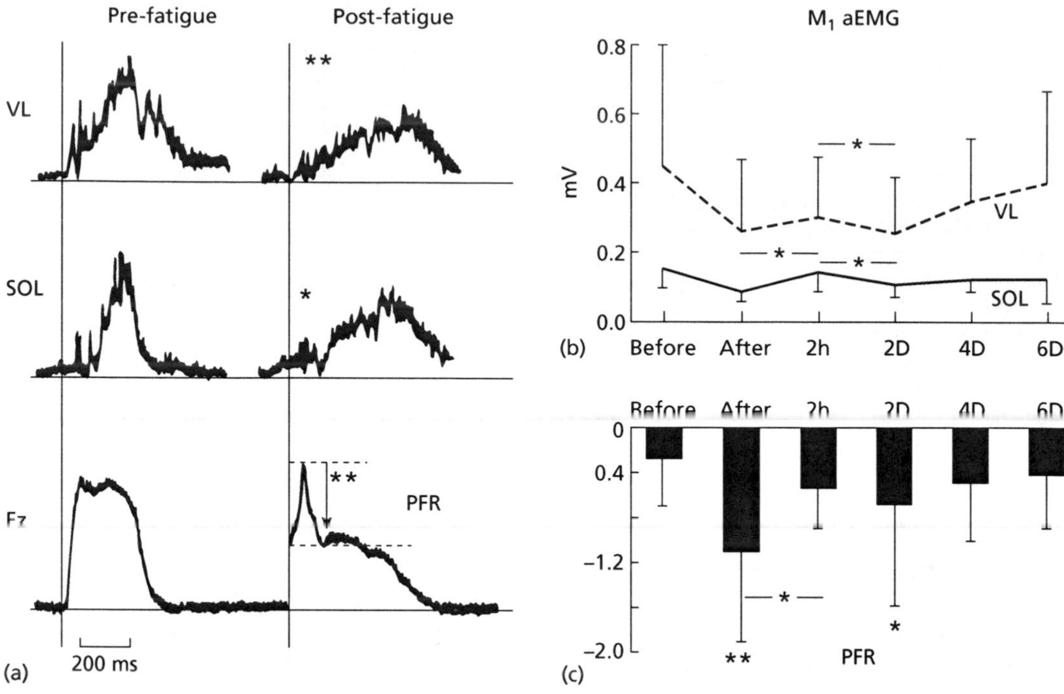

Fig. 11.8 Bimodal trends of recovery observed in 7 subjects after a marathon run: rectified and averaged EMG patterns of the soleus (SOL) and vastus lateralis (VL) muscles, and vertical ground reaction force (Fz)–time curve in 10 successive sledge rebounds performed before and after the run (a). Corresponding active short-latency reflex component (M1 aEMG) of SOL and vastus lateralis (VL) muscles (b), and postlanding stiffness regulation as reflected by the peak force reduction (PFR) measured from Fz record (c). Adapted by permission, from Avela *et al.* (1999b).

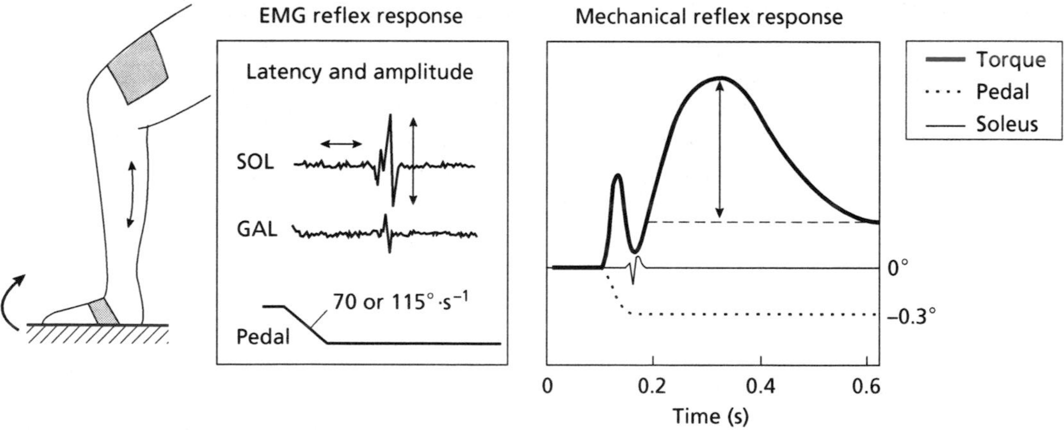

Fig. 11.9 Schematic presentation of the stretch reflex test with the analysis of the associated EMG (left) and mechanical (right) reflex responses.

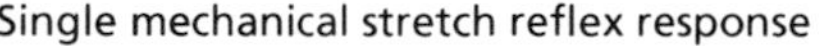

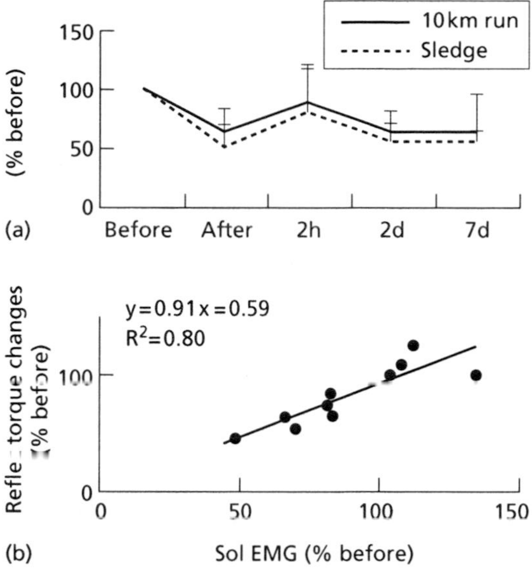

Fig. 11.10 Upper part, acute and delayed fatigue effects of two different SSC exercises on the mechanical reflex response (torque response) of the triceps surae muscle group to a series of single passive stretches. The values are expressed as a percentage of the prefatigue values. Lower part, significant relationship between the relative 2-day delayed fatigue effects on the stretch reflex torque and the respective changes of the reflex EMG response recorded from the soleus (sol) muscle.

et al. 2002) in which fatigue was induced by performing either a 10-km run at a predetermined velocity or a shorter but more intensive rebound exercise on the sledge ergometer. The major influence of the delayed reflex inhibition on the observed torque decrement is demonstrated by the positive relationships, on both days 2 (Fig. 11.10) and 7, between the respective changes in EMG and torque reflex responses.

Figure 11.11 gives further support for the parallelism between different parameters in bimodal recovery after SSC exercise. During recovery from a 10-km run, the 2-day delayed changes in the mechanical reflex response of the triceps surae to passive stretch are significantly related to the respective changes in the muscle activation during the braking phase in a maximal drop-jump (DJ) test. This suggests that the larger the contractile failure is, the more the triceps activation during the braking phase is reduced in maximal DJ. This agrees with 'fatigue-dependent' adjustment of the compensatory neural mechanisms that vary from facilitation to inhibition.

The preceding presentation may give an impression that the fatigue response and subsequent recovery is a very generalized pattern. This is not at all true in all cases, because SSC fatigue responses can be very individual in nature. Figure 11.12 gives examples of these varying responses. In these recent studies (Nicol *et al.* submitted, Kuitunen *et al.* 2002), the pure mechanical reflex response of 12 subjects was divided into three subgroups: G1 presents only acute changes (Fig. 11.12a); G2 follows the expected bimodal trend (Fig. 11.12b); and G3 presents an additional slower rate of relaxation on the 2nd and 4th days post exercise (Fig. 11.12c). The delayed mechanical changes vary in accordance with the respective changes in EMG reflex response and in CK activity. As shown by the limited CK changes, the first subgroup includes the less fatigued subjects of both studies.

These overall results demonstrate that muscle function and stiffness regulation may be disturbed in a delayed but individual manner after exhaustive-type SSC exercise. On the other hand, a clear parallelism exists between the respective changes in performance, in neural (central and peripheral) activation, and in indirect indicators of either metabolic or structural sources of fatigue. This implies the existence of potential coupling between the contractile type of failure and the central and peripheral adjustments that take place during its recovery.

Potential mechanisms

The preceding chapter focused on demonstrating the dominant role of the eccentric phase in SSC fatigue. Intense or prolonged exercises, especially involving unaccustomed eccentric muscle actions, are typically associated with delayed-onset muscle soreness (DOMS). This soreness was suggested as early as in 1902

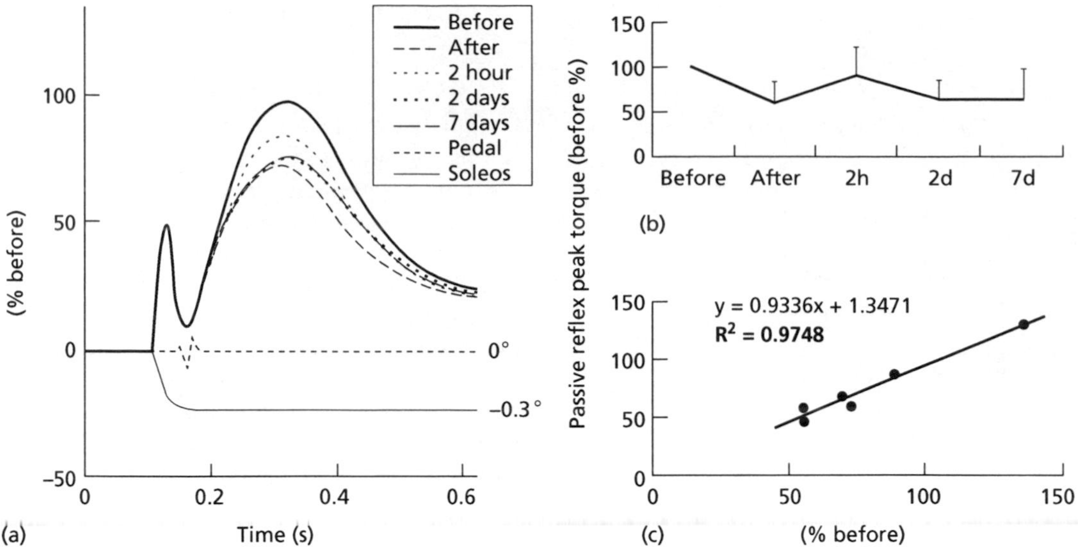

Fig. 11.11 (a,b) Relative changes induced by a fatiguing 10-km run in the passive stretch reflex mechanical response. (c) Relationship on the 2nd day post exercise between the respective fatigue-induced changes in the passive mechanical reflex response from the triceps surae muscle and the lateral gastrocnemius (GAL) activation during the braking phase in maximal drop-jump test (DJ). Data from Nicol *et al.* submitted and Kuitunen *et al.* 2002.

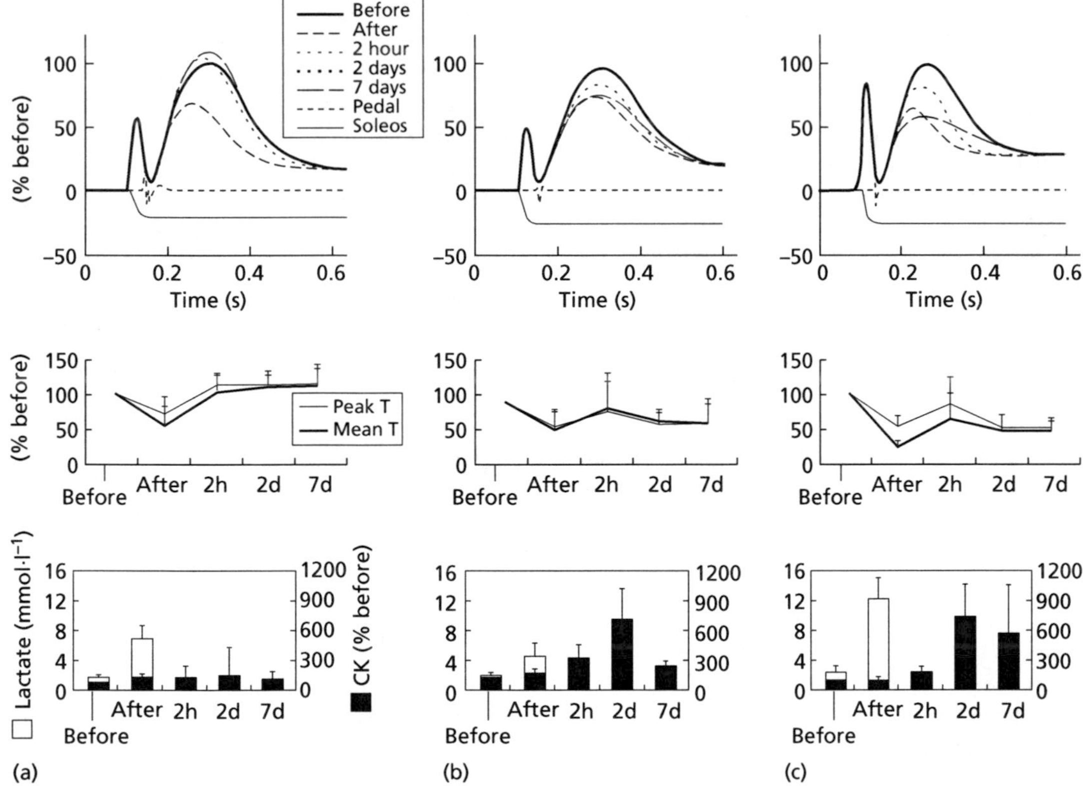

Fig. 11.12 Effects of fatiguing SSC exercises on the passive mechanical reflex response (torque response) (upper 2 lines of graphs) with the respective changes in serum lactate concentration and creatine kinase (CK) activity. The data are presented for 12 subjects divided into three subgroups according to the peak and mean torque (T) reflex responses: G1 with only acute changes (a); G2 with a bimodal trend (b); and G3 with additional slower rate of relaxation on the 2nd and 7th days post exercise (c). (Data from Nicol *et al.* submitted.)

(Hough 1902) to be due to exercise-induced muscle injury. Since these earlier attempts, eccentric exercises have been studied quite extensively, with both animal and human models. The current literature offers many articles and comprehensive reviews on the characteristics of eccentric fatigue. These include muscle damage and DOMS, but also muscle swelling and stiffness, and associated reductions of range of motion and muscle strength as well as altered sense of force and position (Komi & Viitasalo 1977; Waterman-Storer 1991; Kuipers 1994; Clarkson & Newham 1995; MacIntyre *et al.* 1995; Brockett *et al.* 1997; Lieber & Fridén 1999; Grabiner 2000). Delayed increase in tremor amplitude has also been reported after intensive eccentric arm exercise (Saxton *et al.* 1995). The underlying mechanisms of muscle damage and soreness are quite well studied, although the final answers are still to be found.

It has been well documented that the force enhancement by active stretch (eccentric action) results from the combination of several factors (see Chapter 9). This includes the increased strain of attached cross-bridges, probably in combination with a slight increase in their number (Sugi & Tsuchiya 1988; Lombardi & Piazzesi 1990), and the passive resistive force of cytoskeletal proteins found in the intrasarcomeric region, such as titin (Edman & Tsuchiya 1996), desmin (Lieber *et al.* 1996) and nebulin (Patel & Lieber 1997). Eccentric exercises also present the advantage of a lower cost of energy (Asmussen 1956) that could result from the lesser motor unit recruitment at a given force level (Komi 1973) and from the mechanical detachment of cross-bridges by the applied external force (Morgan 1990).

On the other hand, it seems evident from the literature that either intensive or prolonged exercises involving eccentric muscle actions lead to both acute and delayed neuromuscular adjustments to fatigue. When dealing with fatigue induced by SSC-type exercises, one should also consider the involved concentric muscle actions, the loading of which has been shown to increase dramatically in standard exercise during the course of fatigue (Fig. 11.2b) (Nicol *et al.* 1991c; Horita 2000). The increased concentric work observed in parallel with the decreased SSC efficacy with fatigue is expected to lead to a potential metabolic type of fatigue that will vary depending on the intensity and duration of the SSC exercise. This component of fatigue should thus be taken into account when studying the bimodal trend of functional disturbances. After exhaustive SSC exercises, the frequent observation of a rapid partial recovery of the functional parameters in the 2nd hour post exercise tends to suggest that the acute muscle weakness might result from the combined effects of the exercise-induced metabolic changes and ultrastructural damage, whereas the delayed recovery could result from the inflammation process that takes place over a few days after injury. Both intensity and duration of the exercise-induced fatigue are naturally dependent on the type of SSC exercise as well as on the familiarity (adaptation) of the subjects to this task.

The first part of this chapter described in more detail how the neuromuscular adjustments occurred in a bimodal trend during exercise-induced contractile failure. A major question, however, is what the underlying mechanisms could be to explain the observed adjustments to the induced muscle failure, especially in connection with SSC exercises.

Structural and functional changes associated with eccentric-type fatigue

Overall trends

Longlasting, but reversible, ultrastructural muscle damage is the common indicator of injury resulting from exercises involving eccentric muscle actions. Damage has been evidenced directly from histological analysis and indirectly from reductions in strength and range of motion as well as from increases in blood concentration of muscle proteins (for reviews, see e.g. Clarkson & Newham 1995; Fridén & Lieber 2001a,b). It is well documented that the cytoskeletal and myofibrillar abnormalities observed after eccentric

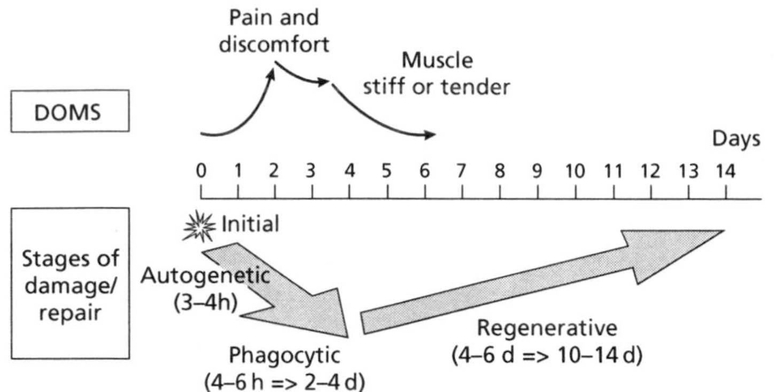

Fig. 11.13 Schematic representation of the four different stages related to (eccentric) exercise-induced muscle damage, and the subjective feelings of pain and discomfort which are associated with the muscular changes in the course of delayed-onset muscle soreness (DOMS).

muscle actions reach a peak 2–3 days after the exercise, with normal muscle architecture being lost from areas adjacent to the damaged sarcomeres and fibres (Fridén *et al.* 1983a,b; Newham *et al.* 1983a). The model proposed by Armstrong (Armstrong 1990; Armstrong *et al.* 1991) which differentiates four subsequent stages: the 'initial', the 'autogenetic', the 'phagocytic' and the 'regenerative', has served as a framework for systematic research on this process (Fig. 11.13). As shown in this figure, unaccustomed and/or intensive exercises involving eccentric-type muscle actions are also associated with DOMS, a typical sensation of dull pain and discomfort that increases in intensity during the first 2 days, remaining symptomatic for 1–2 more days, and disappearing usually 5–7 days after the exercise whereas the muscle regeneration is far from being accomplished. Sore muscles are often stiff and tender, and their ability to produce force is reduced for several days or weeks (Asmussen 1956; Komi & Buskirk 1972; Komi & Rusko 1974; Komi & Viitasalo 1977; Sherman *et al.* 1984; Howell *et al.* 1993; Murayama *et al.* 2000). Even though stiffness was found to increase with a delayed time course that parallels that of muscle soreness (Jones *et al.* 1987), it often lasts much longer (Howell *et al.* 1993; Chleboun *et al.* 1998).

Acute effects

In Armstrong's model (Armstrong 1990; Armstrong *et al.* 1991), the '*initial stage*' includes events that trigger the whole process of further muscle damage and repair. In pure eccentric exercise, much evidence exists that the initial local damage results from mechanical rather than metabolic mechanisms (Evans & Cannon 1991; Lieber & Fridén 1993; Warren *et al.* 1993a; Brooks *et al.* 1995). Histological studies have reported direct evidence of extensive disorganization and even disruption of the myofibrillar structures and intermediate filaments, leading to the classically observed Z-line streaming (Fridén *et al.* 1981, 1984; Waterman-Storer 1991). Indices of sarcolemmal disruption (Hikida *et al.* 1983; McBride *et al.* 2000), swelling and disruption of the sarcotubular system (Armstrong 1990; Fridén & Lieber 1996) and swollen mitochondria (Warhol *et al.* 1985; Stauber 1989) as well as extracellular matrix injury (Myllylä *et al.* 1986; Han *et al.* 1999; Koskinen *et al.* 2001) have also been reported. High tensions can be generated across a given number of recruited fibres under eccentric conditions (Bigland-Ritchie & Woods 1976; Faulkner *et al.* 1993), but it seems that it is not the high stress *per se* that is the primary cause of muscle damage, but the magnitude of the active strain (Lieber & Fridén 1993) or the combination of strain and average force (Brooks *et al.* 1995). Excessive strain is expected to induce extracellular and/or intracellular membrane disruption that may permit hydrolysis of structural proteins leading to myofibrillar disorganization (Lieber & Fridén 1999). The resulting sarcomere and muscle fibre disruptions would then contribute to the common shift of the length–tension relationship towards longer muscle lengths after eccentric exercise (Katz 1939; Wood *et al.* 1993; Jones *et al.* 1997). Interestingly, physical activities involving highly repetitive contraction of relatively small stretches are reported to result in severe muscle injury (Fridén *et al.* 1983b; Newham *et al.* 1983b; Lieber & Fridén 1993). Evidence has also been presented that eccentric exercise is of differing severity in muscles with different architectures (Lieber & Fridén 2000; Fridén & Lieber 2001b) and fibre type specific so that fast-twitch fibres would be more sensitive than slow-twitch fibres to eccentric-induced muscle damage (Fridén *et al.* 1983b, 1988; Fridén & Lieber 2001b; Vijayan *et al.* 2001). In addition to their structural differences, fast-twitch fibres experience a reduced oxidative capacity, which would result during intensive exercises in the failure of cross-bridges to be detached, thus leading to an inhomogeneous resistance to stretch among sarcomeres and muscle fibres (Fridén & Lieber 1992).

On the other hand, excitation–contraction uncoupling has been reported in a recent review (Warren *et al.* 2001) to have the major influence on the eccentric-induced functional failure. Among other parameters, impaired plasmalemmal action potential conduction has been reported in rat muscles 1–2 h after a downhill running exercise (McBride *et al.* 2000). This was suggested to result from an increase in Na^+ permeability in the muscle due to sarcolemmal damage as well as to the activation of stretch-activated ion channels. Magnitude and duration of the postexercise depolarization were found to be related to the intensity (number of eccentric contractions) and to the number of previous exposures to exercise. Differences among protocols are expected to explain partly the opposite results reported by Warren *et al.* (1993b, 1999) after intensive eccentric exercise in rats. Similarly, the review of Warren *et al.* (2001) was based on studies of mouse muscle submitted to maximal electrical stimulation, a model that differs clearly from voluntary eccentric exercises. In voluntary SSC exercises, the hypothesis of an excitation–contraction uncoupling due to exercise-induced sarcolemmal damage is also unlikely due to the partial recovery observed quite systematically when tested around the 2nd hour post exercise (Figs 11.10–11.12).

With regard to the effects of these potential mechanisms on the initial drop in strength after eccentric and SSC exercises, the literature presents equivocal results. According to Morgan and Allen (1999), sarcomere length instabilities would provide the most comprehensive explanation for the early drop in tension. Supporting this hypothesis, the study of Lieber *et al.* (1996) demonstrates significant relationships between the exercise-induced cytoskeletal disruption and the respective loss in strength. Our own findings using different fatiguing protocols emphasize the additional influence of metabolic failure. Considering the similarity of the functional failures induced by either 3 min of intensive rebound exercise or a prolonged marathon run (Fig. 11.10), it is suggested that acidosis induced by the intensive exercise (reflected by 10 and 4 $mmol \cdot l^{-1}$ of blood lactate concentration, respectively) might have favoured the rapid development of inhomogeneous resistance to stretch and muscle damage in connection with the more intensive exercise. This is expected to have enhanced the damaging effect of the high-impact loads experienced during this rebound exercise. On the other hand, excitation–contraction uncoupling is expected to take place, but with an increasing effect, during the subsequent phases of the degrading process. Finally, our results emphasize the role of a reduced maximal activation on the drop in maximal voluntary strength after fatiguing SSC exercises (Nicol *et al.* 1991b; Pullinen *et al.* 1997). The finding of large immediate decreases in the amplitude of both stretch and H-reflex responses (Nicol *et al.* 1996b; Avela *et al.* 1999) tends to support the hypothesis of a reflex inhibition of the activation of the injured muscle that could contribute to the observed functional weakness (Fig. 11.14).

Delayed effects

Armstrong (1990) differentiated this inflammatory period into autogenetic and phagocytic

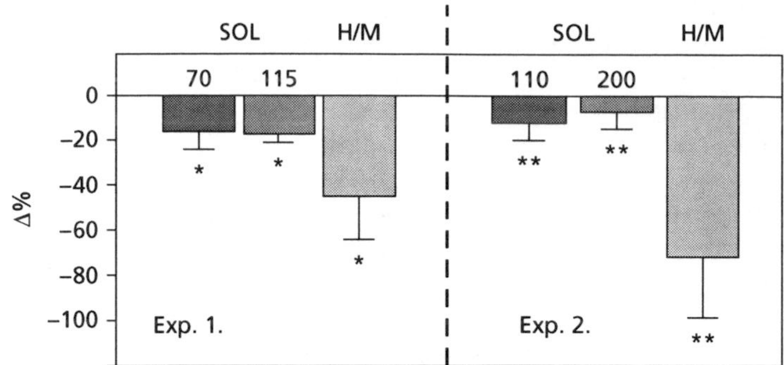

Fig. 11.14 Changes in stretch reflex amplitude measured at different stretching velocities (70, 110, 115 and 120°·s^{-1}) and in H/M-wave ratio of the soleus (SOL) muscle immediately after short- (Exp.1) or long-term (Exp. 2) exhaustive SSC exercises. (Data from Avela *et al.* 1999b; Nicol *et al.* 1996b.)

stages. Both of them are associated with the presence in the blood of indirect indicators of muscle injury, such as muscular protein metabolites (e.g. troponin I, myosin heavy chain) and increased specific muscle enzyme activity (e.g. creatine kinase (CK), lactate dehydrogenase) (for a review see Noakes 1987). CK activity is the most frequently used marker of muscle damage. It should be noted, however, that due to considerable variability in the magnitude of the response of serum enzymes, the peak value does not reflect the amount of muscle damage and is considered as a poor predictor of the functional changes (Ebbeling & Clarkson 1989; Mair *et al.* 1995; Fridén & Lieber 2001a). However, based on the results of several SSC fatigue studies (Nicol *et al.* 1996b; Kyrölainen *et al.* 1998; Avela *et al.* 1999; Horita *et al.* 1999) and illustrated in Fig. 11.12, it is suggested that relative changes in CK might be of some relevance to the detection of tissue inflammation and functional defects associated with SSC fatigue. Other indicators of inflammation include redness, heat and swelling as well as pain and stiffness.

The *'autogenetic stage'* corresponds to the first 3–4 h following the injury and marks the beginning of the degrading process of the membrane structures. The model predicts that exercise-induced damage of the sarcolemma, T-tubule system and sarcoplasmic reticulum (SR) would give rise to a loss of calcium (Ca^{2+}) homeostasis. Following strenuous exercises, gross focal dilatation of SR has been reported to be accompanied by depression in the rate of Ca^{2+} uptake and diminished Ca^{2+} release, resulting in an increase of intracellular free calcium concentration $[Ca^{2+}]_i$ (Byrd 1992). According to the reviews of Ebbeling and Clarkson (1989) and Armstrong (1990), alteration of resting $[Ca^{2+}]_i$ in the injured fibres could result in enhanced calcium-activated endogenous proteases (e.g. calpain) causing further muscle injury. Calpain leads to specific hydrolysis of cytoskeletal proteins such as desmin, but not actin and myosin, whereas other calcium-stimulated proteases act directly on the Z-lines (Reddy *et al.* 1975). Interestingly, Belcastro (1993) demonstrated an increased affinity of calpain for calcium after exercise, suggesting that a given amount of damage could then occur at a lower calcium concentration. Quantitative measurements of resting $[Ca^{2+}]_i$ in skeletal muscles following acute or long-term downhill running exercise have been recently performed in rats (Lynch *et al.* 1997). The results indicated a significant increase in resting $[Ca^{2+}]_i$ which coincided with the functional decrement. It should be mentioned, however, that Lowe *et al.* (1994) reported no immediate changes in $[Ca^{2+}]_i$ and that Lynch *et al.* (1997) observed changes in both $[Ca^{2+}]_i$ and muscle function 48 h, but not 24 h post exercise. According to Lynch *et al.* (1997), these combined results would support the hypothesis that muscles subjected to exercises involving eccentric muscle actions could buffer changes in $[Ca^{2+}]_i$ until the inflammatory phase.

With regard to the relevant functional effects, eccentric and SSC-type exercises are usually associated with larger force reduction at low than at high frequency of stimulation (Edwards *et al.* 1977; Newham *et al.* 1983a; Strojnik & Komi 2000). Reduced Ca^{2+} release by the sarcoplasmic reticulum has been presented as one explanation for the larger reductions of force at low than at high frequencies of stimulation (Davies & White 1981; Newham *et al.* 1983b; Westerblad *et al.* 1993). According to Allen (2001), low frequency fatigue could result also from a slower rate of rise in force of the weakened overstretched sarcomeres. At the present stage, it is not possible to conclude whether one of these mechanisms could have contributed to the slower rate of twitch relaxation observed on the 2nd and 7th days post SSC exercise (Fig. 11.12). More investigations are needed to clarify the underlying mechanisms of the increased intracellular Ca^{2+} concentration and to identify the extent to which raised resting $[Ca^{2+}]_i$ would contribute to the subsequent phases of proteolysis, inflammation and regeneration.

The *'phagocytic stage'* is characterized by a typical inflammatory response in the tissues which may last for 2–4 days or more, with a peak around the 3rd day post exercise (Kihlstrom *et al.* 1984). Several studies have reported greater myofibrillar damage 2 days following eccentric exercise than immediately post exercise (Fridén *et al.* 1981; Newham *et al.* 1983a). After a marathon run, Hikida *et al.* (1983) demonstrated the presence of significant ultrastructural changes that were found to peak on days 1 and 3, some of them persisting on day 7. More precisely, the inflammatory process may be subclassified into acute and chronic. The acute response begins with changes in the vascular wall structure, leading to structural and functional alterations of the basement membrane, and migration of neutrophils and monocytes to the site of injury (Evans & Cannon 1991; Fantone 1993). Mobilization of neutrophils has been reported to be greater after eccentric- than after concentric-type exercises performed by the same subjects at similar levels of oxygen consumption (Smith *et al.* 1989). During inflammation, monocytes accumulate at the site of injury by chemotaxis and undergo morphological and functional differentiation, becoming macrophages. Once activated, neutrophils, monocytes and macrophages are capable of phagocytosis (Faulkner *et al.* 1993) and provide a fresh supply of cytokine mediators and cytotoxic factors which may be partly responsible for amplifying and delaying the inflammation (Adams & Hamilton 1988). In addition, macrophages are the prime sources of cytokines such as interleukin 1 (IL-1) and tumour necrosis factor (TNF) that alter endothelial permeability, leading to leucocyte infiltration and oedema. As reviewed by Evans and Cannon (1991), macrophages secrete fibronectin and proteoglycans that help to stabilize the extracellular matrix, promote cell adhesion, and stimulate fibroblast proliferation and collagen synthesis by means of IL-1. Interestingly, there is strong evidence that supports the hypothesis that following exercise-induced muscle injury regeneration proceeds no further in the absence of macrophages (for a review see Carlson & Faulkner 1983; MacIntyre *et al.* 1995).

Exercise-induced muscle soreness has been suggested, as early as in 1902 by Hough (Hough 1902), to result in its delayed phase from 'some sort of rupture within the muscle'. Hill (1951) suggested that soreness is due to mechanical injury, distributed microscopically throughout the muscle. As referred to by Asmussen (1956), Bøje (1955) was inclined to believe that the pains are located in the intramuscular connective tissues. At present it is known, however, that neither the degree nor the timing of ultrastructural damage correlate well with the respective changes in the DOMS (Newham *et al.* 1983b; Howell *et al.* 1993). In this line, experimental muscle pain induced by intramuscular injections of algogenic substances such as bradykinin, serotonin and substance P did not reveal any dose relation with the induced pain intensity (Babenko *et al.* 1999). Part of this discrepancy may be explained by the fact that when peripheral tissues are damaged, the sensation of pain in response to a given stimulus is enhanced. This phenomenon, termed 'hyperalgesia', may involve lowering of threshold of nociceptors by the presence of locally released chemicals (for a review see Jessel & Kelly 1991; Mizumura 1998; Millan 1999).

Hyperalgesia occurs first at the site of tissue damage before spreading throughout other compartments (Bobbert *et al.* 1986; Fields 1987; Howell *et al.* 1993). In addition, soreness is not constant all the time, being mostly felt when the exercised limbs are extended or fully flexed or when the muscles are palpated deeply (Howell *et al.* 1993).

When comparing the respective recovery of muscle pain and muscle strength, moderate (Talag 1973) or no relationship (Cleak & Eston 1992) has been reported in the literature. Moreover, strength loss and neuromuscular perturbations are well known to start before soreness is perceived and to last for a few days after soreness dissipates (Nicol *et al.* 1996a; Deschesnes *et al.* 2000). It is therefore suggested that this delay could reflect the natural course of the inflammation (Hikida *et al.* 1983; Evans & Cannon 1991; MacIntyre *et al.* 2001) and swelling (Smith 1991) responses of the injured muscle. Referring to the potential muscle pain effect on the EMG activity, the experimental muscle pain study of Graven-Nielsen *et al.* (1997) revealed no increase in the resting EMG level, but a reduced activity in maximal voluntary contraction and changes in coordination during dynamic exercises. In accordance with the pain adaptation model of Lund *et al.* (1991), several other studies reported an increased activity of antagonistic muscles and a decreased activity of agonistic muscles (Arendt-Nielsen *et al.* 1996; Matre *et al.* 1998; Sohn *et al.* 2000). However, considering the delayed EMG recovery after the pain dissipation, it is suggested that DOMS may contribute primarily for the first 2–3 days post exercise to the observed reduction of EMG in maximal effort and increase of EMG during constant submaximal contraction (Komi & Viitasalo 1977).

Stiffness changes have been frequently studied in the case of damaged elbow flexors, which is typically associated with a reduced ability to fully flex the joint (Clarkson *et al.* 1992) and with a more flexed elbow joint when the arm is hanging in a relaxed position (Howell *et al.* 1985; Cleak & Eston 1992; Saxton & Donnelly 1995). This relative flexion is expected to result at least partially from oedema-induced increase of passive stiffness in the injured muscles (Howell *et al.* 1985; Jones *et al.* 1987; Murayama *et al.* 2000). Other explanations have been reported as well. According to Whitehead *et al.* (2001), the rise in passive tension observed in both human and animal muscles after eccentric exercise would result from the development of injury contractures in the damaged muscles. Ebbeling and Clarkson (1989) suggested a potential effect of abnormal accumulation of calcium inside the muscle cell, due to either a loss of sarcolemmal integrity or a dysfunction of the sarcoplasmic reticulum. On the other hand, the 'reflex spasm theory' (De Vries 1966), according to which the skeletal muscle stiffness and pain would result from sustained electrical activity in the damaged muscle, is reported to be unlikely in such a fatigue situation (Howell *et al.* 1985; Bobbert *et al.* 1986; Jones *et al.* 1987).

The '*regenerative stage*' begins on days 4–6 and reflects the regeneration of muscle fibres. Strength recovery has been reported to take place even though the contractile protein content is still decreasing (Lowe *et al.* 1995; Ingalls *et al.* 1998). In the animal study of Lowe *et al.* (1995), protein synthesis rates were found to increase approximately 48 h post injury, remaining elevated by 83% 5 days post injury. By days 10–14, muscle protein degradation and synthesis rates had returned to normal, and phagocytic infiltration was not detected. However, muscle mass, protein content and absolute force production were still lower than before. Based on the review of Warren *et al.* (2001), contractile protein content and strength would recover in parallel towards the end of the recovery (14–28 days). Similar delays in recovery (Hikida *et al.* 1983), but also much longer ones (Warhol *et al.* 1985; Howell *et al.* 1993) have been reported in humans following eccentric-induced muscle damage.

Underlying mechanisms of the neural adaptation to fatigue

During the progressive development of eccentric and SSC-type fatigue, neuromuscular adaptation is likely to vary from neural compensations of the contractile failure to neural protective mechanisms of the damaged muscles (Figs 11.3 & 11.4) (Horita 2000; Strojnik *et al.* 2000, 2001a,b). During and after fatiguing SSC exercises, neural failure and/or adjustments may be expected to affect different parts of the activation pathways. These potential sites have been divided by Bigland-Ritchie and Woods (1984) into three general categories: (i) those which lie within the central nervous system (CNS); (ii) those concerned with neural transmission from the CNS to muscle; and (iii) those within the individual muscle fibres.

Supraspinal fatigue

Despite the uncertainty as to the existence of a supraspinal central fatigue, this hypothesis cannot be ruled out when considering the large reductions in maximal neural activation reported immediately after prolonged (Viitasalo *et al.* 1982; Nicol *et al.* 1991b; Pullinen *et al.* 1997) SSC exercises. During the delayed phase of recovery, this possibility is reinforced by the potential effect of muscle pain. Using transcranial magnetic stimulation techniques, Le Pera *et al.* 2001) demonstrated that tonic muscle pain can inhibit the motor system. During the peak pain, the absence of effects on the H-reflex response suggested that the observed reduction in size of the motor-evoked potentials (MEPs) was probably due to decreased excitability of the motor cortex. Twenty minutes after pain, the MEP amplitude was found to be further depressed and the H-reflex amplitude reduced suggesting an inhibition of the spinal motoneurones' excitability, possibly overlapping the cortical inhibitory process. This observation of a delayed depression of the H-reflex response is supported by the results of Rossi and Decchi (1977), but differs from the absence of change reported by Svensson *et al.* (1998) and Matre *et al.* (1998). It should be mentioned, however, that Matre *et al.* (1998) observed in some of the H-reflex recordings a delayed depression (lasting for more than 40 min after the end of pain) which was then attributed to the potential inhibitory effect originating from group III muscle afferents.

Reflex adjustments of the neural activation

During the delayed phase of the recovery, structural and chemical changes associated with induced damage and inflammation should have logical consequences on the afferent sensory pathways, and consequently on the efferent activities as well. These changes in the activation (either inhibition or facilitation) should then lead to changes or difficulties in the true function of the neuromuscular system.

ACTIVATION OF SMALL-DIAMETER MUSCLE AFFERENTS

The sensation of pain in skeletal muscles is transmitted by nociceptors that belong to two groups of small-diameter groups III (A-delta) and IV (C) muscle afferents (Mense 1977; Kniffki *et al.* 1978). These free nerve endings are particularly dense in the regions of connective tissues, but also between intra- and extrafusal muscle fibres as well as near blood vessels, in the Golgi tendon organs and at the myotendinous junction (Stacey 1969; Kaufman & Rybicki 1987). Small-diameter groups III and IV muscle afferents are mostly polymodal, being sensitive to several parameters associated with either metabolic fatigue and/or muscle injury. Only part of these receptors are of nociceptive type (Mense & Meyer 1985). More specifically, myelinated group III carries sharp, localized pain, whereas unmyelinated group IV carries dull and diffuse pain. Group IV fibres have been suggested by Armstrong (1984) to be primarily responsible for the sensation of DOMS. In humans, the mean conduction velocity for group III and IV fibres has been reported by Simone *et al.* (1994) to vary within the following ranges: (3.1–13.5) and (0.6–1.2) $m \cdot s^{-1}$.

In the case of muscle damage, group III and/or IV metaboceptors are activated by the released biochemical substances, such as bradykinin (Kranz & Mense 1975; Mense & Meyer 1988) and products of cyclooxygenase activation

(Herbaczynska-Cedro *et al.* 1976; Kniffki *et al.* 1978; Rotto & Kaufman 1988). Once activated, the nociceptors release neuropeptides, which cause vasodilatation, oedema and release of histamine. These processes lead then to a further and longlasting activation of some of the sensory endings (Fields 1987). In the case of intense exercise, extracellular increases in potassium, phosphate and lactic acid may constitute acute but additional stimuli of the muscle metaboceptors (Mense 1977; Rybicki *et al.* 1985; Kaufman & Rybicki 1987; Synoway *et al.* 1993; Darques & Jammes 1997; Darques *et al.* 1998; Decherchi *et al.* 1998). According to the review of McMahon and Koltzenburg (1990), unmyelinated primary sensory neurones are particularly responsive to the longlasting changes that can occur with slow tissue perturbations such as inflammation.

CAN ACTIVATION OF SMALL-DIAMETER AFFERENTS HAVE ANY INFLUENCE?

The exact influence of small-diameter muscle afferents on neural activation is not clearly established in fatigue conditions. The literature presents two major and contradictory trends in case of pain and damage.

As early as 1942, Travell and collaborators (Travell *et al.* 1942) proposed the hypothesis of a 'vicious circle' in which group III and IV muscle afferents would activate γ motoneurones, thus leading to subsequent rises in muscle spindle sensitivity, α motoneurone activity and development of fatigue. This hypothesis is based on several works in which an increased fusimotor activity was observed after intra-arterial injection of proinflammatory substances (Ellaway *et al.* 1982; Jovanovic *et al.* 1990; Ljubisavljević *et al.* 1992). A similar trend has been reported after injection of KCl and lactic acid (Johansson *et al.* 1993). Moreover, it has been suggested that increased fusimotor activity evoked by nociceptive afferents of a given muscle might lead to increased activation of muscle spindle afferents (Djupsjöbacka *et al.* 1995) and/or α motoneurone activity (Appelberg *et al.* 1983) of homonymous and heteronymous muscles.

The opposite but currently more convincing hypothesis refers to the sparing and protective effects of the fatigued muscle (Bigland-Ritchie *et al.* 1986; Garland 1991; Enoka & Stuart 1992; Jammes & Balzamo 1992; Garland & Kaufman 1995). The protective effects are expected to act in parallel with the depressed sensitivity of muscle spindle reported in metabolically (Fukami 1988; Lagier-Tessonier *et al.* 1993) as well as in mechanically (Avela *et al.* 2001) stressful conditions. Reduced spindle input to the α motoneurone pool may also be attributed to the indirect effects of small muscle afferents via presynaptic inhibition of the Ia terminals (Duchateau & Hainaut 1993) as well as to the activation of inhibitory spinal interneurones involved in oligosynaptic pathways (Duchateau & Hainaut 1993; Rossi *et al.* 1999). It is known from animal studies that III and IV muscle afferents make a powerful input to inhibitory interneurones (Cleland *et al.* 1982). In case of eccentric-type fatigue, the most convincing evidence for a presynaptic inhibition is supported by the absence of recovery of the H-reflex amplitude while the exercise-induced metabolic accumulation was retained through ischaemia (Avela *et al.* 1999). A bimodal trend of H-reflex recovery has also been clearly demonstrated after 75 min of electrical stimulation combined with mechanically induced stretches (Ogiso *et al.*, in progress) (Fig. 11.15) as well as after exhaustive rebound exercise on the sledge (Nicol *et al.* 1996b). In the latter study, the H-reflex response was found to remain depressed over 15 days during which the subjects performed three exhaustive rebound exercises on days 0, 5 and 10. The secondary decline supports the hypothesis of a potential effect of a prolonged activation of III and IV muscle afferents by the exercise-induced inflammatory process. With regard to the slow conducting velocity of small muscle afferents, their continuous activation supports well their potential role in the inhibition of the short-latency reflex component reported in the SSC (Avela & Komi 1998b; Avela *et al.* 1999) and in passive stretch reflex situations (Nicol *et al.* 1996a,b). In addition to peripheral pathways, however, evidence exists of descending

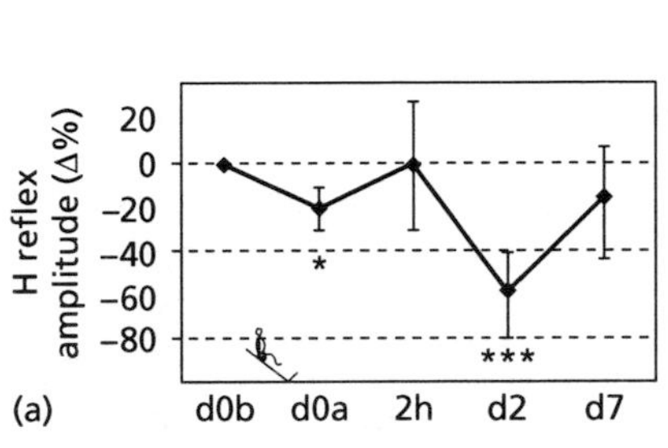

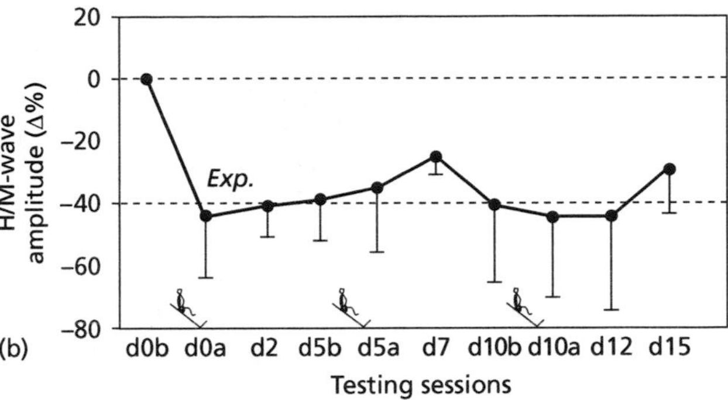

Fig. 11.15 Relative changes in the H-reflex (top) after 75 min of electrical stimulation combined with mechanically induced stretches, and H/M-wave ratio (bottom) in the course of a 15-day follow-up during which an exhaustive short-term SSC exercise was repeated on days 0, 5 and 10. In both experiments the changes are expressed as a percentage of the prefatigue values (d0b, day 0 before). (Data from Ogiso *et al.*, in progress (left) and from Nicol *et al.* 1996b (right).)

influences on the transmission of the sensory information (Hong *et al.* 1979; Alstermark *et al.* 1984; Malmgren & Pierrot-Deseilligny 1987; Cervero *et al.* 1991).

Finally, much less is known about the modulation effects of small muscle afferents on motor cortex excitability. With regard to the inflammation effects, Besson *et al.* (1972, 1975) demonstrated an inhibitory influence of mesencephalitic areas on neurones located in the lamina from the dorsal horn when they were previously sensitized to bradykinin. Andersen *et al.* (1995) reported that a central summation of nociceptive and non-nociceptive afferent activity can occur once secondary hyperalgesia is present. The introduction in humans of a new method of evoking tonic pain discharge may bring new insights to the comprehension of the immediate and delayed pain effects (Rossi & Decchi 1997; Rossi *et al.* 1998, 1999; Sohn *et al.* 2000; Le Pera *et al.* 2001). Despite the limited relevant information available at present on the true central influences, it is very likely that different central and peripheral adjustments may take place depending on the level of the imposed stress to the musculotendinous system (Komi & Gollhofer 1987; Nicol *et al.* 1991a; Horita *et al.* 1999). Variation in receptor types and in the ability to modulate pain at multiple levels in the nervous system could also explain part of the intersubject variability in soreness perception.

Concluding comments

This chapter has attempted to demonstrate that naturally occurring, but exhaustive SSC exercise induces often very dramatic deterioration of muscle force and power production. Although these effects are somewhat similar in mechanisms to those occurring after intensive pure eccentric exercise, the SSC fatigue is much more problematic and complex because the more comprehensive way in which it loads the neuromuscular system: mechanically, metabolically and neurally. All these aspects are responsible for and characteristic of the bimodal trend of fatigue response reflecting their specific roles in characterizing the damage and inflammatory processes in the progress of deterioration and recovery of neuromuscular performance. Because of these factors the neural adjustments, although they are well coupled with the metabolic and mechanical influences, represent the greatest challenges in understanding the detailed mechanisms involved. It is usually understood that the reduced neural input to the muscles, under the influence of SSC fatigue, is at least partly of reflex origin. Different pathways have been suggested, involving both disfacilitation of the muscle spindle sensitivity and presynaptic inhibition of the α motoneurone pool. There are, however, several aspects that need to be explored for further understanding of the nature and the mechanisms of exhaustive and damaging SSC exercise. These include possible structural changes in the proprioceptors (especially in the muscle spindle), and inhibitory/excitatory changes that may take place in the higher centres of the sensory and motor pathways.

References

Adams, D.O. & Hamilton, T.A. (1988) Phagocytic cells: cytotoxic activities of macrophages. In: *Inflammation: Basic Principles and Clinical Correlates* (eds J. I. Gallin, I. M. Goldstein & R. Snyderman), pp. 471–492. Raven Press, New York.

Allen, D.G. (2001) Eccentric muscle damage: mechanisms of early reduction in force. *Acta Physiologica Scandinavica* **171**, 311–319.

Alstermark, B., Lundberg, A. & Sasaki, S. (1984) Integration in descending motor pathways controlling the forelimb in the cat. *Experimental Brain Research* **56**(2), 279–307.

Andersen, O.K., Gracely, R.H. & Arendt-Nielsen, L. (1955) Facilitation of the human nociceptive reflex by stimulation of Aβ-fibres in a secondary hyperalgesia area sustained by nociceptive input from the primary hyperalgesic area. *Acta Physiologica Scandinavica* **155**, 87–97.

Appelberg, B., Hulliger, M., Johansson, H. & Sojka, P. (1983) Actions of γ-motoneurones elicited by electrical stimulation of group III muscle afferent fibres in the hind limb of the cat. *Journal of Physiology (London)* **335**, 275–292.

Arendt-Nielsen, L., Graven-Nielsen, T., Svarrer, H. & Svensson, P. (1996) The influence of low back pain on muscle activity and coordination in gait: a clinical and experimental study. *Pain* **64**, 231–240.

Armstrong, R.B. (1984) Mechanisms of exercise-induced delayed onset muscular soreness: a brief review. *Medicine and Science in Sports and Exercise* **16**, 529–538.

Armstrong, R.B. (1990) Initial events in exercise-induced muscular injury. *Medicine and Science in Sports and Exercise* **22**(4), 429–435.

Armstrong, R.B., Warren, G.L. & Warren, J.A. (1991) Mechanisms of exercise-induced muscle fibre injury. *Sports Medicine* **12**, 184–207.

Asmussen, E. (1956) Observations on experimental muscle soreness. *Acta Rheumatica Scandinavica* **2**, 109–116.

Avela, J. & Komi, P.V. (1998a) Interaction between muscle stiffness and stretch reflex sensitivity after long-term stretch–shortening cycle (SSC) exercise. *Muscle and Nerve* **21**(9), 1224–1227.

Avela, J. & Komi, P.V. (1998b) Reduced stretch reflex sensitivity and muscle stiffness after long-lasting stretch–shortening muscle cycle (SSC) exercise. *European Journal of Applied Physiology* **78**(5), 403–410.

Avela, J., Kyrölainen, H., Komi, P.V. & Rama, D. (1999) Reduced reflex sensitivity persists several days after long-lasting stretch–shortening cycle (SSC) exercise. *Journal of Applied Physiology* **86**(4), 1292–1300.

Avela, J., Kyrölainen, H. & Komi, P.V. (2001) Neuromuscular changes after long-lasting mechanically and electrically elicited fatigue. *European Journal of Applied Physiology* **85**(3–4), 317–325.

Babenko, V., Graven-Nielen, T., Svensson, P., Drewes, A.M., Jensen, T.S. & Arendt-Nielsen, L. (1999) Experimental human muscle pain induced by intramuscular injections of bradykinin, serotonin, and substance P. *European Journal of Pain* **3**(2), 93–102.

Belcastro, A. (1993) Skeletal muscle calcium-activated neural protease (Calpain) with exercise. *Journal of Applied Physiology* **74**, 1381–1386.

Besson, J.M., Conseiller, C., Hamann, K.F. & Maillard, M.C. (1972) Modification of dorsal horn cell activities in the spinal cord, after intra-arterial injection of bradykinin. *Journal of Physiology (London)* **221**, 189–205.

Besson, J.M., Guilbaud, G. & Le Bars, D. (1975) Descending inhibitory influences exerted by the brain stem upon the activities of dorsal horn lamina V cells induced by intra-arterial injection of bradykinin into the limbs. *Journal of Physiology (London)* **248**, 725–739.

Bigland-Ritchie, B. & Woods, J.J. (1976) Integrated EMG and O_2 uptake during positive and negative work. *Journal of Physiology (London)* **260**, 267–277.

Bigland-Ritchie, B. & Woods, J.J. (1984) Changes in muscle contractile properties and neural control during human muscular fatigue. *Muscle and Nerve* **7**, 691–699.

Bigland-Ritchie, B., Dawson, N.J., Johansson, R.S. & Lippold, O.C.J. (1986) Reflex origin for the slowing of motoneurone firing rates in fatigue of human voluntary contractions. *Journal of Physiology (London)* **379**, 451–459.

Bobbert, M.F., Hollander, A.P. & Huijing, P.A. (1986) Factors in delayed onset muscular soreness of man. *Medicine and Science in Sports and Exercise* **18**(1), 75–81.

Brockett, C., Warren, N., Gregory, J.E., Morgan, D.L. & Proske, U. (1997) A comparison of the effects of concentric versus eccentric exercise on force and position sense at the human elbow joint. *Brain Research* **771**, 251–258.

Brooks, S.V., Zerba, E. & Faulkner, J.A. (1995) Injury to muscle fibres after single stretches of passive and maximally stimulated muscles in mice. *Journal of Physiology (London)* **488**(2), 459–469.

Byrd, S.K. (1992) Alterations in the sarcoplasmic reticulum: a possible link to exercise-induced muscle damage. *Medicine and Science in Sports and Exercise* **24**(5), 531–536.

Bøje, O. (1955) *Bevaegelsestaere, Traening og Øvelsesterapi.* Fremad, Copenhagen.

Carlson, B.M. & Faulkner, J.A. (1983) The regeneration of skeletal muscle fibres following injury: a review. *Medicine and Science in Sport and Exercise* **15**(3), 187–198.

Cervero, F., Schaible, H.G. & Schmidt, R.F. (1991) Tonic descending inhibition of spinal cord neurones driven by joint afferents in normal cats and in cats with an inflamed knee joint. *Experimental Brain Research* **83**, 3675–3678.

Chleboun, G.S., Howell, J.N., Conatser, R.R. & Giesey, J.J. (1998) Relationship between muscle swelling and stiffness after eccentric exercise. *Medicine and Science in Sports and Exercise* **30**(4), 529–535.

Clarkson, P.M. & Newham, D.J. (1995) Associations between muscle soreness, damage, and fatigue. In: *Fatigue* (eds S.C. Gandevia, R.M. Enoka, A.J. McComas, D.G. Stuart & C.K. Thomas), pp. 457–469. Plenum Press, New York.

Clarkson, P.M., Nosaka, K. & Braun, B. (1992) Muscle function after exercise-induced muscle damage and rapid adaptation. *Medicine and Science in Sports and Exercise* **24**(5), 512–520.

Cleak, M.J. & Eston, R.G. (1992) Muscle soreness, swelling, stiffness and strength loss after intensive eccentric exercise. *British Journal of Sports Medicine* **26**(4), 267–272.

Cleland, C., Rymer, W. & Edwards, F. (1982) Force-sensitive interneurons in the spinal cord of the cat. *Science* **217**, 652–655.

Darques, J.L. & Jammes, Y. (1997) Fatigue-induced changes in group IV muscle afferent activity: differences between high- and low-frequency induced fatigues. *Brain Research* **750**, 147–154.

Darques, J.L., Decherchi, P. & Jammes, Y. (1998) Mechanisms of fatigue-induced activation of group IV muscle afferents: the roles played by lactic acid and inflammatory mediators. *Neuroscience Letters* **257**, 109–112.

Davies, C.T.M. & White, M.J. (1981) Muscle weakness following eccentric works in man. *Pflügers Archiv* **392**, 168–171.

De Vries, H.A. (1966) Quantitative electromyographic investigation of the spasm theory of muscular pain. *American Journal of Physical Medicine* **45**, 119–134.

Decherchi, P., Darques, J.-L. & Jammes, Y. (1998) Modifications of afferent activities from tibialis anterior muscle in rat by tendon vibrations, increase of interstitial potassium and lactate concentration and electrically-induced fatigue. *Journal of the Peripheral Nervous System* **3**(4), 1–10.

Deschenes, M.R., Brewer, R.E., Bush, J.A., McCoy, R.W., Volek, J.S. & Kraemer, W.J. (2000) Neuromuscular disturbance outlasts other symptoms of exercise-induced muscle damage. *Journal of Neurological Science* **174**(2), 92–99.

Djupsjöbacka, M., Johansson, H., Bergenheim, M. & Wenngren, B.I. (1995) Influence on the γ-muscle spindle system from muscle afferents stimulated by increased intramuscular concentrations of bradykinin and 5-HT. *Neuroscience Research* **22**, 325–333.

Duchateau, J. & Hainaut, K. (1993) Behaviour of short and long latency reflexes in fatigued human muscles. *Journal of Physiology* **471**, 787–799.

Ebbeling, C.B. & Clarkson, P.M. (1989) Exercise-induced muscle damage and adaptation. *Journal of Sports Medicine* 7, 207–234.

Edman, K.A.P. & Tsuchiya, T. (1996) Strain of passive elements during force enhancement by stretch in frog muscle fibres. *Journal of Physiology* **490**(1), 191–205.

Edwards, R.H.T., Hill, D.K., Jones, D.A. & Merton, P.A. (1977) Fatigue of long duration in human skeletal muscle after exercise. *Journal of Physiology* **272**, 769–778.

Ellaway, P.H., Murphy, P.R. & Tripathi, A. (1982) Closely coupled excitation of γ-motoneurones by group III muscle afferents with low mechanical threshold in the cat. *Journal of Physiology (London)* **331**, 481–498.

Enoka, R.M. & Stuart, D.G. (1992) Neurobiology of muscle fatigue. *Journal of Applied Physiology* **72**, 1631–1648.

Evans, W. & Cannon, J.G. (1991) The metabolic effects of exercise-induced muscle damage. In: *Exercise and Sport Sciences Reviews*, Vol. 19 (ed. J.C. Holloszy), pp. 99–125. Williams & Wilkins, Baltimore.

Fantone, J.C. (1993) Basic concepts in inflammation. In: *Sport-Induced Inflammation: Clinical and Basic Science Concepts* (eds W.B. Leadbetter, J.A. Buckwalter & S.L. Gordon), pp. 25–54. American Orthopaedic Society of Sports Medicine, Maryland.

Faulkner, J.A., Brooks, S.V. & Opiteck, J.A. (1993) Injury to skeletal muscle fibres during contractions: conditions of occurrence and prevention. *Physiological Therapy* **73**(12), 911–921.

Fields, H.L. (1987) *Pain*, p. 35. McGraw-Hill, New York.

Franz, M. & Mense, S. (1975) Muscle receptors with group IV afferent fibres responding to application of bradykinin. *Brain Research* **92**(3), 369–383.

Fridén, J. & Lieber, R.L. (1992) Structural and mechanical basis of exercise-induced muscle injury. *Medicine and Science in Sports and Exercise* **24**(2), 521–530.

Fridén, J. & Lieber, R.L. (1996) Ultrastructural evidence for loss of calcium homeostasis in exercised skeletal muscle. *Acta Physiologica Scandinavica* **158**, 381–382.

Fridén, J. & Lieber, R.L. (2001a) Serum creatine kinase level is a poor predictor of muscle function after injury. *Scandinavian Journal of Medicine and Science in Sports* **11**(2), 126–127.

Fridén, J. & Lieber, R.L. (2001b) Eccentric exercise-induced injuries to contractile and cytoskeletal muscle fibre components. *Acta Physiologica Scandinavica* **171**, 321–326.

Fridén, J., Sjöström, M. & Ekblom, B. (1981) A morphological study of delayed muscle soreness. *Experientia* **37**, 506–507.

Fridén, J., Seger, J., Sjöström, M. & Ekblom, B. (1983a) Adaptative response in human skeletal muscle subjected to prolonged eccentric training. *International Journal of Sports Medicine* **4**, 177–183.

Fridén, J., Sjöström, M. & Ekblom, B. (1983b) Myofibrillar damage following intense eccentric exercise in man. *International Journal of Sports Medicine* **4**, 170–176.

Fridén, J., Kjorell, U. & Thornell, L.E. (1984) Delayed muscle soreness and cytoskeletal alterations: an immunocytochemical study in man. *International Journal of Sports Medicine* **5**, 15–18.

Fridén, J., Seger & Ekblom, B. (1988) Sublethal muscle fibre injuries after high-tension anaerobic exercise. *European Journal of Applied Physiology* **57**, 360–368.

Ftaiti, F., Grélot, L., Coudreuse, J.M. & Nicol, C. (2000) Combined effects of heat stress, dehydration and exercise on neuromuscular function in humans. *European Journal of Applied Physiology* **84**, 87–94.

Fukami, Y. (1988) The effects of NH_3 and CO_2 on the sensory ending of mammalian muscle spindles: intracellular pH as a possible mechanism. *Brain Research* **463**, 140–143.

Garland, S.J. (1991) Role of small diameter afferents in reflex inhibition during human muscle fatigue. *Journal of Physiology (London)* **435**, 547–558.

Garland, S.J. & Kaufman, M.P. (1995) Role of muscle afferents in the inhibition of motoneurons during fatigue. In: *Fatigue, Neural and Muscular Mechanisms* (eds S.C. Gandevia, R.M. Enoka, A.J. McComas, D.G. Stuart & C.K. Thomas), pp. 271–278. Plenum, New York.

Gollhofer, A., Komi, P.V., Miyashita & M., Aura, O. (1987a) Fatigue during stretch–shortening cycle exercises: Changes in mechanical performance of human skeletal muscle. *International Journal of Sports Medicine* **8**, 71–78.

Gollhofer, A., Komi, P.V., Fujitsuka, N. & Miyashita, M. (1987b) Fatigue during stretch–shortening cycle exercises. II. Changes in neuromuscular activation patterns of human skeletal muscle. *International Journal of Sports Medicine* **8** (Suppl. 1), 38–47.

Grabiner, M. (2000) Neuromechanics of the initial phase of eccentric-induced muscle injury. In: *Biomechanics in Sport* (ed. V. Zatsiorsky), pp. 588–606. Blackwell Science, Oxford, UK.

Graven-Nielsen, T., Svensson, P. & Arendt-Nielsen, L. (1997) Effects of experimental muscle pain on muscle activity and co-ordination during static and dynamic motor function. *Electroencephalography and Clinical Neurophysiology* **105**, 156–164.

Han, X.Y., Wang, W., Komulainen, J. *et al.* (1999) Increased mRNAs for protocollagens and key regulating enzymes in rat skeletal muscle following downhill running. *Pflügers Archiv* **437**(6), 857–864.

Herbaczynaska-Cedro, K., Staszewska-Barczak, J. & Janczewska, H. (1976) Muscular work and the release of prostaglandin-like substances. *Cardiovascular Research* **10**, 413–420.

Hikida, R.S., Staron, R.S., Hagerman, F.C., Sherman, W.M. & Costill, D.L. (1983) Muscle fiber necrosis associated with human marathon runners. *Journal of Neurological Science* **59**, 185–203.

Hill, A.V. (1951) The mechanics of voluntary muscle. *Lancet* **261**, 947.

Hong, S.K., Kniffki, K.D., Mense, S., Schmidt, R.F. & Wendisch, M. (1979) Descending influences on the responses of spinocervical tract neurones to chemical stimulation of fine muscle afferents. *Journal of Physiology (London)* **290**, 129–140.

Horita, T. (2000) *Stiffness regulation during stretch–shortening cycle exercise.* PhD thesis, Department of Biology of Physical Activity. [Research series published by the University of Jyväskylä, Finland.]

Horita, T., Komi, P.V., Nicol, C. & Kyröläinen, H. (1996) Stretch shortening cycle fatigue: interactions among joint stiffness, reflex, and muscle mechanical performance in the drop jump. *European Journal of Applied Physiology* **73**, 393–403.

Horita, T., Komi, P.V., Nicol, C. & Kyröläinen, H. (1999) Effect of exhausting stretch–shortening cycle exercise on the time course of mechanical behaviour in the drop jump: possible role of muscle damage. *European Journal of Applied Physiology* **79**, 160–167.

Hortobágyi, T., Lambert, N.L. & Kroll, W.P. (1991) Voluntary and reflex responses to fatigue with stretch–shortening cycle exercises. *Canadian Journal of Sports Sciences* **6**, 142–150.

Hough, T. (1902) Ergographic studies in muscle soreness. *American Journal of Applied Physiology* **7**, 76–92.

Howell, J.N., Chila, A.G., Ford, G., David, D. & Gates, T. (1985) A electromyographic study of elbow motion during postexercise muscle soreness. *Journal of Applied Physiology* **58**, 1713–1718.

Howell, J.N., Chleboun, G. & Conatser, R. (1993) Muscle stiffness, strength loss, swelling and soreness following exercise-induced injury in humans. *Journal of Physiology* **464**, 183–196.

Ingalls, C.P., Warren, G.L. & Armstrong, R.B. (1998) Dissociation of force production from MHC and actin contents in muscles injured by eccentric contractions. *Journal of Muscle Research and Cell Motility* **19**, 3215–3224.

Jammes, Y. & Balzamo, E. (1992) Changes in afferent and efferent phrenic activities with electrically-induced diaphragmatic fatigue. *Journal of Applied Physiology* **73**, 894–902.

Jessel, T.M. & Kelly, D.D. (1991) Pain and analgesia. In: *Principles of Neural Science* (eds E.R. Kandel, J.H. Schwartz & T.M. Jessel), pp. 385–399. Elsevier, New York.

Johansson, H., Djupsjobacka, M. & Sjolander, P. (1993) Influences on the gamma-muscle spindle system from muscle afferents stimulated by KCl and lactic acid. *Neuroscience Research* **16**, 49–57.

Jones, D.A., Newham, D.J. & Clarkson, P.M. (1987) Skeletal muscle stiffness and pain following eccentric exercise of the elbow flexors. *Pain* **30**, 233–242.

Jones, C., Allen, T., Talbot, J., Morgan, D.L. & Proske, U. (1997) Changes in the mechanical properties of human and amphibian muscle after eccentric exercise. *European Journal of Applied Physiology and Occupational Physiology* **76**(1), 21–31.

Jovanovic, K., Anastasijevic, R. & Vuco, J. (1990) Reflex effects on gamma fusimotor neurones of chemically induced discharges in small-diameter muscle afferents in decerebrate cats. *Brain Research* **521**, 89–94.

Katz, B. (1939) The relation between force and speed in muscular contraction. *Journal of Physiology (London)* **96**, 45–64.

Kaufman, M.P. & Rybicki, K.J. (1987) Discharge properties of group III and IV muscle afferents: their responses to mechanical and metabolic stimuli. *Circulatory Research* (Suppl.) **61**, 160–165.

Kniffki, K.D., Mense, S. & Schmidt, R.F. (1978) Responses of group IV afferent units from skeletal muscle to stretch, contraction and chemical stimulation. *Experimental Brain Research* **31**, 511–522.

Komi, P.V. (1973) Measurement of the force–velocity relationship in human muscle under concentric and eccentric contraction. In: *Medicine and Sport, Biomechanics III*, Vol. 8 (ed. E. Jokl), pp. 224–229. Karger, Basel.

Komi, P.V. (2000) Stretch–shortening cycle: a powerful model to study normal and fatigued muscle. *Journal of Biomechanics* **33**, 1197–1206.

Komi, P.V. & Buskirk, E.R. (1972) Effect of eccentric and concentric conditioning on tension and electrical activity in human muscle. *Ergonomics* **5**, 417–431.

Komi, P.V. & Gollhofer, A. (1987) Fatigue during stretch–shortening cycle exercise. In: *Muscular Function in Exercise and Training*, Vol. 26. *Medicine and Sport Science* (eds P. Marconnet & P.V. Komi), pp. 119–127. Karger, Basel.

Komi, P.V. & Nicol, C. (2000a) Stretch–shortening cycle fatigue. In: *Biomechanics and Biology of Movement* (eds B. McIntosh, B. Nigg & J. Mester), pp. 385–408. Human Kinetics Publishers, Champaign, IL.

Komi, P.V. & Nicol, C. (2000b) Stretch–shortening cycle of muscle function. In: *Biomechanics in Sport* (ed. V. Zatsiorsky), pp. 87–102. Blackwell Science, Oxford, UK.

Komi, P.V. & Rusko, H. (1974) Quantitative evaluation of mechanical and electrical changes during fatigue loading of eccentric and concentric work. *Scandinavian Journal of Rehabilitation Medicine* (Suppl.) **3**, 121–126.

Komi, P.V. & Viitasalo, J.T. (1977) Changes in motor unit activity and metabolism in human skeletal muscle during and after repeated eccentric and concentric contractions. *Acta Physiologica Scandinavica* **100**, 246–254.

Komi, P.V., Hyvärinen, T., Gollhofer, A. & Mero, A. (1986) Man–shoe–surface interaction. Special problems during marathon running. *Acta University of Oulu* **179**, 69–72.

Koskinen, S.O., Wang, W., Ahtikoski, A.M. *et al.* (2001) Acute exercise induced changes in rat skeletal muscle mRNAs and proteins regulating type IV collagen content. *American Journal of Regulatory and Integrative Comparative Physiology* **280**(5), R1292–R1300.

Kuipers, H. (1994) Exercise induced by muscle damage. *International Journal of Sports Medicine* **15**, 132–152.

Kuitunen, S., Komi, P.V. & Kyrölainen, H. (2002) Knee and ankle joint stiffness in sprint running. *Medicine and Science in Sports and Exercise* **34**, 1.

Kyrölainen, H., Takala, T.E.S. & Komi, P.V. (1998) Muscle damage induced by stretch–shortening cycle exercise. *Medicine and Science in Sports and Exercise* **30**(3), 415–420.

Kyrölainen, H., Pullinen, T., Candau, R., Avela, J., Huttunen, P. & Komi, P.V. (2000) Effects of marathon running on running economy and kinematics. *European Journal of Applied Physiology* **82**(4), 297–304.

Lagier-Tessonier, F., Balzamo, E. & Jammes, Y. (1993) Comparative effects of ischemia and acute hypoxemia on muscle afferents from tibialis anterior in cats. *Muscle and Nerve* **16**, 135–141.

Le Pera, D., Graven-Nielsen, T., Valeriani, M. *et al.* (2001) Inhibition of motor system excitability at cortical and spinal level by tonic muscle pain. *Clinical Neurophysiology* **112**, 1633–1641.

Lieber, R.L. & Fridén, J. (1993) Muscle damage is not a function of muscle force but active muscle strain. *Journal of Applied Physiology* **74**, 520–526.

Lieber, R.L. & Fridén, J. (1999) Mechanisms of muscle injury after eccentric contraction. *Medicine and Science in Sport* **2**(3), 253–265.

Lieber, R.L. & Fridén, J. (2000) Functional and clinical significance of skeletal muscle architecture. *Muscle and Nerve* **23**, 1647–1666.

Lieber, R.L., Thornell, L.E. & Fridén, J. (1996) Muscle cytoskeletal disruption occurs within the first 15 minutes of cyclic eccentric contraction. *Journal of Applied Physiology* **80**, 278–284.

Ljubisavljevic, M., Jovanovic, K. & Anastasijevic, R. (1992) Changes in discharge rate of cat hamstring fusimotor neurones during fatiguing contractions of triceps surae muscles. *Journal of Physiology (London)* **445**, 499–513.

Lombardi, V. & Piazzesi, G. (1990) The contractile response during steady lengthening of stimulated frog muscle fibres. *Journal of Physiology* **431**, 141–171.

Lowe, D.A., Warren, G.L., Hayes, D.A., Farmer, M.A. & Armstrong, R.B. (1994) Eccentric contraction-induced injury of mouse soleus muscle: effect of varying $[Ca^{2+}]_o$. *Journal of Applied Physiology* **76**, 1445–1453.

Lowe, D.A., Warren, G.L., Ingalls, C.P., Boorstein, D.B. & Armstrong, R.B. (1995) Muscle function and protein metabolism after initiation of eccentric contraction-induced injury. *Journal of Applied Physiology* **79**(4), 1260–1270.

Lund, J.P., Donga, R., Widmer, C.G. & Stohler, C.S. (1991) The pain-adaptation model: a discussion of the relationship between chronic musculoskeletal pain and motor activity. *Canadian Journal of Physiology and Pharmacology* **69**, 683–394.

Lynch, G.S., Fary, C.J. & Williams, D.A. (1997) Quantitative measurement of resting skeletal muscle $[Ca^{2+}]_i$ following acute and long-term downhill running exercise in mice. *Cell Calcium* **22**(5), 373–383.

McBride, T.A., Stockert, B.W., Gorin, F.A. & Carlsen, R.C. (2000) Stretch-activated ion channels contribute to membrane depolarization after eccentric contractions. *Journal of Applied Physiology* **88**, 91–101.

MacIntyre, D.L., Reid, W.D. & McKenzie, D.C. (1995) Delayed muscle soreness: the inflammatory response to muscle injury and its clinical implications. *Sports Medicine* **20**(1), 24–40.

McMahon, S. & Koltzenburg, M. (1990) The changing role of primary afferent neurones in pain. *Pain* **43**, 269–272.

Mair, J., Mayr, M., Müller, E. *et al.* (1995) Rapid adaptation to eccentric exercise-induced muscle damage. *International Journal of Sports Medicine* **16**(6), 352–356.

Malmgren, K. & Pierrot-Deseilligny, E. (1987) Inhibition of neurones transmitting non-monosynaptic Ia excitation to human wrist flexor motoneurones. *Journal of Physiology* **405**, 765–783.

Matre, D.A., Sinkjaer, T., Svensson, P. & Arendt-Nielsen, L. (1998) Experimental muscle pain increases the human stretch reflex. *Pain* **75**, 331–339.

Mense, S. (1977) Nervous outflow from skeletal muscle following chemical noxious stimulation. *Journal of Physiology* **267**, 75–88.

Mense, S. & Meyer, H. (1985) Different types of slowly conducting afferent units in cat skeletal muscle and tendon. *Journal of Physiology (London)* **363**, 403–417.

Mense, S. & Meyer, H. (1988) Bradykinin-induced modulation of the response behaviour of different types of feline group III and IV muscle receptors. *Journal of Physiology (London)* **398**, 49–63.

Millan, M.J. (1999) The induction of pain: an integrative review. *Progress in Neurobiology* **57**(1), 1–164.

Mizumura, K. (1998) Natural history of nociceptor sensitization: the search for a peripheral mechanism of hyperalgesia. *Pain Reviews* **5**(2), 59–82.

Morgan, D.L. (1990) New insights into the behavior of muscle during active lengthening. *Biophysical Journal* **57**, 209–221.

Morgan, D.L. & Allen, D.G. (1999) Early events in stretch induced muscle damage. *Journal of Applied Physiology* **87**(6), 2007–2015.

Murayama, M., Nosaka, K., Yoneda, T. & Minamitani, K. (2000) Changes in hardness of the human elbow flexor muscles after eccentric exercise. *European Journal of Applied Physiology* **82**(5–6), 361–367.

Myllylä, R., Salminen, A., Peltonen, L., Takala, T.E.S. & Vihko, V. (1986) Collagen metabolism of mouse skeletal muscle during the repair of exercise injuries. *Pflügers Archiv* **407**, 64–70.

Newham, D.J., McPhail, G., Mills, K.R. & Edwards, R.H.T. (1983a) Ultrastructural changes after concentric and eccentric contractions of human muscle. *Journal of Neurological Science* **61**(109), 122.

Newham, D.J., Mills, K.R., Quigley, B.M. & Edwards, R.H.T. (1983b) Pain and fatigue after concentric and eccentric muscle contractions. *Clinical Science* **64**, 55–62.

Nicol, C., Komi, P.V. & Marconnet, P. (1991a) Fatigue effects of marathon running on neuromuscular performance. I. Changes in muscle force and stiffness characteristics. *Scandinavian Journal of Medicine and Science in Sports* **1**(10), 17.

Nicol, C., Komi, P.V. & Marconnet, P. (1991b) Fatigue effects of marathon running on neuromuscular performance. II. Changes in force: integrated electromyographic activity and endurance capacity. *Scandinavian Journal of Medicine and Science in Sports* **1**, 18–24.

Nicol, C., Komi, P.V. & Marconnet, P. (1991c) Effects of a marathon fatigue on running kinematics and economy. *Scandinavian Journal of Medicine and Science in Sports* **1**, 195–204.

Nicol, C., Komi, P.V., Horita, T., Kyröläinen, H. & Takala, T.E.S. (1996a) Reduced stretch-reflex sensitivity after exhaustive stretch–shortening cycle exercise. *European Journal of Applied Physiology* **72**, 401–409.

Nicol, C., Komi, P.V. & Avela, J. (1996b) Stretch–shortening cycle fatigue reduces stretch reflex response. In: *Abstract Book of the 1996 International Pre-Olympic Scientific Congress*, p. 108, 10–14 July, Dallas, Texas.

Noakes, T.D. (1987) Effect of exercise on serum enzyme activities in humans. *Sports Medicine* **4**, 245–247.

Patel, T.J. & Lieber, R.L. (1997) Force transmission in skeletal muscle. From actomyosin to external tendons. In: *Exercise and Sport Sciences Reviews*, Vol. 25 (ed. J.O. Holloszy), pp. 321–363.

Pullinen, T., Leynaert, M. & Komi, P.V. (1997) Neuromuscular function after marathon. In: *Abstract book of the XIV ISB Congress*, 24–27 August, Tokyo.

Reddy, M.K., Etlinger, J.D., Rabinowitz, M., Fischman, D.A. & Zak, R. (1975) Removal of Z-lines and α-actinin from isolated myofibrils by a calcium-activated neutral protease. *Journal of Biological Chemistry* **250**, 4278–4284.

Rossi, A. & Decchi, B. (1997) Changes in Ib heteronymous inhibition to soleus motoneurones during cutaneous and muscle nociceptive stimulation in humans. *Brain Research* **774**, 55–61.

Rossi, A., Decchi, B., Groccia, della Volpe, R. & Spidalieri, R. (1988) Interactions between nociceptive and non-nociceptive afferent projections to cerebral cortex in humans. *Neuroscience Letters* **248**, 155–158.

Rossi, A., Decchi, B. & Ginanneschi, F. (1998) Presynaptic excitability changes of group Ia fibres to muscle nociceptive stimulation in humans. *Brain Research* **818**(1), 12–22.

Rotto, D.M. & Kaufman, M.P. (1988) Effect of metabolic products of muscular contraction on discharge of group III and IV afferents. *Journal of Applied Physiology* **64**(6), 2306–2313.

Rybicki, K.J., Waldrop, T.G. & Kaufman, M.P. (1985) Increasing gracilis muscle interstitial potassium concentrations stimulate group III and IV afferents. *Journal of Applied Physiology* **58**(3), 936–941.

Saxton, J.M. & Donnelly, A.E. (1995) Light concentric exercise during recovery from exercise-induced muscle damage. *International Journal of Sports Medicine* **16**(6), 347–351.

Saxton, J.M., Clarkson, P.M., James, R. *et al.* (1995) Neuromuscular dysfunction following eccentric exercise. *Medicine and Science in Sports and Exercise* **27**, 1185–1193.

Sherman, W.M., Armstrong, L.E., Murray, T.M. *et al.* (1984) Effect of a 42.2-km footrace and subsequent rest or exercise on muscular strength and work capacity. *Journal of Applied Physiology* **57**, 1668–1673.

Simone, D.A., Marchettini, P., Caputi, G. & Ochoa, J.L. (1994) Identification of muscle afferents subserving sensation of deep pain in humans. *Journal of Neurophysiology* **72**(2), 883–889.

Smith, L.L. (1991) Acute inflammation: the underlying mechanisms in delayed onset muscle soreness? *Medicine and Science in Sports and Exercise* **23**, 542–551.

Smith, L.L., McCammon, M., Smith, S., Chamness, M., Israel, R.G. & O'Brien, K.F. (1989) White blood cell response to uphill walking and downhill jogging at similar metabolic loads. *European Journal of Applied Physiology* **58**, 833–837.

Sohn, M.K., Graven-Nielsen, T., Arendt-Nielsen, L. & Svensson, P. (2000) Inhibition of motor unit firing during experimental muscle pain in humans. *Muscle and Nerve* **23**, 1219–1226.

Stacey, M.J. (1969) Free nerve endings in skeletal muscle of the cat. *Journal of Anatomy* **105**, 231–254.

Stauber, W.T. (1989) Eccentric action of muscles: physiology, injury, and adaptation. *Exercise and Sport Sciences Reviews* **17**, 157–185.

Strojnik, V. & Komi, P.V. (2000) Fatigue after submaximal intensive stretch–shortening cycle exercise. *Medicine and Science in Sports and Exercise* **32**(7), 1314–1319.

Strojnik, V., Komi, P.V. & Nicol, C. (2000) Fatigue during one-week tourist alpine skiing. *Abstract of the 2nd International Congress on Skiing and Science*, pp. 84–85. St Christoph, Arlberg.

Strojnik, V., Nicol, C. & Komi, P.V. (2001a) Fatigue during one-week tourist alpine skiing. In: *Science and Skiing II* (eds E. Müller *et al.*), pp. 599–607. Kovač, Hamburg.

Strojnik, V., Komi, P.V. & Nicol, C. (2001b) Effects of one week of leisure alpine skiing on jumping power. *Abstract Book of the 6th Annual ECSS Congress*, p. 562. Cologne.

Sugi, H. & Tsuchiya, T. (1988) Stiffness changes during enhancement and deficit of isometric force by slow length changes in frog skeletal muscle fibres. *Journal of Physiology* **407**, 215–229.

Svensson, P., De Laat, A., Graven-Nielsen, T. & Arendt-Nielsen, L. (1998) Experimental jaw-muscle pain does not change heteronymous H-reflexes in the human temporal muscle. *Experimental Brain Research* **121**, 311–318.

Synoway, L.I., Hill, J.M., Pickar, J.G. & Kaufman, M.P. (1993) Effects of contraction and lactic acid on the discharge of group III muscle afferents in cat. *Journal of Neurophysiology* **69**, 1053–1059.

Talag, T.S. (1973) Residual muscular soreness as influenced by concentric, eccentric, and static contractions. *Research Quarterly* **44**, 458–468.

Travell, J., Rinzler, S. & Herman, M. (1942) Pain and disability of the shoulder and arm. Treatment by intramuscular infiltration with procaine hydrochloride. *Journal of the American Medical Association* **120**, 417–422.

Viitasalo, J.T., Komi, P.V., Jacobs, I. & Karlsson, J. (1982) Effects of a prolonged cross-counting skiing on neuromuscular performance. In: *Exercise and Sport Biology*, Vol. 12 (ed. P.V. Komi), pp. 191–198. Human Kinetics, Champaign, IL.

Vijayan, K., Thompson, J.L., Norenberg, K.M., Fitts, R.H. & Riley, D.A. (2001) Fiber-type susceptibility to eccentric contraction-induced damage of hindlimb-unloaded rat AL muscles. *Journal of Applied Physiology* **3**, 770–776.

Warhol, M.J., Siegel, A.J., Evans, W.J. & Silverman, L.M. (1985) Skeletal muscle injury and repair in marathon runners after competition. *American Journal of Pathology* **118**(2), 331–339.

Warren, G.L., Hayes, D.A., Lowe, D.A. & Armstrong, R.B. (1993a) Mechanical factors in the initiation of eccentric contraction-induced injury in rat soleus muscle. *Journal of Physiology* **464**, 457–475.

Warren, G.L., Lowe, D.A., Hayes, D.A., Karwoski, C.J., Prior, B.M. & Armstrong, R.B. (1993b) Excitation failure in eccentric contraction-induced injury of mouse soleus muscle. *Journal of Physiology* **468**, 487–499.

Warren, G.L., Ingalls, C.P., Shah, S.J. & Armstrong, R.B. (1999) Uncoupling of vivo torque production from EMG in mouse muscles injured by eccentric contractions. *Journal of Physiology* **515**(2), 609–619.

Warren, G.L., Ingalls, C.P., Lowe, D.A. & Armstrong, R.B. (2001) Excitation–contraction uncoupling: major role in contraction-induced muscle injury. *Exercise and Sport Sciences Reviews* **29**(2), 82–87.

Waterman-Storer, C.M. (1991) The cytoskeleton of skeletal muscle: is it affected by exercise? A brief review. *Medicine and Science in Sports and Exercise* **23**(11), 1240–1249.

Westerblad, H., Duty, S. & Allen, D.G. (1993) Intracellular calcium concentration during low-frequency fatigue in isolated single fibers of mouse skeletal muscle. *Journal of Applied Physiology* **75**, 382–388.

PART 3

MECHANISMS FOR ADAPTATION IN STRENGTH AND POWER TRAINING

Chapter 12

Cellular and Molecular Aspects of Adaptation in Skeletal Muscle

GEOFFREY GOLDSPINK AND STEPHEN HARRIDGE

Skeletal muscle is a tissue that possesses an intrinsic ability to adapt to the type of physical activity it is required to perform. Adaptation takes place during normal growth and as a response to exercise training. This chapter is concerned with the cellular and molecular mechanisms involved in adaptation for increased power output. With the emergence of methods that allow us to study changes in gene expression, we can now begin to understand adaptation in terms of levels of transcription and translation of individual genes and subsets of genes. This will enable us to obtain an understanding that will range from the whole tissue to the gene level and to design athletic training and/or rehabilitation exercise regimes accordingly. Now that the human genome has been sequenced, it may soon be possible to predict which people have the genetic potential to become world-class athletes.

Cellular and molecular basis of muscle power

Means by which muscle shortens and produces force

The process by which muscle converts chemical energy into mechanical work has attracted the attention of many physicists, biochemists and physiologists. This is a brief overview as more detailed accounts can be found in cell biology and physiology textbooks.

Muscle is made up of cellular units called muscle fibres, which are 20–100 μm in diameter. The muscle fibres contain rod like contractile structures, myofibrils, which are about 1 μm in diameter. These are made up of protein filaments arranged in units called sarcomeres (Fig. 12.1). The sarcomere is composed of a number of proteins involved directly in the contraction process or in a structural role. The two most important proteins involved in the contraction process are the 'thin' actin and 'thick' myosin filament. The contraction process involves the sliding of these two interdigitating filaments past one another, a process that is driven by molecular motors. These are part of the cross-bridges that protrude from the myosin filament. Each cross-bridge is an independent force generator, which interacts with a thin filament and pulls it towards the centre of the sarcomere. Recent X-ray crystallographic studies have shown the structure of this molecule, identifying the region of the molecule that binds to the thick filament and that which binds and hydrolyses ATP during the contraction process (Rayment *et al.* 1993a,b). It is now clear that the cross-bridge may bind to the actin filament in more than one state, either weakly or strongly, depending upon whether or not inorganic phosphate is bound. Once detached from the thin filament the cross-bridge has to be reprimed by adenosine triphosphate (ATP) before it can go through another cycle of force generation.

During contraction the thin filaments slide over the thick filaments, which results in the shortening of each sarcomere. This happens all along the length of the myofibrils; hence the

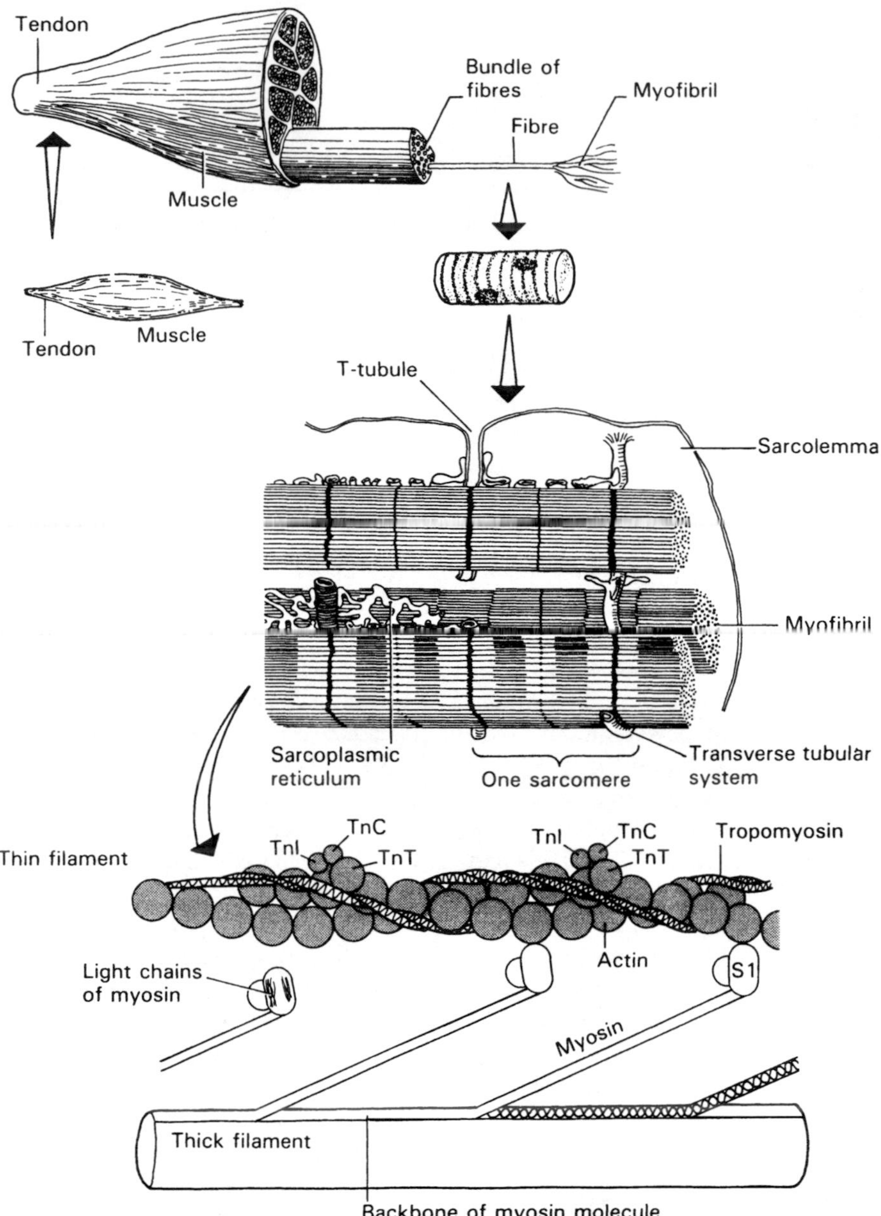

Fig. 12.1 The structure of muscle from the whole tissue to the molecular level. The cellular units or muscle fibres contain contractile elements called myofibrils, which in skeletal and cardiac muscle are striated. The striations are due to the presence of thick (myosin) and thin (actin) filaments. These protein filaments are arranged in units called sarcomeres, which shorten during contraction by the sliding of the thin filaments over the thick filaments. This sliding movement is brought about by the myosin cross-bridges, which act as independent force generators. Movement of the thin filaments commences when calcium binds to the troponin complex (TnI, TnT, TnC), which is believed to pull the tropomyosin to one side to reveal active sites on the actin filament. The other requirement is that the myosin cross-bridges are charged with ATP. The cross-bridge is the part of the myosin heavy chain molecule that projects from the thick filament. The end of the cross-bridge terminates in two globular heads (S1 fragment) that contain ATPase and the actin binding sites. The rate at which the cross-bridge works is mainly determined by the ATPase activity of the type of myosin heavy chain that constitutes the cross-bridge. Also associated with the S1 are two myosin light chains that are believed to modify the cross-bridge cycle time to some extent.

muscle as a whole shortens. The biochemistry of muscular contraction is complex and if we look at the proteins that make up the thick and thin filaments (Fig. 12.1) we find that the system possesses not only a means of generating force but also a mechanism for 'switching on' and 'switching off' the contractile apparatus. The thin actin filaments of the sarcomere are rather like a double pearl necklace that is twisted into a spiral or helix. Decorating these thin filaments are regulatory complexes made up of proteins, tropomyosin and troponins I, T and C. When calcium ions (Ca^{2+}) bind with the troponin complex a conformational change occurs, which results in the tropomyosin being pulled to one side. When the tropomyosin position is changed, active sites are exposed that allow the myosin cross-bridges to interact with thin filaments. The cross-bridges go through repeated cycles of activity until Ca^{2+} is withdrawn.

Ca^{2+} is stored in a network of intracellular sacs surrounding the myofibrils (sarcoplasmic reticulum, SR). The arrival of an action potential results in the depolarization of the sarcolemma and the ultimate release of Ca^{2+} from the SR into the sarcoplasm. This is now believed to result from a charge movement at the junction of the SR with the transverse tubule system. This voltage is sensed by dihydropyrodine receptors, which activate the ryanodine binding channels in the SR, which open and allow Ca^{2+} to diffuse out rapidly. Muscle relaxation occurs through the sequestration of Ca^{2+} back into the SR through the longitudinal vesicles, by an active transport process catalysed by Ca^{2+}-ATPase where 2 ATP molecules are hydrolysed for each Ca^{2+} sequestered.

Ultrastructural and molecular determinants of muscle strength

Strength can be defined as the maximum force that a muscle can develop during a single contraction. Physiologically, this is usually defined where the muscle is tested under isometric or static conditions or where no sarcomere shortening occurs, although it must be borne in mind that at the onset of isometric contractions sarcomeres shorten against the 'slack' of the elastic structures within the muscle and those in the tendon. Hence the contraction is not truly isometric. At the ultrastructural level, the force that can be generated is ultimately related to the number of myosin cross-bridges working in parallel that can interact with the actin filaments. As mentioned earlier, each myosin cross-bridge is an independent force generator; the number of attaching cross-bridges will depend upon the concentration of Ca^{2+} in the sarcoplasm. When primed with ATP and activated by Ca^{2+} these cross-bridges go through a cycle of attachment to the actin filament, force generation and then a detachment phase. Recent advances using laser trap systems (optical tweezers) have allowed the direct measurement of the force and displacement that results from the interaction of a single myosin molecule with a single actin filament. Single force transients of 3–4 pN have been measured under isometric conditions which are consistent with the predictions of the swinging cross-bridge model of contraction (Finer *et al.* 1994).

As muscle force is ultimately a reflection of the number of cross-bridges working in parallel it is convenient to relate the maximum force developed to the muscle fibre cross-sectional area. Fibre cross-sectional area is thus a reasonably accurate way of predicting the force that a muscle fibre can develop. However, from the perspective of a whole muscle this is more complicated. Factors such as the degree to which a muscle is activated and the difficulties in determining accurately physiological cross-sectional area make it impossible to determine specific force generation accurately. The problem is compounded by the lack of any method for determining the percentage of extracellular space within a muscle. Indeed, it is possible that one of the earlier responses to strength training may be the consolidation of the tissue as the muscle fibres increase in girth at the expense of extracellular spaces. That is to say, the initial response may be for the muscle fibre cross-sectional area to increase without a commensurate increase in muscle cross-sectional area, resulting in a more compact and stronger muscle. Furthermore, the fibre arrangements in different muscles differ according to whether the muscle is designed for high force generation or for high shortening speed. In order to increase the effective or 'physiological' cross-sectional area of muscles such as those in the lower leg, the muscle fibres are arranged in a chevron fashion. These are referred to as pennate or multipennate muscles and serve to maximize the physiological cross-sectional area within a given anatomical area of muscle. A necessary consequence of this type of arrangement is that the muscle fibres will be relatively shorter and this means that the muscle will have a lower overall slow rate of shortening.

Ultrastructural and molecular determinants of velocity of shortening

The overall rate of shortening of a muscle is, in contrast to isometric force, determined in part by the number of sarcomeres in series and not those in parallel. When activated, the sarcomeres contract and have an additive effect, so that the more of them there are in series, the more rapid the overall rate of shortening of the fibre. Thus because the overall rate of shortening is partly determined by length, it is necessary to express the maximum velocity of shortening (V_{max}) as the rate of shortening per sarcomeres or per muscle length. In addition to length, V_{max} also depends on the intrinsic velocity of shortening of each sarcomere, which in turn is dependent on the predominant type of myosin cross-bridge expressed.

The individual myosin molecule consists of two heavy chains (molecular weight ~ 220 kDa), which are wound around each other except for their globular heads or S1 regions. Part of the double-stranded region forms the backbone, the light meromyosin (LMM) that is embedded in the myosin filament. The heavy meromyosin (HMM) forms the cross-bridge and terminates in the S1 head region. The S1 part of the myosin heavy chain contains the actin attachment site and the ATPase site, which are the important elements of the contractile mechanism determining the cross-bridge cycle and hence V_{max}. The HMM part of the myosin heavy chain (MyHC) that projects from the filament is hinged so it can swing out and allow the SI head to attach to the active site on the thin filament. The SI heads apparently walk or flick the thin filament along, resulting in sarcomere shortening. The rate of shortening of each sarcomere depends on the number of cross-bridges that can reach the actin filaments; therefore the initial overlap of the filaments (sarcomere length) is important.

Cross-bridges are not homogenous proteins but exist as multiple isoforms (Schiaffino & Reggiani 1996). In contrast to rodents, where there are four, it is apparent that in adult human skeletal muscle there are only three isoforms of myosin heavy chain (MyHC) that may be expressed: MyHC-I, MyHC-IIA and MyHC-IIX (Smerdu *et al.* 1994; Ennion *et al.* 1995). The gene transcript of the latter is homologous to the MyHC-IIX found in rat muscle and not the much faster MyHC-IIB, which is not expressed in human locomotory muscles. This makes sense from a scaling perspective as the appropriate shortening velocities of humans and other larger mammals may by achieved through longer limbs, longer fibres and therefore more sarcomeres in series. Some confusion has arisen as a result of this nomenclature, as the term 'Type IIb' is used by some people for fibres when they are identifying fibres using ATPase histochemistry. These fibres express the MyHC-IIX isoform alone or in combination with MyHC-IIA isoforms (Sant'ana Pereira *et al.* 1994). This multiplicity of isoform expression illustrates the dangers of directly extrapolating data obtained from laboratory rodents to the human.

The reason for this diversity of different myosins (molecular motors) can perhaps best be understood by looking at the mechanical properties of individual muscle fibres. This involves a technique in which membrane systems are removed by a process of chemical skinning, whilst leaving the contractile apparatus intact. These permeablized fibres are then immersed in a solution of high Ca^{2+} concentration ATP to induce contraction. The single-fibre studies performed on human muscle (Fig. 12.2) have

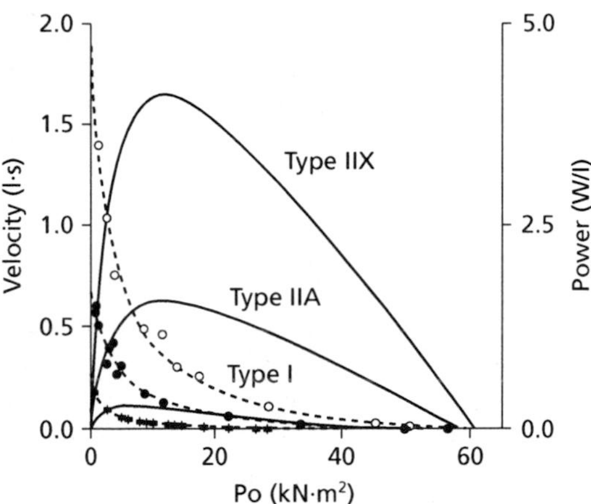

Fig. 12.2 Force–velocity and power–velocity relationships of single human muscle fibre studies at 12° C. Fibres had been chemically skinned and activated in solution with a high concentration of calcium (pCa 4.5) and subjected to isotonic shortening contractions. Three fibres are shown which are identified through gel electrophoresis as expressing MyHC-I, MyHC-IIA and MyHC-IIX. (From Bottinelli *et al.* 1996.)

confirmed earlier animal experiments which show that fibres expressing MyHC-I isoforms are slower to shorten when compared with MyHC-IIA fibres which may be 3 times faster, whilst fibres expressing the MyHC-IIX isoform are faster and more powerful still (Larsson & Moss 1993; Bottinelli *et al.* 1996; Harridge *et al.* 1996; Widrick *et al.* 1999).

In addition to the multiplicity of MyHC isoforms there is also a multiplicity of isoform expression in the ~ 20 kDa myosin light chain proteins. There are two myosin light chains associated with each S1 head and certainly in rodent muscle different isoforms of these proteins modify or 'fine-tune' the rate of shortening in fibres which express the same MyHC isoform (Reisner *et al.* 1985; Bottinelli *et al.* 1994). The fine-tuning effect of the light chains has yet to be established clearly in human single-fibre studies (Larsson & Moss 1993).

The determination of the three-dimensional structure of a myosin S1 using X-ray crystallographic methods (Rayment *et al.* 1993a,b) was a major step forward in elucidating how molecular motors work. By the use of molecular cloning, sequencing methods and computer graphics to compare the fast and slow myosins, it has been shown that they differ only by a few amino acids. The regions where there is some lack of homology are in the flexible surface loops 1 and 2. Loop 1 is over the enzymatic site and by comparing the myosin S1s from different muscles and different animal species it has been suggested that this may act as an electrostatic latch which determines the rate that ATP enters or the rate ADP leaves the active site (Gauvry *et al.* 2000). The other surface loops are associated with the attachment to actin. Thus it seems that the basic molecular motor is the same but it may be fine-tuned by just a few amino acid substitutions in these surface loops. Certain medical conditions such as familial hypertrophic cardiomyopathy (FHMC), sometimes described as sudden death syndrome, is often associated with mutations in the β cardiac (type 1) myosin gene. This has received considerable publicity as it affects some seemingly fit athletes who suddenly collapse and die when they exercise to the limit. The cardiac muscle cells appear to produce more myosin to compensate for the slightly abnormal gene and the myocardium reaches a state of hypertrophy, which becomes life-threatening during extreme exertion. Now that we know that just one or two amino acid substitutions make a difference to the tuning of the molecular motor, other variations in structural genes that result in undesirable or even desirable effects on function will no doubt be elucidated in the near future. This may also explain why some aspects of athletic ability are inherited.

In addition to myosin, other proteins, such as the regulatory proteins troponin and tropomyosin, exist as different fast and slow isoforms and are also involved in the fine-tuning of the contractile system (Schiaffino & Reggiani 1996). However, it is the MyHC isoform which is the prime determinant of contractile character.

Muscle power and fibre phenotype

A common misuse of the term power is to use it when one really means force. Power is the rate of doing work: power = work done (force × distance) per unit time or force × velocity. As mentioned above, muscle strength can be defined as the maximum force produced in a single maximal isometric contraction, but here no power is generated. Muscle power is produced during movement. However, the power requirements of muscles may differ markedly depending upon the nature of the physical activity. The power requirements of weightlifting and sprinting, for example, are clearly different from those of marathon running. The former requires short-duration busts of very high power whilst the latter requires the maintenance of a lower level of power output, but over a prolonged period of time. As has already been mentioned there are different types of muscle fibres, which have evolved for specific roles. For example, fibres which express the MyHC-IIX isoform are adapted for a high power output over a short period, having high rates of cross-bridge cycling and a limited (glycolytic) energy system. The MyHC-IIA fibres may be considered as designed for also generating higher muscle power outputs as they also have a high cross-bridge cycling rate (although lower than the MyHC-IIX isoforms), but over a longer period of time as these possess not only glycolytic, but also oxidative, metabolic potential. Both of these fibre types possess a type of myosin and other contractile proteins such as the fast isoform of SR that produce rapid activation and a high cross-bridge turnover rate. However, as the type MyHC-IIA fibres have more mitochondria and a more oxidative metabolism they are capable of sustaining a high power output over a longer period than the MyHC-IIX fibres.

The MyHC-I type of myosin is homologous to the β cardiac isoform expressed in heart muscle and has a slow cross-bridge cycle rate making these fibres more efficient and more economical for producing slow repetitive movements (He *et al.* 2000) and for sustaining isometric force (Stienen *et al.* 1996), but not for generating a high power output. The MyHC-I fibres are particularly numerous in postural muscle such as the soleus which is a muscle that is activated virtually all the time during standing, walking and running, whilst are expressed least in fibres from muscles that do not have major postural or locomotory functions, such as the triceps brachii (Harridge *et al.* 1996).

Adaptation for increased power

As muscle power is determined by an interaction of the force and velocity of contraction, anything that modifies either of these parameters will also modify power. For clarity, the following has been divided into the mechanisms that may result in force adaptation and those which may affect power by changing velocity of shortening.

Force generation and muscle fibre hypertrophy

As the force of a muscle is more closely related to its cross-sectional area, enlarging a fibre to make it stronger is a major adaptation to increase muscle power output. The number of muscle fibres apparently does not increase during post-natal growth or as a result of exercise training at reasonable intensity levels. However, the mean cross-sectional area of the existing fibres does increase considerably during growth and in adult muscle in response to increased mechanical loading. Studies on laboratory animals indicate that the total number of fibres is genetically determined. It is about the same in males and females but the ultimate muscle fibre size attained in the male is greater than in the female. This is due to the influence of testosterone and other hormones.

The increase in fibre cross-sectional area is associated with a large increase in the myofibrillar content of the fibres. This involves a process by which a myofibril undergoes longitudinal splitting into two or more daughter myofibrils. In this way the myofibrillar mass becomes subdivided as it increases in volume and this allows the sarcoplasmic reticulum and transverse tubular systems to invade the mass and to come into close juxtaposition with the actin and myosin filaments. The longitudinal splitting of existing myofibrils is thought to occur because there is a built-in mismatch between the actin and myosin lattice so that the actin filaments are slightly displaced as they run from the Z-disc (square lattice) to the A-band (hexagonal lattice). This displacement or oblique pull of the actin filaments causes a mechanical stress to occur in the centre of each Z-disc that results in splitting of the myofibril (Goldspink 1971) (Fig. 12.3). Splitting tends to be more complete in fast-contracting fibres and therefore the myofibrils in these fibres are small and punctate. In slow-contracting fibres splitting is often incomplete and therefore the myofibrils appear branched in longitudinal section. An increase in the total number of myofibrils within existing fibres occurs during growth and during hypertrophy in response to overload. The maximum force production of a muscle is related to the myofibril cross-sectional area so that the physiological significance of this type of adaptation is apparent.

Hypertrophy, protein synthesis and the importance of stretch

There are two main ways in which proteins are accumulated during growth or exercise training. One way is to increase the rate at which proteins are synthesized. The other is to decrease the rate at which they are broken down. Even in adult muscle, proteins are constantly being synthesized and broken down and the turnover, or half-life, of the contractile proteins is probably of the order of 7–15 days. The soluble sarcoplasmic proteins have an even shorter half-life. A process in which more than half of the contractile proteins are broken down and replaced every 7 days or so would seem to be rather wasteful. However, the process enables the muscle to replace damaged proteins and confers a certain adaptability for changing the type of protein at certain stages of development and under certain physiological conditions. Also, reutilization of amino acids takes place so the process is expensive in terms of energy but not in the supply of amino acids.

All types of muscle fibres are capable of undergoing hypertrophy but they do not usually undergo hypertrophy to the same extent. Also, it appears that they use different strategies for the secretion of protein. With fast fibres of animals the synthesis rate is increased, and with slow fibres the degradation rate is decreased. The very limited data available in humans suggest that there is no difference in the rate of protein turnover between fibre types (Rennie & Tipton 2000). The fast-contracting fibres are recruited only infrequently (for rapid power movements or high-intensity isometric contractions) but when they are recruited and 'overloaded' they tend to undergo hypertrophy very readily. Selective hypertrophy of the fast fibres can be regarded as an adaptation for increased power production under situations when all or most of the fibres are being recruited. Slow fibres may also increase in size as a response to frequent recruitment, but to a lesser extent than the fast fibres. In repetitive low-intensity exercise and postural activity the fast fibres in some muscles may hardly ever be recruited. Under these conditions they may atrophy at the same time as the slow fibres are undergoing some hypertrophy, for example during long-distance running or cycling. Thus, there is a selective response depending on the type of training.

The question is often asked as to whether hyperplasia (increase in cell number) occurs as well as hypertrophy (increase in cell size) in response to strenuous exercise training. In general, animal experiments using normal types of exercise have not shown any change in the total number of fibres (Goldspink & Ward 1979; McCall *et al.* 1996). However, partially splitting muscle fibres, not to be confused with splitting myofibrils, are observed in surgically overloaded muscle (Vaughan & Goldspink 1979). It is therefore possible that muscle fibre splitting may lead to hyperplasia, e.g. under conditions of repeated, incremental exercise. For this to be regarded as an adaptive phenomenon rather than a pathological change, the splitting would have to be complete and resulting fibres innervated.

The degree of atrophy in disused muscle is affected by the degree of stretch the muscle is subjected to. Stretching the soleus muscle of rabbits for 3 or 5 days produces marked changes

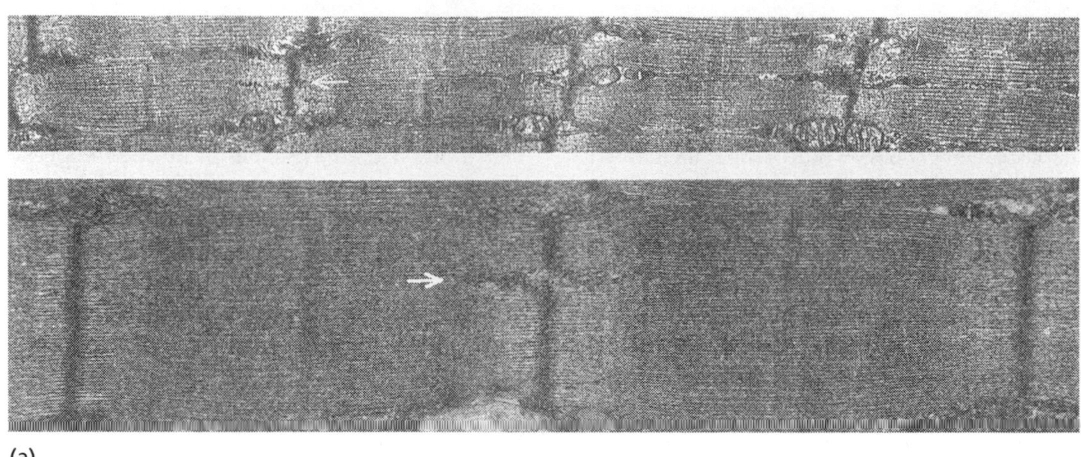

(a)

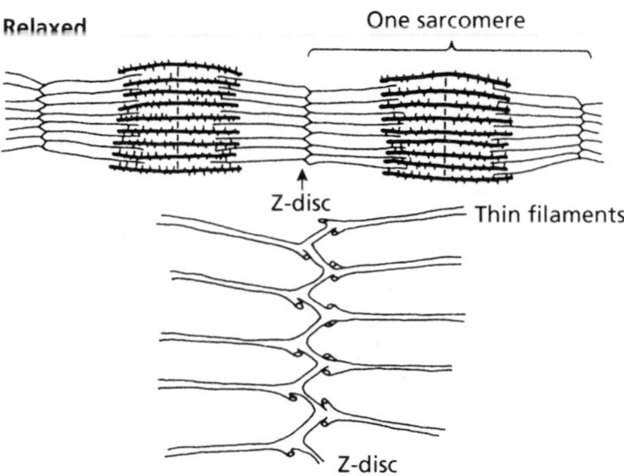

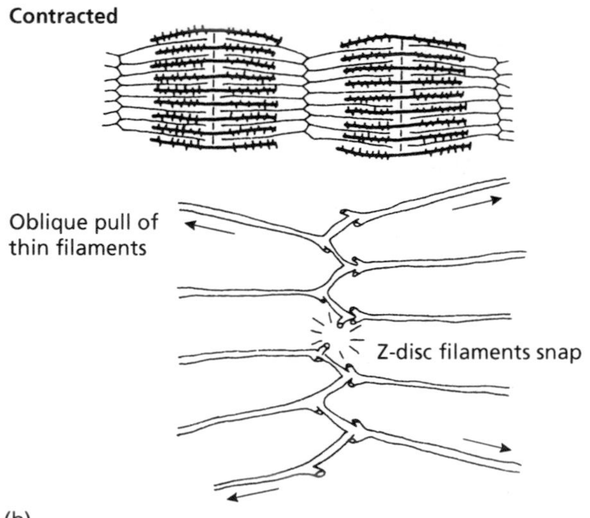

(b)

Fig. 12.3 (a) Longitudinal sections showing myofibrils in the process of splitting as seen under the electron microscope. The top section shows a myofibril that has just commenced to split with intact Z-discs on each side of the ripped disc. Already elements of the SR and T systems can be seen in the fork of the split. (b) The mechanism of longitudinal splitting appears to depend on the oblique pull of peripheral actin filaments. This arises because of a mismatch in the actin and myosin filament lattices. The obliqueness increases as the myofibrils grow and increase in girth. When force is developed, this oblique pull of the actin filaments results in a mechanical stress being set up in the centre of the Z-disc, which causes it to rip. This is repeated all along the myofibril resulting in two daughter myofibrils.

in protein turnover. Increases in protein synthesis have been found in stretched and immobilized muscle when measured *in vivo* (Booth & Seider 1979; Goldspink *et al.* 1983; Goldspink & Goldspink 1986) or *in vitro* (Goldspink 1977). Such changes have been detected as early as 6 h after the imposition of stretch in both normally innervated and denervated muscles, the latter pointing to a passive myogenic response rather than any active component triggered by sensory receptors within the stretched muscle. Thus the effect of stretch is to significantly increase the rate of muscle protein synthesis as well as to increase the number of sarcomeres in series. The therapeutic applications of stretch should therefore be borne in mind when designing regimes for rehabilitation or improved athletic performance.

Molecular regulation of muscle fibre hypertrophy

Muscle is a tissue in which gene expression is regulated to a large extent by mechanical signals. Changes in gene expression can be detected by analysing RNA in hybridization studies employing cDNA probes specific for fast and slow myosin heavy chain genes (Goldspink & Scutt 1989; Goldspink *et al.* 1991). The skeletal MyHC genes belong to a family of genes that are arranged in tandem on chromosome 17 in humans. The cardiac muscle myosin genes, for which there are two isoforms (α and β) are on chromosome 14 in humans. There are at least five isoform genes for the skeletal MyHCs and these are expressed in the sequence: embryonic, neonatal, adult fast, adult fast oxidative, and adult slow.

As a result of overload in the stretched position, the fast-contracting tibialis anterior muscle in an adult rabbit is induced to synthesize a lot of protein and to grow by as much as 30% within a period as short as 4 days. This very rapid hypertrophy was found to be associated with a 250% increase in the RNA content of the muscle and a change in the species of mRNA produced (Goldspink *et al.* 1983). Both stretch alone and electrical stimulation alone caused some activation of the slow-type and repression of the fast-type genes. However, a more complete switch in MyHC gene expression was achieved when these mechanical stimuli were combined and when higher frequencies of stimulation were used. This leads to the conclusion that muscle fibre adult phenotype is determined by stretch and force generation (passive plus active tension) and that this is controlled at the level of gene transcription. The regulation of growth, however, is probably limited by the rate of translation of the message into protein. In this context it is interesting to note that the ribosomal density is increased very significantly during hypertrophy. It also decreases significantly during postnatal growth in line with the slowing of muscle development. It therefore appears that the translational process, which is known to be much slower than the transcriptional process, is the rate-determining step in hypertrophy. Certainly, the 250% increase in ribosomal RNA during the rapid hypertrophy of an adult muscle means that extra ribosomes are available to translate the message, whatever it may be. Therefore, the rapid synthesis of more ribosomes seems to be the first step in producing muscle fibre hypertrophy.

Local and systemic growth factors involved in hypertrophy

It has long been appreciated that there is local as well as systemic regulation of muscle growth. The growth hormone/insulin growth-like factor I (GH/IGF-I) axis is the main regulator of tissue growth during early life although there is also local control of tissue growth, repair and remodelling. The cDNA of two growth factors which are expressed by muscle when it is subjected to activity that are derived from the IGF-I gene by alternative splicing have been cloned (Yang *et al.* 1996). One (L.IGF-I) is very similar to the liver endocrine type of IGF-IEa. The other is a new growth factor and is detected in exercised/overloaded muscle. For this reason, and to distinguish it from the liver IGF-I which has a systemic mode of action, it has been called mechanogrowth factor (MGF). The structure of the cDNA of this isoform indicates that it has different exons to the liver type and unlike the latter, MGF is not glycosylated. Therefore it is expected to be smaller and have a shorter half-life than the systemic IGF-Is. Both muscle isoforms were found to be up-regulated by stretch and overload (McKoy *et al.* 1999), and the evidence indicates that during exercise the muscle L.IGF-I contributes significantly to circulating levels of IGF-I. This would explain the findings of Brahm *et al.* 1997) who reported that during intensive cycling exercise most of the circulating IGF-I was being produced by the muscles rather than the liver. MGF, on the other hand, appears to be designed for local action and probably does not enter the bloodstream in any quantity. It has a 49-base insert in the E domain in the human and a 52-base insert in the rat which alters the reading frame of the 3′ end. This end codes for the carboxy terminal end of the peptide which recognizes the binding protein, and hence MGF binds to a binding protein which is specific to muscle and neuronal tissue. This would be expected to localize its action as it would be unstable in the unbound form, which is important as its production would not unduly perturb glucose homeostasis. Specific antibodies have been generated to these muscle IGF-I isoforms, and using a proteomics approach involving two-dimensional Western blotting and mass spectrometry the specific binding protein for MGF appears to be creatine kinase (the MM type in skeletal muscle and the BB type in the central nervous system). Creatine kinase (CK) is bound to the myofibrils but detaches when the pH falls below 7 and when the myofibrils are stretched (Kraft *et al.* 2000). MGF binds strongly to CK, which when the muscle is damaged, exits from the fibres through the damaged and leaky membrane. This indicates that MGF can be regarded as a repair factor and that it is over-expressed when a muscle is overloaded, which then results in hypertrophy. Recent work has shown that muscles in old rats do not respond to mechanical overload by expressing as much MGF as those in young animals and that MGF and IGF-IEa are regulated differently even though they are derived from the same gene (Owino *et al.* 2001). These two growth factors have different kinetics of expression as following damage by stretch combined with electrical stimulation of the rat tibialis anterior muscle, it was found that MGF expression peaked at 1 day and IGF-IEa peaked at 5 days following the induced local damage (Hill and Goldspink, unpublished findings). Experiments in which muscle cells in culture were subjected to different types of stretch revealed that MGF is expressed in response to a single ramp stretch and IGF-I to cyclical stretches of lower amplitude (Chema *et al.*, unpublished findings). The dependence on different types of mechanical signals may help explain why some training regimes such as forceful eccentric contractions result in an increase in muscle mass whilst others do not.

Gene transfer of IGF-I has been used but in these cases this has involved the systemic Ea type of IGF-I (Mathews *et al.* 1988; Barton-Davies *et al.* 1998). A transgenic mouse which over-expresses this form (Ea) of IGF-I (which they termed m.IGF-I) has also been developed which shows considerable general muscle hypertrophy (Mathews *et al.* 1988; Musaro *et al.* 2001). Recently, Yang and Goldspink (2001) introduced the MGF cDNA in a plasmid vector by direct intramuscular injection into mouse muscle. In the latter case it was found that a single injection of MGF cDNA resulted in a 25% increase in muscle mass with a commensurate increase in muscle fibre size within 2 weeks. Therefore there seems to be little doubt that MGF is very potent. The cloning and sequencing of the cDNAs of the autocrine as well as the systemic muscle IGF-I splice variants (Yang *et al.* 1996) made it possible to develop probes to measure changes in their expression using RNase protection assays (McKoy *et al.* 1999) and more recently real-time quantitative PCR. This latter approach can be used to determine the mRNA levels of the different IGF-I isoforms in small muscle biopsy samples. Clearly there is much more work which needs to be carried out on the local and systemic growth factors in order to define the mechano-transduction mechanism and the upstream signalling involved in the production of these and other growth factors.

The mechanotransduction mechanism is not known but a clue emerged with the finding that dystrophic muscles apparently cannot respond to mechanical strain by producing MGF. Local repair is important in postmitotic tissue, and both muscle and neuronal tissue have a complex cytoskeletal system, which involves the dystrophin complex. The function of dystrophin is not known although there is evidence that it stiffens the membrane. Because of its structure and its connection to the extracellular matrix and because there is a tyrosine kinase and neuronal nitric acid synthase (nNOS) as integral parts of dystrophin complex, it has been suggested that it does more than just stabilize the membrane. Indeed, it appears that the dystrophin complex may act as a mechanotransducer. The cytoskeleton is defective in the sex-linked Duchenne muscular dystrophy as dystrophin is missing, and in autosomal dystrophies it is also one of the other cytoskeletal/extracellular matrix proteins that is defective or missing. This appears to result in the inability to produce MGF and thus carry out the ongoing local tissue repair in these muscles, which are more susceptible to damage leading to muscle cell death. This cell damage results in the over-expression of collagen I and III genes resulting in fibrosis which in turn causes more damage. The build-up of hard inextensible collagen causes more muscle fibre damage which helps explain the progressive nature of this disease. The challenge is to break this vicious cycle of damage and fibrosis and promote the ongoing repair of the tissue.

Satellite cells

The mechanism by which increased growth factor expression results triggers hypertrophy is unclear, but it is likely that it involves in some way in the differentiation and proliferation of satellite cells (muscle stem cells). Muscle fibres are postmitotic cells, and once embryonic differentiation is complete there is no further cell division taking place. In mice, satellite cells account for about 30% of the muscle nuclei at birth, which drops to about 5% in adult animals. Satellite cells provide the nuclei for postnatal growth and are also involved in repair and regeneration following local injury of muscle fibres. In normal, undamaged muscle the satellite cells are quiescent and are usually detected beneath the basal lamina expressing m-cadherin. When activated they express m-cadherin, c-met as well as MyoD and myf5 and later myogenin (Cornelison & Wold 1997). These cells are believed to remain mitotically inactive, but are mobilized by increased mechanical loading or damage, playing a role in both adaptation and repair of muscle. Recent work by Yang and Goldspink (2002) has shown that MGF when added to muscle cells in culture causes mononucleated myoblasts (satellite cells) to proliferate whilst IGF-I Ea causes them to fuse to form myotubes. As satellite cells are derived from residual myoblasts and also pluripotent stem cells which differentiate into myoblasts, it seems that one of the roles of MGF is to activate the satellite cells following mechanical overload and local damage. It is believed that these cells proliferate and then fuse with existing fibres providing new nuclei to maintain the DNA to protein ratios of fibres undergoing hypertrophy. In this regard it has recently been demonstrated that the number of myonuclei and the number of satellite cells is higher in weight-trained individuals with hypertrophied muscle fibres when compared to untrained subjects (Kadi & Thornell 2000). Once a satellite cell has divided each daughter cell can either undergo terminal differentiation into a myoblast, or remain a stem cell to provide new nuclei for the next cycle of division and differentiation. Weight-trained athletes who also use anabolic steroids exhibit larger muscle fibres and also a higher number of myonuclei with fibres (Kadi *et al.* 1999), providing evidence that maintaining a constant nuclear to cytoplasmic ratio is a fundamental mechanism for muscle fibre growth.

Satellite cells have also received considerable attention not only for the reasons given, but also because they represent a way of transferring genes. Myoblasts and satellite cells have been used to transfer the dystrophin gene (Partridge 1993). However, the realization that pluripotent stem cells can develop into muscle, liver or neuronal tissue presents the possibility not just of transferring genes but of rebuilding tissue *in situ*. This therefore brings us into the era of tissue engineering and it is highly probable that within the next decade or so muscle will be reconstituted following physical trauma and in children with congenital and hereditary problems of muscle growth.

Optimization of sarcomere length for force development

During postnatal development there is a considerable increase in the length of muscles and this results from the constituent fibres adding on sarcomeres serially. Studies with radioactive precursors have shown that the new sarcomeres are added on at the ends of the existing myofibrils (Williams & Goldspink 1971). The functional significance of the sarcomere addition is apparent since the velocity of contraction and the force developed by a muscle are dependent on the number of cross-bridges that can be engaged between actin and myosin filaments. As stated above, this depends on the overlap of these filaments within the sarcomere and the only way initial sarcomere length can be adjusted is by changing the sarcomere number in series (Fig. 12.4). As the limb bones grow, the fibres are apparently stretched out to a point where there would be no overlap of the thick and thin filaments, were it not for the addition of new sarcomeres. The number of sarcomeres in series is important in determining not only the distance through which the muscle can shorten but also the sarcomere length at which it can produce maximum power. Sarcomere number is not fixed, even in adult muscle, being capable of either increasing or decreasing (Tabary *et al.* 1972; Williams & Goldspink 1973) (Fig. 12.4). Regulation of sarcomere number is considered to be an adaptation to changes in the functional length of the muscle. These length-associated changes can be induced when the working length of the muscle is experimentally altered (Oudet & Petrovic 1981) or where there is postural misalignment (Kendall *et al.* 1952). Similar effects are observed during immobilization. In muscle immobilized in the shortened position, sarcomeres are lost and the remaining sarcomeres are altered to a length that enables the muscle to develop its maximum tension at the length that corresponds to the immobilized position (Williams & Goldspink 1978). In muscles immobilized in the lengthened position, sarcomeres are added on and this results in sarcomere length being reduced as compared with non-adapted muscle fixed in a similar position. Maximum tension again is found to be developed at an increased functional length, which corresponds to the immobilized position. When the cast is removed sarcomere number returns to normal within a few days.

The regulation of sarcomere number to allow adjustment of sarcomere length would imply that the muscle fibre monitors sarcomere length in some way, either at a particular joint angle or over a range of angles. The sarcomere length would then be adjusted by adding or subtracting sarcomeres, resulting in a decrease or increase in sarcomere length, respectively. The significant factor for the monitoring of sarcomere length may be the amount of tension along the myofibril and/or the myotendon junction, with high tension leading to an addition of sarcomeres and low tension to a subtraction of sarcomeres (Herring *et al.* 1984). The internal tension sensing may involve the cytoskeletal elements that form the scaffold on which the thick and thin filaments are assembled and in particular the protein titin, which is believed to transmit force through the sarcomere. It has been likened to a bungee rope as its compliance decreases markedly with stretch and its elasticity would mean that the sarcomeres return to their optimum overlap position leaving a space at the ends where the new sarcomeres are added. Normal muscle functions at many lengths and obviously sarcomere length can be optimum for force production at only one joint angle. It seems likely that sarcomere number is regulated so as to achieve optimum sarcomere length at the muscle length at which most force (active and passive) is normally exerted.

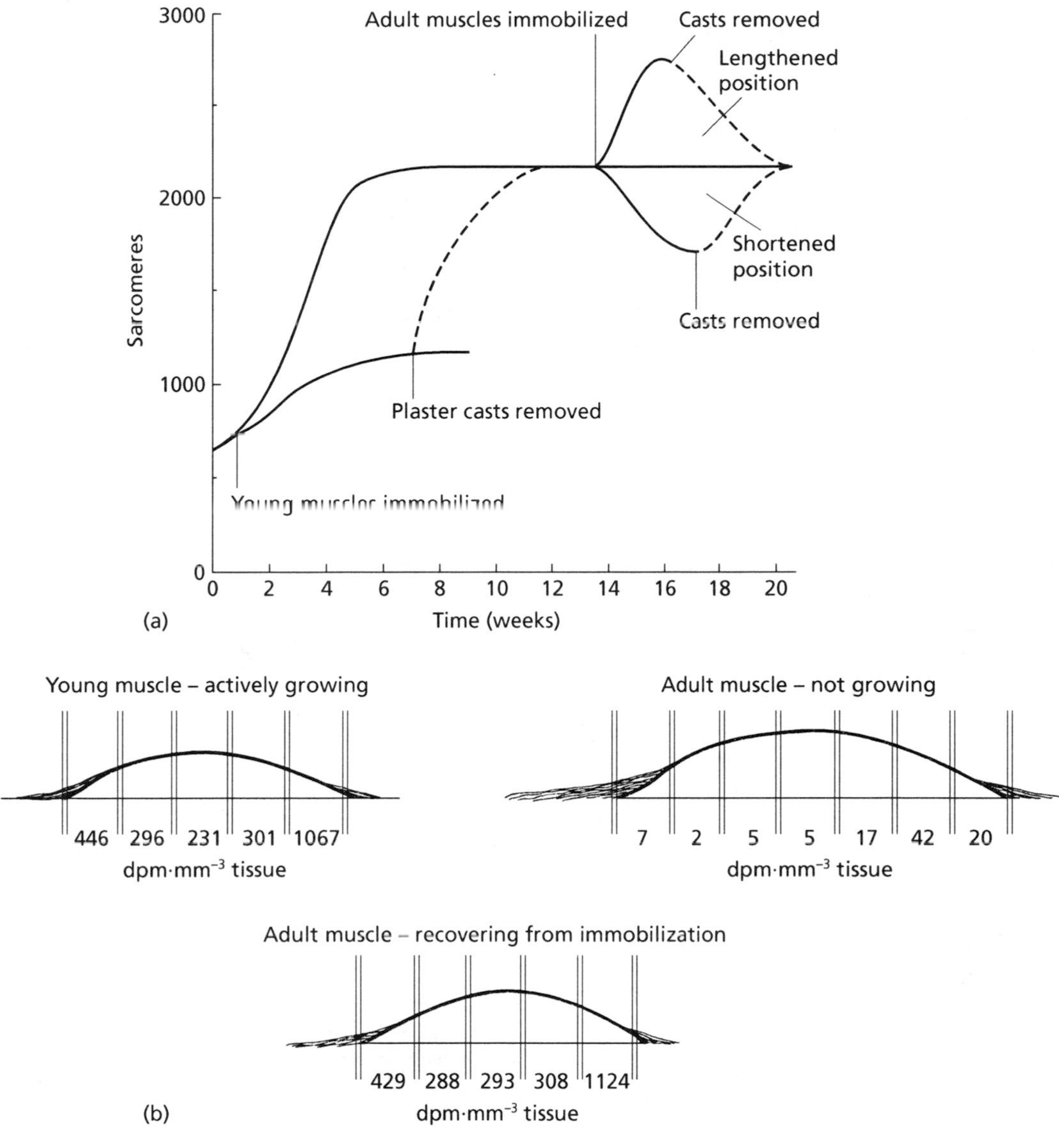

Fig. 12.4 (a) Summarizes data for the addition of sarcomeres along existing myofibrils during the normal growth of a muscle (mouse soleus). Also given are data for immobilization of a muscle in a young animal where the production of sarcomeres is suppressed. However, when the plaster cast is removed sarcomeres are produced at a very rapid rate until the normal number is attained within a week or so. In the adult animal, immobilization of the muscle in its lengthened position results in 20% loss of sarcomeres in series. This adaptation to a new functional length is reversible and when the plaster cast is removed the sarcomere number in series soon returns to normal. (b) The incorporation of radioactively labelled adenosine into the newly formed actin filaments in a young actively growing muscle, in an adult muscle that is not growing in length or in girth, and in an adult muscle that is recovering from a period of immobilization in the shortened position. The data were obtained by sectioning the muscle from end to end and placing batches of sections in a scintillation counter. Some sections were mounted on microscope slides and used to estimate the volume of tissue in each batch so that the radioactivity could be expressed as disintegrations per minute (dpm) per mm^3 of tissue. Note that the end regions of the fibres are the most heavily labelled in young and adult muscle recovering from the shortened position. This and other evidence indicates that the new sarcomeres are added onto the ends of the existing myofibrils.

Adaptation for increased velocity or economy

Adjustment to optimum sarcomere length

The velocity of contraction of a muscle is dependent on the length of a muscle or muscle fibre, the temperature of the muscle, and the type of myosin cross-bridge expressed. In addition, there may also be short-term mechanisms which fine-tune the speed at which a muscle may shorten; these include the role of nitric oxide (Maréchel & Gailly 1999). The way sarcomere length and sarcomere number are adjusted during growth has been described above. These adjustments are all in scale with the changes in skeleton dimensions. In the adult there seems to be little scope for adjustment during normal athletic training. However, if the muscle is not habitually put through its normal range of excursion then problems may arise. For instance, the wearing of high-heeled shoes can cause the gastrocnemius and soleus muscles to shorten by losing sarcomeres and remodelling their connective tissue. This may result in the Achilles tendon being pulled off the bone when the adapted shortened muscle is then required to go through the normal range of lengthening (eccentric) actions.

Determination of muscle fibre phenotype

As mentioned above, there are fast-contracting fibres that are adapted for high power output and slow-contracting fibres that are adapted for performing slow movements efficiently and developing isometric force economically. Recent measurements (Stienen *et al.* 1996) on human single fibres have shown that as molecular motors the MyHC-I fibres are more economical at maintaining isometric force, in other words may maintain a given tension at a lower cost per ATP utilized. More recently, He *et al.* (2000) determined the ATP hydrolysis rate during shortening in muscle fibres using a fluorescently labelled phosphate binding protein. The peak mechanochemical/thermodynamic efficiencies (mechanical power/rate of energy release) were

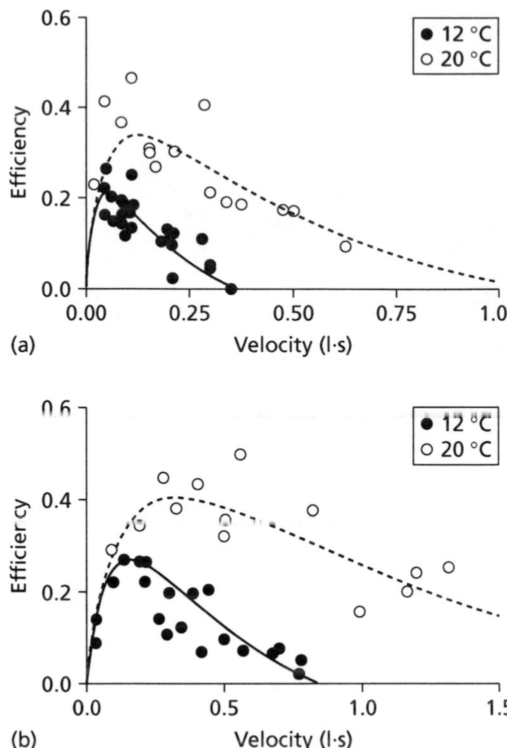

Fig. 12.5 Thermodynamic efficiency of muscle shortening in fibres expressing MyHC-I (a) and MyHC-IIA fibres (b) determined from chemically skinned preparations at 12 and 20 °C. Thermodynamic efficiency was calculated by dividing mechanical power by the rate of energy release. The ATP hydrolysis rate in the muscle fibres was determined with a fluorescently labelled phosphate binding protein. At 12 °C the ATP consumption rate was similar for both fibre types (0.21–0.27) but was reached at a higher speed of shortening for the faster fibres. (From He *et al.* 2000.)

similar for the MyHC-I and MyHC-IIA fibres, but the velocity at which peak efficiency occurred was higher in the MyHC-IIA fibres (Fig. 12.5). Thus in order for the slow fibres or the fast fibres to achieve their maximum efficiency, their intrinsic rate of shortening has to be matched to the rate to which they are required to shorten. Therefore, the slow fibres with the slow myosin cross-bridges are much more efficient for producing the slow repetitive contractions required for, say, long-distance running. They are also more economical for developing and maintaining isometric force as their slow cross-bridge cycle time means that the attachment phase (when no ATP is being used) is much longer than it is for fast muscle. Thus for maximizing performance in power events it is preferred to have molecular motors that will deliver high levels of power (e.g. MyHC-IIA/MyHC-IIX isoforms), but for endurance events it would be more appropriate to have molecular motors that are more economical (e.g. MyHC-I isoforms).

Plasticity of muscle

Animal studies

Based on the force–velocity relationship of skeletal muscle, power may be altered by varying the speed of shortening. Without a change in muscle length this would mean an alteration of the type of myosin expressed. Is it therefore possible to alter muscle fibre types through training? The interconvertibility of fibre types has been demonstrated in animal studies through nerve cross-innervation and chronic stimulation experiments (see Pette & Vrbová 1992). It has become generally accepted that in some animals (e.g. rabbits), but not others (e.g. rats) it is possible to alter both phenotypic and mechanical properties of a 'fast' muscle to those of a 'slow' muscle by delivering a pattern of neural input normally delivered to a slow muscle. It is often believed that the frequency of stimulation (i.e. low, such as 10 Hz) is the important factor in determining fibre type transition. However, it was shown that higher stimulation frequencies were just as effective in producing the fast to slow switch (Streter *et al.* 1982). Using plaster cast limb immobilization stretch without any stimulation at all was also found to induce fast fibres to lay down slow-type sarcomeres (Williams *et al.* 1986a), and under these conditions virtually no electromyograph (EMG) signal can be detected (Hnik *et al.* 1985). Therefore it is not possible that stimulation frequency *per se* is the sole or primary cause of muscle phenotype determination. As mentioned above, more complete reprogramming of the muscle was obtained when stretch was combined with electrical stimulation irrespective of the frequency. This suggests that the signal for the fast to slow change is mechanical strain rather than stimulation frequency *per se*. This makes physiological sense as it can be argued that the muscle cells, by responding to isometric overload, are adapting to an increased postural role.

When a muscle is subjected to stretch and/or electrical stimulation not only is the slow type 1 myosin expressed but the fast myosin genes are turned off, thus demonstrating complete reprogramming (Goldspink *et al.* 1992). Indeed, it seems that all muscle fibres stay phenotypically fast unless they are subjected to repeated stretch and isometric force development. This is shown by the soleus muscle which, when immobilized in the shortened position (Loughna *et al.* 1990), subjected to surgical overload (Gregory *et al.* 1986) or subjected to hypogravity (Oganov & Popatov 1976), reverts to expressing fast myosin genes. More recent work in rabbits strongly indicates that the determination of muscle phenotype is controlled at the level of gene transcription and initially this involves relatively rapid switches from MyHC-IIX to MyHC-IIA mRNA (Goldspink *et al.* 1992). However, muscle fibre hypertrophy, which is also related to mechanical signals, apparently involves a different mechanism with regulation at the level of translation rather than transcription (although the latter is important for the production of more ribosomal RNA and protein). The induction of hypertrophy seems to have a shorter time window than the induction of the slow type I genes. Therefore for adaptation for sprinting short intensive bouts of exercise are required as these result in increase in mass without the up-regulation of slow myosin.

Other subsets of genes are also involved in the interconversion of fibre types, including mitochondrial and cytoplasmic enzyme genes and those that induce changes in the vascularity of the tissue. These are apparently not coordinated, and indeed the signals involved in switching of myosin isoform gene expression are probably different from those that induce mitochondrial or sarcoplasmic enzyme expression but under most training conditions the directions happen to coincide. Sanders Williams *et al.* (1986b) reported that 10-Hz chronic stimulation of the rabbit tibialis anterior muscle for 21 days, which is known to increase type 1 myosin expression, resulted in a fivefold increase in cytochrome b mRNA but a fourfold reduction in the levels of aldolase mRNA. These three subgroups of genes have a different time course for expression, which illustrates that duration as well as the intensity of the mechanical signals is important. It is known from EMG studies that postural muscle fibres, such as those of the soleus, are activated about 90% of the time during standing or walking whilst the fibres in other skeletal muscles are activated only 5% of the time (Hnik *et al.* 1985). Therefore slow postural muscles are subjected to stretch and stimulation long enough for the full transition to the slow type I phenotype to be achieved.

Human studies

It is clear from the cross-sectional data on athletes that those who excel in the power events have the appropriate muscles dominated by faster fibres, whilst top endurance athletes have muscles with a higher distribution of slow muscle fibres (Costill *et al.* 1976). The extent to which this is a product of genetic predisposition or the result of years of specific training remains unknown. A study by Andersen and Henriksson (1975) reported that endurance training in the form of cycling exercise for 8 weeks progressively decreased the proportion of Type IIb fibres (expressing the MyHC-IIX myosin), increased the relative proportion of Type IIa fibres, but had no effect on the relative proportion of Type I fibres. Over the last three decades numerous training studies have been performed, whether they be strength and power or endurance based, which have essentially reported similar findings, albeit with more sophisticated techniques (Harridge 1996). For example 12 weeks of strength training was found to decrease the proportion of MyHC-IIX isoforms as determined by electrophoresis. The proportion of MyHC-IIA isoforms was increased, but there was no change in the proportion of MyHC-I isoforms (Adams *et al.* 1993). It now seems clear that disuse or inactivity of human muscle down-regulates the slow muscle genes and that fast muscle genes are up-regulated as is the case in animal experiments. For example, in the vastus lateralis muscle of spinal cord injured individuals 80% of fibres may express MyHC-IIX isoforms either alone or in combination with MyHC-IIA (Andersen *et al.* 1996). In agreement with studies on able-bodied individuals, electrically evoked cycle training (3 times a week for 1 year) decreased dramatically the number of fibres expressing MyHC-IIX in these subjects, but did not result in an increase in the proportion of MyHC-I fibres. Thus the majority of the fibres after training were MyHC-IIA. Using *in situ* hybridization techniques Andersen and Schaiffino (1997) demonstrated that an uncoupling or mismatch may exist between the MyHC proteins in a muscle fibre and the predominant myosin gene transcript within that fibre. These fibres are thus likely to be in a state of transition. Using this technique it was demonstrated that the gene for MyHC-IIX may be down-regulated after a couple of days following a bout of exercise. This contrasts with a similar approach taken by Harridge *et al.* (2002) who chronically stimulated the tibialis anterior muscle of spinal cord injured subjects and showed that it takes considerably longer for the MyHC-I gene to be up-regulated in fast fibres (see Fig. 12.6). Indeed, this longer time scale may explain why traditionally exercise training studies (usually performed over a 12-week period) have apparently failed to increase the proportion of Type I fibres.

Thus, whereas the conversion from the MyHC-IIX to the MyHC-IIA takes place very readily, it appears that the switch from the fast Type II fibres to the slow Type I is much more difficult to achieve. The *MyHC-I* and *MyHC-II* genes are on different chromosomes and it is clear that a much longer time window is required for this conversion. However, recent evidence has suggested that muscle fibre damage results in expression of the slow-type myosin (Yang *et al.* 1997). This may be a prerequisite for a relatively rapid conversion to the slow Type 1 fibres, e.g.

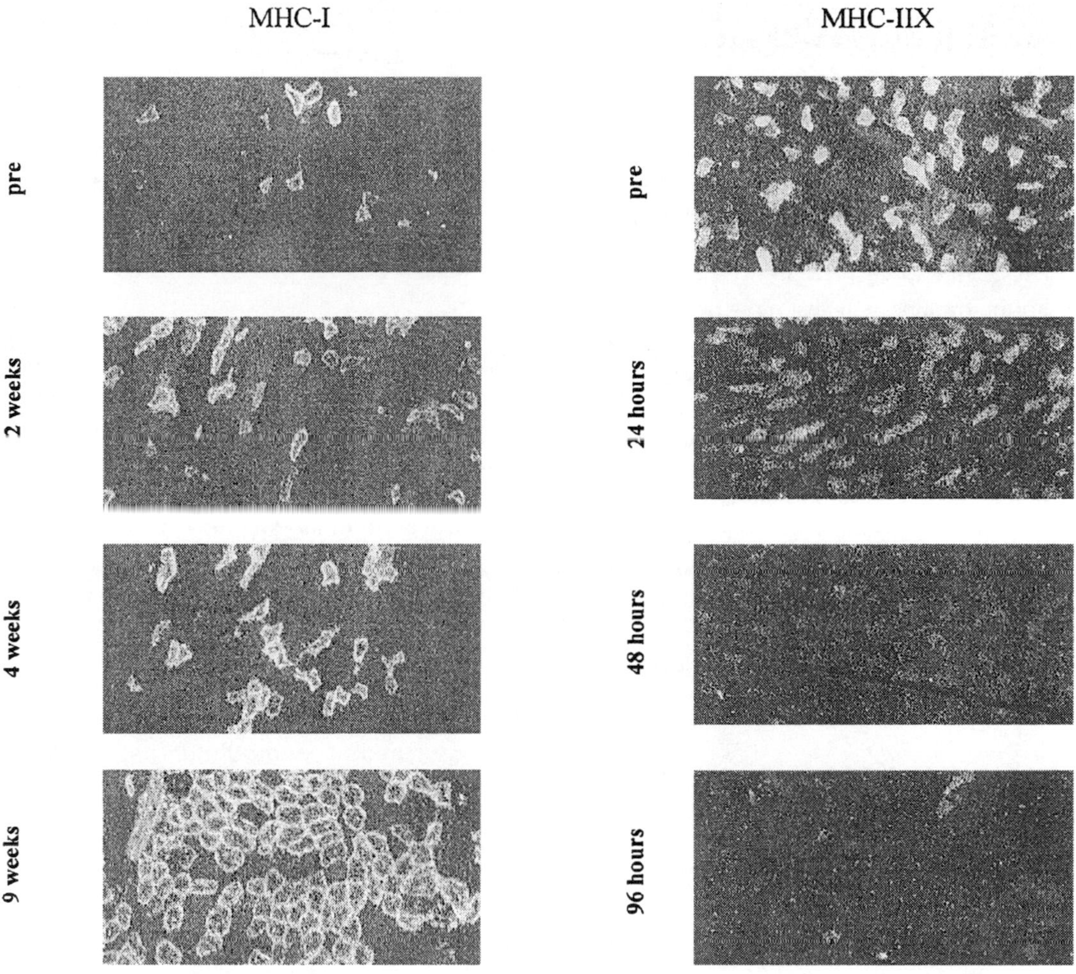

Fig. 12.6 Sections of human muscle processed using *in situ* hybridization. Sections were hybridized with ^{35}S-labelled probes specific for the mRNA transcripts for MyHC-I (a) and MyHC-IIX (b) isoforms processed for autoradiography and visualized by dark-field microscopy. (a) Sections from the tibialis anterior muscles of a subject with a spinal cord injury who had undergone a daily muscle conditioning programme involving chronic low-frequency electrical stimulation for 9 weeks. (b) Sections taken from the vastus lateralis muscle of an able-bodied young male subject at intervals up to 96 h following a single bout of exercise. The data from two separate studies indicate the rapid (hours and days) down-regulation of the MyHC-IIX gene following a single bout of exercise (Andersen, unpublished) which contrasts to the slower up-regulation (weeks and months) of the slow MyHC-I gene as a result of a prolonged stimulus (Harridge *et al.* 2002).

running several hours a day on hard surfaces. There may be a minimum time window needed for switching on the slow genes so that they are only switched on by long periods of activity. The cellular signals for the muscle gene switching are not understood. Recent evidence suggests that the increased cell calcium concentration may serve as a messenger by a signalling pathway that involves the activation of calcineurin. This is a cyclosporin-sensitive, calcium-regulated serine/threonine phosphatase which up-regulates specific slow-fibre-specific promoters in a mechanism involving the NFAT and MEF2 protein families (Chin *et al.* 1998).

Contractile change without fibre switching

The chemically skinned fibre technique has allowed the mechanical properties of single human muscle fibres to be studied from individuals before and after training. Harridge *et al.* (1998) reported no difference in the V_{max} of MyHC-I and MyHC-IIA fibres after 6 weeks of sprint training, suggesting a tight coupling between myosin expression and contractile function. More recently however, longitudinal studies of older men undergoing strength training (Trappe *et al.* 2000) and astronauts following 17 days of space flight (Widrick *et al.* 1999) have shown increased speed of muscle fibre shortening in fibres which express the same MyHC isoform. No change was observed in light chain composition in these studies and it was suggested that a geometric alteration in myofilament spacing might be partly responsible for changes in fibre mechanical properties.

Mechanisms of increased power

It is clear from an analysis of the factors that influence both force and velocity of contraction that muscle power can be influenced most significantly by manipulating muscle size. Furthermore, a preferential hypertrophy of the faster fibres will result in relatively more of a muscle being occupied by fast myosin motors. These, however, are likely of be of the MyHC-IIA phenotype rather than the faster and more powerful MyHC-IIX, as it is clear that the genes for these fast isoforms are, unfortunately for power athletes, rapidly repressed with exercise. One interesting study in this regard showed that following a period of detraining the relative proportion of MyHC-IIX isoforms was found to increase to values higher than those observed prior to training (Andersen & Aargaard 2000). Such an 'overshoot' or 'boost' might provide a physiological rationale for the tapering of training of sprint athletes to undertaking relatively light exercise prior to competition.

In contrast, the principal mechanisms of adaptation for sustaining power output are through increasing the metabolic potential of the muscle (increased number and volume of mitochondria, increased mitochondrial enzyme activity, increased capillary density, etc.), whilst it remains possible that the development of more economical molecular motors, i.e. MyHC-I isoforms, remains a possible long-term (months and years) adaptive response to endurance training.

The future

The scope for misuse of peptides and proteins based on legitimate medical applications is predicted to increase. Indeed certain steroids and more recently certain peptides when combined with exercise training are known to be very effective when used for altering the mass and phenotype of muscle in order to enhance performance. This will also no doubt be extended to gene doping which will have longer-lasting effects and will be difficult to detect when engineered genes containing human cDNA are introduced. Hopefully, the methods used to detect the foreign gene products or the vectors used to introduce the exogenous cDNAs will stay ahead of 'gene cheats'.

New ethical issues will emerge relating to the sequencing of the human genome. This has provided a powerful database for obtaining gene sequences and with the commensurate developments in automated technology, the possibility now exists for screening athletes for site-specific sequence differences in certain signalling as well as in structural genes. Once these have been identified as being related to athletic performance it is probable that the data will be used to select potential athletes. A ban on this type of activity would probably be difficult to sustain on a worldwide basis.

Rather surprisingly the human genome has fewer genes than previously expected. There are about 6 times more proteins than there are genes. Therefore the complexity of expression of the hereditary information is believed to be controlled by the signalling pathways. As muscle cells like several other cell types respond to mechanical as well as chemical signals, it is likely that exercise regimes will become more scientifically based using genomic and proteomic methods to optimize regimes for achieving the appropriate muscle mass and phenotype for a particular activity. However, these will probably only fine-tune rather than replace the training procedures derived in an *ad hoc* manner over many decades. Nevertheless as 1 or 2% often makes a difference between an Olympic medal or failing to qualify, we can anticipate that this new biomedical technology will be used increasingly to enhance athletic performance.

Acknowledgements

Whilst this chapter was being written Professor Goldspink was in receipt of grants from the EU for respiratory muscle function and from the Wellcome Trust for expression of local growth factors. Dr Harridge was in receipt of a Wellcome Trust Fellowship.

References

Adams, G.R., Hather, B.M., Baldwin, K.M. & Dudley, G.A. (1993) Skeletal muscle myosin heavy chain composition and resistance training. *Journal of Applied Physiology* **74**, 911–915.

Andersen, J.L. & Aagaard, P. (2000) Myosin heavy chain IIX overshoot in human skeletal muscle. *Muscle and Nerve* **23**, 1095–1004.

Andersen, P. & Henriksson, J. (1975) Training induced changes in the subgroups of human type II skeletal muscle fibres. *Acta Physiologica Scandinavica* **99**, 123–125.

Andersen, J.L. & Schaiffino, S. (1997) Mismatch between myosin heavy chain mRNA and protein distribution in human skeletal muscle fibers. *American Journal of Physiology* **272**, C1881–C1889.

Andersen, J.L., Mohr, T., Biering-Sørenson, F., Galbo, H. & Kjær, M. (1996) Myosin heavy chain isoform transformation in single fibres from m. vastus lateralis in spinal cord injured individuals: Effects of long term functional electrical stimulation (FES). *Pflügers Archiv* **431**, 513–518.

Barton-Davis, E.R., LaFrambroise, W.A. & Kushmerick, M.J. (1996) Activity-dependent induction of slow myosin gene expression in isolated fast-twitch mouse muscle. *American Journal of Physiology* **271**, C1409–1419.

Barton-Davis, E.R., Shoturma, D.I., Musaro, A., Rosenthal, N. & Sweeney, H.L. (1998) Viral mediated expression of insulin-like growth factor I blocks the aging-related loss of skeletal muscle function. *Proceedings of the National Academy of Sciences of the United States of America* **95**, 15603–15607.

Booth, F.W. & Seider, M.J. (1979) Early changes in skeletal muscle protein synthesis after immobilization of rats. *Journal of Applied Physiology* **49**, 974–977.

Bottinelli, R., Betto, R., Schiaffino, S. & Reggiani, C. (1994) Unloaded shortening velocity and myosin heavy and alkali light chain isoform composition in rat skeletal muscle fibres. *Journal of Physiology* **478**(2), 341–349.

Bottinelli, R., Canepari, M., Pelligrino, M.A. & Reggiani, C. (1996) Force–velocity properties of human skeletal muscle fibres: myosin heavy chain isoform and temperature dependence. *Journal of Physiology* **495**, 573–586.

Brahm, H., Piehl-Aulin, K., Saltin, B. & Ljunghall, S. (1997) Net fluxes over working thigh of hormones, growth factors and biomarkers of bone metabolism during short lasting dynamic exercise. *Calcified Tissue International* **60**, 175–180.

Chin, E.A., Olson, E.N., Richardson, J.A. *et al.* (1998) A calcineurin-dependent transcriptional pathway controls skeletal muscle fiber type. *Genes and Development* **12**, 2499–2509.

Cornelison, D.D. & Wold, B.J. (1997) Single-cell analysis of regulatory gene expression in quiescent and activated mouse skeletal muscle satellite cells. *Developmental Biology* **191**(2), 270–283.

Costill, D.L., Daniels, W., Fink, W., Krahenbuhl, G. & Saltin, B. (1976) Skeletal muscle enzymes and fibre composition in male and female track athletes. *Journal of Applied Physiology* **40**, 149–154.

Ennion, S., Sant'ana Pereira, J.A.A., Sargeant, A.J., Young, A. & Goldspink, G. (1995) Characterization of human skeletal muscle fibres according to the myosin heavy chains they express. *Journal of Muscle Research and Cell Motility* **16**, 35–43.

Finer, J.T., Simmons, R.M. & Spudich, J.T. (1994) Single myosin molecule mechanics: piconewton forces and nanometre steps. *Nature* **10**; 368 (6467), 113–119.

Gauvry, L., Ennion, S., Ettelaie, C. & Goldspink, G. (2000) Characterisation of red and white muscle myosin heavy chain coding sequences from antarctic and tropical fish. *Comparative Biochemistry and Physiology*, Part B **127**, 575–588.

Goldspink, G. (1971) Ultrastructural changes in striated muscle fibres during contraction and growth with particular reference to the mechanism of myofibril splitting. *Journal of Cell Science* **9**, 123–138.

Goldspink, D.F. (1977) The influence of immobilization and stretch on protein turnover of rat skeletal muscle. *Journal of Physiology* **264**, 267–282.

Goldspink, D.F. & Goldspink, G. (1986) The role of passive stretch in retarding muscle atrophy. In: *Electrical Stimulation and Neuromuscular Disorders* (eds W. A. Nix & G. Vrbova), pp. 91–100. Springer Verlag, Berlin.

Goldspink, D.F., Garlick, P.J. & McNurlan, M.A. (1983) Protein turnover measured in vivo and in vitro in muscles undergoing compensatory growth and subsequent denervation atrophy. *Biochemical Journal* **210**, 89–98.

Goldspink, G. & Scutt, A. (1989) Stretch and isometric tension induce rapid changes in gene expression in adult skeletal muscle. *Journal of Physiology* **415**, 129.

Goldspink, G. & Ward, P.S. (1979) Changes in rodent muscle fibre types during post-natal growth, undernutrition and exercise. *Journal of Physiology* **296**, 453–469.

Goldspink, G., Scutt, A., Martindale, J., Jaenicke, T., Turay, L. & Gerlach, G.-F. (1991) Stretch and force generation induce rapid hypertrophy and isoform gene switching in adult skeletal muscle. *Biochemical Society Transactions* **19**, 368–373.

Goldspink, G., Scutt, A., Loughna, P.T., Wells, D.J., Jaenicke, T. & Gerlach, G.F. (1992) Gene expression in skeletal muscle in response to stretch and force generation. *American Journal of Physiology* **262**, R356–R363.

Gregory, P., Low, R. & Stirewalt, W.S. (1986) Changes in skeletal-muscle myosin isoenzymes with hypertrophy and exercise. *Journal of Biochemistry* **238**, 55–63.

Harridge, S.D.R. (1996) The contractile system and its adaptation and training. In: *Human Muscular Function during Dynamic Exercise* (eds P. Marconnet, B. Saltin, P. V. Komi & J. Poortmans), **41**, 82–94. Medicine Sports Science, Karger, Basel.

Harridge, S.D.R., Bottinelli, R., Reggiani, C. *et al.* (1996) Whole muscle and single fibre contractile properties and myosin isoforms in humans. *Pflügers Archiv* **432**, 913–920.

Harridge, S.D.R., Bottinelli, R., Reggiani, C. *et al.* (1998) Sprint training, in vitro and in vivo muscle function and myosin heavy chain expression. *Journal of Applied Physiology* **84**(2), 442–449.

Harridge, S.D.R., Andersen, J.L. & Hartkopp, A. *et al.* (2002) Training by low-frequency of tibialis anterior in spinal cord-injured men. *Muscle and Nerve* **25**, 685–694.

He, H.-Z., Bottinelli, R., Pellegrino, M.A., Ferenczi, M.A. & Reggiani, C. (2000) ATP consumption and efficiency of human single fibers with different myosin isoform composition. *Biophysical Journal* **79**, 945–961.

Herring, S.W., Grimm, A.F. & Grimm, B.R. (1984) Regulation of sarcomere number in skeletal muscle: a comparison of hypotheses. *Muscle and Nerve* **7**, 161–173.

Hnik, P., Vejsada, R., Goldspink, D.F., Kasicki, S. & Krekule, I. (1985) Quantitative evaluation of electromyogram activity in rat extensor and flexor muscles immobilized at different lengths. *Experimental Neurology* **88**, 515–528.

Kadi, F. & Thornell, L.-E. (2000) Concomitant increases in myonuclear and satellite cell content in female trapezius muscle following strength training. *Histochemistry and Cell Biology* **113**, 99–103.

Kadi, F., Eriksson, A., Holmner, S. & Thornell, L.E. (1999) Effects of anabolic steroids on the muscle cells of strength trained athletes. *Medicine and Science in Sports and Exercise* **31**, 1528–1534.

Kendall, H.O., Kendall, F.P. & Boynton, D.A. (1952) In: *Posture and Pain* (ed. M. D. Baltimore), pp. 103–124. Williams & Wilkins, Baltimore.

Kraft, T., Hornemann, T., Stolz, M., Nier, V. & Wallimann, T. (2000) Coupling of creatine kinase to glycolytic enzymes at the sarcomeric I-band of skeletal muscle: a biochemical study in situ. *Journal of Muscle Research and Cell Motility* **21**, 691–703.

Larsson, L. & Moss, R. (1993) Maximum velocity of shortening in relation to myosin isoform composition in single fibres from human skeletal muscle fibres. *Journal of Physiology* **472**, 595–614.

Loughna, P.T., Izumo, S., Goldspink, G. & Nadal-Ginard, B. (1990) Rapid changes in sarcomeric myosin heavy chain gene and alpha-actin expression in response to disuse and stretch. *Development* **109**, 217–223.

McCall, G.E., Byrnes, W.C., Dickinson, A., Pattany, P.M. & Fleck, S.J. (1996) Muscle fiber hypertrophy, hyperplasia and capillary density in college men after resistance training. *Journal of Applied Physiology* **81**, 2004–2201.

McKoy, G., Ashley, W., Mander, J. *et al.* (1999) Expression of insulin growth factor-1 splice variants and structural genes in rabbit skeletal muscle induced by stretch and stimulation. *Journal of Physiology* **516**, 583–592.

Maréchel, G. & Gailly, P. (1999) Effects of nitric oxide on the contraction of skeletal muscle. *Cellular and Molecular Life Sciences* **55**(8–9), 1088–1102.

Mathews, L.S., Hammer, R.E., Behringer, R.R. *et al.* Growth enhancement of transgenic mice expressing human insulin-like growth factor I. *Endocrinology* **123**(6), 2827–2833.

Musaro, A.K., McCollagh, W.J., Paul, A. *et al.* (2001) Localized IGF-I transgene expression sustains hypertrophy and regeneration in senescent muscle. *Nature Genetics* **27**(1), 195–200.

Oganov, V.S. & Popatov, A.N. (1976) The mechanism of the change in skeletal muscles in the weightless environment. *Life Science Space Research* **19**, 137–143.

Oudet, C.L. & Petrovic, A.G. (1981) Regulation of the anatomical length of the lateral pterygoid muscle in the growing rat. *Advances in Physiological Sciences* **24**, 115–121.

Owino, V., Yang, S-Y. & Goldspink, G. (2001) Age-related loss of skeletal muscle function and the inability to express the autocrine form of insulin-like growth factor-1 (MGF) in response to mechanical overload. FEBS Letts **505**, 259–263.

Partridge, T. (1993) *Molecular and Cell Biology of Muscular Dystrophy*. Chapman & Hall, London.

Pette, D. & Vrbová, G. (1992) Adaptation of mammalian skeletal muscle fibers to chronic electrical stimulation. *Reviews in Physiology, Biochemistry and Pharmacology* **120**, 115–202.

Rayment, I., Rypniewski, W.R., Schmidt-Base, K. *et al.* (1993a) Three-dimensional structure of myosin subfragment-1: a molecular motor. *Science* **261**, 50–58.

Rayment, I., Holden, H.M., Whitaker, M. *et al.* (1993b) Structure of the actin-myosin complex and its implications for muscle contraction. *Science* **261**, 58–65.

Reisner, P.J., Moss, R.L. & Giuliam, G.C. *et al.* (1985) Shortening velocity and myosin heavy chains of developing rabbit muscle fibres. *Journal of Biological Chemistry* **206**, 14403–14405.

Rennie, M.J. & Tipton, K.D. (2000) Protein and amino acid metabolism during and after exercise and the effects of nutrition. *Annual Review of Nutrition* **20**, 457–483.

Sant'ana Pereira, J.A.A., Wessels, A., Nijtmans, L., Moorman, A.F.M. & Sargeant, A.J. (1994) New method for the accurate characterization of single human skeletal muscle fibres demonstrates a relation between mATPase and MyHC expression in pure and hybrid fibre types. *Journal of Muscle Research and Cell Motility* **16**, 21–34.

Schiaffino, S. & Reggiani, C. (1996) Molecular diversity of myofibrillar proteins: gene regulation and functional significance. *Physiological Reviews* **76**, 371–423.

Smerdu, V., Karschizrachi, I., Campione, M., Leinwand, L. & Schiaffino, S. (1994) Type IIX myosin heavy chain transcripts are expressed in type IIb fibers of human skeletal muscle. *American Journal of Physiology* **36**, 1723–1728.

Stienen, G.J.M., Kiers, J.L., Bottinelli, R. & Reggiani, C. (1996) Myofibrillar ATPase activity in skinned human skeletal muscle fibres: fibre type and temperature dependence. *Journal of Physiology* **293**(2), 229–307.

Streter, F.A., Pinter, K., Jolesz, F. & Mabauchi, A. (1982) Fast to slow transformation of fast muscles in reponse to longterm phasic stimulation. *Experimental Neurology* **75**, 95–102.

Tabary, I.C., Tabary, C., Tardieu, C., Tardieu, G. & Goldspink, G. (1972) Physiological and structural changes in the cat's soleus muscle due to immobilization at different lengths by plaster cast. *Journal of Physiology* **224**, 231–244.

Trappe, S., Williamson, D., Godard, M., Porter, D., Rowden, G. & Costill, D. (2000) Effect of resistance training on single muscle fiber contractile function in older men. *Journal of Applied Physiology* **89**, 143–152.

Vaughan, H.S. & Goldspink, G. (1979) Fibre number and fibre size in a surgically overloaded muscle. *Journal of Anatomy* **129**, 293–303.

Widrick, J.J., Knuth, S.T., Norenberg, K.M. *et al.* (1999) Effect of a 17 day spaceflight on contractile properties of human soleus muscle fibres. *Journal of Physiology* **516**, 915–930.

Williams, P.E. & Goldspink, G. (1971) Longitudinal growth of striated muscle fibres. *Journal of Cell Science* **9**, 751–767.

Williams, P.E. & Goldspink, G. (1973) The effect of immobilization on the longitudinal growth of striated muscle fibres. *Journal of Anatomy* **116**, 45–55.

Williams, P.E. & Goldspink, G. (1978) Changes in sarcomere length and physiological properties in immobilized muscle. *Journal of Anatomy* **127**, 459–468.

Williams, P.E., Watt, P., Bicik, V. & Goldspink, G. (1986a) Effect of stretch combined with electrical stimulation on the type of sarcomeres produced at the ends of muscle fibres. *Experimental Neurology* **93**, 500–509.

Williams, R.S., Salmons, S., Newsholme, E.A., Kaufman, R.E. & Mellor, J. (1986b) Regulation of nuclear and mitochondrial gene expression by contractile activity in skeletal muscle. *Journal of Biological Chemistry* **261**(1), 376–380.

Yang, S.Y. & Goldspink, G. (2000) US patent 09/142583.

Yang, S.Y. & Goldspink, G. (2002) Different roles of the IGF-I Ec peptide (MGF) and mature IGF-I in myoblast proliferation and differentiation. *FEBS Lett* **522**, 156–160.

Yang, S., Alnaqeeb, M., Simpson, H. & Goldspink, G. (1996) Cloning and characterization of an IGF-1 isoform expressed in skeletal muscle subjected to stretch. *Journal of Muscle Research and Cell Motility* **17**, 487–495.

Yang, S.Y., Alnaqeeb, M., Simpson, H. & Goldspink, G. (1997) Changes in muscle fibre type, muscle mass and IGF-1 gene expression in rabbit skeletal muscle subjected to stretch. *Journal of Anatomy* **190**, 613–622.

Chapter 13

Hypertrophy and Hyperplasia

J. DUNCAN MACDOUGALL

Introduction

Skeletal muscle is an extremely dynamic tissue with a remarkable capacity for adapting, both structurally and physiologically, to different forms of functional overload. A functional overload occurs when a muscle is required to contract more forcibly (as in resistance training), or more frequently (as in endurance training) than normal. These two forms of training elicit very different adaptive responses in the muscle. Endurance training typically results in enhanced mitochondrial and capillary densities with little or no change in muscle size, whereas strength training normally results in increased size (hypertrophy) and strength. The focus in this chapter will be those factors that contribute to the muscle hypertrophy that occurs in response to resistance training.

In theory, an increase in muscle size could occur as a result of an increase in fibre size, an increase in fibre numbers (hyperplasia), and/or an increase in the amount of connective tissue in the muscle. The fact that resistance training and other forms of mechanical loading causes an increase in cross-sectional fibre area has been well established in humans (MacDougall *et al.* 1979, 1980; McDonagh & Davies 1984; Tesch 1987) and other mammals (Gonyea & Ericson 1976; Timson *et al.* 1985). Likewise, it is well known that the major contributor to muscle growth up until early infancy is an increase in fibre numbers (Goldspink 1974; Mastaglia 1981; Malina 1986). Whether or not hyperplasia contributes to the hypertrophy response in adults, however, remains controversial. Relative to contractile protein, connective tissue comprises only a small proportion of the total muscle volume and is thus limited in its capacity to significantly affect muscle size.

A number of experimental models have been used to induce muscle enlargement. These include animal models involving ablation of synergistic muscles (Goldberg *et al.* 1975; Gollnick *et al.* 1981) or chronic suspension of weights from one limb (Ashmore & Summers 1981). In such instances, however, the stimulus for hypertrophy probably differs from that derived from the brief maximal voluntary contractions performed by human weightlifters or bodybuilders (Timson 1990). Alternative models in which the intact animal performs brief voluntary (Goldspink & Howells 1974; Gonyea & Ericson 1976) or involuntary (Wong & Booth 1988; Tamaki *et al.* 1992) contractions are restricted to certain muscles and have obvious limitations in isolating a given joint movement or applying progressive overload through the variety of techniques available to the human subject. As a result, direct application of the findings in such studies to humans is often difficult. Discussion in this chapter will, for the most part, be confined to the hypertrophy response to resistance training as would be performed by the adult strength and power athlete or bodybuilder.

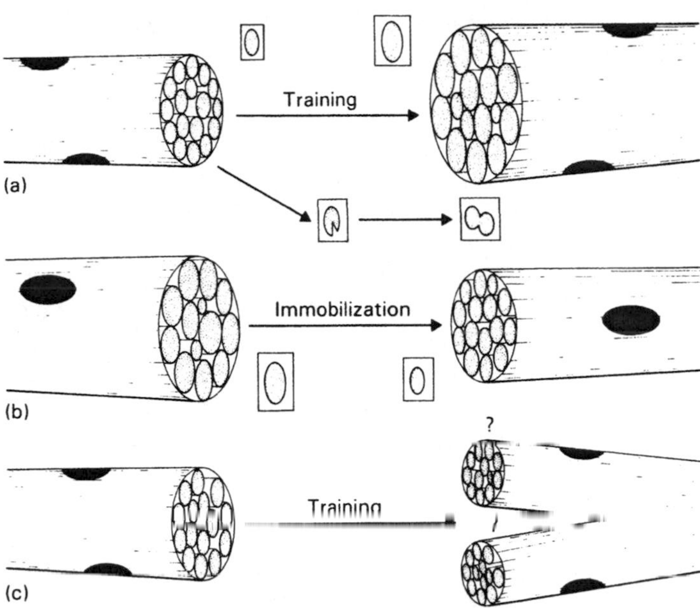

Fig. 13.1 An illustration of the structural adaptations that cause changes in fibre area in response to strength training or immobilization. (a) With training, cross-sectional fibre area increases (hypertrophy) in direct proportion to the increases in myofibrillar size and myofibrillar number. (b) With immobilization, fibre area decreases (atrophy) in proportion to the decrease in myofibrillar size. (c) Training-induced fibre splitting has been [illegible] hyperplasia in certain species, but does not occur in humans. (From MacDougall 1986b.)

Hypertrophy of muscle fibres in response to strength training

A bout of heavy-resistance exercise results in a rapid increase in myofibrillar protein synthesis in the exercised muscles (Chesley *et al.* 1992). The response appears to peak at approximately 24 h following the training session but remains elevated for 36–48 h (MacDougall *et al.* 1995; Phillips *et al.* 1997). This increased synthesis is accompanied by a proportionally smaller increase in protein degradation rate (Biolo *et al.* 1995; Phillips *et al.* 1997), such that the net effect is an increase in protein balance. The increased protein synthetic rate is apparently mediated by a more efficient translation of mRNA, since it occurs in the absence of any change in total RNA or contractile protein mRNA (Chesley *et al.* 1992; Welle *et al.* 1999).

With repeated bouts of resistance exercise (training), the increased protein synthesis manifests itself as an increase in both myofibrillar area and myofibrillar number, with no change in myofibrillar packing density (Fig. 13.1). Myosin and actin filaments are added to the periphery of each myofibril, thus creating larger myofibrils without altering filament packing density or cross-bridge spacing (MacDougall 1986b). Since the increase in total fibre area proportionally exceeds the average increase in myofibrillar area, it is apparent that an increase in the number of myofibrils must also occur. The increase in myofibrillar numbers is thought to be the result of longitudinal 'splitting', as has been shown to occur with normal postnatal growth in young animals (Goldspink 1970, 1974). This splitting may be a mechanical process that results from discrepancies between the A- and I-band lattice spacing. When the myofibril achieves a critical size and force-generating capacity, forceful contractions are thought to cause tearing or rupturing of the connective tissue in the Z-discs, which is transmitted along the myofibril to result in two or more 'daughter myofibrils' of the same length (Goldspink 1992) (Fig. 13.1).

Changes in fibre area

Fibre areas increase in direct proportion to the increases in myofibrillar size and number. The magnitude of this increase varies considerably and is dependent upon a number of factors including the individual's responsiveness to training (MacDougall 1986a), the intensity and duration of the training programme and the training status of the individual prior to the commencement of the programme. Following training studies that have been conducted in our laboratory, changes in fibre area have ranged from no significant change in either fibre type in vastus lateralis of active young men and women after 6 months of training (Sale *et al.* 1990), to an increase of 33% in Type II and 27% in Type I fibre area in a group of untrained young men who trained their triceps brachii for 6 months (MacDougall *et al.* 1979). In a study where 14 older men (60–70 years) performed resistance training for 3 months, Type II fibre area in biceps brachii was found to increase by 30% and Type I by 14% (Brown *et al.* 1988). In a cross-comparison study, fibre areas for biceps brachii in a group of elite bodybuilders were approximately 58% (Type II) and 39% (Type I) larger than those of untrained age-matched controls (MacDougall *et al.* 1984).

CHANGES IN FIBRE AREA ACCORDING TO FIBRE TYPE

Resistance training results in an increase in cross-sectional area of all fibre types; however, most studies indicate that a greater relative hypertrophy occurs in the Type II units (Thorstensson 1976; MacDougall *et al.* 1979; Tesch *et al.* 1985; Staron *et al.* 1990). Since all fibre types are thought to be activated in the performance of maximal and near-maximal contractions, the greater hypertrophy of the Type II fibres may reflect the greater *relative* involvement of these high-threshold units than would normally occur during daily living.

CONVERSION OF FIBRE TYPES WITH TRAINING

Whether classified as to their myosin ATPase characteristics (Staron *et al.* 1990, 1994), or their myosin heavy chain content (Adams *et al.* 1993; Carroll *et al.* 1998; Andersen & Aagaard 2000), it is apparent that resistance training results in an increase in the percentage of Type IIA fibres and a proportional decrease in the percentage of IIB (or IIX) fibres. In humans, however, such conversions in fibre type seem to be confined to the Type II subtypes and it is unlikely that conventional resistance training affects the proportion of Type I fibres. This conclusion is based on our finding of no change in the percentage of Type I fibres in a group of young men following 6 months of intensive resistance training (MacDougall *et al.* 1980), as well as our finding of the same percentage of Type I fibres in triceps and biceps of elite bodybuilders as that of untrained subjects, despite 6–8 years of training by the bodybuilders (MacDougall *et al.* 1982, 1984) (see Fig. 13.2). The topic of alteration of fibre types with training is presented in more detail in Chapter 14 (Tesch & Alkner).

The functional significance of the reduction in IIB fibres and down-regulation of fast IIX myosin heavy chain (Baldwin & Haddad 2001) is not readily apparent, since there is no 'slowing' of con-tractile properties following a period of heavy-resistance training (Alway *et al.* 1989a). One possible explanation is that the resultant preferential hypertrophy in the Type II subtypes serves to counterbalance the effect. It also appears that, when subjects cease training, the conversion of Type II subtypes is reversed and may even overshoot, such that, after a few months, the proportion of IIB (IIX) fibres may exceed original pretraining levels (Andersen & Aagaard 2000).

Other changes

The proportion of interstitial connective tissue remains quite constant over a wide range of muscle sizes, as indicated in biopsies from biceps of elite and novice bodybuilders and untrained controls. We have estimated the volume density of non-contractile tissue to be approximately 13% of the total muscle volume. Of this, approximately 6% is collagen and 7% other tissue (MacDougall *et al.* 1984). These data indicate that increases in fibre size caused by resistance

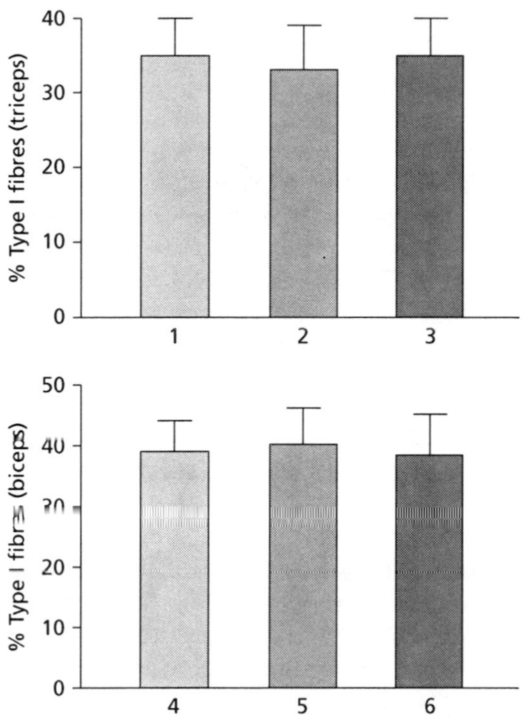

Fig. 13.2 (Upper panel) Percentage Type 1 fibres in triceps brachii of nine young male subjects before (1) and after (2) 6 months of heavy-resistance training and after 6 weeks of immobilization of the elbow joint (3). Note no change in fibre type. (Lower panel) Percentage Type 1 fibres in biceps brachii in a group of 13 untrained controls (4), a group of seven intermediate-calibre bodybuilders (5) and a group of five elite bodybuilders (6). Note no difference in fibre type between groups. Values are means and SD. (From MacDougall 1986a.)

training are accompanied by a proportional increase in interstitial connective tissue. Thus, while the absolute amount of connective tissue increases with training, the relative amount stays the same and can only be considered as making a minor contribution to the increase in total muscle size.

At the ultrastructural level, the increase in contractile protein dilutes the mitochondrial proportion of the fibre, resulting in a significant decrease in mitochondrial volume density (MacDougall *et al.* 1979; Lüthi *et al.* 1986; Chilibeck *et al.* 1999) and oxidative enzyme activity (Tesch 1987; Masuda *et al.* 1999). Sarcoplasmic reticulum and T-tubule volume density, on the other hand, increase in proportion to the changes in myofibrillar volume, so that their relative volume density remains constant in both fibre types and the electrically induced twitch properties are unaltered (Alway *et al.* 1989a).

Unlike endurance training, it is unclear whether or not the increased fibre areas caused by resistance training are accompanied by sufficient angiogenesis to preserve normal capillary density in the muscle. Several studies have reported a decrease in capillary density (Tesch *et al.* 1984; MacDougall 1986b), while others have noted no change or even a slight increase (Green *et al.* 1999; McCall *et al.* 1996) following training. Differences in the magnitude of the hypertrophy response and in training protocols may, in part, account for such variations in findings.

Hyperplasia of skeletal muscle fibres

Fibre proliferation during development

Mammalian skeletal muscle develops embryonically from the mesoderm. Repeated mitotic division gives rise to millions of mononucleated cells known as myoblasts. By approximately the 4th week of gestation, groups of myoblasts align and begin to fuse together to form the multinucleated myotubes that will eventually become mature muscle fibres. The process continues until birth, and perhaps a few months after birth. Since the peripherally located nuclei of the myotubes are incapable of further mitotic division at this stage, it is generally thought that, by birth (or shortly thereafter), total muscle fibre number is fully established (Fischman 1972; Mastaglia 1981; Malina 1986).

Postnatal muscle growth is the result of an increase in fibre area and length. The increase in muscle length is the result of the addition of sarcomeres to the ends of the fibre and continues until bone growth is complete. The increase in fibre area and length is accompanied by a proportional increase in the number of myonuclei. These nuclei are thought to be derived from satellite (stem) cells (Moss & LeBlond 1971; Goldspink 1974; Malina 1986), which in turn are considered to be derived from populations of myoblasts that did not fuse to form myotubes during development (White & Esser 1989).

Several early investigators have reported numerical increases in muscle fibres during early neonatal growth in certain species, such as the rat (Chiakulus & Pauly 1965; Rayne & Crawford 1975) and various mechanisms have been proposed to account for such hyperplasia.

1 *De novo* formation of fibres from residual myoblasts.

2 Longitudinal splitting of, or budding from, existing fibres.

3 Lengthening of short fibres that did not previously traverse the full length of the muscle.

4 Separation and further growth of immature fibres, previously enclosed within the basement membrane of fibres at a more advanced stage of development (Mastaglia 1981).

Electron microscopic evidence in developing neonatal muscle in rats indicates that the first two mechanisms probably do not occur, and what appears to be an addition of fibre numbers can be accounted for by the latter two processes (Ontell & Dunn 1978; Mastaglia 1981).

Hyperplasia in adult muscle?

Since the work by Morpurgo (1897) who trained dogs on a running wheel, it had generally been accepted that the fibre content of adult mammalian muscle does not increase and that muscle growth occurs exclusively through enlargement of the existing fibres. In the 1970s, however, a series of studies appeared which suggested that compensatory and training-induced growth in several animal species was the result of both hypertrophy of existing fibres and the addition of new fibres (Reitsma 1969; Hall-Craggs 1970; Gonyea *et al.* 1977; Sola *et al.* 1973; Gonyea 1980).

In 1981, Gollnick and colleagues challenged these latter studies and suggested that methodological errors associated with the method of estimation of fibre numbers from histological sections may have biased their interpretation. Utilizing a technique by which all of the fibres in a muscle were isolated and counted, these authors (Gollnick *et al.* 1981) concluded that, in rats, muscle enlargement caused by ablation of a synergist and treadmill running could be totally accounted for by hypertrophy of the existing fibres, without the addition of more fibres. This was corroborated by a subsequent study using mice (Timson *et al.* 1985). Use of running as a training mode differs considerably, however, from the heavy-resistance training that was used in many of the studies that have reported hyperplasia. Indeed, using the same fibre counting technique as Gollnick and coworkers, a significant 9% increase in fibre numbers has been found in cats, following a programme of progressive weightlifting, whereby the animals were taught to perform near-maximal voluntary contractions in order to receive a food reward (Gonyea *et al.* 1986). In addition, there have also been several subsequent studies offering indirect evidence for fibre hyperplasia following weightlifting training in cats (Giddings & Gonyea 1992) and rats (Tamaki *et al.* 1997).

It is well known that the application of chronic stretch is a very potent model for inducing muscle enlargement. Stretch is usually imposed by suspending a heavy weight from one wing of an avian species such as the quail or chicken, with the muscles of the opposite wing serving as a control. In such studies, after several weeks, the increase in muscle mass is clearly the result of both increased fibre area and fibre numbers (Sola *et al.* 1973; Alway *et al.* 1989b, 1990; Antonio & Gonyea 1993a), with one study reporting an 82% increase in fibre number in response to 37 days of progressive stretch (Antonio & Gonyea 1993a). Based on a meta-analysis of studies that have investigated fibre hyperplasia in animals subjected to mechanical loading, Kelley (1996) concluded that stretch overload was the most effective intervention, and that hyperplasia was more likely to occur in avian than in mammalian species. For further discussion of the effects of chronic stretch on muscle fibre hyperplasia, readers are referred to the review by Antonio and Gonyea (1993b).

Fibre hyperplasia in humans

The extent to which fibre hyperplasia might occur in muscles of humans who participate in heavy-resistance training remains controversial. Indirect evidence based on measurement of fibre size (MacDougall *et al.* 1982; Tesch & Larsson 1982) and estimations of fibre numbers per motor unit (Larsson & Tesch 1986) suggests that some bodybuilders possess more muscle fibres than untrained subjects. In such instances, however, it must be recognized that the greater fibre numbers may have been inherited rather than the result of training-induced hyperplasia. Because of the methodological difficulties in determining muscle fibre numbers in humans it is difficult to resolve this issue.

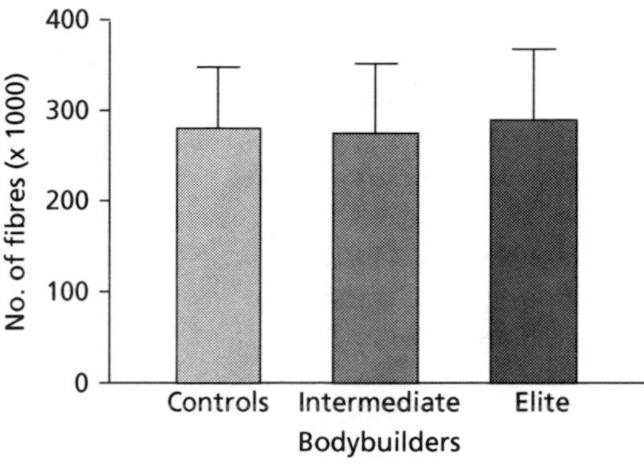

Fig. 13.3 Estimated fibre numbers in biceps brachii of a group of 13 untrained controls, a group of seven intermediate-calibre bodybuilders and a group of five elite bodybuilders. Values are means and SD. (From MacDougall 1986a.)

Using an *in vivo* method for estimating fibre numbers, we examined biceps brachii in 25 young males, of whom five were elite bodybuilders, seven were intermediate-calibre bodybuilders and 13 were age-matched untrained controls (MacDougall *et al.* 1984). Muscle fibre numbers were determined from measurements of total muscle area (computed tomography scanning) and fibre area (from needle biopsies) with the assumption that, since most fibres of biceps extend from origin to insertion, measurement of cross-sectional area at the belly of the muscle includes all fibres. Since biceps is a muscle that is trained by bodybuilders to achieve maximum hypertrophy (biceps area in some bodybuilders was more than threefold greater than that of some controls), it is particularly suited for investigation of possible hyperplasia. It was our hypothesis that, if heavy-resistance training induces an increase in fibre number, the biceps of such individuals should show evidence of hyperplasia in comparison to control subjects.

The data indicated that while total fibre numbers in biceps brachii ranged from approximately 172 000 to 419 000 fibres, the average number of fibres was the same for each group (Fig. 13.3). Since both groups of bodybuilders had trained their biceps to achieve maximum hypertrophy for a minimum of 6 years and yet had the same number of fibres as the untrained control subjects, we concluded that such training does not result in a significant net increase in fibre numbers. We also found that, within each group, there was a tendency for the subjects with the largest muscles also to have a higher than average number of fibres. Thus, although muscle size is primarily determined by the size of the individual fibres, it is also affected by the genetically determined number of fibres.

In the only longitudinal investigation of hyperplasia in human subjects, McCall *et al.* (1996) observed no change in fibre numbers in biceps brachii of young men, following 12 weeks of intense resistance training. In this study, the method for estimating fibre numbers was the same as that used by MacDougall *et al.* (1984) and its validity is based on the assumption that the average fibre area in the biopsy sample is representative of the whole muscle. We examined the precision of this technique by comparing our estimates of fibre number in the biceps of one arm with that of the other arm in each subject, and concluded that the standard error of estimate was approximately ± 11% (MacDougall *et al.* 1984). As such, one must accept that this method is not as precise as, for example, direct fibre counting following nitric acid digestion of the whole muscle, and that small changes in total fibre numbers might not be detected.

In an autopsy investigation of right and left anterior tibialis muscles of previously right-handed young men, Sjostrom *et al.* (1991) detected larger cross-sectional muscle areas on the left side, but no difference in fibre area between the two sides. They concluded that the larger muscles of the lower left leg were due to compensatory hypertrophy associated with long-term asymmetrical usage of that leg by right-handed individuals. In addition, they interpreted their data as indicating that the enlarged muscle was due to an approximate 9.8% increase in fibre numbers (Sjostrom *et al.* 1991).

From the existing literature, it thus appears that net increases in fibre numbers do not occur in healthy adult human muscle in response to resistance exercise, or, if they do, that they are of little numerical significance. How then does one reconcile the clear evidence for abundant fibre hyperplasia in certain animal models, with its lack in the human model? One possible explanation is that hyperplasia occurs only in response to a significant stretch overload that also causes muscle lengthening, and that conventional resistance training does not impose such a stimulus. Let us examine the rationale for this explanation.

Some investigators have reported small net increases in fibre numbers in mammals following weightlifting training or synergistic ablation (Ho *et al.* 1980; Gonyea *et al.* 1986), but most have not (Gollnick *et al.* 1981; Timson *et al.* 1985; Snow & Chortkoff 1987; Yarasheski *et al.* 1990). In contrast, most investigators who have used chronic stretch of wing muscles in avians report large increases in total fibre number (Alway *et al.* 1989b; Sola *et al.* 1973; Antonio & Gonyea 1993a). In addition, the magnitude of the increase in fibre number appears related to the magnitude of the stretch stimulus as well as to its duration (Antonio & Gonyea 1993a). Unlike the avian model, it is difficult to impose chronic stretch on a muscle of a quadruped. Thus, the tendency for hyperplasia to occur to a greater extent in avians than in mammals may be due to the effectiveness of the experimental model, rather than to species differences *per se*.

It is also doubtful whether conventional resistance training subjects the muscle to a high degree of stretch. Most weightlifting movements begin with the muscle at (or slightly beyond) its resting length, followed by a shortening of sarcomeres throughout the concentric phase of the lift. Although some stretching of sarcomeres occurs towards the end of the eccentric or lowering phase, the structure of most human joints is such that only moderate lengthening of sarcomeres is permitted. A possible exception is the ankle joint, where a considerable range of dorsiflexion can be achieved, thus imposing stretch on the calf muscles. In a recent study (Fowles *et al.* 2000) we examined the effects of a bout of maximal tolerated passive stretch on muscle protein synthetic rate of soleus. Using a foot- and leg-holding device instrumented to strain gauges (described by Sale *et al.* 1982), eight young men endured ~ 30 min of passive stretch of the calf muscles of one leg with the other leg serving as control. The procedure began with the subject's foot locked into the maximal tolerable dorsiflexed position without pain and thereafter, every 2 min, the magnitude of the stretch was increased and a new maximal joint angle established, as limited by the tolerance of the subject. On average, this protocol resulted in a 6–7° increase in joint angle, beyond the original maximal tolerable stretch. Fractional protein synthetic rate was then measured in soleus of both legs, by quantifying the incorporation rate of L-[1–13C] leucine into needle biopsy samples. In spite of the intervention, no difference in protein synthetic rate occurred between the two muscles. Since the magnitude and the duration of the stretch in this experiment vastly exceeded that encountered during a typical resistance training session, and yet were still not sufficient to stimulate protein synthesis, it is apparent that minimal muscle stretch occurs during weightlifting.

Muscle satellite cells and the hypertrophy process

The process for the exercise-induced increase in fibre number in adult animals was once

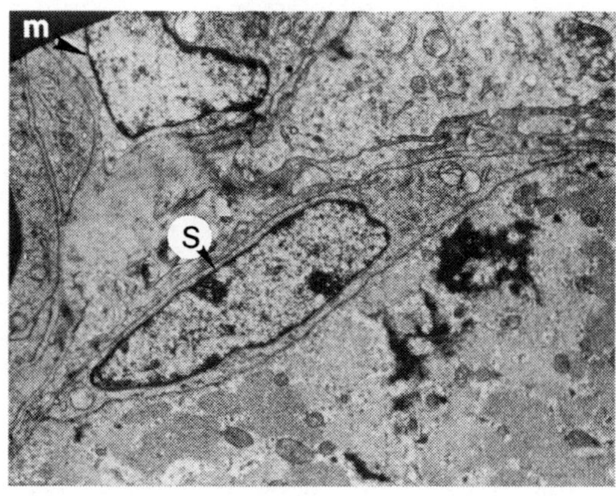

(a)

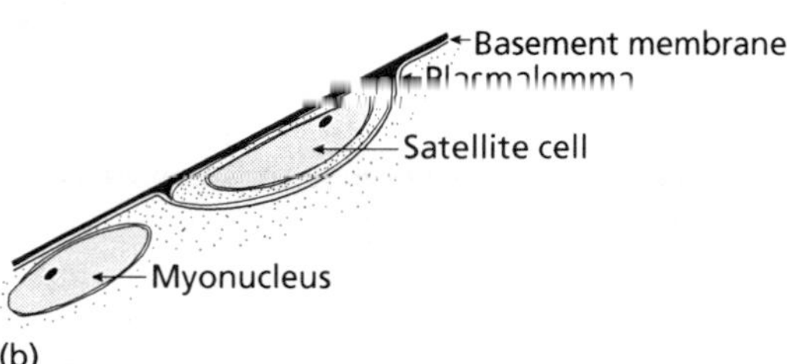

(b)

Fig. 13.4 (a) An electron micrograph showing two satellite cells in wing muscle of a quail that has been subjected to stretch overloading. S indicates a typical satellite cell, while m indicates a satellite cell on an adjacent fibre, at the presumptive myoblast stage and probably in the process of migration. Courtesy of S.E. Alway, West Virginia University. (b) A schematic illustration of a typical satellite cell. The satellite cell can be distinguished from other myonuclei because it lies outside the plasma membrane (plasmalemma). Courtesy of A.J. McComas, McMaster University.

hypothesized to be longitudinal splitting of existing fibres (Hall-Craggs 1970; Gonyea *et al.* 1977), but it is now generally accepted that this is not the mechanism (Snow & Chortkoff 1987) and that new fibres develop from satellite cells (Kennedy *et al.* 1988; Antonio & Gonyea 1993a; Kadi & Thornell 2000). The term 'satellite cell' was first used by Mauro (1961) to describe a type of non-functioning reserve cell that occurs outside the muscle fibre plasma membrane but within the basal lamina (Fig. 13.4). At the light microscope level such cells appear as normal myonuclei, but can be identified at the electron microscope level since myonuclei lie within the plasma membrane. It is thought that these satellite cells are derived from a population of myoblasts that did not fuse to form myotubes and functional fibres during embryonic development (White & Esser 1989).

Satellite cells appear to occur more frequently in the muscles of younger animals and to decrease in frequency as the animal ages (Schultz 1989; White & Esser 1989). In healthy adult humans, satellite cell nuclei constitute approximately 2–4% of all myonuclei detected in electron micrographs (Schmalbruch & Hellhammer 1976; Roth *et al.* 2000) and do not seem to decrease in frequency (Roth *et al.* 2000) or responsiveness (Hikida *et al.* 2000) with ageing. The cells remain quiescent until muscle homeostasis is altered to the point where they become stimulated to undergo rapid proliferation through mitotic division.

Satellite cells are the source for adding myonuclei to muscle fibres as they increase in area and length with maturation or with exercise-induced hypertrophy, thus maintaining their myonuclei to cytoplasmic volume ratio (Kadi & Thornell 2000). Moreover, it appears that their activation is, in fact, necessary for the hypertrophy process to occur in the first place (Rosenblatt *et al.* 1994; Phelan & Gonyea 1997), although not all studies support this concept (Lowe & Alway 1999). A second important function of satellite cells is their role in the regeneration of injured fibres (Bischoff 1989; Schultz 1989). When a traumatic injury such as a crush lesion occurs to a muscle fibre, satellite cells on the injured fibre are activated to undergo mitotic proliferation and to migrate along the length of the fibre to the site of the injury. They then enter the cell and differentiate to repair the damage by forming new myofibrils in the existing fibre, while the debris is removed by macrophages (Chambers & McDermott 1996). If the injury to the fibre is severe, the satellite cells fuse with themselves to form a multinucleated myotube. The myotube then matures into a new muscle fibre through a process similar to that which occurs during fetal development and replaces the necrotic fibre (Bischoff 1989; Schultz 1989). It also appears that, when a fibre is injured, activation of satellite cells is confined to those on the damaged fibre, with little or no recruitment of satellite cells occurring from non-damaged fibres (Schultz *et al.* 1986). If this is the case, and if only one myotube develops per necrotic fibre, then the process is one of *replacement* with no net increase in fibre numbers.

Satellite cell activation with exercise and training

Satellite cell activation has been observed to occur in animals following an acute bout of eccentric (Darr & Schultz 1987), or level (Jacobs *et al.* 1995) treadmill running, as well as chronic resistance training (Giddings *et al.* 1985; Tamaki *et al.* 1997). In these studies, the exercise protocols were also associated with various degrees of fibre damage and the investigators hypothesized that this may have been the mechanism for activation. In humans, satellite cell activation has been documented following a period of cycling (Appell *et al.* 1988) and resistance training (Kadi & Thornell 2000). Although no measurement of tissue damage was made in the latter two studies, it is likely to have occurred, and especially with resistance training. We have quantified electron microscopic evidence of contractile protein damage following a typical weight training session, in both untrained and strength-trained young men. Immediately following the exercise, approximately 80% of the fibres examined in the untrained subjects demonstrated some degree of myofibrillar disruption, with more than 40% displaying what was considered to be extreme disruption (Gibala *et al.* 1995). In the trained subjects, approximately 45% of the fibres showed some degree of disruption, of which only 3% was classified as severe (Gibala *et al.* 2000). In addition, in both investigations it was apparent that greater damage occurred during the lowering or eccentric phase of lifting. It is thus apparent that varying degrees of damage to contractile protein is an inevitable consequence of heavy-resistance training. This damage may result in the activation and proliferation of the satellite cells observed following such training (Kadi & Thornell 2000) for the purpose of fibre repair or replacement. Kadi *et al.* (1999) have observed that approximately 3% of the fibres in needle biopsies of trapezius muscle of elite power lifters were abnormally small in diameter and expressed markers for early myogenesis. This suggests that a constant cycle of muscle damage and repair occurs in athletes undergoing heavy-resistance training. Relatively mild damage is repaired by incorporation of satellite cells into existing fibres, while severely damaged fibres are replaced by fusion of satellite cells to form new fibres. Moreover if, at any one time, 3% of the fibres in strength athletes are 'new' developing fibres (Kadi *et al.* 1999), the process is probably one of replacement, with no net addition of fibre numbers. If this were not the case, then, after several years of resistance training, there would be massive increases in fibre numbers that would be clearly evident.

It is also possible that satellite cells may be activated by processes other than injury (Irintchev & Wernig 1987; Yan 2000) and that they may play an important role in muscle adaptation and fibre type transformation with endurance exercise (Yan 2000). In support of this, there is evidence that they respond to various growth factors that are not necessarily related to muscle injury (Chambers & McDermott 1996; Miller *et al.* 2000).

Summary

Heavy-resistance exercise stimulates an increase in muscle contractile protein synthesis. With repeated bouts of exercise (training), this manifests itself as an increase in cross-sectional fibre and muscle area. The increased fibre area is the result of an increase in myofibrillar area and number. There is also an increase in interstitial connective tissue, that is proportional to the increase in fibre area.

Muscle satellite cells play an important (and perhaps essential) role in the hypertrophy process by maintaining the normal cytoplasmic volume to nuclei ratio as the fibre increases in size, as well as by repairing or replacing fibres that are damaged in training. In some species, and with certain perturbations, such as passive chronic stretch of the wing muscles of the quail, the satellite cells will fuse to form *additional* new fibres, so that there is a net increase in fibre numbers. There is, however, little evidence to indicate that, in humans, heavy-resistance training results in an increase in muscle fibre numbers. One is therefore left to conclude that the new fibres that are formed from satellite cells, in the human training model, replace necrotic fibres, such that little or no net addition occurs in number.

References

Adams, G.R., Hather, B.M., Baldwin, K.M. & Dudley, G.A. (1993) Skeletal muscle myosin heavy chain composition and resistance training. *Journal of Applied Physiology* **74**, 911–915.

Alway, S.E., MacDougall, J.D. & Sale, D.G. (1989a) Contractile adaptations in the human triceps surae after isometric exercise. *Journal of Applied Physiology* **66**, 2725–2732.

Alway, S.E., Winchester, P.K., Davis, M.E. & Gonyea, W.J. (1989b) Regionalized adaptations and muscle fiber proliferation in stretch-induced enlargement. *Journal of Applied Physiology* **66**, 771–781.

Alway, S.E., Gonyea, W.J. & Davis, M.E. (1990) Muscle fiber formation and fiber hypertrophy during the onset of stretch-overload. *American Journal of Physiology* **259**, C92–102.

Andersen, J.L. & Aagaard, P. (2000) Myosin heavy chain IIX overshoot in human skeletal muscle. *Muscle and Nerve* **23**, 1095–1104.

Antonio, J. & Gonyea, W.J. (1993a) Progressive stretch overload of skeletal muscle results in hypertrophy before hyperplasia. *Journal of Applied Physiology* **75**, 1263–1271.

Antonio, J. & Gonyea, W.J. (1993b) Skeletal muscle fiber hyperplasia. *Medicine and Science in Sports and Exercise* **25**, 1333–1345.

Appell, H.J., Forsberg, S. & Hollmann, W. (1988) Satellite cell activation in human skeletal muscle after training: evidence for muscle fiber neoformation. *International Journal of Sports Medicine* **9**, 297–299.

Ashmore, C.R. & Summers, P.J. (1981) Stretch-induced growth in chicken wing muscles: myofibrillar proliferation. *American Journal of Physiology* **241**, C93–C97.

Baldwin, K.M. & Haddad, F. (2001) Effects of different activity and inactivity paradigms on myosin heavy chain gene expression in striated muscle. *Journal of Applied Physiology* **90**, 345–557.

Biolo, G., Maggi, S.P., Williams, B.D., Tipton, K.D. & Wolfe, R.R. (1995) Increased rates of muscle protein turnover and amino acid transport after resistance exercise in humans. *American Journal of Physiology* **268**, E514–E520.

Bischoff, R. (1989) Analysis of muscle regeneration using single myofibers in culture. *Medicine and Science in Sports and Exercise* **21** (Suppl.), S164–S172.

Brown, A.B., McCartney, N., Moroz, D., Sale, D. & MacDougall, J.D. (1988) Strength training effects in aging. *Medicine and Science in Sports and Exercise* **20**, S80.

Carroll, T.J., Abernethy, P.J., Logan, P.A., Barber, M. & McEniery, M.T. (1998) Resistance training frequency: strength and myosin heavy chain responses to two and three bouts per week. *European Journal of Applied Physiology and Occupational Physiology* **78**, 270–275.

Chambers, R.L. & McDermott, J.C. (1996) Molecular basis of skeletal muscle regeneration. *Canadian Journal of Applied Physiology* **21**, 155–184.

Chesley, A., MacDougall, J.D., Tarnopolsky, M.A., Atkinson, S.A. & Smith, K. (1992) Changes in human muscle protein synthesis after resistance exercise. *Journal of Applied Physiology* **73**, 1383–1388.

Chiakulus, J.J. & Pauly, J.E. (1965) A study of post-natal growth of skeletal muscle in the rat. *Anatomical Record* **152**, 55–62.

Chilibeck, P.D., Syrotuik, D.G. & Bell, G.J. (1999) The effect of strength training on estimates of mitochondrial density and distribution throughout muscle fibres. *European Journal of Applied Physiology and Occupational Physiology* **80**, 604–609.

Darr, K.C. & Schultz, E. (1987) Exercise-induced satellite cell activation in growing and mature skeletal muscle. *Journal of Applied Physiology* **63**, 1816–1821.

Fischmann, D.A. (1972) Development of striated muscle. In: *The Structure and Function of Muscle: Structure*, Part 1, Vol. 1 (ed. G.H. Bourne), pp. 75–148. Academic Press, New York.

Fowles, J.R., MacDougall, J.D., Tarnopolsky, M.A., Sale, D.G., Roy, B.D. & Yarasheski, K.E. (2000) The effects of acute passive stretch on muscle protein synthesis in humans. *Canadian Journal of Applied Physiology* **25**, 165–180.

Gibala, M.J., MacDougall, J.D., Tarnopolsky, M.A., Stauber, W.T. & Elorriaga, A. (1995) Changes in human skeletal muscle ultrastructure and force production after acute resistance exercise. *Journal of Applied Physiology* **78**, 702–708.

Gibala, M.J., Interisano, S.A., Tarnopolsky, M.A. *et al.* (2000) Myofibrillar disruption following acute concentric and eccentric resistance exercise in strength-trained men. *Canadian Journal of Physiology and Pharmacology* **78**, 656–661.

Giddings, C.J., Neaves, W.B. & Gonyea, W.J. (1985) Muscle fiber necrosis and regeneration induced by prolonged weight-lifting exercise in the cat. *Anatomical Record* **211**, 133–141.

Giddings, C.J. & Gonyea, W.J. (1992) Morphological observations supporting muscle fiber hyperplasia following weight-lifting exercise in cats. *Anatomical Record* **233**, 178–195.

Goldberg, A.L., Etlinger, J.D., Goldspink, D.F. & Jablecki, C. (1975) Mechanism of work-induced hypertrophy of skeletal muscle. *Medicine and Science in Sports and Exercise* **7**, 185–198.

Goldspink, G. (1970) The proliferation of myofibrils during muscle fiber growth. *Journal of Cell Science* **6**, 593–603.

Goldspink, G. (1974) Development of muscle. In: *Growth of Cells in Vertebrate Tissues* (ed. G. Goldspink), pp. 69–99. Chapman & Hall, London.

Goldspink, G. (1992) Cellular and molecular aspects of adaptation in skeletal muscle. In: *Strength and Power in Sport* (ed. P.V. Komi), pp. 211–229. Blackwell Scientific Publications, Oxford.

Goldspink, G. & Howells, K.F. (1974) Work-induced hypertrophy in exercised normal muscles of different ages and the reversibility of hypertrophy after cessation of exercise. *Journal of Physiology* **239**, 179–193.

Gollnick, P.D., Timson, B.F., Moore, R.L. & Reidy, M. (1981) Muscle enlargement and number of fibers in skeletal muscle of rats. *Journal of Applied Physiology* **50**, 939–943.

Gonyea, W.J. (1980) Role of exercise in inducing increases in skeletal muscle fiber number. *Journal of Applied Physiology* **48**, 421–426.

Gonyea, W.J. & Ericson, G.C. (1976) An experimental model for the study of exercise-induced skeletal muscle hypertrophy. *Journal of Applied Physiology* **40**, 630–633.

Gonyea, W., Ericson, G.C. & Bonde-Peterson, F. (1977) Skeletal muscle fiber splitting induced by weight lifting exercise in cats. *Acta Physiologica Scandinavica* **99**, 105–109.

Gonyea, W.J., Sale, D., Gonyea, Y. & Mikesky, A. (1986) Exercise induced increases in muscle fiber number. *European Journal of Applied Physiology* **55**, 137–141.

Green, H., Goreham, C., Ouyang, J., Ball-Burnett, M. & Ranney, D. (1999) Regulation of fiber size, oxidative potential, and capillarization in human muscle by resistance exercise. *American Journal of Physiology* **276**, R591–R596.

Hall-Craggs, E.C.B. (1970) The longitudinal division of overloaded skeletal muscle fibers. *Journal of Anatomy* **107**, 459–470.

Hikida, R.S., Staron, R.S., Hagerman, F.C. *et al.* (2000) Effects of high-intensity resistance training on untrained older men. II. Muscle fiber characteristics and nucleo-cytoplasmic relationships. *Journals of Gerontology Series A: Biological Sciences and Medical Sciences* **55**, B347–B354.

Ho, K.W., Roy, R.R., Tweedle, C.D., Heusner, W.W., Van Huss, W.D. & Carrow, R.E. (1980) Skeletal muscle fiber splitting with weight-lifting exercise in rats. *American Journal of Anatomy* **157**, 433–440.

Irintchev, A. & Wernig, A. (1987) Muscle damage and repair in voluntarily running mice: strain and muscle differences. *Cell and Tissue Research* **249**, 509–521.

Jacobs, S.C., Wokke, J.H., Bar, P.R. & Bootsma, A.L. (1995) Satellite cell activation after muscle damage in young and adult rats. *Anatomical Record* **242**, 329–336.

Kadi, F. & Thornell, L.E. (2000) Concomitant increases in myonuclear and satellite cell content of female trapezius muscle following strength training. *Histochemistry and Cell Biology* **113**, 99–103.

Kadi, F., Eriksson, A., Holmner, S., Butler-Browne, G.S. & Thornell, L.E. (1999) Cellular adaptation of the trapezius muscle in strength-trained athletes. *Histochemistry and Cell Biology* **111**, 189–195.

Kelley, G. (1996) Mechanical overload and skeletal muscle fiber hyperplasia: a meta analysis. *Journal of Applied Physiology* **81**, 1584–1588.

Kennedy, J.M., Eisenberg, B.R., Reid, S.K., Sweeney, L.J. & Zak, R. (1988) Nascent muscle fiber appearance in overloaded chicken slow-tonic muscle. *American Journal of Anatomy* **181**, 203–215.

Larsson, L. & Tesch, P.A. (1986) Motor unit fiber density in extremely hypertrophied skeletal muscles in man. *European Journal of Applied Physiology* **55**, 130–136.

Lüthi, J.M., Howald, H., Classen, H., Rosler, K., Vock, P. & Hoppeler, H. (1986) Structural changes in skeletal muscle tissue with heavy-resistance exercise. *International Journal of Sports Medicine* **7**, 123–127.

Lowe, D.A. & Alway, S.E. (1999) Stretch-induced myogenin, MyoD, and MRF4 expression and acute hypertrophy in quail slow-tonic muscle are not dependent upon satellite cell proliferation. *Cell and Tissue Research* **296**, 531–539.

McCall, G.E., Byrnes, W.C., Dickinson, A., Pattany, P.M. & Fleck, S.J. (1996) Muscle fiber hypertrophy, hyperplasia, and capillary density in college men after resistance training. *Journal of Applied Physiology* **81**, 2004–2012.

McDonagh, M.J.N. & Davies, C.T.M. (1984) Adaptive response of mammalian muscle to exercise with high loads. *European Journal of Applied Physiology* **52**, 139–155.

MacDougall, J.D. (1986a) Adaptability of muscle to strength training—a cellular approach. In: *Biochemistry of Exercise VI*, Vol. 16 (ed. B. Saltin), pp. 501–513. Human Kinetics, Champaign, Illinois.

MacDougall, J.D. (1986b) Morphological changes in human skeletal muscle following strength training and immobilization. In: *Human Muscle Power* (eds N. L. Jones, N. McCartney & A.L. McComas), pp. 269–288. Human Kinetics, Champaign, Illinois.

MacDougall, J.D., Sale, D.G., Moroz, J.R., Elder, G.C.B., Sutton, J.R. & Howald, H. (1979) Mitochondrial volume density in human skeletal muscle following heavy resistance training. *Medicine and Science in Sports* **11**, 164–166.

MacDougall, J.D., Elder, G.C.B., Sale, D.G., Moroz, J.R. & Sutton, J.R. (1980) Effects of strength training and immobilization on human muscle fibers. *European Journal of Applied Physiology* **43**, 25–34.

MacDougall, J.D., Sale, D.G., Elder, G.C.B. & Sutton, J.R. (1982) Muscle ultrastructural characteristics of elite powerlifters and bodybuilders. *European Journal of Applied Physiology* **48**, 117–126.

MacDougall, J.D., Sale, D.G., Alway, S.E. & Sutton, J.R. (1984) Muscle fiber number in biceps brachii in bodybuilders and control subjects. *Journal of Applied Physiology* **57**, 1399–1403.

MacDougall, J.D., Gibala, M.J., Tarnopolsky, M.A., MacDonald, J.R., Interisano, S.A. & Yarasheski, K.E. (1995) The time course for elevated muscle protein synthesis following heavy resistance exercise. *Canadian Journal of Applied Physiology* **20**, 480–486.

Malina, R.M. (1986) Growth of muscle tissue and muscle mass. In: *Human Growth A Comprehensive Treatise*, Vol. 2 (eds F. Falkner & J. M. Tanner), pp. 77–99. Plenum Press, New York.

Mastaglia, F.L. (1981) Growth and development of the skeletal muscles. In: *Scientific Foundations of Paediatrics* (eds J.A. Davis & J. Dobbing), pp. 590–620. Heinemann, London.

Masuda, K., Choi, J.Y., Shimojo, H. & Katsuta, S. (1999) Maintenance of myoglobin concentration in human skeletal muscle after heavy resistance training. *European Journal of Applied Physiology and Occupational Physiology* **79**, 347–352.

Mauro, A. (1961) Satellite cells of skeletal muscle fibers. *Journal of Biophysical and Biochemical Cytology* **9**, 493–495.

Miller, K.J., Thaloor, D., Matteson, S. & Pavlath, G.K. (2000) Hepatocyte growth factor affects satellite cell activation and differentiation in regenerating skeletal muscle. *American Journal of Physiology—Cell Physiology* **278**, C174–C181.

Morpurgo, B. (1897) Überaktivitäts-Hypertrophie der Willkürlichen Muskeln. *Virchows Archives fur Pathologische Anatomie und Physiologie* **15**, 522–554.

Moss, F.P. & LeBlond, C.P. (1971) Satellite cells as the source of nuclei in muscles of growing rats. *Anatomical Record* **170**, 421–436.

Ontell, J. & Dunn, R.F. (1978) Neonatal muscle growth: a quantitative study. *American Journal of Anatomy* **152**, 539–556.

Phelan, J.N. & Gonyea, W.J. (1997) Effect of radiation on satellite cell activity and protein expression in overloaded mammalian skeletal muscle. *Anatomical Record* **247**, 179–188.

Phillips, S.M., Tipton, K.D., Aarsland, A., Wolf, S.E. & Wolfe, R.R. (1997) Mixed muscle protein synthesis and breakdown after resistance exercise in humans. *American Journal of Physiology* **273**, E99–E107.

Rayne, J. & Crawford, G.N.C. (1975) Increase in fiber numbers of the rat pterygoid muscles during postnatal growth. *Journal of Anatomy* **118**, 347–357.

Reitsma, W. (1969) Skeletal muscle hypertrophy after heavy exercise in rats with surgically reduced muscle function. *American Journal of Physical Medicine* **48**, 237–259.

Rosenblatt, J.D., Yong, D. & Parry, D.J. (1994) Satellite cell activity is required for hypertrophy of overloaded rat muscle. *Muscle and Nerve* **17**, 608–613.

Roth, S.M., Martel, G.F., Ivey, F.M. *et al.* (2000) Skeletal muscle satellite cell populations in healthy young and older men and women. *Anatomical Record* **260**, 351–358.

Sale, D., Quinlan, J., Marsh, E., McComas, A.J. & Belanger, A.Y. (1982) Influence of joint position on ankle plantarflexion in humans. *Journal of Applied Physiology* **52**, 1636–1642.

Sale, D.G., MacDougall, J.D., Jacobs, I. & Garner, S. (1990) Interaction between concurrent strength and endurance training. *Journal of Applied Physiology* **68**, 260–270.

Schmalbruch, H. & Hellhammer, U. (1976) The number of satellite cells in normal human tissue. *Anatomical Record* **185**, 279–288.

Schultz, E. (1989) Satellite cell behavior during skeletal muscle growth and regeneration. *Medicine and Science in Sports and Exercise* **21** (Suppl.), S181–S186.

Schultz, E., Jaryszak, D.L., Gibson, M.C. & Albright, D.J. (1986) Absence of exogenous satellite cell contribution to regeneration of frozen skeletal muscle. *Journal of Muscle Research and Cell Motility* **7**, 361–367.

Sjostrom, M., Lexell, J., Eriksson, A. & Taylor, C.C. (1991) Evidence of fibre hyperplasia in human skeletal muscles from healthy young men? A left–right comparison of the fibre number in whole anterior tibialis muscles. *European Journal of Applied Physiology and Occupational Physiology* **62**, 301–304.

Snow, M.H. & Chortkoff, B.S. (1987) Frequency of bifurcated muscle fibers in hypertrophic rat soleus muscle. *Muscle and Nerve* **10**, 312–317.

Sola, O.M., Christensen, D.L. & Martin, A.W. (1973) Hypertrophy and hyperplasia of adult chicken anterior latissimus dorsi muscles following stretch with and without denervation. *Experimental Neurology* **41**, 76–100.

Staron, R.S., Malicky, E.S., Leonardi, M.J., Falkel, J.E., Hagerman, F.C. & Dudley, G.A. (1990) Muscle hypertrophy and fast fiber type conversions in heavy resistance-trained women. *European Journal of Applied Physiology and Occupational Physiology* **60**, 71–79.

Staron, R.S., Karapondo, D.L., Kraemer, W.J. *et al.* (1994) Skeletal muscle adaptations during early phase of heavy-resistance training in men and women. *Journal of Applied Physiology* **76**, 1247–1255.

Tamaki, T., Uchiyama, S. & Nakano, S. (1992) A weight-lifting exercise model for inducing hypertrophy in the hindlimb muscle of rats. *Medicine and Science in Sports and Exercise* **24**, 881–886.

Tamaki, T., Akatsuka, A., Tokunaga, M., Ishige, K., Uchiyama, S. & Shiraishi, T. (1997) Morphological and biochemical evidence of muscle hyperplasia following weight-lifting exercise in rats. *American Journal of Physiology* **273**, C246–C256.

Tesch, P.A. (1987) Acute and long-term metabolic changes consequent to heavy-resistance exercise. *Medicine and Science in Sports and Exercise* **26**, 67–87.

Tesch, P.A. & Larsson, L. (1982) Muscle hypertrophy in bodybuilders. *European Journal of Applied Physiology* **49**, 301–306.

Tesch, P.A., Thorrson, A. & Kaiser, P. (1984) Muscle capillary supply and fiber type characteristics in weight and power lifters. *Journal of Applied Physiology* **56**, 35–38.

Tesch, P.A., Häkinen, K. & Komi, P.V. (1985) The effect of strength training and detraining on various enzyme activities. *Medicine and Science in Sports and Exercise* **17**, 245.

Thorstensson, A. (1976) Muscle strength, fiber types and enzyme activities in man. *Acta Physiologica Scandinavica* **433** (Suppl.), 1–44.

Timson, B.F. (1990) Evaluation of animal models for the study of exercise-induced muscle enlargement. *Journal of Applied Physiology* **69**, 1935–1945.

Timson, B.F., Bowlin, B.K., Dudenhoeffer, G.A. & George, J.B. (1985) Fiber number, area and composition of mouse soleus muscle following enlargement. *Journal of Applied Physiology* **58**, 619–624.

Welle, S., Bhatt, K. & Thornton, C.A. (1999) Stimulation of myofibrillar synthesis by exercise is mediated by more efficient translation of mRNA. *Journal of Applied Physiology* **86**, 1220–1225.

White, T.P. & Esser, K.A. (1989) Satellite cell and growth factor involvement in skeletal muscle growth. *Medicine and Science in Sports and Exercise* **21** (Suppl.), S158–S163.

Wong, T.S. & Booth, F.W. (1988) Skeletal muscle enlargement with weight-lifting exercise by rats. *Journal of Applied Physiology* **65**, 950–954.

Yan, Z. (2000) Skeletal muscle adaptation and cell cycle regulation. *Exercise and Sport Sciences Reviews* **28**, 24–26.

Yarasheski, K.E., Lemon, P.W. & Gilloteaux, J. (1990) Effect of heavy-resistance exercise training on muscle fiber composition in young rats. *Journal of Applied Physiology* **69**, 434–437.

Chapter 14

Acute and Chronic Muscle Metabolic Adaptations to Strength Training

PER A. TESCH AND BJÖRN A. ALKNER

Strength exercise is always performed intermittently. Training with very heavy loads (close to or at one repetition maximum) and performed with few (one to three) repetitions is usually followed by relatively long (more than 5 min) rest periods. This is a strategy practised by power lifters and athletes aimed at developing maximum force and power. The majority of resistive exercise programmes employ a sequence or a set of consecutive coupled concentric and eccentric muscle actions (6–15 repetitions), typically followed by a rest period and then repeated two to four or perhaps even more times. In exercise sessions utilizing less heavy loads and where sets comprise approximately 12–15 repetitions carried out until muscular failure, the rest period between sets is typically less than 2 min. A complete exercise session emphasizing several muscle groups may comprise up to 10–12 different exercises. It is imperative that the acute metabolic stress and the subsequent chronic muscular adaptations are impacted by the design of the exercise task being performed. Thus, the myriad of possible programme variations and hence exercise stimulus should be appreciated.

Acute adaptations to strength exercise

During an exercise session involving the large muscle groups of the lower limbs while performing the leg press or the squat, oxygen uptake is about 50–60% of maximal aerobic power in strength-trained or untrained men (Fig. 14.1; Dudley *et al.* 1991). The seated, one-joint knee extension, which isolates the quadriceps muscle, is carried out at a considerably lower oxygen cost than the squat that uses additional muscle groups. The energy turnover for exercises involving less muscle mass, e.g. upper body exercises, is much lower. Moreover, because the energy turnover during eccentric exercise is only about one-eighth of the energy required to perform the task by means of a concentric action (Asmussen 1953), resistance exercise emphasizing eccentric actions is carried out at a very low oxygen uptake. Although it is evident that eccentric actions are essential in order to optimize muscle growth and increases in strength in response to strength training, it appears they contribute little to enhancement of oxidative capacity of muscle.

Despite the apparently low oxygen uptake all available major energy sources are mobilized during an exercise session aimed at increasing muscle mass. Thus, in resistive exercise, typically performed by bodybuilders, adenosine triphosphate (ATP), creatine phosphate and glycogen decreased in response to 30 min of exercise performed at a calculated power output of approximately 200 W. There were also marked increases in the concentration of blood lactate and intramuscular lactate, glucose, glucose 6-phosphate and glycerol 3-phosphate, indicating a high rate of anaerobic glycolysis (Table 14.1; Tesch *et al.* 1986). Although anaerobic non-glycolytic and glycolytic energy sources were utilized, there was evidence of lipids being mobilized as substrate as well. This was evident in that plasma

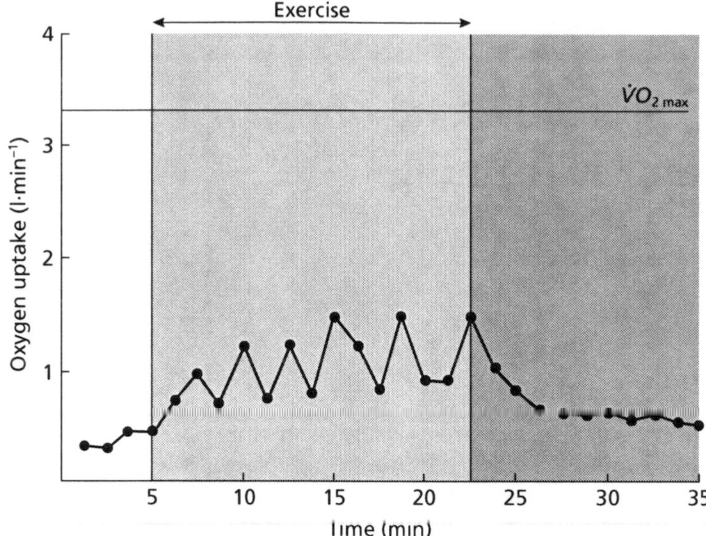

Fig. 14.1 Oxygen uptake before, during and after supine leg press exercise in untrained men ($n = 8$). Subjects performed 5 sets of 6–12 repetitions per set. Each set was followed by 3 min of rest. Expired gas was collected continuously and oxygen uptake analysed using an on-line system. Each data point represents the mean value for every 2.5-min period. (From Dudley *et al.* 1991.)

Table 14.1 Muscle metabolite contents (mmol·kg^{-1} d.w.) and plasma metabolite concentrations (mmol·l^{-1}) before (after warm-up) and at cessation of 30 min of strength exercise comprising 4 sets (6–12 repetitions per set) each of front and back squat, leg press and leg extension. Subjects were male bodybuilders ($n = 9$). Differences ($P < 0.05$) between mean values are denoted by *. (From Tesch *et al.* 1986 and Essén-Gustavsson & Tesch 1990.)

	Pre-exercise	Postexercise	Difference
Muscle			
ATP	24.8	19.7	*
Creatine phosphate	89.5	45.8	*
Creatine	50.8	100.0	*
Glucose	1.5	8.2	*
Glucose 6-phosphate	1.8	16.7	*
Glycerol 3-phosphate	5.7	14.1	*
Lactate	22.7	79.5	*
Glycogen	690	495	*
Triglyceride	23.9	16.7	$P > 0.05$
Plasma			
Free fatty acids	0.22	0.22	$P > 0.05$
Glycerol	0.02	0.1	*
Glucose	4.2	5.5	*
Lactate	3.8	11.7	*

glycerol concentration increased and, surprisingly, most individuals showed decreased muscle triglyceride content after exercise (Table 14.1; Essén-Gustavsson & Tesch 1990).

It seems plausible though that resistance exercise, simulating competition, can be executed solely at the expense of the available ATP and creatine phosphate stores (Keul *et al.* 1978) providing very few muscle actions are performed in a sequence, and that there is ample time allowed for during the recovery that follows. A marked drop in creatine phosphate occurs after only one set of 12 arm curls to failure (MacDougall *et al.* 1999), with no measurable decrease in ATP

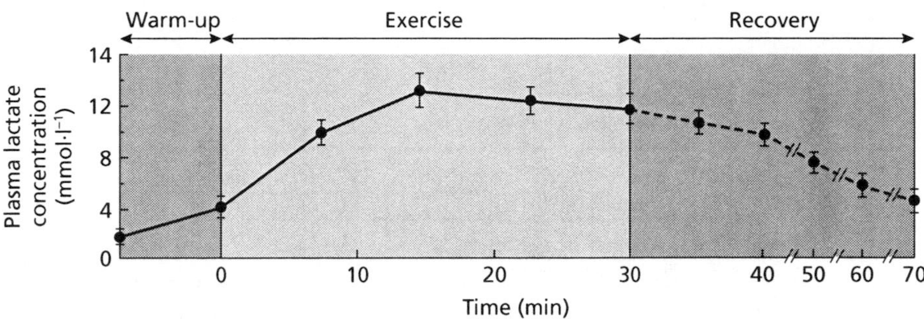

Fig. 14.2 Plasma lactate concentration before and during strength exercise and the subsequent recovery. Values are mean ± SD. (From Tesch *et al.* 1986.)

content. A single set is, however, sufficient to stress glycogenolysis as well, because glycogen decreased 12 and 24% after 2 additional sets. There was a 25% drop in muscle glycogen content 6 h after exhaustive resistance exercise comprising about 9 sets of 6 repetitions of knee extensions until failure (Pascoe *et al.* 1993); and four consecutive elbow extensor exercises, each performed using 4 sets of 8–12 repetitions to failure, decreased the glycogen stores of the long head of triceps brachii about 25% (Yström & Tesch 1996, unpublished results). The results of these studies provide evidence that the intramuscular glycogen store is the most important energy source in resistance exercise. One would expect that regimens relying on lower resistance, higher number of repetitions and short recovery periods would call for greater reliance upon anaerobic glycolytic and oxidative meta-bolism (Fig. 14.2; Tesch *et al.* 1986). Hence, plasma lactate levels are higher during such an exercise regimen compared to that carried out with a higher load and lower number of repetitions (Kraemer *et al.* 1987). However, glycogen decreased and lactate increased at similar rates using programmes at set work but using different number of repetitions and load, i.e. 35 or 70% of one repetition maximum (1 RM) (Robergs *et al.* 1991).

It should be recalled that it is not known whether metabolic stress *per se* influences increases in muscle mass, or maximal strength or power. From classical studies of the selective glycogen depletion pattern, using semiquantitative histochemical (periodic acid–Schiff, PAS) staining procedures, it appears that forces below 20% of maximum voluntary isometric force are sustained by recruitment of Type I muscle fibres only (Gollnick *et al.* 1974). To produce higher forces Type II fibres must be brought into play, as evidenced by a progressively greater rate of glycogen loss when the level of sustained tension is increased. In support, Type I and IIa were depleted, yet not voided, after 5 sets of 10 knee extensions at 30 and 45% of 1 RM (Tesch *et al.* 1998). At 60% there was greater depletion and glycogen levels dropped in Type IIb and IIab fibres as well, as evidenced from analyses of the optical density of PAS-stained fibres. This would infer these fibres are involved at loads lower than what is generally believed.

As a consequence, in resistance exercise typical for weight trainees and carried out with loads equal to about 70% of the maximum load lifted, Type II fibres show greater depletion than Type I fibres. Indeed, after performing 20 sets of 6–12 repetitions each of four different quadriceps exercises (see Tesch *et al.* 1986), Type II fibres showed greater glycogen loss than Type I fibres. At cessation of exercise, no Type I fibres, but 15% of the Type II fibres examined were glycogen voided. Although strenuous strength training appears not to exhaust the glycogen stores, the high rate of glycogen utilization may be sufficient to deplete certain muscle fibres. This in turn may limit the ability to perform in single or multiple daily exercise sessions.

Table 14.2 Fibre type composition, assessed by means of histochemical ATPase stains, in different categories of strength-trained athletes. Myosin heavy chain (MHC) content was analysed in single fibres* or whole-muscle homogenates†. Some studies also incorporated control subjects. Muscles studied are shown as: VL, vastus lateralis; Delt, deltoid; Lat Gast, lateral gastrocnemius; M Gast, medial gastrocnemius; Sol, soleus; BicBr, biceps brachii; Trap, trapezius.

				Fibre type composition (%)				
Author	Year	Subjects: *n*; gender; category; age	Muscle	I	I/IIa	IIa	IIa/b	IIb/x
Prince *et al.*	1976	4; M; power lifters	VL	45		11		33
		5; ctrl (no training)	VL	36		38		26
Tesch *et al.*	1984	8; M; weight-/ power lifters; 27 yrs	VL				59	
		8; M; ctrl (pilots); 26 yrs	VL				61	
Staron *et al.*	1984	7; M; weightlifters; 24 yrs, > 3 yrs training, 4–6 days/week	VL	38	0.3	40		22
		5; M; untrained ctrl; 29 yrs	VL	23	0	34		43
Larsson & Tesch	1986	4; M; bodybuilders; 30 yrs	VL				48	
		8; M; ctrl; 26 yrs	VL				51	
Gollnick *et al.*	1972	4; M; weightlifters; 25 yrs	VL	46				
		12; M; untrained; 27 yrs	VL	36				
Tesch & Larsson	1982	3; M; bodybuilders; 25 yrs	VL			40		4
		50; ctrl (students); 23 yrs	VL				53	
Tesch & Karlsson	1985	7; M; weight-/power lifters	VL	44				
		12; M; PE students; 22 yrs	VL	43				
Gollnick *et al.*	1972	4; M; weightlifters; 25 yrs	Delt	53				
		12; M; untrained; 27 yrs	Delt	46				
Tesch & Larsson	1982	3; M; bodybuilders; 25 yrs	Delt			33		3
		12; ctrl (PE students); 23 yrs	Delt				50	
Tesch & Karlsson	1985	7; M; weight-/power lifters	Delt	54				
		12; M; PE students; 22 yrs	Delt	50				
Schantz & Källman	1989	12; M; strength-trained; 25 yrs	Delt	67		21		12
		12; M; untrained; 26 yrs	Delt	59		23		18
Alway	1991	6; M; bodybuilders; 27 yrs	Lat Gast	53			47	
		6; M; active; 28 yrs	Lat Gast	53			47	
		6; M; sedentary; 25 yrs	Lat Gast	51			49	
Alway	1991	6; M; bodybuilders; 27 yrs	M Gast	56			44	
		6; M; active; 28 yrs	M Gast	65			35	
		6; M; sedentary; 25 yrs	M Gast	57			43	
Alway	1991	6; M; bodybuilders, 27 yrs	Sol	74			27	
		6; M; active; 28 yrs	Sol	73			27	
		6; M; sedentary; 25 yrs	Sol	80			19	
Klitgaard *et al.*	1990	4; M; bodybuilders; 25 yrs, > 6yrs training	BicBr	51	0	31		18
		4; M; sedentary ctrl; 28 yrs	BicBr	48	0	25		26
		4; M; bodybuilders; 25 yrs, * > 6 yrs training	BicBr	41	6	36	16	1
		4; M; sedentary ctrl; 28 yrs	BicBr	36	6	12	34	12
Kadi *et al.*	1999	10; M; power lifters; 28 yrs	Trap	55	2	39	4	0
		6; M; ctrl; 23 yrs	Trap	64	0.2	26	10	0.2
		† 10; M; power lifters; 28 yrs	Trap	47		44		9
		6; M; ctrl; 23 yrs	Trap	54		27		19

Chronic adaptations to strength exercise

Most effective strength training programmes produce increased muscle cross-sectional area and hence muscle mass, mainly due to an increase in myofibrillar protein content (see Chapter 13). In response to short-term training programmes, however, appreciable increases in muscle strength and strength-related performances are possible with no or minute concomitant muscle hypertrophy (see Chapter 15). This is important to keep in mind when discussing the specific metabolic adaptations that occur in response to strength training because some of the changes described below occur secondary to training-induced muscle hypertrophy. Moreover, one should bear in mind that the magnitude, but also specifics of adaptations to resistance exercise, or any other type of exercise, are impacted by factors such as age, initial fitness level and past training history.

Fibre type composition

Endurance training induces a shift in fibre type composition, at least temporarily, promoting transformation of fast-twitch to slow-twitch fibres (cf. Saltin & Gollnick 1983). It appears that trained muscles of successful Olympic weightlifters and power lifters and other power athletes do not necessarily possess a predominance of fast-twitch fibres (Table 14.2; Gollnick *et al.* 1972; Prince *et al.* 1976; Staron *et al.* 1984; Tesch *et al.* 1984; Tesch & Karlsson 1985; Kadi *et al.* 1999). If they do, this is unlikely to be the result of the specific training carried out by these athletes. More likely this reflects the success of athletes with the genetics to build muscle and develop speed, power and strength. Since resistance exercise clearly promotes preferential fast-twitch fibre hypertrophy, a typical characteristic of these athletes is that perhaps 80–90% of the trained muscle comprises fast contractile protein. In bodybuilders of various calibres, a wide range in fibre type composition of vastus lateralis, deltoid, biceps brachii and triceps brachii muscles has been reported (MacDougall *et al.* 1982; Schantz 1982; Tesch & Larsson 1982; Dudley *et al.* 1986; Larsson & Tesch 1986; Essén-Gustavsson & Tesch 1990; Klitgaard *et al.* 1990). It has been repeatedly shown in a large number of studies of men or women (Table 14.3), that resistance training programmes induce no change in Type I percentage (Frontera *et al.* 1988; Brown *et al.* 1990; Staron *et al.* 1990; Alway 1991; Charette *et al.* 1991; Hather *et al.* 1991; Staron *et al.* 1991; Adams *et al.* 1993; Fry *et al.* 1994; Ploutz *et al.* 1994; Kraemer *et al.* 1995; Lexell *et al.* 1995; Jürimäe *et al.* 1996; McCall *et al.* 1996; Hepple *et al.* 1997; Carroll *et al.* 1998; Bishop *et al.* 1999; Green *et al.* 1999; King *et al.* 1999; Masuda *et al.* 1999; Andersen & Aagaard 2000; Hikida *et al.* 2000).

The finding of a decrease (Kadi & Thornell 1999) in the Type I fibre percentage of trapezius muscle following a resistance exercise regimen comprising 3 sets of 10–12 repetitions of various upper-body and shoulder exercises and performed by middle-aged women is in frank contrast, and the results are not readily explained. Further, two studies implementing 12 weeks of resistance training in older men (Williamson *et al.* 2000), and in men who had previously been immobilized by means of casting (Hortobágyi *et al.* 2000), respectively, reported increased Type I fibre percentages. The results of these studies merely demonstrate the plasticity of skeletal muscle in that there is a shift from Type II to Type I fibres in response to resistance training employed following months or years of muscle disuse.

Using standard histochemical staining procedures for ATPase (Staron *et al.* 1990; Hather *et al.* 1991; Wang *et al.* 1993; Ploutz *et al.* 1994; Kraemer *et al.* 1995), or measuring myosin heavy chain isoform content or pattern (Carroll *et al.* 1998; Kadi & Thornell 1999), or by employing both techniques (Adams *et al.* 1993; Fry *et al.* 1994; Andersen & Aagaard 2000; Hikida *et al.* 2000; Hortobágyi *et al.* 2000), several studies have shown or inferred a shift from Type IIb/IIx to Type IIa fibres or that fibres expressing MHC IIb/IIx isoforms decreased after strength training programmes of varying intensity and duration. Thus either the percentage of Type IIa increased or that of Type IIb/IIx decreased or

Table 14.3 (a) Resistance training studies reporting fibre type composition in the vastus lateral is muscle, assessed using either ATPase stains or single-fibre myosin heavy chain (MHC) content. Only studies that examined subgroups of Type II fibres are listed. ↑, increase in percentage of that fibre type; ↓, decrease in percentage; →, unchanged percentage; ⇑, increase in fibre area; ⇓, decrease in fibre area; ⇒, unchanged fibre area; >, increased relative area occupied by this fibre type, <, decreased relative area occupied by this fibre type; =, no change in relative area occupied by this fibre type. con, concentric; ecc, eccentric.

Author	Year	Subjects: *n*; gender; age	Duration, frequency and sets/repetitions	Fibre type (%) I	I/IIa	IIa	IIa/b	IIb/x	Comment
Lüthi *et al.*	1986	8; M; 18 yrs	6 weeks, 3/week, 1 × 8–9	→		→		→	'Healthy'
Staron *et al.*	1990	24; F; 23 yrs	20 weeks, 2/week, 3 × 6–8	→	→	↑	→	↓	10 active, 14 inactive
Staron *et al.*	1991	6; F; 21 yrs; previously trained, 30 weeks detrained	6 weeks, 2/week, 3 × 6–8	→ ⇒	→	→ ⇑	→	↓ ⇑	Students
		7; F; 21 yrs; not previously trained	6 weeks, 2/week, 3 × 6–8	↑ ⇑	→	→ ⇑	→	↓ ⇑	
Hather *et al.*	1991	34 (8 + 8 + 10 + 8 ctrl), M; middle-aged	19 weeks training, 2/week, 4–5 × 6–12 (con/ecc, con, con/con)	→ ⇑		↑	⇑	↓	Untrained
Adams *et al.*	1993	17 (13 + 4 ctrl); M; 36 yrs	19 weeks, 2/week, 3–5 × 6–12 RM	→		↑		↓	'Healthy'
Wang *et al.*	1993	12; F	20 weeks, 2/week, 3 × 6–8	⇑		↑⇑	⇑	↓⇑	Students
Andersen *et al.*	1994	14; M; 25 yrs strength + ctrl	12 weeks, 3/week, 4 × 8	→ ⇒		↓ ⇒	↑	↑ ⇒	Soccer players, off-season*
				→		→		→	MHC
Andersen *et al.*	1994	6; M; 23 yrs	3 months training, 6/week, strength 2.5/week, 1–8 RM	↓		↑		↓	Sprinters, sprint and strength training*
				↓	→	↑	↓	→	MHC
Staron *et al.*	1994	13 + 8 (7 + 5 ctrl); M + F; 21 yrs	8 weeks, 2/week, 3 × 6–12	→	→	→	→	↓	Untrained
Ploutz *et al.*	1994	9; M	9 weeks, 2/week, 3–6 × 12	→ ⇒		→ ⇒	↑ ⇒	↓ ⇒	Sedentary
Kraemer *et al.*	1995	35 (9 + 5 ctrl); M; 23 yrs	12 weeks, 4/week	→ ⇑		↑ ⇑	→ ⇑	↓ ⇒	Trained (militaries)
Green *et al.*	1998	6; M; 19 yrs	12 weeks, 3/week, 3 × 6–8	→ ⇑		→ ⇑	→ ⇑	↓ ⇑	Sedentary
Masuda *et al.*	1999	11 (5 + 6); M; 28 yrs	8 weeks, 2/week 5 × 90% 1 RM	→ ⇑		→ ⇑		→ ⇑	Untrained
			9 × 80–40%	→ ⇑		→ ⇑		→ ⇑	
Bishop *et al.*	1999	21 (14 + 7 ctrl); F; 18–42 yrs	12 weeks, 2/week, 3 × 5–15 (15: 50%, 8: 70%, 5: 80%)	→ ⇒		→	⇒	→	Cyclists
Andersen & Aagaard	2000	9; M; 27 yrs	3 months, 3/week, 4–5 × 6–15	→ ⇒	→	↑ ⇑	→	↓ ⇑	Sedentary
Hortobágyi *et al.*	2000	24 + 24 (12 + 12 + 12 + 6 + 6); M + F; 22 yrs	12 weeks, 3/week, 4–6 × 8–12 (con, con/ecc, ecc)	↑↑ ⇑⇑		↑ ⇑⇑		↓↓ ⇑⇑	Active students
Williamson *et al.*	2000	7; M; 74 yrs	12 weeks, 3/week, 3 × 10	→ ↑	↓	→ →	↓	→ →	Untrained MHC
Trappe *et al.*	2000	7; M; 74 yrs	12 weeks, 3/week, 3 × 10	↑ ⇑⇑		→ ⇑		→	MHC Untrained
Hikida *et al.*	2000	9 + 9 ctrl; M; 65 yrs	16 weeks, 2/week, 3 × 6–8	→ ⇑ =		↑ ⇑>	→	↓ ⇑<	

Table 14.3 (b) Resistance training studies reporting myosin heavy chain (MHC) isoform content. Unless otherwise indicated the vastus lateralis muscle was examined. ↑, increase in percentage; ↓, decrease in percentage; →, unchanged percentage.

Author	Year	Subjects: *n*; gender; age	Duration, frequency and sets/repetitions	MHC isoforms			Comment
				I	IIa	IIa/x	
Adams *et al.*	1993	17 (13 + 4 ctrl); M; 36 yrs	19 weeks, 2/week, 3–5 × 6–12	→	↑	↓	'Healthy'
Fry *et al.*	1994	21 + 14 (1/2 ctrl); M + F; 21 yrs	8 weeks, 2/week, 3 × 6–12	→	↑	↓	Untrained; F showed no ↑
Carroll *et al.*	1998	8 + 9 (11 + 6 ctrl); M + F; 18 yrs	6 weeks, 3/week, 3 × 10, 9 weeks, 2/week, 3 × ca 10	→ →	↑ →	→ →	Students
Welle *et al.*	1999	5 + 3; M + F; 62–75 yrs	Day 1 and 4: 4 × 10, day 6: 5 × 10	→	→	→	mRNA, biopsy day 7
Andersen & Aagaard	2000	[illegible]	[illegible]	[illegible]	↑	↓	[illegible]
Hortobágyi *et al.*	2000	24 + 24 (12 + 12 + 12 + 6 + 6); M + F; 22 yrs	12 weeks, 3/week, 4–6 × 8–12 (1 con, 2 con/ecc, 3 ecc)	↑	→	↓	After limb unloading
Hikida *et al.*	2000	9 + 9 ctrl; M; 65 yrs	16 weeks, 2/week, 3 × 6–8	→	↑	↓	
Jürimäe *et al.*	1996	15 (11 + 4 ctrl); 22 yrs	12 weeks, 3/week, 4 × 12	→	→	↓	Triceps brachii; students
Kadi & Thornell	1999	30; F; 39 yrs	10 weeks, 3/week, 3 × 10–12	↓	↑	↓	Trapezius; health care and social workers

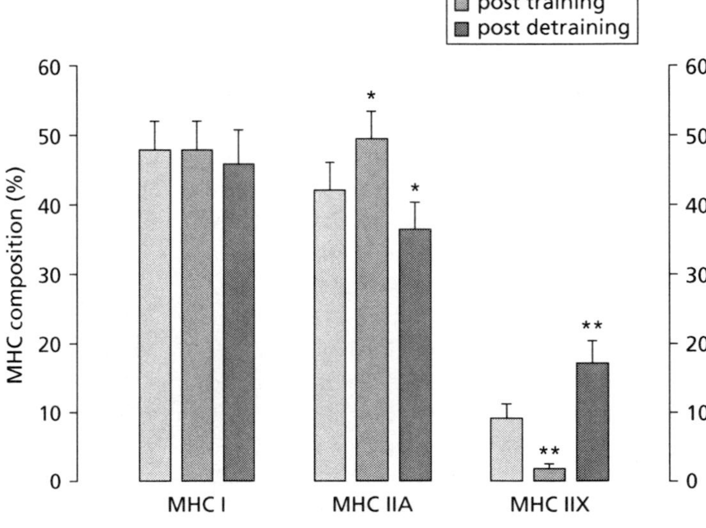

Fig. 14.3 The relative distribution of MHC isoforms before and after chronic resistance exercise. Open bars, pretraining; hatched bars, postresistance training; solid bars, post-detraining. Asterisk (*) denotes MHC IIa distribution is different ($p < 0.05$) such that post-detraining < pretraining < post-training; double asterisk (**) denotes a difference ($p < 0.01$) in MHC IIx distribution: post-detraining > pretraining > postresistance training. Values are mean ± SE ($n = 9$). (From Andersen & Aagaard 2000, with permission of John Wiley & Sons, Inc.)

both events occurred simultaneously. Other studies (Staron *et al.* 1991; Jürimäe *et al.* 1996; Green *et al.* 1999; Williamson *et al.* 2000), have reported similar, yet not significant, trends (Table 14.3). These are responses similar to those known to occur following chronic endurance exercise. When examining those training studies of healthy subjects that show a marked increase, i.e. greater than 7%, in overall muscle or fibre cross-sectional area, with the exception of one report (Trappe *et al.* 2000), there was no increase in Type I fibre percentage (Staron *et al.* 1990; Alway 1991; Charette *et al.* 1991; Hather *et al.* 1991; Staron *et al.* 1991; Wang *et al.* 1993; Hickson *et al.* 1994; Kraemer *et al.* 1995; Lexell *et al.* 1995; Hepple *et al.* 1997; Green *et al.* 1999; Masuda *et al.* 1999; Andersen & Aagaard 2000; Hikida *et al.* 2000). In the studies that produced significant hypertrophy, the percentage of Type IIb/IIx fibres decreased (Staron *et al.* 1990; Hather *et al.* 1991; Staron *et al.* 1991; Wang *et al.* 1993; Kraemer *et al.* 1995; Green *et al.* 1999; Andersen & Aagaard 2000; Hikida *et al.* 2000). Two studies failed to show such a response (Masuda *et al.* 1999; Trappe *et al.* 2000).

In bodybuilders the vastus lateralis muscle (Essén-Gustavsson & Tesch 1990) and the deltoid muscle (Schantz & Källman 1989) possess very few Type IIb/IIx fibres. In fact, bodybuilders and power lifters show higher Type IIa and lower IIb/IIx percentages than controls (Klitgaard *et al.* 1990; Kadi *et al.* 1999). Further, the relative number of fibres classified as Type IIb fibres by means of ATPase stains, and expressing both myosin heavy chain (MHC) IIb and MHC IIa isoforms, decreases following resistance training (Williamson *et al.* 2000). In concert, whole-muscle MHC IIb/IIx content decreased after resistance training (Adams *et al.* 1993; Fry *et al.* 1994; Kadi & Thornell 1999). The decrease in MHC IIb/IIx fibres with either endurance or resistance training may simply be explained by the MHC IIb/IIx being the 'default gene' that is expressed with no training (for example; Adams *et al.* 1993; Andersen *et al.* 1994). Thus, subjects who resumed a sedentary lifestyle following a resistance training programme, showed an increase in MHC IIx content to above 'normal' levels (Andersen & Aagaard 2000), suggesting an 'overshoot' in expressing this isoform, triggered by abrupt withdrawal from resistance training (Fig. 14.3).

The finding of an increase in Type I percentage following resistance training in elderly men (see above; Williamson *et al.* 2000) is not a consistent finding. Hence, in support of studies examining younger and more active populations, the results of several reports suggest no increase or decrease in Type I percentage in elderly people subjected to resistance training (Frontera *et al.* 1988; Brown *et al.* 1990; Charette *et al.* 1991; Lexell *et al.* 1995). Likewise, and similar to what has been reported in younger populations, the relative proportion of IIb fibres decreased and that of IIa fibres increased (Hikida *et al.* 2000). In the light of these findings, the increase in Type I fibre percentage, with no change in Type IIa or IIb percentage, yet a decrease in hybrid fibres (Williamson *et al.* 2000), is not readily explained. It also appears that the response to resistance training does not vary between men and women, regardless of age (Staron *et al.* 1991, 1994; Lexell *et al.* 1995; Kadi & Thornell 1999).

In summary, although muscles of high-calibre strength or power athletes may display a preponderance of Type II fibres and certainly a high content of fast protein due to preferential Type II fibre hypertrophy, all evidence suggests resistance exercise does not produce a shift from Type I to Type II fibres. Indeed, and similar to endurance exercise, resistance exercise promotes an increase in the relative proportion of Type IIa fibres at the expense of Type IIb/IIx fibres. The functional significance and implications of these changes for strength- and power-related performance remain to be proven.

Capillary supply

Numerous studies have shown that the capillary supply, expressed either as capillaries per fibre or as capillaries per mm^2, increases in response to endurance training. Likewise, endurance-trained athletes show greater capillary density than sedentaries (see Saltin & Gollnick 1983).

In contrast to strength training, endurance training does not produce muscle hypertrophy. An increase in muscle fibre size *per se* will therefore decrease capillary density. Most effective strength training regimens are associated with increases in muscle cross-sectional area as a result of increases in individual muscle fibre size. Assuming no capillary neoformation one would expect capillary density to decrease in proportion to the increase in muscle fibre size in response to strength training. In agreement with this, successful Olympic weightlifters and power lifters show lower capillary density than non-trained subjects (Tesch *et al.* 1984; Kadi *et al.* 1999). Thus, whereas the number of capillaries per fibre of vastus lateralis muscle is similar in lifters and non-athletes, capillaries per unit muscle area is markedly lower in lifters (Fig. 14.4). In the trapezius muscles of power lifters, Type I but not Type II fibres displayed more capillaries per fibre than in muscles of control subjects (Kadi *et al.* 1999). This response in the rarely examined trapezius muscle could very well reflect different adaptive responses between weightbearing and non-weightbearing muscles. Bodybuilders relying on a different training regimen, however, show somewhat greater numbers of capillaries per fibre and similar capillaries per unit area as non-athletes (Schantz 1982; Tesch *et al.* 1984; Schantz & Källman 1989; Essén-Gustavsson & Tesch 1990). Thus, in the light of the greater capillaries per fibre, a certain capillary proliferation of the quadriceps femoris muscle may occur in these athletes. In the non-postural triceps brachii of bodybuilders, however, a pattern similar to that observed in the vastus lateralis of lifters (Tesch *et al.* 1984) has been demonstrated. Lifters and bodybuilders have been compared with regard to the capillary supply of the vastus lateralis and triceps brachii muscles (Dudley *et al.* 1986). In both muscles bodybuilders showed greater capillaries per fibre than lifters, indicating that capillary proliferation may occur in both postural and non-postural muscles in response to strength training emphasizing high repetition training systems. No changes in capillary density were observed following strength training programmes of 6–12 weeks' duration (Tesch *et al.* 1983; Lüthi *et al.* 1986; Tesch *et al.* 1990; McCall *et al.* 1996; Hepple *et al.* 1997; Green *et al.* 1999).

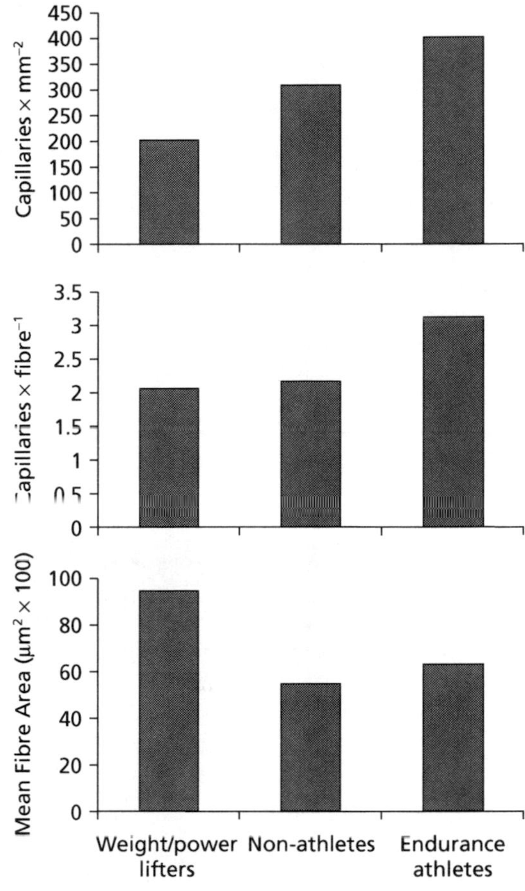

Fig. 14.4 Mean fibre area, capillaries per fibre and capillary density of vastus lateralis muscle in weight- and power lifters, non-athletes and endurance athletes. (Modified from Tesch *et al.* 1984.)

Training programmes ranging from 16 to 24 weeks in duration have produced either no increase (Wang *et al.* 1993; Hagerman *et al.* 2000) or a small increase (Hather *et al.* 1991) in capillary density. Overwhelming evidence, however, suggests intense resistance training carried out for that duration promotes capillary proliferation. Yet, the increase in capillaries per fibre is less than the increase in muscle fibre size (Frontera *et al.* 1990; Hather *et al.* 1991; Wang *et al.* 1993;

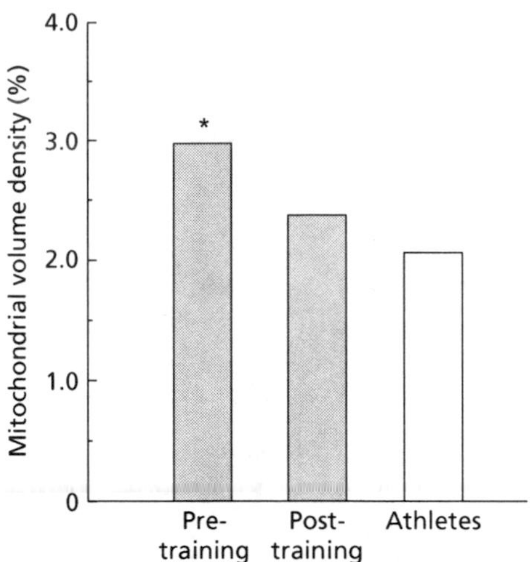

Fig. 14.5 Mitochondrial volume density of triceps brachii muscle before and after 6 months of strength training; muscle fibre size increased by 30%. Values for athletes (bodybuilders and power lifters) are shown for comparison. Asterisk (*) denotes a difference from values obtained after short-term (post-training) or long-term (athletes) heavy-resistance training. (From MacDougall *et al.* 1979.)

McCall *et al.* 1996; Hepple *et al.* 1997; Green *et al.* 1999). This may suggest that adaptations similar in nature, but not magnitude, to those attained by endurance training, are possible with resistance exercise.

Altogether, it appears that strength training emphasizing high-load, low-repetition exercises will not result in capillary neoformation. When pronounced hypertrophy of individual muscle fibres occurs, the capillary density rather decreases. More intense training regimens, emphasizing moderately high load and a larger number of repetitions per set, may induce capillary proliferation, but not necessarily increased capillary density.

Mitochondrial density

In lower mammals exercise-induced muscle hypertrophy seems to be associated with a proportional increase in mitochondrial volume (Seiden 1976). Studies of strength-trained athletes have, however, demonstrated reduced mitochondrial density of trained muscles (MacDougall *et al.* 1982; Alway *et al.* 1988). This finding, albeit not being a consistent observation (Staron *et al.* 1984), has found support in that mitochondrial volume density decreased in parallel with increases in muscle mass in subjects performing strength training over 6–8 weeks (Fig. 14.5; MacDougall *et al.* 1979; Lüthi *et al.* 1986). In other studies (Alway 1991; Wang *et al.* 1993) mitochondrial volume density remained unchanged after 20 weeks of training despite an increase in mean fibre area. If a decrease in mitochondrial density occurs secondary to exercise-induced muscle hypertrophy, this is commensurate with the observations referred to below, of attenuated oxidative enzyme content in muscles of athletes trained for strength or power.

Enzyme content

AEROBIC OXIDATIVE ENZYMES

Strength training using heavy loads does not enhance the activity of enzymes involved in oxidative metabolism (Komi *et al.* 1982; Houston *et al.* 1983; Tesch *et al.* 1987, 1990; Ploutz *et al.* 1994; Green *et al.* 1999). Thus, contents of succinate dehydrogenase, malate dehydrogenase or citrate synthase or 3-hydroxyacyl-CoA dehydrogenase (HAD), favouring lipid oxidation, remained unchanged or even decreased somewhat in response to programmes that induced substantial increases in muscle strength. These results are supported by the demonstration of normal or 'subnormal' activities of oxidative enzymes in strength- or power-trained athletes (Gollnick *et al.* 1972; Apple & Tesch 1989; Schantz & Källman 1989; Tesch *et al.* 1989a; Essén-Gustavsson & Tesch 1990). Yet, resistance training in elderly (Frontera *et al.* 1990) or sedentary populations (Wang *et al.* 1993) may evoke a differential response, e.g. an increase in oxidative enzyme activity.

The difference in enzyme activity between fast- and slow-twitch fibres, typically observed in untrained or endurance-trained populations, was also present in strength-trained athletes. In these individuals, however, the citrate synthase and HAD activity of slow-twitch fibres was lower than in sedentaries. Interestingly, bodybuilders displayed higher citrate synthase activity of fast-twitch fibres than Olympic weightlifters or power lifters. Hence, the high repetition strategy practised by bodybuilders obviously produces more favourable adaptations with regard to aerobic metabolism than the heavy-resistance, low-repetition regimens often practised by lifters (Tesch 1992).

ANAEROBIC NON-GLYCOLYTIC ENZYMES

A high content of enzymes favouring contractility or fast ATP replenishment, for example ATPase, creatine kinase or myokinase, may have physiologically important implications in athletic events requiring speed, strength or power; hence, strength training provoking meaningful increases in anaerobic non-glycolytic enzyme content. Although not being a consistent finding, myokinase increases somewhat in response to explosive or strength training (Thorstensson *et al.* 1976a; Komi *et al.* 1982). These studies reported that no increase in ATPase or creatine kinase content could enhance performance. Several studies however, show no evidence of enhanced content of anaerobic non-glycolytic enzymes in response to strength training (Thorstensson *et al.* 1976b; Häkkinen *et al.* 1981; Houston *et al.* 1983; Tesch *et al.* 1987, 1990; Wang *et al.* 1993). Myokinase activity of Type II fibres was higher in lifters/bodybuilders than in controls. Myokinase activity of Type I fibres, however, was comparable in the two groups (Tesch *et al.* 1989a). Interestingly, bodybuilders showed higher enzyme content of Type II fibres compared with lifters. These results provide evidence that some metabolic adaptations are sensitive to the type of resistance exercise protocol employed.

ANAEROBIC GLYCOLYTIC ENZYMES

Endurance training programmes typically do not enhance anaerobic glycolytic enzyme activity, and to produce such changes exercise has to be carried out at work loads exceeding maximal aerobic power (see Saltin & Gollnick 1983). The activities of phosphofructokinase or lactate dehydrogenase are unaffected by heavy-resistance training (Thorstensson *et al.* 1976a; Komi *et al.* 1982; Houston *et al.* 1983; Tesch *et al.* 1987, 1990; Wang *et al.* 1993; Bishop *et al.* 1999). Strength-trained athletes, however, show slightly higher glycolytic activity, e.g. lactate dehydrogenase, of fast-twitch fibres than sedentaries (Tesch *et al.* 1989a). This difference may simply reflect the limited use of fast-twitch fibres in sedentaries, not a specific training response, because strength- or endurance trained athletes and moderately active 'non-athletes' (Apple & Tesch 1989) show similar lactate dehydrogenase activity of fast- and slow-twitch fibres. Likewise, phosphofructokinase activity of mixed tissue samples from a non-postural muscle, e.g. the deltoid, was similar in bodybuilders, swimmers and physically active students (Schantz & Källman 1989).

Muscle substrate levels

GLYCOGEN CONTENT

Muscle glycogen concentration at rest increases in response to endurance training, and this adaptation appears to occur following strength training as well. Thus, in the triceps brachii muscle of individuals who trained for 5 months using variable resistance, the glycogen content increased by 35% (MacDougall *et al.* 1977). Also, the vastus lateralis muscle of bodybuilders showed more than 50% higher glycogen content than that typically noticed in non-athletes (Tesch *et al.* 1986). In contrast to these observations, glycogen content was not enhanced in response to 3 months of quadriceps training (Tesch *et al.* 1990; Goreham *et al.* 1999). Although it may require more robust and longlasting exercise regimens to promote an increase in glycogen stores in the resting state, a glycogen-sparing effect, as a result of resistance training, has been reported (Goreham *et al.* 1999). Thus, less glycogen was utilized during a standardized bout of aerobic exercise following 3 months of resistance training.

ATP AND CREATINE PHOSPHATE CONTENT

Bouts of strength exercise lower ATP and creatine phosphate stores (see above) with partial or complete resynthesis between bouts (Tesch *et al.* 1989b). It remains to be shown whether this acute metabolic response provides the adaptive stimuli for increased storage capacity of high-energy phosphate compounds. Substantial increases in the resting phosphagen levels of the triceps brachii muscle have been shown after 5 months of strength training that produced marked increases in elbow extensor strength and fibre size (MacDougall *et al.* 1977, 1979). In contrast, 3 months of quadriceps training 3 times a week and comprising 48–60 maximal voluntary muscle actions per session did not alter resting ATP and creatine phosphate stores (Tesch *et al.* 1990). Results in support of this notion have subsequently been reported following training programmes of similar duration and intensity (Goreham *et al.* 1999; Volek *et al.* 1999). It appears that this lack of increase in phosphagen content occurs regardless of whether hypertrophy takes place (Tesch *et al.* 1990; Goreham *et al.* 1999; Volek *et al.* 1999). Moreover, normal levels of ATP and creatine phosphate were observed in athletes possessing marked muscle hypertrophy of the vastus lateralis (Tesch *et al.* 1986). It could only be speculated whether these conflicting findings reflected different responses between postural (Goreham *et al.* 1999) and non-postural muscles (MacDougall *et al.* 1977, 1979). Nevertheless, if changes in ATP and creatine phosphate content are consequences of chronic resistance exercise, these changes are subtle.

LIPID CONTENT

There is uncertainty as to whether endurance training promotes increased content of lipids stored in the muscle (see Saltin & Gollnick 1983). Likewise, it is not clear whether or not strength training stimulates an increase in lipid content. The triglyceride content of the quadriceps muscle of bodybuilders and untrained populations is not different (Essén-Gustavsson & Tesch 1990), and bodybuilders showed a similar lipid volume fraction to that of sedentary or active controls (Alway *et al.* 1988). The findings of lower lipid content in the quadriceps of lifters (Staron *et al.* 1984) and the observation of an increase in lipid volume density of the triceps muscle (MacDougall *et al.* 1979), but not of the quadriceps muscle (Lüthi *et al.* 1986; Wang *et al.* 1993) in response to heavy-resistance training, may imply different responses between muscles. Alternatively, the type of resistance training employed may affect the subsequent adaptations.

Myoglobin content

Myoglobin has an important role for oxygen transport within skeletal muscle. Thus myoglobin facilitates oxygen extraction. Although slow-twitch muscle fibres typically contain more myoglobin than fast-twitch fibres, endurance training does not promote increased myoglobin content of human skeletal muscle (see Saltin & Gollnick 1983). Because myoglobin content increased in parallel with a decrease in oxidative enzyme content, secondary to muscle atrophy induced by immobilization (Jansson *et al.* 1988), it appears that myoglobin content decreases following strength training. Hence, short-term programmes using either bodybuilding or weight-lifting loading strategies, and carried out by sedentary men over 8 weeks, tended to attenuate myoglobin content (Masuda *et al.* 1999). In another study (P. Tesch *et al.* unpublished observations) myoglobin content was measured in the vastus lateralis muscle before and after a 16-week strength training programme that induced a 20% increase in muscle fibre size. Data suggest that muscle hypertrophy was paralleled by a corresponding decrease in myoglobin content. Muscle fibre size decreased following detraining, and this effect was accompanied by an increase in myoglobin content. Provided there is an increase in muscle fibre size these results suggest that long-term resistance exercise may reduce the potential for skeletal muscle to extract oxygen. Such an effect would probably decrease aerobic work capacity.

Conclusions

Strength training promotes hypertrophy. Yet few if any favourable metabolic adaptations take place in response to chronic training. The occurrence and magnitude of these effects are influenced by the type, intensity and duration of training. It is clear, for example, that the metabolic adaptations are different when comparing programmes comprising high-load low repetitions or light-load high repetitions, or whether or not the programme is of such a duration and intensity that it will induce muscle hypertrophy.

Likewise, the initial state of training will influence training responses. Therefore, results obtained in studies examining, for example, prepubertal children, untrained women or aged populations, should be interpreted with caution and not be regarded as reflecting 'classical' responses to heavy-resistance training. Similarly, the adaptations shown in weight-trained athletes may not necessarily apply to short-term strength training programmes.

Some of the confusion concerning skeletal muscle adaptations taking place in response to strength training stems from the fact that results have been reported from studies where the training performed had been termed 'strength', 'weight' or 'heavy-resistance' training although it had not induced meaningful increases in strength or muscle mass. Exercise prescriptions for athletes, physically active or inactive or aged populations, or those undergoing rehabilitation, must consider such information.

References

Adams, G.R., Hather, B.M., Baldwin, K.M. & Dudley, G.A. (1993) Skeletal muscle myosin heavy chain composition and resistance training. *Journal of Applied Physiology* **74**(2), 911–915.

Alway, S.E. (1991) Is fiber mitochondrial volume density a good indicator of muscle fatigability to isometric exercise? *Journal of Applied Physiology* **70**(5), 2111–2119.

Alway, S.E., MacDougall, J.D., Sale, D.G., Sutton, J.R. & McComas, A.J. (1988) Functional and structural adaptations in skeletal muscle of trained athletes. *Journal of Applied Physiology* **64**(3), 1114–1120.

Andersen, J.L. & Aagaard, P. (2000) Myosin heavy chain IIX overshoot in human skeletal muscle. *Muscle and Nerve* **23**(7), 1095–1104.

Andersen, J.L., Klitgaard, H. & Saltin, B. (1994) Myosin heavy chain isoforms in single fibres from m. vastus lateralis of sprinters: influence of training. *Acta Physiologica Scandinavica* **151**(2), 135–142.

Apple, F.S. & Tesch, P.A. (1989) CK and LD isozymes in human single muscle fibers in trained athletes. *Journal of Applied Physiology* **66**(6), 2717–2720.

Asmussen, E. (1953) Positive and negative muscular work. *Acta Physiologica Scandinavica* **28**(4), 364–382.

Bishop, D., Jenkins, D.G., Mackinnon, L.T., McEniery, M. & Carey, M.F. (1999) The effects of strength training on endurance performance and muscle characteristics. *Medicine and Science in Sports and Exercise* **31**(6), 886–891.

Brown, A.B., McCartney, N. & Sale, D.G. (1990) Positive adaptations to weight-lifting training in the elderly. *Journal of Applied Physiology* **69**(5), 1725–1733.

Carroll, T.J., Abernethy, P.J., Logan, P.A., Barber, M. & McEniery, M.T. (1998) Resistance training frequency: strength and myosin heavy chain responses to two and three bouts per week. *European Journal of Applied Physiology* **78**(3), 270–275.

Charette, S.L., McEvoy, L., Pyka, G. *et al.* (1991) Muscle hypertrophy response to resistance training in older women. *Journal of Applied Physiology* **70**(5), 1912–1916.

Dudley, G.A., Tesch, P.A., Fleck, S.J., Kraemer, W.J. & Baechle, T.R. (1986) Plasticity of human muscle with resistance training. *Anatomical Record* **214**(4), 451.

Dudley, G.A., Tesch, P.A., Harris, R.T., Golden, C.L. & Buchanan, P. (1991) Influence of eccentric actions on the metabolic cost of resistance exercise. *Aviation Space and Environmental Medicine* **62**(7), 678–682.

Essén-Gustavsson, B. & Tesch, P.A. (1990) Glycogen and triglyceride utilization in relation to muscle metabolic characteristics in men performing heavy-resistance exercise. *European Journal of Applied Physiology and Occupational Physiology* **61**(1–2), 5–10.

Frontera, W.R., Meredith, C.N., O'Reilly, K.P., Knuttgen, H.G. & Evans, W.J. (1988) Strength conditioning in older men: skeletal muscle hypertrophy and improved function. *Journal of Applied Physiology* **64**(3), 1038–1044.

Frontera, W.R., Meredith, C.N., O'Reilly, K.P. & Evans, W.J. (1990) Strength training and determinants of $\dot{V}O_{2\,max}$ in older men. *Journal of Applied Physiology* **68**(1), 329–333.

Fry, A.C., Allemeier, C.A. & Staron, R.S. (1994) Correlation between percentage fiber type area and myosin heavy chain content in human skeletal muscle. *European Journal of Applied Physiology* **68**(3), 246–251.

Gollnick, P.D., Armstrong, R.B., Saubert, C.W., Piehl, K. & Saltin, B. (1972) Enzyme activity and fiber composition in skeletal muscle of untrained and trained men. *Journal of Applied Physiology* **33**(3), 312–319.

Gollnick, P.D., Karlsson, J., Piehl, K. & Saltin, B. (1974) Selective glycogen depletion in skeletal muscle fibres of man following sustained contractions. *Journal of Physiology* **241**(1), 59–67.

Goreham, C., Green, H.J., Ball-Burnett, M. & Ranney, D. (1999) High-resistance training and muscle metabolism during prolonged exercise. *American Journal of Physiology* **276**(3 Part 1), E489–E496.

Green, H., Goreham, C., Ouyang, J., Ball-Burnett, M. & Ranney, D. (1999) Regulation of fiber size, oxidative potential, and capillarization in human muscle by resistance exercise. *American Journal of Physiology* **276**(2 Part 2), R591–R596.

Hagerman, F.C., Walsh, S.J., Staron, R.S. *et al.* (2000) Effects of high-intensity resistance training on untrained older men. I. Strength, cardiovascular, and metabolic responses. *Journal of Gerontological A Biol Science Medical Science* **55**(7), B336–B346.

Häkkinen, K., Komi, P.V. & Tesch, P.A. (1981) Effect of combined concentric and eccentric strength training and detraining on force-time, muscle fiber and metabolic characteristics of leg extensor muscles. *Scandinavian Journal of Sports Science* **3**, 50–58.

Hather, B.M., Tesch, P.A., Buchanan, P. & Dudley, G.A. (1991) Influence of eccentric actions on skeletal muscle adaptations to resistance training. *Acta Physiologica Scandinavica* **143**(2), 177–185.

Hepple, R.T., Mackinnon, S.L., Thomas, S.G., Goodman, J.M. & Plyley, M.J. (1997) Quantitating the capillary supply and the response to resistance training in older men. *Pflügers Archiv* **433**(3), 238–244.

Hickson, R.C., Hidaka, K., Foster, C., Falduto, M.T. & Chatterton, R.T. (1994) Successive time courses of strength development and steroid hormone responses to heavy-resistance training. *Journal of Applied Physiology* **76**(2), 663–670.

Hikida, R.S., Staron, R.S., Hagerman, F.C. *et al.* (2000) Effects of high-intensity resistance training on untrained older men. II. Muscle fiber characteristics and nucleo-cytoplasmic relationships. *Journal of Gerontological A Biological Science Medical Science* **55**(7), B347–B354.

Hortobágyi, T., Dempsey, L., Fraser, D. *et al.* (2000) Changes in muscle strength, muscle fibre size and myofibrillar gene expression after immobilization and retraining in humans. *Journal of Physiology (London)* **524** (Part 1), 293–304.

Houston, M.E., Froese, E.A., Valeriote, S.P., Green, H.J. & Ranney, D.A. (1983) Muscle performance, morphology and metabolic capacity during strength training and detraining: a one leg model. *European Journal of Applied Physiology and Occupational Physiology* **51**(1), 25–35.

Jansson, E., Sylven, C., Arvidsson, I. & Eriksson, E. (1988) Increase in myoglobin content and decrease in oxidative enzyme activities by leg muscle immobilization in man. *Acta Physiologica Scandinavica* **132**(4), 515–517.

Jürimäe, J., Abernethy, P.J., Blake, K. & McEniery, M.T. (1996) Changes in the myosin heavy chain isoform profile of the triceps brachii muscle following 12 weeks of resistance training. *European Journal of Applied Physiology* **74**(3), 287–292.

Kadi, F. & Thornell, L.E. (1999) Training affects myosin heavy chain phenotype in the trapezius muscle of women. *Histochemistry and Cell Biology* **112**(1), 70–78.

Kadi, F., Eriksson, A., Holmner, S., Butler-Browne, G.S. & Thornell, L.E. (1999) Cellular adaptation of the trapezius muscle in strength-trained athletes. *Histochemistry and Cell Biology* **111**(3), 189–195.

Keul, J., Haralambie, G., Bruder, M. & Gottstein, H.J. (1978) The effect of weight lifting exercise on heart rate and metabolism in experienced weight lifters. *Medicine and Science in Sports* **10**(1), 13–15.

King, D.S., Sharp, R.L., Vukovich, M.D. *et al.* (1999) Effect of oral androstenedione on serum testosterone and adaptations to resistance training in young men: a randomized controlled trial. *Journal of the American Medical Association* **281**(21), 2020–2028.

Klitgaard, H., Zhou, M. & Richter, E.A. (1990) Myosin heavy chain composition of single fibres from m. biceps brachii of male body builders. *Acta Physiologica Scandinavica* **140**(2), 175–180.

Komi, P.V., Karlsson, J., Tesch, P.A., Suominen, H. & Heikkinen, E. (1982) Effects of heavy resistance and explosive-type strength training methods on mechanical, functional and metabolic aspects of performance. In: *Exercise and Sport Biology: International Series on Sports Sciences* (ed. P.V. Komi) Vol. 12, 90–102. Human Kinetics, Champaign, Illinois.

Kraemer, W.J., Noble, B.J., Clark, M.J. & Culver, B.W. (1987) Physiologic responses to heavy-resistance exercise with very short rest periods. *International Journal of Sports Medicine* **8**(4), 247–252.

Kraemer, W.J., Patton, J.F., Gordon, S.E. *et al.* (1995) Compatibility of high-intensity strength and endurance training on hormonal and skeletal muscle adaptations. *Journal of Applied Physiology* **78**(3), 976–989.

Larsson, L. & Tesch, P.A. (1986) Motor unit fibre density in extremely hypertrophied skeletal muscles in man. Electrophysiological signs of muscle fibre hyperplasia. *European Journal of Applied Physiology and Occupational Physiology* **55**(2), 130–136.

Lexell, J., Downham, D.Y., Larsson, Y., Bruhn, E. & Morsing, B. (1995) Heavy-resistance training in older

Scandinavian men and women: short- and long-term effects on arm and leg muscles. *Scandinavian Journal of Medicine and Science in Sports* **5**(6), 329–341.

Lüthi, J.M., Howald, H., Claassen, H., Rosler, K., Vock, P. & Hoppeler, H. (1986) Structural changes in skeletal muscle tissue with heavy-resistance exercise. *International Journal of Sports Medicine* **7**(3), 123–127.

McCall, G.E., Byrnes, W.C., Dickinson, A., Pattany, P.M. & Fleck, S.J. (1996) Muscle fiber hypertrophy, hyperplasia, and capillary density in college men after resistance training. *Journal of Applied Physiology* **81**(5), 2004–2012.

MacDougall, J.D., Ward, G.R., Sale, D.G. & Sutton, J.R. (1977) Biochemical adaptation of human skeletal muscle to heavy resistance training and immobilization. *Journal of Applied Physiology* **43**(4), 700–703.

MacDougall, J.D., Sale, D.G., Moroz, J.R., Elder, G.C., Sutton, J.R. & Howald, H. (1979) Mitochondrial volume density in human skeletal muscle following heavy resistance training. *Medicine and Science in Sports* **11**(2), 164–166.

MacDougall, J.D., Sale, D.G., Elder, G.C. & Sutton, J.R. (1982) Muscle ultrastructural characteristics of elite powerlifters and bodybuilders. *European Journal of Applied Physiology and Occupational Physiology* **48**(1), 117–126.

MacDougall, J.D., Ray, S., Sale, D.G., McCartney, N., Lee, P. & Garner, S. (1999) Muscle substrate utilization and lactate production. *Canadian Journal of Applied Physiology* **24**(3), 209–215.

Masuda, K., Choi, J.Y., Shimojo, H. & Katsuta, S. (1999) Maintenance of myoglobin concentration in human skeletal muscle after heavy resistance training. *European Journal of Applied Physiology and Occupational Physiology* **79**(4), 347–352.

Pascoe, D.D., Costill, D.L., Fink, W.J., Robergs, R.A. & Zachwieja, J.J. (1993) Glycogen resynthesis in skeletal muscle following resistive exercise. *Medicine and Science in Sports and Exercise* **25**(3), 349–354.

Ploutz, L.L., Tesch, P.A., Biro, R.L. & Dudley, G.A. (1994) Effect of resistance training on muscle use during exercise. *Journal of Applied Physiology* **76**(4), 1675–1681.

Prince, F.P., Hikida, R.S. & Hagerman, F.C. (1976) Human muscle fiber types in power lifters, distance runners and untrained subjects. *Pflügers Archiv* **363**(1), 19–26.

Robergs, R.A., Pearson, D.R., Costill, D.L. *et al.* (1991) Muscle glycogenolysis during differing intensities of weight-resistance exercise. *Journal of Applied Physiology* **70**(4), 1700–1706.

Saltin, B. & Gollnick, P.D. (1983) Skeletal muscle adaptability: significance for metabolism and performance. In: *Handbook of Physiology* (eds L. Peachy, R. Adrian & S.R. Gerzer), pp. 555–631. American Physiological Society, Bethesda.

Schantz, P. (1982) Capillary supply in hypertrophied human skeletal muscle. *Acta Physiologica Scandinavica* **114**(4), 635–637.

Schantz, P.G. & Källman, M. (1989) NADH shuttle enzymes and cytochrome b5 reductase in human skeletal muscle: effect of strength training. *Journal of Applied Physiology* **67**(1), 123–127.

Seiden, D. (1976) Quantitative analysis of muscle cell changes in compensatory hypertrophy and work-induced hypertrophy. *American Journal of Anatomy* **145**(4), 459–465.

Staron, R.S., Hikida, R.S., Hagerman, F.C., Dudley, G.A. & Murray, T.F. (1984) Human skeletal muscle fiber type adaptability to various workloads. *Journal of Histochemistry and Cytochemistry* **32**(2), 146–152.

Staron, R.S., Malicky, E.S., Leonardi, M.J., Falkel, J.E., Hagerman, F.C. & Dudley, G.A. (1990) Muscle hypertrophy and fast fiber type conversions in heavy resistance-trained women. *European Journal of Applied Physiology* **60**(1), 71–79.

Staron, R.S., Leonardi, M.J., Karapondo, D.L. *et al.* (1991) Strength and skeletal muscle adaptations in heavy-resistance-trained women after detraining and retraining. *Journal of Applied Physiology* **70**(2), 631–640.

Staron, R.S., Karapondo, D.L., Kraemer, W.J. *et al.* (1994) Skeletal muscle adaptations during early phase of heavy-resistance training in men and women. *Journal of Applied Physiology* **76**(3), 1247–1255.

Tesch, P.A. (1992) Training for Bodybuilding. In: *Strength and Power in Sport* (ed. P.V. Komi), 1st edn, pp. 370–380. Blackwell Science Ltd, Oxford.

Tesch, P.A. & Karlsson, J. (1985) Muscle fiber types and size in trained and untrained muscles of elite athletes. *Journal of Applied Physiology* **59**(6), 1716–1720.

Tesch, P.A. & Larsson, L. (1982) Muscle hypertrophy in bodybuilders. *European Journal of Applied Physiology and Occupational Physiology* **49**(3), 301–306.

Tesch, P.A., Hjort, H. & Balldin, U.I. (1983) Effects of strength training on G tolerance. *Aviation Space and Environmental Medicine* **54**(8), 691–695.

Tesch, P.A., Thorsson, A. & Kaiser, P. (1984) Muscle capillary supply and fiber type characteristics in weight and power lifters. *Journal of Applied Physiology* **56**(1), 35–38.

Tesch, P.A., Colliander, E.B. & Kaiser, P. (1986) Muscle metabolism during intense, heavy-resistance exercise. *European Journal of Applied Physiology and Occupational Physiology* **55**(4), 362–366.

Tesch, P.A., Komi, P.V. & Häkkinen, K. (1987) Enzymatic adaptations consequent to long-term strength training. *International Journal of Sports Medicine* **8** (Suppl. 1), 66–69.

Tesch, P.A., Thorsson, A. & Essén-Gustavsson, B. (1989a) Enzyme activities of FT and ST muscle fibers in heavy-resistance trained athletes. *Journal of Applied Physiology* **67**(1), 83–87.

Tesch, P.A., Thorsson, A. & Fujitsuka, N. (1989b) Creatine phosphate in fiber types of skeletal muscle before and after exhaustive exercise. *Journal of Applied Physiology* **66**(4), 1756–1759.

Tesch, P.A., Thorsson, A. & Colliander, E.B. (1990) Effects of eccentric and concentric resistance training on skeletal muscle substrates, enzyme activities and capillary supply. *Acta Physiologica Scandinavica* **140**(4), 575–580.

Tesch, P.A., Ploutz-Snyder, L.L., Yström, L., Castro, M.J. & Dudley, G.A. (1998) Skeletal muscle glycogen loss evoked by resistance exercise. *Journal of Strength and Conditioning Research* **12**(2), 67–73.

Thorstensson, A., Hultén, B., von Döbeln, W. & Karlsson, J. (1976a) Effect of strength training on enzyme activities and fibre characteristics in human skeletal muscle. *Acta Physiologica Scandinavica* **96**(3), 392–398.

Thorstensson, A., Karlsson, J., Viitasalo, J.H., Luhtanen, P. & Komi, P.V. (1976b) Effect of strength training on EMG of human skeletal muscle. *Acta Physiologica Scandinavica* **98**(2), 232–236.

Trappe, S., Williamson, D., Godard, M., Porter, D., Rowden, G. & Costill, D. (2000) Effect of resistance training on single muscle fiber contractile function in older men. *Journal of Applied Physiology* **89**(1), 143–152.

Volek, J.S., Duncan, N.D., Mazzetti, S.A. *et al.* (1999) Performance and muscle fiber adaptations to creatine supplementation and heavy resistance training. *Medicine and Science in Sports and Exercise* **31**(8), 1147–1156.

Wang, N., Hikida, R.S., Staron, R.S. & Simoneau, J.A. (1993) Muscle fiber types of women after resistance training—quantitative ultrastructure and enzyme activity. *Pflügers Archiv* **424**(5–6), 494–502.

Williamson, D.L., Godard, M.P., Porter, D.A., Costill, D.L. & Trappe, S.W. (2000) Progressive resistance training reduces myosin heavy chain coexpression in single muscle fibers from older men. *Journal of Applied Physiology* **88**(2), 627–633.

Yström, L. & Tesch, P.A. (1996) Effect of acute endurance exercise on muscle glycogen content and performance during subsequent resistance exercise. *Medicine and Science in Sports and Exercise* **28** (5 Suppl.), S22, no. 128.

Chapter 15

Neural Adaptation to Strength Training

DIGBY G. SALE

Introduction

Strength performance is the product of a partnership between muscles and the nervous system. The muscles provide the 'engine' that can actually generate force, whereas the nervous system provides the engine controller (Fig. 15.1). The increase in strength seen during a training programme could be the result of changes (adaptations) in the muscles, the engine, or in the nervous system, the engine controller. The latter training-induced changes, referred to as neural adaptations, are the subject of this chapter (for other reviews on neural adaptation, see e.g. Bawa 2002; Moritani 1993; Enoka 1997; see also Chapters 16 & 17 in this volume).

Strength performance is a motor act, which challenges the nervous system. One challenge is to fully activate the prime mover muscles (agonists). A second challenge is to appropriately activate assisting muscles (synergists) and muscles which oppose the action of the agonists (antagonists). These two challenges must be met against a background of sensory feedback from muscles and joints, acting in the form of reflexes or as conscious perception. The challenges may range in severity. An example of a relatively easy challenge would be performing a unilateral (one limb only), single-joint, isometric action of the elbow extensors in the seated position. An example of a more difficult challenge would be a standing overhead barbell press, which is a bilateral, multijoint, dynamic (concentric) action, requiring activation of muscles in the upper and lower limbs and trunk. The more severe the challenges to the nervous system as the engine controller, the greater the probability of initial failure to meet the challenges. On the other hand, more difficult challenges probably lend greater scope for neural adaptations to increase the probability of success. The ultimate goal of training in meeting these challenges is to generate the greatest possible force and/or rate of force development in the intended direction of movement (Fig. 15.2). This chapter will focus on the scheme shown in Fig. 15.2. Other forms of neural adaptation, such as changes in motor nerve conduction velocity (e.g. Kamen *et al.* 1984; Sleivert *et al.* 1995) and reflex function (e.g. Häkkinen & Komi 1983; Casabona *et al.* 1990; see Enoka 1997 for a review, and Chapters 10, 17 and 24), will not be covered in this chapter.

Increased activation of agonists

The most obvious neural adaptation to consider is increased activation of agonist muscles (Fig. 15.3). Increased activation could occur in three ways. First, training would allow recruitment or a more consistent recruitment of the highest-threshold motor units (Fig. 15.3, top panel). In accordance with the size principle of motor unit recruitment (Henneman *et al.* 1965), the high-threshold motor units would consist of large motoneurones innervating Type II (fast-twitch) muscle fibres. It is important to recruit these motor units in a maximal contraction because they contain the largest number of muscle fibres.

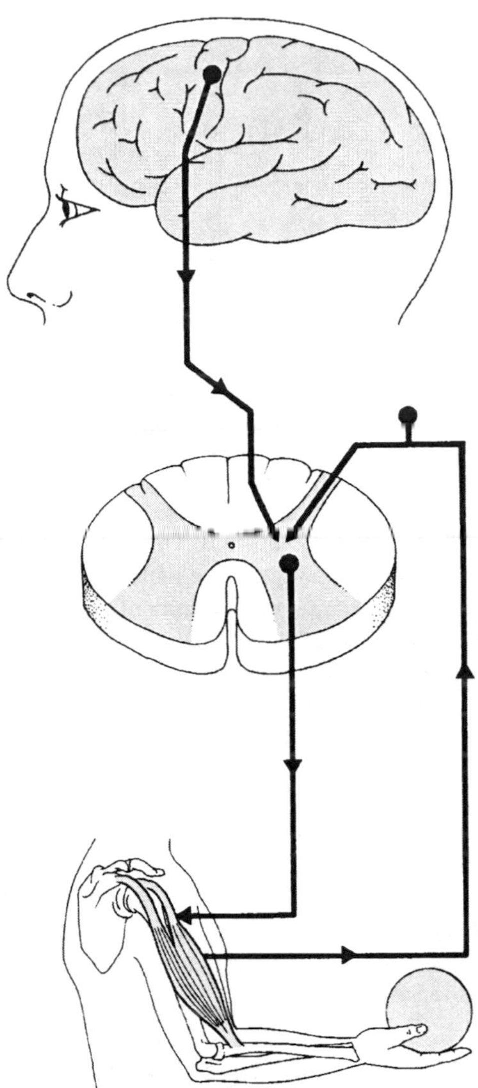

Fig. 15.1 Control of muscle by the nervous system. Voluntary strength performance is determined not only by the quantity and quality of the involved muscle mass, the 'engine', but also by the ability of the nervous system, the engine controller, to effectively activate the muscles. Nervous system adaptations to strength training may improve the control of muscles to increase maximum force (strength). These 'neural' adaptations may occur in higher brain centres or within the spinal cord.

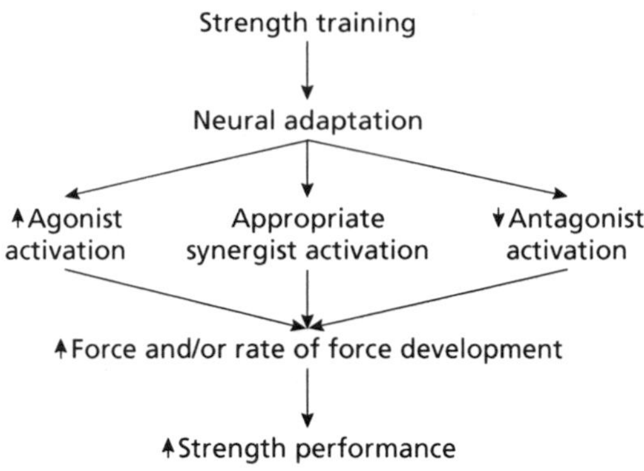

Fig. 15.2 Neural adaptations to strength training may take the form of increased activation of agonist muscles, more appropriate activation of synergist muscles ('coordination'), and decreased (relative) activation of antagonist muscles. These adaptations would act to increase maximum force (strength) and/or rate of force development.

For example, it has been estimated that in triceps brachii, only about 5% of the motor units are Type IIb (IIx), but this small number of units contains about 20% of the total number of muscle fibres in the muscle (Enoka & Fuglevand 2001). The second way increased activation could occur is through increased motor unit firing rates (Fig. 15.3, middle panel). By increasing or decreasing firing rate (also referred to as discharge rate or rate coding), a motor unit can vary its force output over an approximately 10-fold range, known as the force–frequency relationship. The motor unit firing rates observed in maximal voluntary contractions appear to be lower than needed for maximum force output (Enoka & Fuglevand 2001; cf. Bellemare *et al.* 1983). Training may allow for firing rates consistently high enough to be on the plateau of the force–frequency relationship, where force is maximal. The third way increased activation could occur is also through increased motor unit firing rates (Fig. 15.3, bottom panel). When the intent is to contract the muscle as fast as possible with maximum rate of force development (so-called 'ballistic' contractions), motor units begin firing at a very high frequency, followed by a rapid decline in frequency (Zehr & Sale 1994). The peak firing rates attained

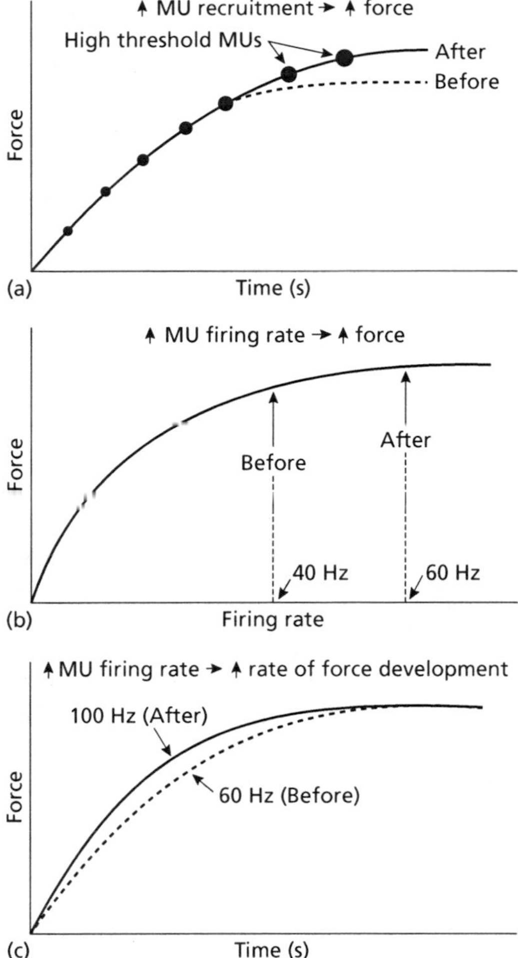

Fig. 15.3 Depiction of how training-induced increased agonist activation could increase strength performance. In the top panel training (a maximal isometric action before and after training) is shown to increase the recruitment of high-threshold motor units. Since these units contain a relatively large number of fast-contracting muscle fibres, there is a large benefit from being able to consistently recruit these units. The middle panel shows how an increase in maximum motor unit firing rate could increase the force produced by a motor unit. A higher firing rate after training allows the muscle fibres to operate farther up on their force–frequency relation. The bottom panel illustrates the effect of increased motor unit firing rate at the onset of an isometric action with the intent to develop force as rapidly as possible. A higher initial firing rate may not increase the peak force but may allow the peak force to be attained more quickly.

are in excess of those needed to achieve maximum force in a sustained contraction. What the high initial firing rates do provide, even if only sustained for a few discharges (Stein & Parmiggiani 1979), is an increase in rate of force development (Miller *et al.* 1981). If training were to increase the peak firing rates attained at the onset of ballistic contractions, the rate of force development and speed of contraction would increase (see Fig. 15.3, bottom panel and Fig. 15.7; see also Chapter 16).

Electromyographic studies

Most of the evidence for increased agonist activation after training has come from electromyographic studies. Electromyography is a method of recording and quantifying the electrical activity (muscle fibre action potentials) produced by the muscle fibres of activated motor units. In a typical training study, electromyographic (EMG) recordings are made from selected agonist muscles during maximal voluntary contractions before and after training. Most commonly, EMG recordings are made using surface electrodes applied to the skin overlying the muscle or muscles of interest. The recorded EMG can be quantified in different ways, and reflects a combination of the number of motor units recruited and their firing rates. The combination of motor unit recruitment and firing rates is often referred to as motor unit activation. If training causes an increase in the quantified EMG during a maximal voluntary contraction, it is concluded that an increase in motor unit activation (and hence neural adaptation) has occurred. With surface EMG it is usually not possible to distinguish between increased recruitment and firing rates, although an EMG technique called power density spectral analysis has been used to make this distinction (Solomonow *et al.* 1990). Less commonly, EMG recordings have been made with needle or fine wire electrodes inserted into the muscle. The advantage of this EMG technique is that it allows the recruitment and firing rate patterns of individual motor units to be monitored. The difficulty with this technique is that it is very difficult, if not impossible, to identify and record the same motor units before and after training, or to record from a large number of motor units. Instead, the behaviour of samples of the motor unit population are compared before and after training. The surface and intramuscular techniques can be compared with the following analogy. A surface electrode is like a microphone placed over the centre of a soccer field. It can record and quantify the roar of the crowd but cannot register what individual crowd members (motor units) are saying. The intramuscular electrode can be likened to a microphone placed close to the mouth of a single crowd member. Although the background roar can still be heard, it is possible to hear what the single crowd member is saying (i.e. record the activity of individual motor units).

SURFACE EMG STUDIES

An example of the surface EMG technique is shown in Fig. 15.4. In this study (Rabita *et al.* 2000) isometric training of the knee extensor

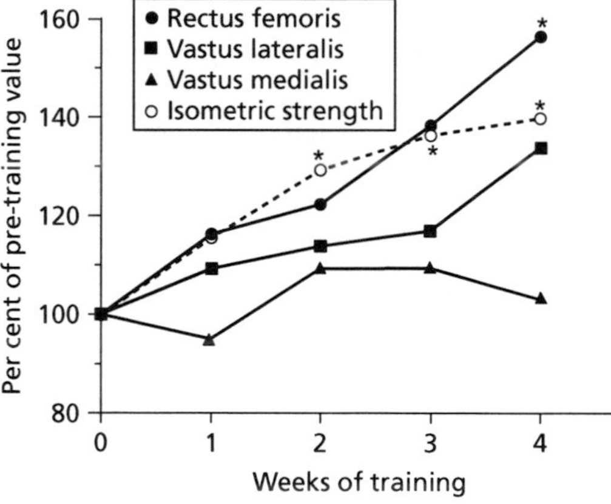

Fig. 15.4 Effect of isometric training of the knee extensor muscles on maximum isometric strength and activation of three of the four heads of the quadriceps femoris. Four weeks of training increased strength, but increased activation (measured by surface electromyography, EMG) occurred in only one (rectus femoris) of the three muscles monitored. (Based on Rabita *et al.* 2000.)

muscles was done for 4 weeks. EMG was recorded from three of the four heads of the quadriceps while the subjects did brief maximal isometric test action. Only one head, the rectus femoris, showed a significant increase in EMG to accompany the increase in isometric strength after training. This study is but one of many training studies which have assessed the effect of strength training on possible increases in motor unit activation (e.g. increased integrated EMG (iEMG) or similar measurement) in the quadriceps muscle, by far the most frequently studied muscle group. The types of training have included isometric exercise (Komi *et al.* 1978; Carolan & Cafarelli 1992; Garfinkel & Cafarelli 1992; Bandy & Hanten 1993; Weir *et al.* 1994, 1995; Rabita *et al.* 2000), weight training (Thorstensson *et al.* 1976; Häkkinen & Komi 1983; Häkkinen *et al.* 1985a,b, 1996, 1998a,b, 2000, 2001; Häkkinen & Häkkinen 1995; Narici *et al.* 1996; Hortobágyi & DeVita 2000) and isokinetic concentric or eccentric exercise (Higbie *et al.* 1996; Narici *et al.* 1989; Hortobágyi *et al.* 1996a; Hortobágyi *et al.* 1996b; Hortobágyi *et al.* 1997; Aagaard *et al.* 2000; Rutherford *et al.* 2001). The studies have ranged in duration from as brief as 1 week (Hortobágyi & DeVita 2000) to as long as 48 weeks (Häkkinen *et al.* 2000). Some studies, for example the one depicted in Fig. 15.4, adhered strictly to mode 'specificity' in that the type of action (isometric, concentric or eccentric), movement pattern and apparatus were the same for both training and testing. Other studies involved training with one mode and testing with another; for example, training by weightlifting and testing with isokinetic (velocity-controlled) concentric and eccentric actions (e.g. Aagaard *et al.* 2000), or isometric actions (e.g. Häkkinen & Komi 1983). Some studies have used both specific and non-specific EMG tests (e.g. Häkkinen *et al.* 1998a).

Viewed collectively, some general observations can be made about the effect of training on motor unit activation in the quadriceps femoris. First, a majority of the studies show increased EMG with training. Second, it cannot be assumed that all heads of the quadriceps respond in the same way to training (e.g. Fig. 15.4; Häkkinen &

Komi 1983; Aagaard *et al.* 2000). Thus, caution should be exercised in extrapolating the results in one head of the quadriceps to the other three heads. As examples in addition to the study depicted in Fig. 15.4, in which an increase in EMG was observed in only one of three heads monitored, two studies assessed only the vastus lateralis and found no increase in EMG after training (Carolan & Cafarelli 1992; Garfinkel & Cafarelli 1992). Changes may have occurred in one or more of the other three heads. Similarly, another study assessed only the rectus femoris and found an increase in EMG (Komi *et al.* 1978). There may have been no changes in the remaining heads. Third, in all studies the results could have been influenced by several factors, including the intensity, volume, frequency and duration of training, the movement pattern and type of muscle action used in training, and similarity (specificity) between the training and test modes. An example of specificity, in terms of both test vs. training mode, and type of muscle action, is illustrated in Fig. 15.5. In the study shown in Fig. 15.5 (Hortobágyi *et al.* 1996a), the test and training modes were the same (isokinetic concentric and eccentric actions). Specificity of training with either concentric or eccentric actions was examined. The major findings were that EMG increased in the two heads of the quadriceps monitored, the magnitude of increases was training mode (concentric vs. eccentric) specific, and that eccentric training produced the greatest specific increases.

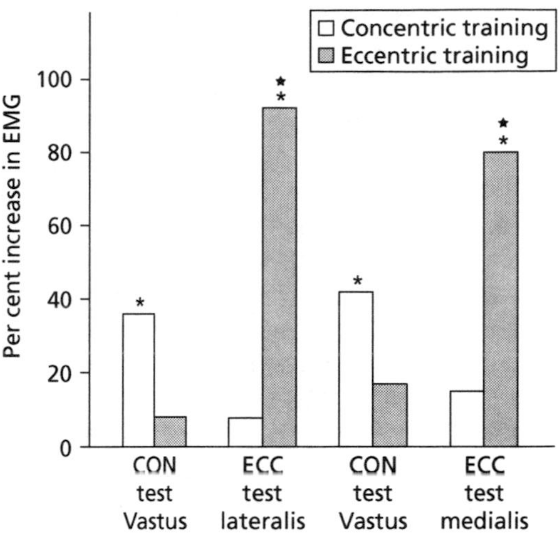

Fig. 15.5 Effects of either concentric or eccentric isokinetic knee extension training on the activation (from surface EMG) of two of four heads of the quadriceps femoris. Specificity in the training effect was observed in both muscles. Eccentric training produced the greatest increases in activation in the eccentric test, and concentric training produced the greatest increases in the concentric test. In respective specific tests, eccentric training caused the greatest increase. *, significant increase pre- to post training; ★, increase in the eccentric test with eccentric training was significantly greater than the increase in the concentric test with concentric training. Pattern of strength increases was similar (not shown). (Based on Hortobágyi *et al.* 1996a.)

Other muscle groups trained include ankle dorsiflexors (Van Cutsem *et al.* 1998), elbow flexors (Moritani & deVries 1979; Thépaut-Mathieu *et al.* 1988; Ozmun *et al.* 1994; Martin *et al.* 1995; Colson *et al.* 1999; Macaluso *et al.* 2000), adductor pollicis (Cannon & Cafarelli 1987), first dorsal interosseus (Keen *et al.* 1994) and hypothenar muscles (Yue & Cole 1992). As with the studies of the quadriceps, these studies vary in the features of training, application of specificity and number of muscles monitored within an agonist group. All but one (Cannon & Cafarelli 1987) found an increase in EMG with training. A few studies have observed increased EMG early in training programmes followed by a decrease (Häkkinen & Komi 1983; Keen *et al.* 1994; Narici *et al.* 1996). Unique among the studies, regardless of muscle group, is that of Yue and Cole (1992), which compared the effect of actual and 'imagined' isometric training. Imagined training consisted of subjects imagining making a series of maximal isometric actions in each training session, the number being identical to another group who actually made the isometric actions. Imagined (and actual) training produced significant increases in strength and EMG. It is notable that muscles displayed EMG 'silence' during the imagined training, suggesting that a supraspinal neural mechanism was responsible for the increased strength and EMG in test contractions (Yue & Cole 1992). The presence of a supraspinal mechanism was further supported by functional magnetic resonance imaging, which showed activation of the prefrontal association cortex during imagined muscle contractions (Yue *et al.* 1995).

Most studies have focused on the relationship between increased maximum EMG and increased maximum force (strength). In two studies, the emphasis in the training was to develop force as rapidly as possible. The rate of rise in EMG increased along with rate of force development (Häkkinen *et al.* 1985b; Van Cutsem *et al.* 1998; see also Fig. 15.6). In a study (Narici *et al.* 1996) in which the emphasis in training was not rapid force development (conventional weight training), the rate of rise in EMG in the one head of quadriceps monitored (vastus lateralis) was not altered by training, although isometric rate of force development increased.

The conclusion that increased surface EMG represents increased motor unit activation requires the assumption that training does not produce other changes that might alter the quantity of the recorded motor unit activity. Changes in subcutaneous fat and fibre pennation angle, or changes in the amplitude of the muscle fibre action potentials, could conceivably increase EMG independently of any change in motor unit activation. The best control for these possibilities is to record in a test session maximal evoked (by electrical stimulation) EMG (e.g. M-wave) as well as voluntary contraction EMG. If the evoked EMG remains unchanged but voluntary EMG increases (Van Cutsem *et al.* 1998), or if the voluntary EMG is normalized to the evoked EMG (Yue & Cole 1992; Keen *et al.* 1994) and the normalized value increases, then it can be reasonably concluded that an increase in motor unit activation has occurred. Furthermore, the increased surface EMG of test contractions of untrained contralateral limbs ('cross-training' effect; see Zhou 2000 for a review) after training (Moritani & deVries 1979; Yue & Cole 1992; Hortobágyi *et al.* 1997, 1999), or the increased EMG after imagined training (Yue & Cole 1992) could not be ascribed to changes in the muscle. Finally, specific training effects, such as greater EMG increases in bilateral than in unilateral actions after bilateral training (Häkkinen *et al.* 1996), point to an actual increase in motor unit activation.

Another surface EMG method that has been applied to strength training studies is called *reflex potentiation*. In this method reflex EMG responses are elicited during maximal voluntary contractions. The greater the voluntary effort and hence the motor unit activation, the greater the potentiation of the reflex response. Strength training studies have demonstrated an increase in reflex potentiation after training (Milner-Brown *et al.* 1975; Sale *et al.* 1983a). Cross-sectional studies have shown reflex potentiation to be enhanced in weightlifters (Milner-Brown *et al.* 1975; Sale *et al.* 1983b) and sprinters (Upton & Radford 1975). The reflex potentiation method cannot distinguish between the relative contributions of increased recruitment and increased firing rates to the increase in motor unit activation.

INTRAMUSCULAR EMG

The training-induced increase in surface EMG reviewed in the preceding section could result from some combination of increased recruitment and firing rates of motor units. There have been a few studies that have used intramuscular recording electrodes to monitor recruitment and firing rates of motor units before and after training. These studies have shown increased motor unit firing rates during maximal contractions after training (Kamen *et al.* 1998; Van Cutsem *et al.* 1998; Patten *et al.* 2001). Isometric training of abductor digiti minimi resulted in an increase in maximal motor unit firing rates during maximal contractions after only 2 days of training; curiously, firing rates then reverted towards pre-training values as training progressed (Patten *et al.* 2001). Isometric and dynamic training of knee extensor muscles increased the maximum motor unit firing rates of vastus lateralis in maximal isometric actions (Kamen *et al.* 1998). 'Ballistic' training of ankle dorsiflexors, which increased peak isometric force and surface EMG, was also associated with increased rate of force

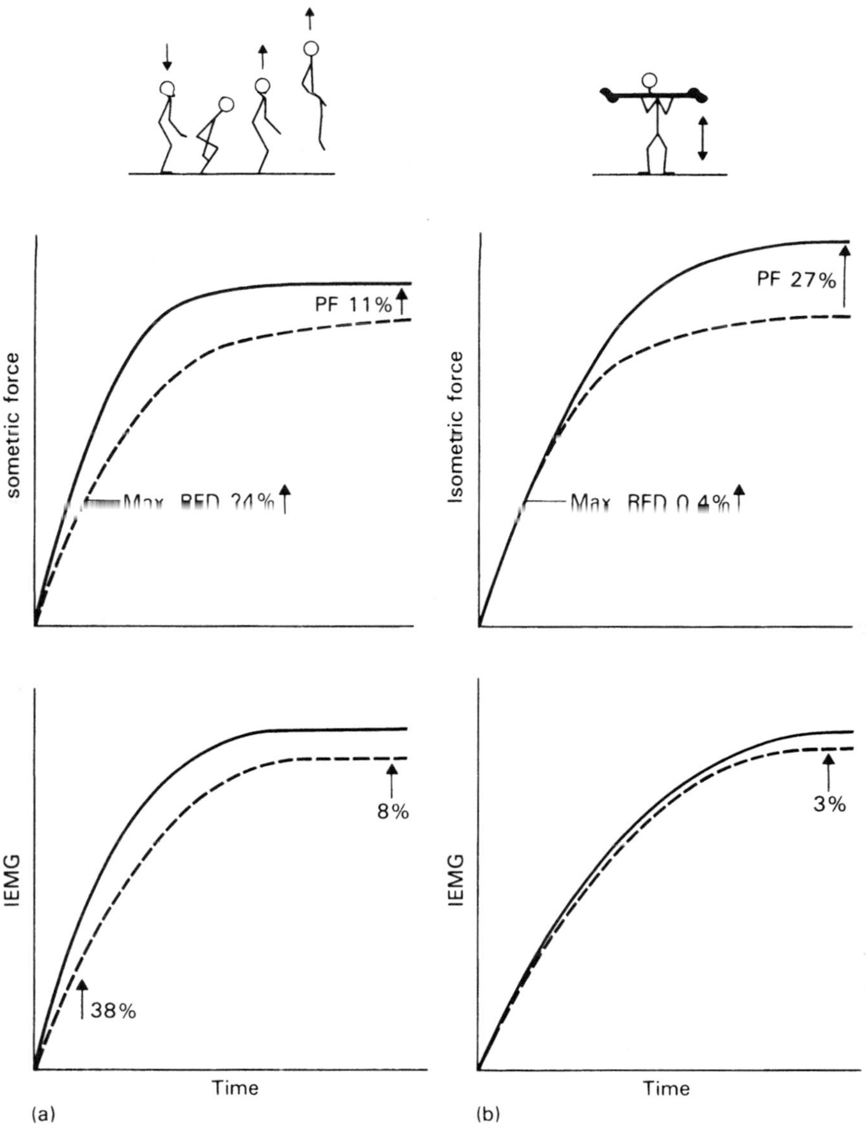

Fig. 15.6 Left, effect of explosive jump training on isometric strength and motor unit activation (surface EMG quantified as integrated EMG, iEMG). The top panel shows that rate of force development (max RFD) increased more (24%) than peak force (PF, 11%). Similarly, the bottom panel shows that the maximum rate of onset of EMG increased more (38%) than the peak EMG (8%). The greater increases related to rate of force development may reflect specific neural adaptations to explosive training. Right, by comparison heavy-resistance weight training produced the opposite pattern of results. (Based on Häkkinen *et al.* (1985a,b and reproduced by permission from Sale 1988.)

development and increased peak motor unit firing rates (in tibialis anterior) at the onset of isometric actions in which the intent was the highest possible rate of force development (Fig. 15.7; Van Cutsem *et al.* 1998). Training also reduced the rate of decline in firing rate during the ballistic contractions (actually isometric actions with rapid rate of force development).

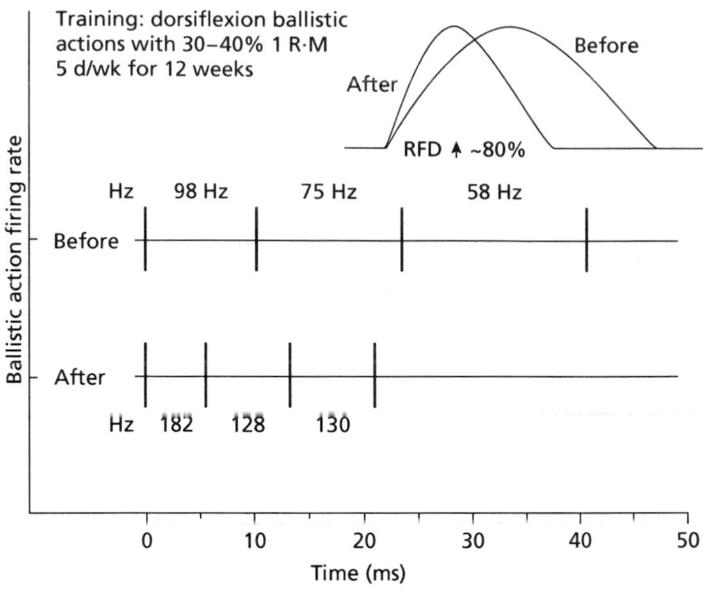

Fig. 15.7 Effect of 'ballistic' training on rate of force development and motor unit firing rates. The ankle dorsiflexor muscles were trained by maximal effort (for speed) ballistic actions with loads corresponding to 30–40% of the maximum single weight lift (one repetition maximum, 1 R·M). Test actions were isometric with the intent to develop force as rapidly as possible. The top right of the figure shows, schematically, the ~ 80% increase in rate of force development (RFD) that occurred with training. The peak forces were set to the same level. The remainder of the figure shows the increase in motor unit firing brought about by training. From a sample of motor units monitored before and after training, the average firing rates (measured as discharges per second, i.e. hertz, Hz) over the first four discharges at the onset of a ballistic (isometric) contraction are illustrated. Thus, over the first three interdischarge intervals, firing rate decreased (on average) from 98 to 58 Hz before training but from 182 to 130 Hz after training. The increased firing rates after training should have contributed to the increase in rate of force development (see Fig. 15.3, bottom panel). See text for further discussion. (Based on Van Cutsem *et al.* 1998.)

Training increased the percentage of motor units exhibiting 'doublets' in these isometric actions (Van Cutsem *et al.* 1998). (Doublets are very short (2–5 ms) interspike (interaction potential) intervals corresponding to very high instantaneous firing rates (200–500 Hz).) The magnitude of changes in discharge behaviour was not related to the recruitment threshold of the motor units, indicating the involvement of both low- and high-threshold motor units in the adaptation to training.

Although not strictly a training study, in a fatigue study (Grimby *et al.* 1981) some subjects were unable to fire high-threshold units in the short toe extensor muscles at rates necessary for maximum force output. After repeated experiments these subjects were then able to achieve higher firing rates; at this point their voluntary force matched the force evoked by tetanic (high-frequency) stimulation. The repeated experiments, which consisted of sustaining maximal contractions, could be considered a form of strength training. This training also increased the time (from a few to about 20 s) that the highest-threshold motor units could be kept active (recruited) in sustained maximal contractions. A 'drop-out' (cessation of firing) of motor units during sustained maximal contractions has been recently confirmed (Peters & Fuglevand 1999). Delay of motor unit drop-out would contribute to increased 'strength endurance' after training.

In addition to these longitudinal studies, a cross-sectional study found that weightlifters, compared to untrained subjects, had greater maximum motor unit firing rates in maximum isometric actions of the quadriceps (Leong *et al.* 1999). A comparison among untrained subjects, sprinters and long-distance runners indicated that sprinters had the highest motor unit firing rates in tibialis anterior (an ankle dorsiflexor) at the onset of rapidly developing isometric actions (Saplinskas *et al.* 1980). It will be recalled from Fig. 15.3 (middle and bottom panels) that increased motor unit firing rates could increase either maximum force or rate of force development.

Intramuscular EMG records from only a sample of motor units within a muscle; therefore, it is difficult to estimate whether training has increased motor unit recruitment. Nevertheless, Patten *et al.* (2001) found that after isometric training there was a trend of an increased number of active motor units in abductor digiti minimi during maximal isometric actions. Ballistic training caused a leftward shift in the recruitment thresholds of motor units in slowly developing 'ramp' contractions; that is, the average threshold, expressed as a percentage of maximal strength (MVC), decreased (Van Cutsem *et al.* 1998). There was no change in the recruitment order of motor units in the ramp contractions after training; thus, the size principle of recruitment was preserved. Thresholds during ballistic contractions were not measured (Van Cutsem *et al.* 1998). A cross-sectional study indicated that sprinters, in comparison to untrained subjects and long-distance runners, recruited motor units of tibialis anterior at lower force thresholds in isometric actions with rapid rate of force development. Sprinters also exhibited a greater incidence of recruitment reversals in these fast actions; that is, motor units which had lower thresholds in slow actions had higher thresholds in fast actions (Saplinskas *et al.* 1980).

The relative roles of increased motor unit recruitment and increased firing rates as adaptations to training may depend on their relative roles in grading the force of contraction (Fig. 15.8). In small hand muscles few if any

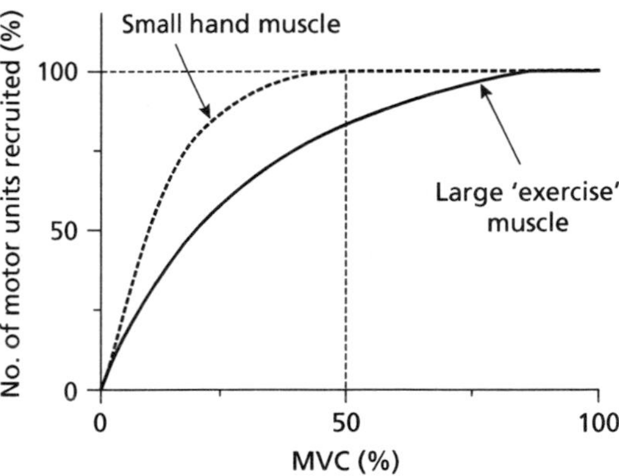

Fig. 15.8 Relative roles of motor unit recruitment and increased firing rates in increasing the force of an isometric action. In some muscles, for example some small hand muscles, all motor units are recruited by about 50% of maximum strength (MVC, maximal voluntary contraction). This means that increased motor unit firing rates are solely responsible for increasing force beyond 50% MVC. In other larger muscles, more typically involved in sport training programmes, motor units are recruited up to about 80–90% MVC. Note, however, that even in these muscles the majority of units are recruited by 50% MVC; therefore, increased firing rates appears to play the major if not exclusive role. This predominance of firing rates is offset to some extent by the later recruited units having more muscle fibres (see Enoka & Fuglevand 2001). It is possible that muscles with high-threshold units are more difficult to fully activate. See text for further discussion.

motor units are recruited beyond about 50% of maximum strength (Milner-Brown *et al.* 1973; Kukulka & Clamann 1981; DeLuca *et al.* 1982). Untrained people should be able to recruit all motor units in a maximal voluntary effort, but they may not be able to bring all units to maximal firing rates; hence, increased firing rates would be a possible training adaptation. In larger muscles such as the tibialis anterior (Hannerz 1974; Van Cutsem *et al.* 1998), biceps (Kukulka & Clamann 1981) and deltoid (DeLuca *et al.* 1982), motor units are recruited up to about 80–90% of maximum strength, although the majority of motor units are recruited by 50% of maximum strength (Fig. 15.8). This may also be true for other large muscles associated with strength training (e.g. latissimus dorsi, pectoralis major, gluteus maximus). In muscles such as these untrained people may have difficulty in both recruiting the highest-threshold motor units and bringing all units to their optimum firing rate. This may be especially true when the training exercise requires coordination. It should be noted that for a given muscle, the range of contraction strength over which motor unit recruitment occurs can be influenced by the task performed and the rate at which force is developed (see Bernardi *et al.* 1995, 1996, 1997).

MOTOR UNIT SYNCHRONIZATION

A special aspect of altered or increased agonist activation is motor unit synchronization. There are reports, in both longitudinal (Milner-Brown *et al.* 1975) and cross-sectional studies (Milner-Brown *et al.* 1975; Semmler & Nordstrom 1998; Felici *et al.* 2001), and with both surface and intramuscular EMG methods, of increased motor unit synchronization (of firing or discharge) associated with strength training. While this undoubtedly represents a neural adaptation to training, it is not yet clear how increased synchronization, usually assessed with submaximal contractions, could increase the peak force of a maximal voluntary contraction. Studies with animal nerve–muscle preparations indicate that at low stimulation frequencies, corresponding to low motor unit firing rates, force output is actually greater with asynchronous than synchronous stimulation; at high stimulation frequencies corresponding to maximal motor unit firing rates in maximal voluntary contractions, synchronous and asynchronous stimulation are equally effective (Rack & Westbury 1969; Lind & Petrofsky 1978). A more synchronous *onset* of discharge of recruited motor units might conceivably increase rate of force development (Felici *et al.* 2001), but once discharge has commenced, the recruited motor units would almost immediately be firing asynchronously because of different firing rates. Asynchronous firing at this stage may not be a disadvantage, since it has been shown that synchronous stimulation at supraphysiological frequencies cannot match the rate of force development achieved by a voluntary contraction (Miller *et al.* 1981). This comparison may not be entirely fair, however, because it is not possible to replicate, in a stimulated contraction, the coordination of synergists present in a voluntary contraction.

Magnetic resonance imaging

A relatively recent technique for assessing training-induced changes in muscle activation is a form of magnetic resonance imaging (MRI). Exercise causes 'contrast shifts' (increases in muscle proton spin–spin relaxation time, T_2) in MR images of muscles (Yue *et al.* 1994). The images can be used to indicate which muscles have been activated in a particular exercise, and the extent of their activation (Adams *et al.* 1992). Assessments of muscle activity with MRI correlate well with EMG measurements (Adams *et al.* 1992) and have the advantage that muscles inaccessible to EMG can be readily examined, such as all four heads of the quadriceps (Ploutz *et al.* 1994) or superficial and deep neck (head) extensor muscles (Conley *et al.* 1997a). One study using the MRI technique estimated that untrained subjects can activate only ~ 70% of the quadriceps in a maximal voluntary contraction (Adams *et al.* 1993).

The MRI technique was used in a study in which the neck extensor muscles were trained (weight training) for 12 weeks (Conley *et al.* 1997a). In a maximal test, consisting of three sets of 10 repetitions with the heaviest possible weight, muscle activation, expressed as the relative cross-sectional area of muscle showing activation, increased in some neck muscles but not others after training (Fig. 15.9). These results are in agreement with the previously discussed EMG studies showing that some but not all muscles in an agonist group may increase their activation after strength training (e.g. Fig. 15.4). Another study showed increased activation of the quadriceps after 2 weeks of isokinetic knee extension training (Akima *et al.* 1999).

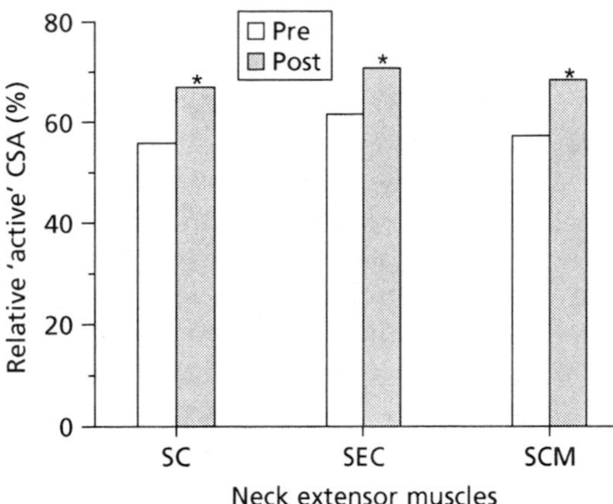

Fig. 15.9 Effect of training on muscle activation assessed by magnetic resonance imaging. Neck (head) extensor muscles were trained with a weight training neck extension exercise. In a maximal exercise test (three sets of 10 repetitions with maximum weight) pre- and post training, the relative active proportion of muscle cross-sectional area (% CSA) increased after training in three of six neck extensor muscles/muscle pairs: SC, splenius capitis; SEC, semispinalis capitis; SCM, semispinalis cervicis and multifidus. These results indicated greater neural activation in some but not all muscles involved in neck extension. (Based on Conley *et al.* (1997a.)

Voluntary vs. evoked contractions

STIMULATION SUPERIMPOSED ON VOLUNTARY CONTRACTIONS

There have been two approaches to using (electrically) evoked contractions to assess the extent of motor unit activation during maximal voluntary contractions, in addressing the issue of whether untrained subjects can fully activate their muscles (agonists). One approach consists of superimposing, via the motor nerve, a single stimulus (interpolated twitch; e.g. Belanger & McComas 1981; Bulow *et al.* 1993; Allen *et al.* 1995; Yue *et al.* 2000), a pair of stimuli (interpolated 'doublet'; e.g. Gandevia & McKenzie 1988; Kent-Braun & Le Blanc 1997) or a train of stimuli (interpolated tetanus; e.g. Westing *et al.* 1990; Strojnik 1995; Kent-Braun & Le Blanc 1997) during a maximal voluntary contraction. If an increment in force is caused by the interpolated stimulus or stimuli, voluntary activation is considered to be less than maximal. There has been some debate over the relative validity of these variations of interpolation, and whether one indicates a greater activation deficit than the other (Dowling *et al.* 1994; Herbert *et al.* 1997; Kent-Braun & Le Blanc 1997; Allen *et al.* 1998; Herbert & Gandevia 1999; Kent-Braun 1999; Yue *et al.* 2000). The assessments of motor unit activation have been conducted in a variety of muscle groups, usually in unilateral isometric actions. The results of various studies include full activation being achieved in untrained subjects (e.g. Carolan & Cafarelli 1992), a small (5–10%) deficit of activation (e.g. Yue *et al.* 2000), and a more substantial (~ 20%) activation deficit (e.g. Bulow *et al.* 1995). Across several attempts over several days, subjects are not consistent in the extent of activation achieved (Allen *et al.* 1995). Factors which may affect the extent of motor unit activation are muscle group tested (Belanger & McComas 1981; McKenzie *et al.* 1992; Allen *et al.* 1998), joint angle/muscle length (may or may not: Gandevia & McKenzie 1988; Huber *et al.* 1998; Becker & Awiszus 2001), and whether activation is related to peak force vs. rate of force development (Strojnik 1995, 1998; Yue *et al.* 2000). Of special note is the effect of the type of muscle action. Interpolating a tetanus has a greater augmenting effect on eccentric than concentric or isometric voluntary actions (Westing *et al.* 1990; Amiridis *et al.* 1996). On the other hand, activation of elbow flexors (biceps) is similar in isometric actions and concentric actions at a variety of velocities (Gandevia *et al.* 1998). In addition to increasing peak force, interpolated tetani have increased isometric rate of force development (Strojnik 1995, 1998), and the peak velocity and power of concentric actions (Strojnik 1998). These latter observations indicate an activation deficit related to speed and power.

A more recent method than stimulating the motor nerve is to stimulate the motor cortex via transcranial magnetic stimulation during a maximal isometric action (for reviews see Taylor *et al.* 2000; Taylor & Gandevia 2001). This method also reveals a small deficit in motor unit activation (Herbert & Gandevia 1996) that increases as a maximal contraction is sustained (Gandevia *et al.* 1996). The fact that cortical stimulation can augment force indicates that the deficit is 'upstream' from both the spinal cord and the motor cortex.

COMPARISON OF SEPARATE EVOKED AND VOLUNTARY CONTRACTIONS

The second approach to using evoked contractions to assess the extent of motor unit activation has been to compare the force attained with evoked vs. voluntary contractions separately (Westing *et al.* 1990), or to compare the 'shape' of the force–velocity relationship (Dudley *et al.* 1990; Westing *et al.* 1990) and force–joint angle relationships (Koh & Herzog 1995) obtained with evoked vs. voluntary contractions. This approach indicates, in agreement with the results of the interpolated stimulation method, that the greatest activation deficit exists, at least for knee extensors, in the low-velocity concentric region and generally in the eccentric region of the force–velocity relationship (Dudley *et al.* 1990; Westing *et al.* 1990; Harris & Dudley 1994). The evoked and voluntary force–joint angle/muscle length relationships of ankle dorsiflexors have been compared (Marsh *et al.* 1981; van Schaik *et al.* 1994; Koh & Herzog 1995). The results of these studies are not consistent, but suggest that muscle length/joint angle has little influence on the ability to activate muscle. This is in accord with one of the interpolated stimulation studies cited previously, which examined ankle dorsiflexors, fifth finger abductors and elbow flexors (Gandevia *et al.* 1988), but is in disagreement with two studies of knee extensors, which also disagree with each other, one showing greater activation at short muscle lengths (Huber *et al.* 1998) and the other showing the opposite (Becker & Awiszus 2001).

There are limitations to the evoked contraction techniques. One is that it is not always possible to stimulate all muscles of an agonist group, making it difficult to equate voluntary and evoked contraction force. In stimulation, muscles not stimulated remain relaxed, whereas in a voluntary contraction synergistic muscles likely contribute to the contraction. Indeed, voluntary force may exceed stimulated force because of this contribution (Herbert & Gandevia 1999). A second limitation is that it may be difficult to avoid inadvertently stimulating antagonists along with agonists. Thirdly, it is difficult to replicate, with stimulating electrodes, the central nervous system's expertise in activating muscles. In particular, it is difficult to apply the method to relatively complex, bilateral movements involving several joints. For example, superimposed tetanic stimulation of one of the muscles (quadriceps) acting during the vertical jump actually impaired performance, perhaps by interfering with the coordination of the action (Strojnik 1998). In activities like these, EMG is more suitable for uncovering an activation deficit and its modification by training (see Fig. 15.10).

In summary, the stimulation methods indicate some deficit in motor unit activation in maximal voluntary contractions. The untapped activation potential that can be realized by neural adaptations to training is perhaps less than would be expected, based on the increases in EMG that have been reported in some training studies, and the amount by which strength increases exceed observable muscle adaptations. However, in the case of eccentric actions, there appears to be good correspondence between the size of the activation deficit (relatively large) and the increase in EMG with training (see section 'Electromyographic studies' and Fig. 15.5). It should also be noted that the activation deficit and therefore the potential for neural adaptation may be greater in more complex movements to which the stimulation methods cannot be easily applied. For example, it would difficult to determine whether the pectoralis major is completely activated in a single maximal barbell bench press (1 RM), or whether the deltoid is fully activated in an overhead press. It is possible that fully activating muscles under these conditions is more challenging than in the unilateral, single-joint actions so often studied. Relevant here is the frequent observation of a bilateral 'deficit' in strength and

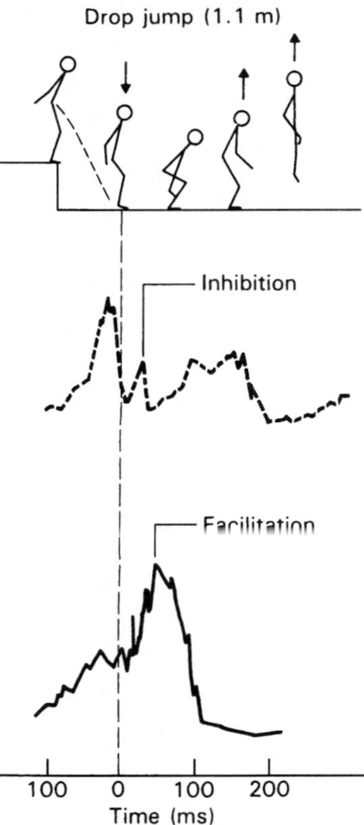

Fig. 15.10 EMG recordings from the gastrocnemius muscle during drop jumps in an untrained subject (top) and in a trained jumper (bottom). During the eccentric phase of high stretch load (to immediate right of vertical dashed line at time 0), the untrained subject responded with a period of inhibition. In contrast the trained jumper responded with a period of facilitation. The facilitation in the jumper may reflect a neural adaptation to training that is related to reflex responses. (Based on Schmidtbleicher and Gollhofer 1982 as cited in Komi 1986 and reproduced by permission from Sale 1988.)

activation when bilateral vs. unilateral actions are attempted (see Jakobi & Chilibeck 2001 for a review).

TRAINING STUDIES

In contrast to the number of studies using evoked contractions to assess the extent of motor unit activation in untrained subjects, there have been relatively few longitudinal training studies, or cross-sectional studies comparing trained and untrained groups. In two longitudinal training studies (Carolan & Cafarelli 1992; Garfinkel & Cafarelli 1992), knee extensors were trained with isometric actions. In both studies subjects achieved complete activation assessed by the interpolated twitch method in the pretests, so there was no change in activation with training. There was also no change in EMG. In one study strength and muscle cross-sectional area increased 28% and 15%, respectively; a non-hypertrophic adaptation was not identified (Garfinkel & Cafarelli 1992). In the other study, a 33% increase in strength was accompanied by no change in agonist EMG, but there was a decrease in antagonist EMG early in the training that accounted for some of the increase in strength. Possible hypertrophic adaptations were not assessed (Carolan & Cafarelli 1992). In another study (Harridge *et al.* 1999), elderly subjects trained knee extensors and flexors with weightlifting exercise. Motor unit activation, assessed by the interpolated twitch method, was 81% and 85% pre- and post-training, respectively (non-significant change). However, activation was measured in a strength test (isometric knee extension at a joint angle of 90°), which also showed no significant increase in strength. If activation had been measured in one of the tests that did show a significant increase in strength, perhaps a significant increase in activation would have been found (Fig. 15.11). Similarly, weight training of elbow flexors (Brown *et al.* 1990) and knee extensors (Sale *et al.* 1992) increased weightlifting but not isometric strength. Correspondingly, there was no change in motor unit activation assessed with the interpolated twitch technique in the isometric test. One study compared the effects of real and imagined training of the elbow flexor muscles. Activation based on the interpolated twitch method was close to maximal before training (96%), and was unaltered by 8 weeks of isometric training. Only actual training produced a significant increase in strength (Herbert *et al.* 1998). (This study contrasts with a study reviewed earlier, Yue & Cole 1992, in which imagined training of a small hand

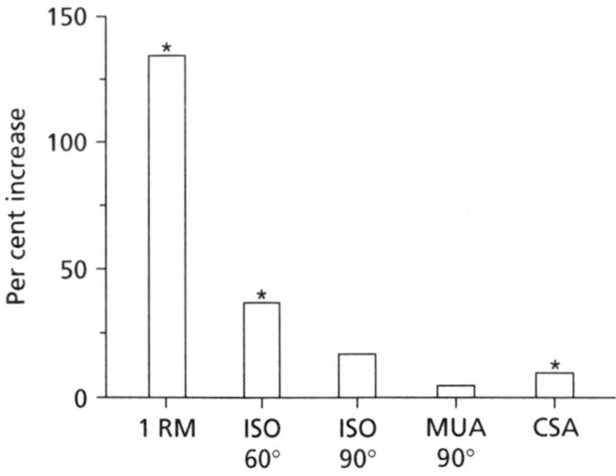

Fig. 15.11 Specificity in the response to strength training. The knee extensor muscles were trained with weight training exercises. Specific strength, that is, one repetition maximum (1 RM), increased greatly. In contrast, isometric strength measured at a joint angle of 60° increased to a much lesser degree, and isometric strength at 90° did not increase significantly. At this angle motor unit activation (MUA)was also assessed with the interpolated twitch method, and no increase was found. Perhaps if the method had been applied to the 60° isometric test or to the weightlifting test, an increase in MUA might have been observed. There was a significant increase in muscle cross-sectional area (CSA), but the amount of increase failed to account for all of the increase in specific strength and failed to increase one measure of non-specific strength. Based on Harridge *et al.* (1999).

muscle increased strength and EMG to levels similar to those of actual training.) Twenty days of bed rest decreased the activation of knee extensors from 86 to 80%, whereas specific isometric knee extension training during the bed rest prevented the loss of activation (Kawakami *et al.* 2001). A cross-sectional study indicated that volleyball players who had undergone strenuous (rehabilitation) training of knee extensors following injury, had less inhibition (greater activation as assessed by interpolated twitch) than players who had never sustained an injury (Huber *et al.* 1998). The reduction in inhibition was greatest at the joint angle at which greater torque could be generated, which was also the joint angle at which the inhibition was greatest in uninjured athletes. A study comparing high jumpers with sedentary subjects found that superimposed tetanic stimulation augmented knee extensor eccentric torque in the sedentary subjects but not the athletes, suggesting that training had increased the activation achieved in these actions (Amiridis *et al.* 1996).

In summary, some studies have shown training-induced increases in activation using stimulation techniques. The lack of consistent results can be attributed to the same factors likely responsible for the varied results of EMG studies (specificity, muscle group, nature of training programme, etc.).

Decreased activation of agonists?

With all the attention placed on increased agonist activation as a neural adaptation to training, it might be overlooked that there is evidence of *decreased* agonist activation after strength training. This observation is made when trainees exercise at the same absolute intensity (e.g. 10 repetitions with 50 kg) before and after training. The given absolute load may represent maximal relative intensity (e.g. 100% 10 RM) before training but submaximal intensity (e.g. 75% 10 RM) after training. One line of evidence for decreased agonist activation is the decrease in EMG seen when exercising at the same absolute load or force after training, causing a decrease in the ratio of EMG to force (Komi *et al.* 1978; Moritani & deVries 1979; Häkkinen *et al.* 1985a; Garfinkel & Cafarelli 1992). A second line of evidence comes from MRI studies showing a decreased activation of muscle cross-sectional area after training (Ploutz *et al.* 1994; Conley *et al.* 1997a).

The traditional interpretation of the EMG studies is that hypertrophy of muscle fibres results in fewer fibres (motor units) required for a given force, hence reduced motor unit activation (EMG). An underlying assumption is that the same *absolute* muscle mass or cross-sectional area (CSA) is active after training, whereas the *relative* CSA is reduced. In contrast, the important observation of the MRI studies is that both the relative *and* absolute CSA needed for a given absolute force decreases with training. This implies that for the smaller number of active muscle fibres, the generated force per unit CSA is increased. One explanation could be that the specific tension (force per unit CSA) of trained muscle fibres has increased, allowing fewer to be activated; however, there is little evidence that strength training increases specific tension (measured with evoked contractions). Another possible explanation is that with training the nervous system 'forces' a smaller number of fibres to produce greater force by having them operate further up on their force–frequency relation; that is, the motoneurones innervating the muscle fibres would be required to discharge at higher rates. Yet another possible explanation is altered synchronization of active motor units (see Ploutz *et al.* 1994 for discussion). Evidence that a neural mechanism is partly involved is the observation of decreased absolute muscle activation in both trained and untrained contralateral limbs (Ploutz *et al.* 1994). Muscle adaptations could not account for the reduced activation per unit force in the untrained limb. (It should be noted, however, that in the EMG study by Moritani & deVries 1979, the decreased EMG/force slope was found only in the trained limb.)

Another interpretation of the decreased absolute agonist activation at a given absolute intensity is that a neural adaptation, in the form of synergists being relatively more active after training, allows the prime agonist to become less active. However, studies which measured activation of the entire quadriceps (Ploutz *et al.* 1994) and neck extensor complex (Conley *et al.* 1997a) found decreased activation or no change in activation in all muscles that could have contributed to the action.

Another neural adaptation that would have to be accounted for is decreased antagonist coactivation after training, which would also reduce the required level of agonist activation for a given absolute force (Carolan & Cafarelli 1992). The MRI studies of knee and neck extensor muscles did not report specifically on changes in activation in antagonists; however, a change in antagonist activity would likely make only a small, if any, contribution to the decreased agonist activation per unit muscle force (Ploutz *et al.* 1994; Conley *et al.* 1997a).

Activation of synergists

Muscles that contribute to a movement are called synergists (Jamison & Caldwell 1993). This expansive definition implies that agonists, 'fixators' and even antagonists (Basmajian 1974) qualify as synergists. Thus, it can be argued that all muscles that are engaged in performing a strength task are acting as synergists. The previous section dealt with increased agonist activation, and the subsequent section will consider antagonist coactivation. Therefore, this section will focus on a narrower definition of synergists —groups of separate agonist muscles, compartments within a muscle or subpopulations of motor units within a muscle that act together to perform a function. For example, the biceps, brachialis and brachioradialis are agonists for elbow flexion. Each is considered a synergist for the other two; however, their relative activation may vary depending on the action performed. The long and short heads of the biceps may act synergistically, but their relative activation may be task dependent. Finally, within a head of biceps, subpopulations of motor units may be more or less active depending on the task. In this latter case, the muscle fibres of some motor units may be more strategically situated to deliver force in a particular action. Another aspect of coordination among active motor units is that their collective force delivery is dependent on the in-series and in-parallel connections among the muscle fibres (Sheard 2000). Finally, in some movements muscles may act as fixators. Fixators may not cause a joint action directly, but they may assist by preventing unwanted movement at other joints; in this sense they could be referred to as synergists. Fixators may also provide a stable 'platform' for a joint action, for example stabilizing the trunk in an overhead lift.

In strength performance, the goal of appropriate activation or coordination of synergists is the greatest possible force in the intended direction of movement. That training enhances this coordination by neural adaptations is strongly suggested by many studies that have demonstrated specificity in the training response. Specificity may be related to the movement pattern, type of muscle action (eccentric, isometric, concentric) and velocity employed in training (Sale & MacDougall 1981). A general manifestation of specificity is much greater strength increases when the strength test is identical to the training exercise, and much smaller increases when the strength test of the same muscle group is not identical to the training exercise (Kanehisa & Miyashita 1983; Rutherford & Jones 1986; Rutherford *et al.* 1986; Rutherford 1988; Morrisey *et al.* 1995; Aagaard *et al.* 1996; Almasbakk & Hoff 1996; Häkkinen *et al.* 1996; Narici *et al.* 1996; Wilson *et al.* 1996; see also Fig. 15.11). Only rarely is this type of specificity not seen (Laidlaw *et al.* 1999). At the extreme, training that causes a large increase in specific strength and hypertrophy may actually fail to increase strength in a non-specific strength test of the same muscle group (Brown *et al.* 1990; Sale *et al.* 1992; Higbie *et al.* 1996; Harridge *et al.* 1999; see Fig. 15.11).

Electromyographic studies

EVIDENCE OF TASK-DEPENDENT SYNERGIST COORDINATION

Most of the evidence showing varied activation of synergists in specific tasks comes from electromyographic studies. Many synergist groups have been monitored while performing varied movements or tasks. In the elbow flexors, for example, the brachioradialis assists the biceps in flexion but not supination (Caldwell *et al.* 1993). The relative activation of the biceps is affected by joint angle during maximal concentric and isometric actions, whereas the activation of the brachioradialis is affected by joint angle only during maximal eccentric actions (Kasprisin & Grabiner 2000). The ratio of brachioradialis to biceps activation is greater at flexed than extended joint angles in isometric and eccentric actions, but in concentric actions the ratio is unaffected by joint angle. At extended angles, the ratio is greater in eccentric than concentric actions (Nakazawa *et al.* 1993). Within the biceps, increasing the length of the muscle (extended joint angle) promoted increased activation of the long head in relation to the short head in producing supination (Brown *et al.* 1993). Greater activation is attained in both heads of the biceps in combined (flexion plus supination) actions than in either action alone (Caldwell *et al.* 1993; Perot *et al.* 1996), and greater activation of the biceps is achieved in maximal supination than flexion efforts (Jamison & Caldwell 1993). Within the long head of the biceps, laterally located motor units are preferentially activated in flexion whereas medially located units are preferentially activated in supination (ter Harr Romeny *et al.* 1984; see Fig. 15.12).

The relative activation of the four heads of the quadriceps may vary in different actions. Medial and lateral vasti were most active during the last 15° of knee extension (Gryzlo *et al.* 1994). In the knee extension weightlifting exercise, the relative activation of the vastus lateralis, vastus medialis and rectus femoris is similar in the concentric phase of each repetition, but in the eccentric phase the rectus femoris shows the greatest activation (Narici *et al.* 1996). In the same exercise, the rectus femoris is more active with the tibia laterally rotated than in the neutral or inwardly rotated position (Signorile *et al.* 1995). The ratio of vastus medialis to vastus lateralis activation is greater when knee extension is combined with tibial medial rotation than when combined with hip adduction (Laprade *et al.* 1998).

The relative activation of the components of the triceps surae (the soleus and lateral and medial gastrocnemius) is affected by movement pattern, type of muscle action and velocity. In plantarflexion concentric actions at low velocities (submaximal efforts), the soleus is relatively more active than the gastrocnemius in the flexed than in extended knee positions. At the highest velocities (maximal efforts), the soleus/gastrocnemius activation ratio is unaffected by knee joint position. In the flexed position, the gastrocnemius is relatively more active than the soleus at higher velocities, whereas the opposite is true

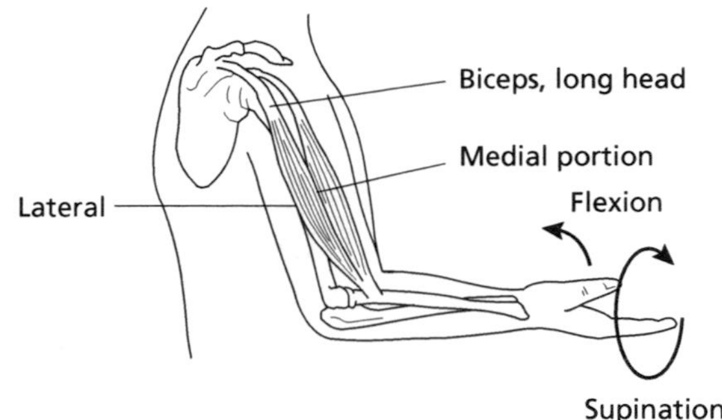

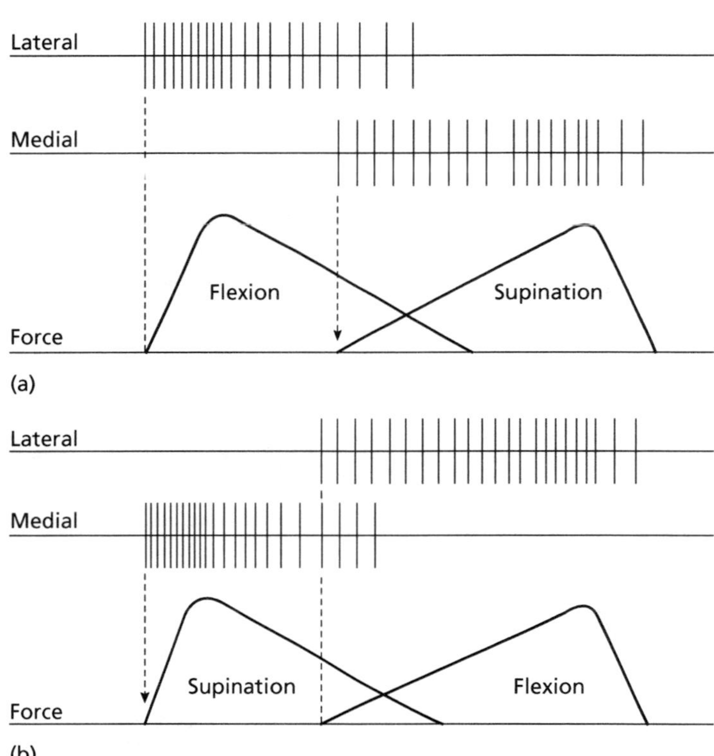

Fig. 15.12 Effect of movement pattern on motor unit recruitment. The biceps can act as an agonist in elbow flexion and forearm supination. In the top panel it is shown that when a flexion force is first developed the motor unit in the lateral (LAT) portion of the long head of the biceps is preferentially recruited over the unit in the medial (MED) portion. As the subject reduces the flexion force and begins to develop a supination force, the medial unit is preferentially activated. The bottom panel shows that when the order of producing flexion and supination forces is reversed, so is the order of preferential activation. Selective activation of motor units within a muscle, depending on the task, may be related to the specificity of movement pattern that has been observed in strength training. (Based on ter Harr Romeny *et al*. 1984.)

with the extended knee. A general observation is earlier onset of gastrocnemius than soleus activity in faster actions (Carpentier *et al*. 1996). The soleus is relatively more active than the gastrocnemius in submaximal concentric actions against resistance, whereas the gastrocnemius is relatively more active in eccentric actions (Nardone & Schieppati 1988; see Fig. 15.13). Within the gastrocnemius, slow-twitch motor units are preferentially activated in the concentric phase whereas fast-twitch units are more active in the eccentric phase (Nardone *et al*. 1989; see also Fig. 15.14). In stationary cycling, the gastrocnemius is preferentially activated over the soleus at higher pedalling speeds (Duchateau *et al*. 1986; see Fig. 15.15). The gastrocnemius is also preferentially activated in hopping (Moritani *et al*. 1990).

'Pressing' exercises are often used in strength training programmes. The relative activation of several muscles is influenced by the orientation of the trunk when doing these exercises (Barnett

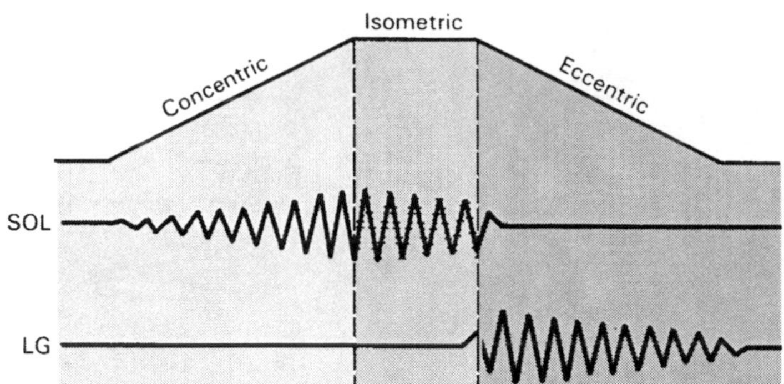

Fig. 15.13 Effect of action type on muscle activation. Recordings are made from soleus (SOL) and lateral gastrocnemius (LG) muscles of the calf when the muscles are acting as agonists in a shortening (concentric) action to raise a weight, an isometric contraction to hold the weight still briefly, and a lengthening (eccentric) action to lower the weight back down again. This movement pattern is typical of weight training exercises. Note that the soleus was preferentially activated during the concentric and isometric phases, whereas the lateral gastrocnemius was preferentially activated during the eccentric phase. The selective activation of the LG was most pronounced when the eccentric action was done relatively quickly. (Based on Nardone & Schieppati 1988.)

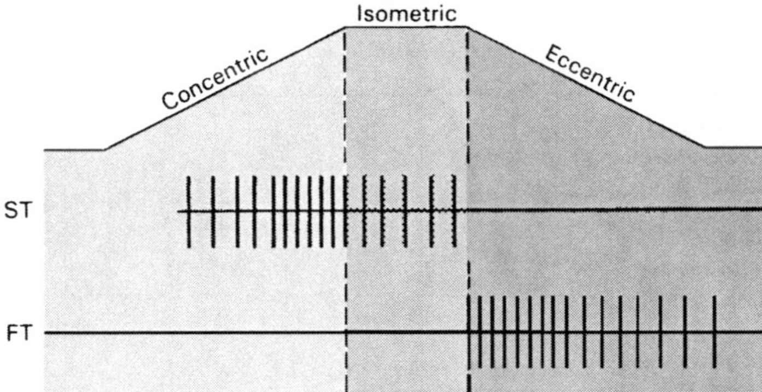

Fig. 15.14 Effect of action type on motor unit recruitment pattern. Recordings are made from a low-threshold slow-twitch (ST) and a high-threshold fast-twitch (FT) motor unit in the gastrocnemius muscle when the muscle is acting as an agonist in a shortening (concentric) action to raise a weight, an isometric action to hold the weight still briefly, and a lengthening (eccentric) action to lower the weight back down again. This movement pattern is typical of weight training exercises. Note that the ST unit is preferentially activated during the concentric and isometric phases, whereas the FT unit was preferentially activated during the eccentric phase. The selective activation of the FT unit was most pronounced when the eccentric action was done relatively quickly. (Based on Nardone *et al.* 1989.)

et al. 1995; see Fig. 15.16). For example, the sternocostal head of the pectoralis major is highly activated when the trunk is horizontal ('flat' bench press) but minimally active when the trunk is vertical (overhead or 'military' press). The anterior head of the deltoid becomes progressively more active as the trunk orientation moves from the decline (head down) to incline (head up) position (Barnett *et al.* 1995). The activation of muscles in pressing exercises is also influenced by hand spacing on the bar; for example, the activation of the sternocostal head but not the clavicular of pectoralis major was affected by hand spacing in some exercises (100% vs. 200% of biacromial diameter; Barnett *et al.* 1995).

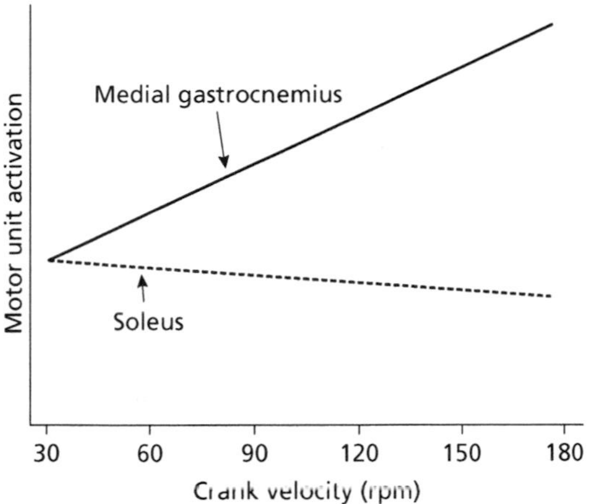

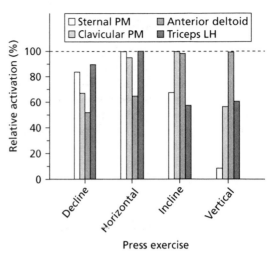

Fig. 15.15 Effect of velocity on muscle activation. EMG was recorded from two calf muscles during cycling at constant load but at different velocities. The medial gastrocnemius increased its activity greatly as velocity increased. In contrast, the soleus became slightly less active as velocity increased. One interpretation of these results is that the nervous system preferentially activated the gastrocnemius at high velocities because this muscle has a higher percentage of fast-twitch fibres than the soleus. Such a selective activation of muscles at certain speeds of movement may partly explain the specificity of velocity in training that has been observed. (Based on Duchateau *et al.* 1986.)

Fig. 15.16 Activation of some muscles acting at the shoulder joint in four versions of the 'press' exercise: decline bench press (head down), horizontal or 'flat' bench press, incline press (head up), and (trunk) vertical press. Surface EMG of sternal and clavicular heads of pectoralis major (PM), anterior deltoid, and long head (LH) of triceps was monitored. For display, the EMG of each muscle has been normalized to the value obtained in the exercise in which it was most active. It can be seen that these muscles are much more active in some exercises than others (see text for details). Training with a particular exercise is likely to evoke specific neural and muscular adaptations related to the pattern of muscle use. (Based on Barnett *et al.* 1995.)

TRAINING STUDIES

In contrast to the many EMG studies indicating varied task-dependent synergist activation, few studies have monitored possible changes in the relative activation of synergists after training.

The most relevant observations are the previously discussed preferential increases in EMG seen after training (e.g. Fig. 15.4). These studies show that increases in EMG may be restricted to one head of the quadriceps after knee extension training. It is not certain whether such findings indicate that EMG increases were restricted to a particular synergist because it was more extensively activated in the training exercises, or whether the synergist could not be activated as well before training and therefore had more scope for adaptation (increased activation). For example, in maximal isometric elbow flexion actions activation is less complete in the brachioradialis than the biceps (Allen *et al.* 1998); therefore, a larger training-induced increase in activation (EMG) might be expected in the brachioradialis.

One cross-sectional study has shown that trained subjects (correct performers) activate abdominal muscles differently from untrained subjects (incorrect performers). In correct performers, the curl-up exercise produces greater activity in the upper rectus abdominis, whereas in the pelvic tilt exercise the lower rectus abdominis is relatively more active. The upper and lower portions are less distinctly activated in untrained subjects (Sarti *et al.* 1996).

Magnetic resonance imaging

As discussed previously, magnetic resonance imaging can be used to indicate which muscles are active in an exercise and the extent of activation. Thus this method can be used to assess activation of synergists acutely, and to assess possible changes in patterns of activation after training.

EVIDENCE OF TASK-DEPENDENT SYNERGIST COORDINATION

In the common dumbbell curl (elbow flexion) exercise with forearm supinated, at a given intensity, fewer repetitions were needed to show activation in the short vs. long head of the biceps, indicating that the short head is more active in the exercise (Yue *et al.* 1994). These results agree with EMG findings showing relatively greater activation of the short head in a variety of flexion tasks (Jamison & Caldwell 1993). Isokinetic concentric knee extension actions involved activation of all four heads of the quadriceps but the rectus femoris appeared to be most active (Akima *et al.* 1999). Six muscles or muscle pairs can act in neck extension; however, only three muscles are largely active even in high-intensity resistance exercise (Conley *et al.* 1995). The MRI method has been used to assess the relative activation of several upper and lower limb muscles in common weight training exercises (Tesch 1999). A limitation of the method is that it cannot be readily applied to muscles of the trunk (e.g. pectoralis major, latissimus dorsi).

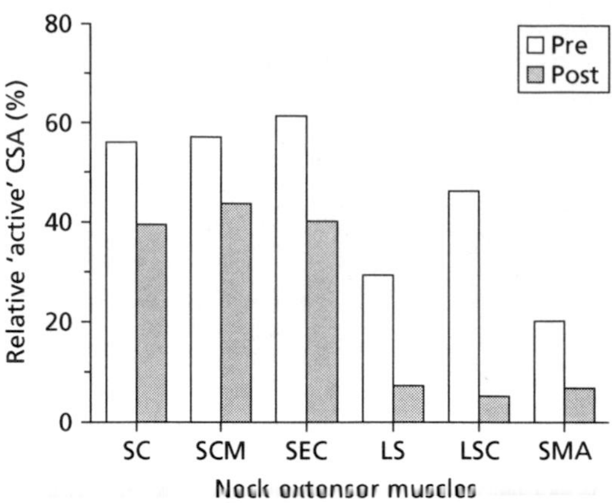

Fig. 15.17 Effect of training on muscle activation assessed by magnetic resonance imaging. Neck (head) extensor muscles were trained with a weight training neck extension exercise. Nine muscle regions were monitored, including the following six muscles/muscle pairs: SC, splenius capitis; SCM, semispinalis cervicis and multifidus; SEC, semispinalis capitis; LS, levator scapulae; LSC, longissimus capitis; SMA, scalenus medius and anterior. The figure shows the indicated relative use (percentage of muscle CSA active) of each muscle/muscle pair before training following three sets of 10 RM, and after training with the same absolute weight but now a smaller percentage (~ 75%) of the 10 RM. All muscles/muscle pairs showed less activation after training, but the greatest decrease occurred in the muscles that were less active before training (three muscles/muscle pairs to the right in the figure). Thus, an apparent neural adaptation consisted of not only a general decrease in activation for the same absolute load, but a redistribution of the load across the group of synergists. (Based on Conley *et al.* 1997a.)

TRAINING STUDIES

In relation to the activation of neck extensor muscles noted above, training could act to accentuate, attenuate or reverse the pattern of synergist activation. A training study indicated that the muscles most active in neck extension before training showed even greater relative (compared to less active muscles) activation after training in exercise with the same absolute load (maximal intensity before training but submaximal after training) (Conley *et al.* 1997a; see Fig. 15.17). Moreover, the muscles that showed the greatest relative activation in submaximal exercise displayed the greatest increase in activation in maximal exercise post training (Fig. 15.9). In response to isokinetic concentric training of knee extensors, increased activation was especially (i.e. significantly) marked in the vastus lateralis and intermedius. It was also found that increased activation was uniform along the length of the muscle; on the other hand, there was an indication of greater increased activation in the anterior portions of some quadriceps heads (Akima *et al.* 1999).

Preferential hypertrophy

PREFERENTIAL HYPERTROPHY AMONG SYNERGISTS

An indirect indication that some muscles in a group of synergists are preferentially activated in particular training exercises, or that their activation is preferentially amplified after a period of training, would be corresponding preferential hypertrophy of these muscles. Training of knee extensor muscles with isokinetic concentric actions caused preferential hypertrophy of the vastus intermedius and medialis compared to the other two heads of the quadriceps; correspondingly, EMG recordings indicated greater relative activation of these muscles in the training exercise (Narici *et al.* 1989). On the other hand, a later study using a very similar training protocol found the greatest hypertrophy in the rectus femoris (Housh *et al.* 1992). Weight training exercise (coupled eccentric–concentric actions of knee extensors) produced preferential hypertrophy of the vastus lateralis and rectus femoris compared to vastus medialis and intermedius (Hisaeda *et al.* 1996). With similar training another study showed a more balanced hypertrophy response but the response was nevertheless greatest in the rectus femoris. EMG monitoring during the training exercise indicated that all heads of the quadriceps were about equally active in the concentric phase of each repetition, but the rectus femoris bore a disproportionate load during the eccentric phase, which may have accounted for the preferential hypertrophy of this muscle (Narici *et al.* 1996).

Two studies of elbow flexors gave opposite results, one showing greater hypertrophy of the biceps than the brachialis (McCall *et al.* 1996), the other showing the reverse (O'Hagan *et al.* 1995). The different hypertrophy response likely reflected the use of different training exercises. One study used four unspecified elbow flexor exercises (McCall *et al.* 1996), while the other used a combination of a weight training exercise and an exercise on an accommodating resistance device (O'Hagan *et al.* 1995).

Training of the neck extensor muscles resulted in preferential hypertrophy in three of six muscles or muscle pairs (Conley *et al.* 1997b). These were the same muscles that increased their activation in maximal exercise, and their relative (to other muscles) activation in submaximal exercise (Conley *et al.* 1997a; see Figs 15.9 & 15.17).

PREFERENTIAL HYPERTROPHY WITHIN REGIONS OF A MUSCLE

Some training regimens may cause non-uniform hypertrophy along the length of muscles. One research group found that in the quadriceps the relative (percentage increase in CSA) hypertrophy was generally greater in the proximal than in the distal region after isokinetic training (Narici *et al.* 1989) but more uniform along muscle (femur) length following weight training (Narici *et al.* 1996). However, other groups found a trend of greater distal hypertrophy with isokinetic training (Housh *et al.* 1992), and greater proximal hypertrophy with weight training (Smith & Rutherford 1995).

Proximal vs. distal hypertrophy of the quadriceps may be head specific. For example, weight training produced preferential proximal hypertrophy of the vastus medialis but distal hypertrophy in the rectus femoris and vastus lateralis (Narici *et al.* 1996). Results with isokinetic training have not been consistent (Narici *et al.* 1989; Housh *et al.* 1992).

Regional hypertrophy in upper limb muscles has received little attention. One study indicated that training with the overhead elbow extension exercise caused uniform relative (percentage) increases in CSA along the entire length of the long head of triceps, except for the extreme proximal and distal ends at the tendon (Kawakami *et al.* 1995).

NEURAL VS. MUSCLE ADAPTATIONS?

Preferential hypertrophy of synergists within a group or subregions within a muscle encourages the interpretation that neural adaptations, in the form of preferential activation of synergists or muscle subregions in training, are responsible for the preferential hypertrophy. In some instances there is corroborating EMG (Narici *et al.* 1996) or MRI evidence (Conley *et al.* 1997a) to support this interpretation. There are other possible interpretations, however. For example, some muscles within a group of synergists may be less active in a sedentary lifestyle. Simply activating them more regularly in a training programme would stimulate hypertrophy to 'catch up' to the generally more active muscles. The same argument could apply to a region of a muscle that for the first time becomes regularly active as a result of training. No profound neural adaptation is at work. The nervous system has just been called upon to perform unaccustomed neuromuscular tasks.

Coactivation of antagonists

Prevalence and functions

Contraction of agonists (prime movers in a task) may be associated with simultaneous contraction of their antagonists (muscles that produce force and movement in the opposite direction), referred to as antagonist cocontraction or coactivation. Usually, agonist/antagonist muscles are distinct (e.g. elbow flexors and extensors), but may involve different portions of the same muscle (e.g. anterior and posterior heads of the deltoid). There are several factors that could affect the presence and extent of antagonist coactivation, and its opposing (to agonists) effects, such as muscle group (physiological cross-sectional area and moment arm), velocity and type of muscle action, intensity of effort, joint position and injury status (Osternig *et al.* 1986, 1995; Carpentier *et al.* 1996; Kellis & Baltzopoulos 1997, 1998; Kellis 1998). Motor unit recruitment strategy of a muscle may vary depending on whether it is acting as an agonist or an antagonist (Bernardi *et al.* 1997; Carpentier *et al.* 1999).

Coactivation of antagonists would seem to be counterproductive, particularly in a strength task, because the opposing torque developed by the antagonists would decrease the net torque in the intended direction of movement. For example, in maximal concentric knee extensions, the antagonist knee flexors will generate (opposing) torque ranging from 10 to 75% of total extensor torque, depending on the point in the range of movement (Baratta *et al.* 1988; Kellis & Baltzopoulos 1997; Aagaard *et al.* 2000). These estimates of opposing torque took into account the activation level of the knee flexors, together with the type of muscle action (eccentric for knee flexors), velocity and range of motion. There is also evidence that antagonist coactivation may impair, by reciprocal inhibition, the ability to fully activate agonists (Tyler & Hutton 1986; Milner *et al.* 1995). As discussed previously with regard to agonist activation, antagonists of a functional group may not participate equally in coactivation. For example, in relatively slow isokinetic concentric knee extension, coactivation is greater in lateral (biceps femoris) than medial (semitendinosus) hamstrings (Aagaard *et al.* 2000).

Set against the apparent disadvantage of antagonist coactivation (opposing torque) are potential advantages. Antagonist coactivation may assist in maintaining joint stability (Carpentier *et al.* 1996; Kellis 1998; Kellis & Baltzopoulos 1999; Aagaard *et al.* 2000; Solomonow & Krogsgaard 2001) and coordinating a movement (Jongen *et al.* 1989; Van Zuylen *et al.* 1988). For example, much research has addressed the issue of antagonist coactivation and stability of the knee joint (Kellis 1998). An example related to coordination is that when the biceps acts to supinate the forearm, the triceps must be activated to eliminate unwanted elbow flexion. Antagonist coactivation is prominent in high-velocity (ballistic) actions (Corcos *et al.* 1989; Carpentier *et al.* 1996), where it may provide stabilization, precision and a braking mechanism (Lestienne 1979; Marsden *et al.* 1983; Wierzbicka *et al.* 1986). In rapid actions with the intention of stopping the movement (e.g. reaching a target position), a three-phase activation pattern occurs (agonist–antagonist–agonist) (Marsden *et al.* 1983), whereas when there is no intention to stop, the agonist and antagonist bursts are concurrent (Carpentier *et al.* 1996).

Finally, the apparently detrimental inhibition of agonists caused by antagonist coactivation may be a protective mechanism in activities involving strong or rapid actions (Tyler & Hutton 1986). Related to this point, it is of interest that the antagonist activation (Kellis & Baltzopoulos 1998) and antagonistic moment of knee flexors are apparently greater in eccentric than in concentric knee extension actions (Kellis & Baltzopoulos 1997, 1999).

Effects of training

Alteration of antagonist coactivation poses a dilemma for the central nervous system. On the one hand, a neural adaptation in the form of decreased antagonist coactivation would contribute to increased strength (net torque at a joint). On the other hand, a maintained balance between agonist and antagonist activation may be all the more important for joint stability as forces acting at joints increase in the course of training. The dilemma is sometimes resolved by allowing some decrease in antagonist coactivation (Bernardi *et al.* 1996). In terms of actual muscle activation, two patterns of results have been observed in longitudinal training studies: a decrease in absolute antagonist activation in conjunction with either an increase (Häkkinen *et al.* 1998a, 2000) or no change in agonist (Carolan & Cafarelli 1992) activation; secondly, unchanged absolute antagonist activation but increased agonist activation, decreasing the antagonist/agonist activation ratio (Colson *et al.* 1999; Hortobágyi & DeVita 2000; Häkkinen *et al.* 2001). Two studies that made frequent measurements found that decreased antagonist activation occurred early in the training programme (Carolan & Cafarelli 1992; Häkkinen *et al.* 1998a). An example of the contribution that decreased coactivation can make to increased strength is shown in Fig. 15.18. In this study (Carolan & Cafarelli 1992) the knee extensors were trained with isometric actions for 8 weeks. After 1 week of training, it was estimated that decreased antagonist (knee flexors) coactivation had contributed about one-third of the increase in knee

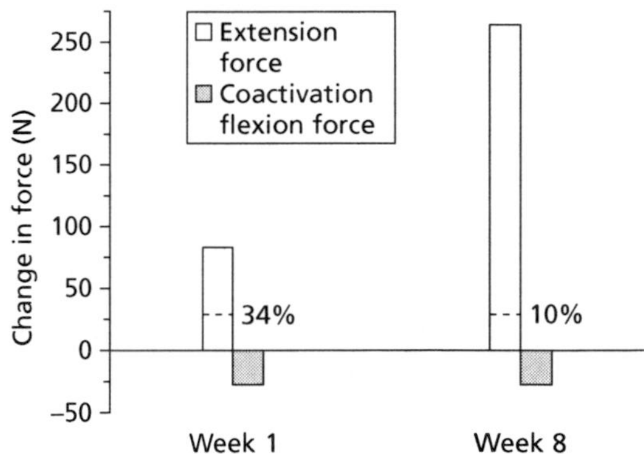

Fig. 15.18 Evidence of decreased antagonist activation in strength training. The knee extensor muscles were trained with isometric actions. After 1 week of training isometric strength had increased. Based on surface EMG, agonist (vastus lateralis) activation had not changed; however, a decrease in antagonist (knee flexor) coactivation was observed. It was estimated that decreased antagonist activation contributed 34% to the total increase in strength after 1 week of training. In the following 7 weeks of training strength increased much more (33% after 8 weeks), but no changes were detected in agonist or antagonist activation. Therefore, the contribution of decreased antagonist activation to the total increase in strength had dropped to 10%. The contributor(s) to the remaining 90% of strength increase was left unaccounted for. There may have been some hypertrophy (not measured) or activation may have increased in the heads of the quadriceps not monitored. (Based on Carolan & Cafarelli 1992.)

extension strength. After 8 weeks, however, there had been no further decrease in antagonist coactivation, so its relative contribution had dropped to about 10% (Fig. 15.18). A final point to consider is that even if exclusive training of agonists resulted in no change in antagonist coactivation, no matter how measured or expressed, the opposing torque offered by antagonists, relative to the increasing agonist torque, could decrease because of non-neural (e.g. hypertrophy) adaptations in agonists. It could thus be argued that in the event of exclusive agonist training, antagonist coactivation would actually have to *increase* to maintain the pretraining 'balance of power' at the joint, with its implications for joint stability. It is advisable to consider this point in the design of specific training

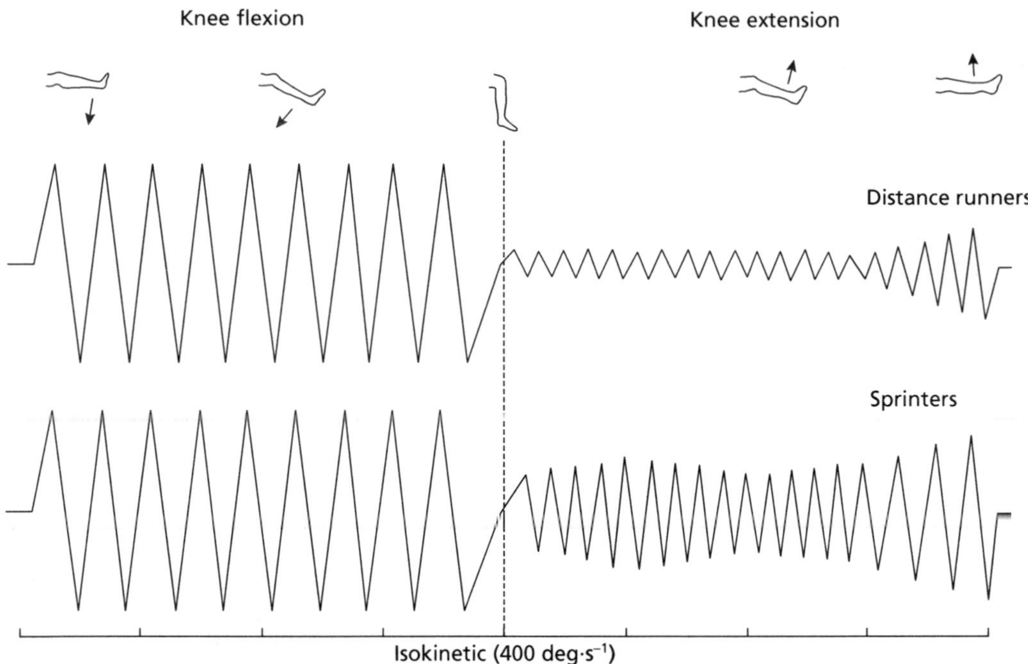

Fig. 15.19 Schematic representation of knee flexor EMG during alternate rapid knee extension and flexion (concentric actions) on an isokinetic dynamometer. In the extension phase when the flexors were acting as antagonists, flexor activity was greater in sprinters than in distance runners. The difference in flexor activity may reflect specific neural adaptation to training. (Based on Osternig *et al.* 1986 and reproduced by permission from Sale 1988.)

programmes; that is, specificity carried to the extreme might jeopardize joint stability. In contrast, equitable training of agonist/antagonist pairs may preserve joint stability (e.g. Aagaard *et al.* 1996).

Cross-sectional studies have shown varied results. Sprinters showed a greater degree of antagonist coactivation than distance runners when performing high-velocity knee extensions (concentric actions) on an isokinetic dynamometer (Fig. 15.19). In contrast, strength and power athletes vs. endurance athletes had less knee flexor coactivation during slow knee extensions designed to stretch the knee flexors (Osternig *et al.* 1990). High jumpers had less knee flexor coactivation than untrained subjects when performing concentric and eccentric isokinetic knee extension actions at a range of velocities (Amiridis *et al.* 1996). Athletes with hypertrophied quadriceps showed less coactivation of knee flexors during low-velocity isokinetic knee extensions than control subjects, but athletes given specific knee flexion training exercises increased flexor coactivation to control levels within a few weeks (Baratta *et al.* 1988).

Interaction of neural and muscular adaptations

The concept of neural adaptation probably arose from three principal observations. One was the almost immediate increase in strength at the onset of training, in the absence of (measurable) hypertrophy. The second was the overall magnitude of (specific) strength increase, which could only be partly accounted for by hypertrophy. The third was the cross-training effect, wherein training of one limb increases strength in the contralateral untrained limb. The classic study of Moritani and deVries (1979) set out to quantify

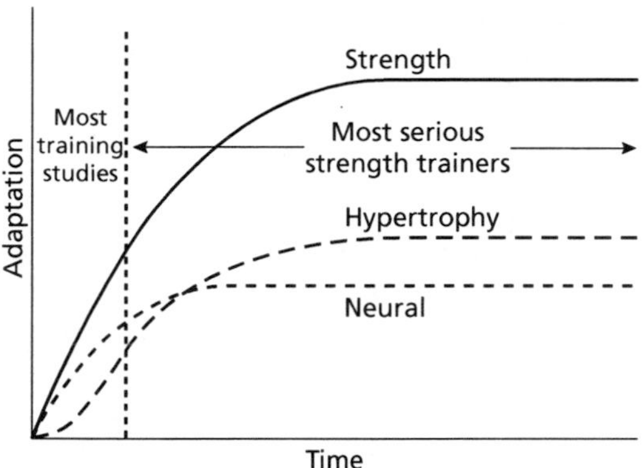

Fig. 15.20 The relative roles of neural and muscular adaptation to strength training. In the early phase of training neural adaptation predominates but may not be the sole contributor to increased strength (see discussion in text and Fig. 15.21). This phase also encompasses most training studies. In intermediate and advanced training progress is limited to the extent of muscular adaptation that can be achieved. Long-term advanced trainees spend much of their career on a plateau, and become increasingly susceptible to the enticement of using food supplements and anabolic drugs. The figure implies that hypertrophy is the only muscle adaptation that increases strength; however, adaptations that might increase the specific force (force per unit muscle cross-sectional area) of muscle cannot be excluded.

the contributions of neural and muscular adaptations, and to chart the time course of the two forms of adaptation. What this and subsequent studies have found is summarized in Fig. 15.20. Neural adaptation dominates early in the training programme. Later, as neural adaptations reach a plateau, muscular adaptation (hypertrophy) dominates. Eventually adaptation of any type reaches a limit and strength increases cease—a plateau in strength performance is reached. At this stage, with advanced trainees, intensive training brings little or no further improvement (Häkkinen *et al.* 1988, 1991; Alway *et al.* 1992). In frustration, trainees may look to food supplements or anabolic drugs in a desperate bid to rise above the plateau. There is no lack of purveyors of these items. For trainees who have spent some time on a plateau, perhaps partly due to overtraining, reduced rather than increased training will increase strength, neural activation and even muscle fibre size (Häkkinen *et al.* 1991; Gibala *et al.* 1994; Trappe *et al.* 2000).

The time course and magnitude of contributions made by neural and muscular adaptations may be affected by the neuromuscular challenge posed by the training exercises. It has been observed that hypertrophy but not strength increase is delayed in muscle groups participating in more complex, multijoint exercises like the bench press and leg press, in comparison to simpler single-joint movements like the arm curl (Chilibeck *et al.* 1998). Hypertrophy is also delayed when training the non dominant compared to the dominant limb (Moritani & deVries 1979), perhaps because the former presents a greater challenge. Based on the specificity principle, a change in the training programme, such as different exercises involving the same muscles, could trigger a transient burst of neural and muscular adaptations. For the trainee in the gym, one sign of a changed programme is muscle soreness after the first 'new' training session. In time another plateau is reached.

One difference in the scheme depicted in Fig. 15.20, compared to its previous version (Sale 1988; Sale *et al.* 1992), is that muscle adaptation (hypertrophy) is shown rising above the baseline at an earlier time point. Indeed, muscle adaptation may be induced by the first training session. The first training session in untrained subjects is known to induce muscle fibre damage (Gibala *et al.* 2000) and stimulate protein synthesis and degradation, leading to a net gain in myofibrillar proteins (Phillips 2000). The question is how quickly the net gain can produce measurable increases in fibre or whole-muscle size, and contribute to increased strength. A review of several studies suggests that about 6 weeks of training is needed to produce *significant* increases in fibre area, given the sample sizes used and the precision of the measurement (Phillips 2000); however, hypertrophy could conceivably be contributing at an earlier time point. Two examples of studies in which serial biopsies (from vastus lateralis) were taken over intervals as frequent as 2–4 weeks are shown in Fig. 15.21. The data

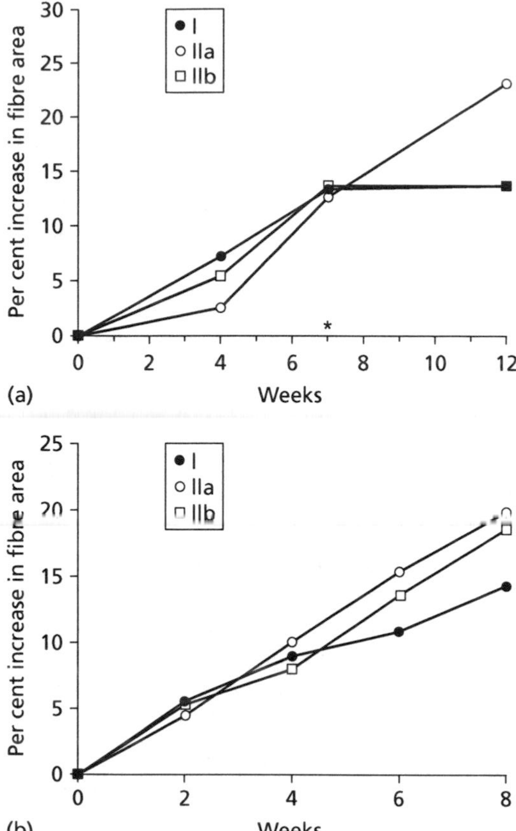

Fig. 15.21 Time course of vastus lateralis muscle fibre area increase during a strength training programme. (a) Measurements of Type I, IIa and IIb fibre area made at 4, 7 and 12 weeks of weight training in six young men. *, increases in fibre area were statistically significant by 7 weeks. (Based on Green *et al.* 1998.) (b) Measurements of fibre area at 2, 4, 6 and 8 weeks of weight training in eight young women and 13 young men (results combined in figure). Apparently substantial increases in fibre area were not significant even after 8 weeks. (Based on Staron *et al.* 1994.) In both studies, relatively small sample sizes compared to the variability in the fibre area measurement (i.e. lack of statistical power) contributed to the failure to find significant increases in fibre area at early time points in training.

in Fig. 15.21(a) do not show a significant increase in fibre area until week 7, although it appears some hypertrophy has occurred by 4 weeks. In Fig. 15.21(b) the apparently substantial increases in fibre area were not significant even at 8 weeks, but again it appeared that hypertrophy was beginning already at 2 weeks. Adding to the difficulty of interpreting biopsy data is the variable hypertrophy that occurs along the length of the muscle; the biopsy site may be where the least hypertrophy has occurred (Narici *et al.* 1996; see also section on preferential hypertrophy of synergists). Another complication is that the synergist sampled may not have shown the greatest hypertrophy. Magnetic resonance imaging has the advantage of measuring whole-muscle CSA along its entire length. One study used this method to assess possible hypertrophy after only 2 weeks (nine training sessions) of isokinetic concentric knee extension training. Voluntary peak torque at the training velocity, and muscle activation, measured by exercise-induced contrast shift MR imaging, increased significantly. The small increase (~ 3%) in whole-quadriceps CSA was not significant. However, a previous study with the same type of training had shown preferential hypertrophy of two of the four heads of the quadriceps (Narici *et al.* 1989). Therefore, it is possible that one or two heads underwent greater than ~ 3% hypertrophy.

A final consideration is the assumption, depicted in Fig. 15.20, that hypertrophy (increased muscle fibre or whole-muscle CSA) is the only muscular adaptation that could contribute to increased strength. If training could in the short term increase the specific force or tension of muscle fibres (i.e. force per unit CSA), strength could increase without actual hypertrophy. One proposed scheme by which this could occur is an increase in the number and size of myofibrils within a muscle fibre without an increase in fibre area (Phillips 2000). However, myofibrils make up 80–85% of fibre volume, so there may be limited room for myofibrillar expansion at the expense of other cellular components such as the sarcoplasmic reticulum. In the long term, training may actually decrease myofibrillar volume density (MacDougall *et al.* 1982). Another possibility is that 'packing' density of myofilaments may be quickly altered to increase the specific tension of myofibrils and by extension muscle fibres. However, whereas disuse is associated with both a decrease in filament lattice spacing and a decrease in specific tension (Widrick *et al.* 1999), long-term strength training does not change myofilament packing density (MacDougall *et al.* 1986; see also Chapter 13). Training at a particular muscle length/joint angle could increase (or decrease) strength at a point in the range of motion by altering muscle fibre length (sarcomere addition or deletion) rather than fibre area or neural activation (Koh 1995; Rassier *et al.* 1999). The remaining possibility is a training-induced increase in the force generated by each myosin head in its interaction with actin; however, there has been no demonstration of such an adaptation.

In summary, it is still reasonable to conclude that in many types of strength training programmes neural adaptations play the major role in increasing strength in the first weeks of training. Whether and for how long neural changes are the *exclusive* contributors to increased strength are questions that await more precise measurements of changes in muscle fibre size (CSA and/or length) and strength. After about a month or so of training some muscle adaptations (hypertrophy) are clearly evident and play the dominant role. It should be recognized, however, that if the training exercises are changed, even if they involve the same muscles, neural adaptations will reassert themselves in response to a new neuromuscular challenge.

Future considerations

The acceptance of and evidence for neural adaptations to strength training have advanced in stages. First, neural adaptations were simply deduced by default on the basis of increases in strength that could not be accounted for by muscle adaptations. Second, a large number of electromyographic studies accumulated, the majority of which indicated increased muscle activation as an adaptation. Most of the EMG studies have used surface recordings, which can tell what the whole 'crowd' of motor units is doing, and in some cases distinguish between increases in motor unit recruitment and increases in firing rates. More recently, studies employing relatively challenging intramuscular single motor unit recording techniques have begun to describe changes in motor unit behaviour in response to training. The future is likely to see a lot more of this type of research. Third, the development of magnetic resonance imaging techniques to monitor muscle activation has allowed study of muscles inaccessible by EMG. These studies, which have produced novel findings, should stimulate continued research with this technique.

The next stage will be to uncover the mechanisms responsible for the observed changes in muscle activation and motor unit behaviour. Changes in the motor cortex, other brain areas acting on the motor cortex, spinal circuits, reflex pathways and the motoneurones themselves are potential sites of morphological adaptations leading to functional changes. One example is identification of the important role of spinal mechanisms and afferent feedback from muscles in the cross-training effect, based on electrical stimulation experiments (Zhou 2000; cf. Lyle & Rutherford 1998). Another challenge of future research will be to relate changes in motor unit behaviour to the mechanical effects of their constituent muscle fibres. Fibres from different motor units are mechanically 'connected' in series and in parallel. The appropriate activation of these neighbouring fibres could markedly affect the collective force output attained (Sheard 2000).

References

Aagaard, P., Simonsen, E.B., Trolle, M., Bangsbo, J. & Klausen, K. (1996) Specificity of training velocity and training load on gains in isokinetic knee joint strength. *Acta Physiologica Scandinavica* **156**, 123–129.

Aagaard, P., Simonsen, E.B., Andersen, J.L., Magnusson, S.P., Bojsen-Moller, F. & Dyhre-Poulsen, P. (2000) Antagonist muscle coactivation during isokinetic knee extension. *Scandinavian Journal of Medicine and Science in Sports* **10**, 58–67.

Adams, G.R., Duvoisin, M.R. & Dudley, G.A. (1992) Magnetic resonance imaging and electromyography as indexes of muscle function. *Journal of Applied Physiology* **73**, 1578–1583.

Adams, G.R., Harris, R.T., Woodard, D. & Dudley, G.A. (1993) Mapping of electrical muscle stimulation using MRI. *Journal of Applied Physiology* **74**, 532–537.

Akima, H., Takahashi, H., Kuno, S.Y. *et al.* (1999) Early phase adaptations of muscle use and strength to isokinetic training. *Medicine and Science in Sports and Exercise* **31**, 588–594.

Allen, G.M., Gandevia, S.C. & McKenzie, D.K. (1995) Reliability of measurements of muscle strength and voluntary activation using twitch interpolation. *Muscle and Nerve* **18**, 593–600.

Allen, G.M., McKenzie, D.K. & Gandevia, S.C. (1998) Twitch interpolation of the elbow flexor muscles at high forces. *Muscle and Nerve* **21**, 318–328.

Almasbakk, B. & Hoff, J. (1996) Coordination, the determinant of velocity specificity? *Journal of Applied Physiology* **81**, 2046–2052.

Alway, S.E., Grumbt, W.H., Stray-Gundersen, J. & Gonyea, W.J. (1992) Effects of resistance training on elbow flexors of highly trained competitive bodybuilders. *Journal of Applied Physiology* **72**, 1512–1521.

Amiridis, I.G., Martin, A., Morlon, B. *et al.* (1996) Coactivation and tension-regulating phenomena during isokinetic knee extension in sedentary and highly skilled humans. *European Journal of Applied Physiology* **73**, 149–156.

Bandy, W.D. & Hanten, W.P. (1993) Changes in torque and electromyographic activity of the quadriceps femoris muscles following isometric training. *Physical Therapy* **73**, 455–467.

Baratta, R., Solomonow, M., Zhou, B.H., Letson, D., Chuinard, R. & D'Ambrosia, R. (1988) Muscular coactivation. The role of the antagonist musculature in maintaining knee stability. *American Journal of Sports Medicine* **16**, 113–122.

Barnett, C., Kippers, V. & Turner, P. (1995) Effects of variations of the bench press exercise on the EMG activity of five shoulder muscles. *Journal of Strength and Conditioning Research* **9**, 222–227.

Basmajian, J.V. (1974) *Muscles Alive*, 3rd edn. Williams and Wilkins, Baltimore.

Bawa, P. (2002) Neural control of motor output: Can training change it? *Exercise and Sport Sciences Reviews* **30**, 59–63.

Becker, R. & Awiszus, F. (2001) Physiological alterations of maximal voluntary activation by changes in knee joint angle. *Muscle and Nerve* **24**, 667–672.

Belanger, A.Y. & McComas, A.J. (1981) Extent of motor unit activation during effort. *Journal of Applied Physiology* **51**, 1131–1135.

Bellemare, F., Woods, J.J., Johansson, R. & Bigland-Ritchie, B. (1983) Motor-unit discharge rates in maximal voluntary contractions of three human muscles. *Journal of Neurophysiology* **50**, 1380–1392.

Bernardi, M., Solomonow, M., Sanchez, J.H., Baratta, R.V. & Nguyen, G. (1995) Motor unit recruitment strategy of knee antagonist muscles in a step-wise, increasing isometric contraction. *European Journal of Applied Physiology* **70**, 493–501.

Bernardi, M., Solomonow, M., Nguyen, G., Smith, A. & Baratta, R. (1996) Motor unit recruitment strategy changes with skill acquisition. *European Journal of Applied Physiology* **74**, 52–59.

Bernardi, M., Solomonow, M. & Baratta, R.V. (1997) Motor unit recruitment strategy of antagonist muscle pair during linearly increasing contraction. *Electromyography and Clinical Neurophysiology* **37**(1), 3–12.

Brown, A.B., McCartney, N. & Sale, D.G. (1990) Positive adaptations to weightlifting training in the elderly. *Journal of Applied Physiology* **69**, 1725–1733.

Brown, J.M., Solomon, C. & Paton, M. (1993) Further evidence of functional differentiation within biceps brachii. *Electromyography and Clinical Neurophysiology* **33**, 301–309.

Bulow, P.M., Norregaard, J., Danneskiold-Samsøe, B. & Mehlsen, J. (1993) Twitch interpolation technique in testing maximal muscle strength: influence of potentiation, force level, stimulus intensity and preload. *European Journal of Applied Physiology* **67**, 462–466.

Bulow, P.M., Norregaard, J., Mehlsen, J. & Danneskiold-Samsøe, B. (1995) The twitch interpolation technique for the study of fatigue of human quadriceps muscle. *Journal of Neuroscience Methods* **62**, 103–109.

Caldwell, G.E., Jamison, J.C. & Lee, S. (1993) Amplitude and frequency measures of surface electromyography during dual task elbow torque production. *European Journal of Applied Physiology* **66**, 349–356.

Cannon, R.J. & Cafarelli, E. (1987) Neuromuscular adaptations to training. *Journal of Applied Physiology* **63**, 2396–2402.

Carolan, B. & Cafarelli, E. (1992) Adaptations in coactivation after isometric resistance training. *Journal of Applied Physiology* **73**, 911–917.

Carpentier, A., Duchateau, J. & Hainaut, K. (1996) Velocity-dependent muscle strategy during plantarflexion in humans. *Journal of Electromyography and Kinesiology* **6**, 1–11.

Carpentier, A., Duchateau, J. & Hainaut, K. (1999) Load-dependent muscle strategy during plantarflexion in humans. *Journal of Electromyography and Kinesiology* **9**, 1–11.

Casabona, A., Polizzi, M.C. & Perciavalle, V. (1990) Differences in H-reflex between athletes trained for explosive contractions and non-trained subjects. *European Journal of Applied Physiology* **61**(1–2), 26–32.

Chilibeck, P.D., Calder, A.W., Sale, D.G. & Webber, C.E. (1998) A comparison of strength and muscle mass increases during resistance training in young women. *European Journal of Applied Physiology* **77**, 170–175.

Colson, S., Pousson, M., Martin, A. & Van Hoecke, J. (1999) Isokinetic elbow flexion and coactivation following eccentric training. *Journal of Electromyography and Kinesiology* **9**, 13–20.

Conley, M.S., Meyer, R.A., Bloomberg, J.J., Feeback, D.L. & Dudley, G.A. (1995) Non-invasive analysis of human neck muscle function. *Spine* **23**, 2505–2512.

Conley, M.S., Stone, M.H., Nimmons, M. & Dudley, G.A. (1997a) Resistance training and human cervical muscle recruitment plasticity. *Journal of Applied Physiology* **83**, 2105–2111.

Conley, M.S., Stone, M.H., Nimmons, M. & Dudley, G.A. (1997b) Specificity of resistance training responses in neck muscle size and strength. *European Journal of Applied Physiology* **75**, 443–448.

Corcos, D.M., Gottlieb, G.L. & Agarwal, G.C. (1989) Organizing principles for single-joint movements II. A speed sensitive strategy. *Journal of Neurophysiology* **62**, 358–368.

DeLuca, C.J., LeFever, R.S., McCue, M.P. & Xenakis, A.P. (1982) Behaviour of human motor units in different muscles during linearly varying contractions. *Journal of Physiology* **329**, 113–128.

Dowling, J.J., Konert, E., Ljucovic, P. & Andrews, D.M. (1994) Are humans able to voluntarily elicit maximum muscle force? *Neuroscience Letters* **179**, 25–28.

Duchateau, J., Le Bozec, S. & Hainaut, K. (1986) Contributions of slow and fast muscles of triceps surae to a cyclic movement. *European Journal of Applied Physiology* **55**, 476–481.

Dudley, G.A., Harris, R.T., Duvoisin, M.R., Hather, B.M. & Buchanan, P. (1990) Effect of voluntary vs artificial activation on the relationship of muscle torque to speed. *Journal of Applied Physiology* **69**, 2215–2221.

Enoka, R.M. (1997) Neural adaptations with chronic physical activity. *Journal of Biomechanics* **30**, 447–455.

Enoka, R.M. & Fuglevand, A.J. (2001) Motor unit physiology: some unresolved issues. *Muscle and Nerve* **24**, 4–17.

Felici, F., Rosponi, A., Sbriccoli, P., Filligoi, G.C., Fattorini, L. & Marchetti, M. (2001) Linear and nonlinear analysis of surface electromyograms in weightlifters. *European Journal of Applied Physiology* **84**, 337–342.

Gandevia, S.C. & McKenzie, D.K. (1988) Activation of human muscles at short muscle lengths during maximal static efforts. *Journal of Physiology* **407**, 599–613.

Gandevia, S.C., Allen, G.M., Butler, J.E. & Taylor, J.L. (1996) Supraspinal factors in human muscle fatigue: evidence for suboptimal output from the motor cortex. *Journal of Physiology* **490**, 529–536.

Gandevia, S.C., Herbert, R.D. & Leeper, J.B. (1998) Voluntary activation of human elbow flexor muscles during maximal concentric contractions. *Journal of Physiology* **512**, 595–602.

Garfinkel, S. & Cafarelli, E. (1992) Relative changes in maximal force, EMG, and muscle cross-sectional area after isometric training. *Medicine and Science in Sports and Exercise* **24**, 1220–1227.

Gibala, M.J., MacDougall, J.D. & Sale, D.G. (1994) The effects of tapering on strength performance in trained athletes. *International Journal of Sports Medicine* **15**, 492–497.

Gibala, M.J., Interisano, S.A., Tarnopolsky, M.A. *et al.* (2000) Myofibrillar disruption following acute concentric and eccentric resistance exercise in strength-trained men. *Canadian Journal of Physiology and Pharmacology* **78**, 656–661.

Green, H., Goreham, C., Ouyang, J., Ball-Burnett, M. & Raney, D. (1998) Regulation of fiber size, oxidative potential, and capillarization in human muscle by resistance exercise. *American Journal of Physiology* **276** (*Regulatory, Integrative, and Comparative Physiology* 45) R591–R596.

Grimby, L., Hannerz, J. & Hedman, B. (1981) The fatigue and voluntary discharge properties of single motor units in man. *Journal of Physiology* **316**, 545–554.

Gryzlo, S.M., Patek, R.M., Pink, M. & Perry, J. (1994) Electromyographic analysis of knee rehabilitation exercises. *Journal of Orthopaedic and Sports Physical Therapy* **20**, 36–43.

Häkkinen, K. & Häkkinen, A. (1995) Neuromuscular adaptations during intensive strength training in middle-aged and elderly males and females. *Electromyography and Clinical Neurophysiology* **35**, 137–147.

Häkkinen, K. & Komi, P.V. (1983) Electromyographic changes during strength training and detraining. *Medicine and Science in Sports and Exercise* **15**, 455–460.

Häkkinen, K., Alen, M. & Komi, P.V. (1985a) Changes in isometric force- and relaxation-time, electromyographic and muscle fibre characteristics of human skeletal muscle during strength training and detraining. *Acta Physiologica Scandinavica* **125**, 573–585.

Häkkinen, K., Komi, P.V. & Alen, M. (1985b) Effect of explosive type strength training on isometric force- and relaxation-time, electromyographic and muscle fibre characteristics of leg extensor muscles. *Acta Physiologica Scandinavica* **125**, 587–600.

Häkkinen, K., Pakarinen, A., Alen, M., Kauhanen, H. & Komi, P.V. (1988) Neuromuscular and hormonal adaptations in athletes to strength training for two years. *Journal of Applied Physiology* **65**, 2406–2412.

Häkkinen, K., Kallinen, M., Komi, P.V. & Kauhanen, H. (1991) Neuromuscular adaptations during short-term 'normal' and reduced training in strength athletes. *Electromyography and Clinical Neurophysiology* **31**, 35–42.

Häkkinen, K., Kallinen, M., Linnamo, V., Pastinen, U.M., Newton, R.U. & Kraemer, W.J. (1996) Neuromuscular adaptations during bilateral versus unilateral strength training in middle-aged and elderly men and women. *Acta Physiologica Scandinavica* **158**, 77–88.

Häkkinen, K., Kallinen, M., Izquierdo, M. *et al.* (1998a) Changes in agonist–antagonist EMG, muscle CSA, and force during strength training in middle-aged and older people. *Journal of Applied Physiology* **84**, 1341–1349.

Häkkinen, K., Newton, R.U., Gordon, S.E. *et al.* (1998b) Changes in muscle morphology, electromyographic activity, and force production characteristics during progressive strength training in young and older men. *Journals of Gerontology Series A: Biological Sciences and Medical Sciences* **53**, B415–B423.

Häkkinen, K., Alen, M., Kallinen, M., Newton, R.U. & Kraemer, W.J. (2000) Neuromuscular adaptation during prolonged strength training, detraining and re-strength-training in middle-aged and elderly people. *European Journal of Applied Physiology* **83**, 51–62.

Häkkinen, A., Häkkinen, K., Hannonen, P. & Alen, M. (2001) Strength training induced adaptations in neuromuscular function of premenopausal women with fibromyalgia: comparison with healthy women. *Annals of the Rheumatic Diseases* **60**, 21–26.

Hannerz, J. (1974) Discharge properties of motor units in relation to recruitment order in voluntary contraction. *Acta Physiologica Scandinavica* **91**, 374–384.

ter Harr Romeny, B.M., Denier van der Gon, J.J. & Gielen, C.A.M. (1984) Relation between location of a motor unit in the human biceps brachii and its critical firing levels for different tasks. *Experimental Neurology* **85**, 631–650.

Harridge, S.D., Kryger, A. & Stensgaard, A. (1999) Knee extensor strength, activation, and size in very elderly people following strength training. *Muscle and Nerve* **22**, 831–839.

Harris, R.T. & Dudley, G.A. (1994) Factors limiting force during slow, shortening actions of the quadriceps femoris muscle group in vivo. *Acta Physiologica Scandinavica* **152**, 63–71.

Henneman, E., Somjen, G. & Carpenter, D.C. (1965) Functional significance of cell size in spinal motoneurons. *Journal of Neurophysiology* **28**, 560–580.

Herbert, R.D. & Gandevia, S.C. (1996) Muscle activation in unilateral and bilateral efforts assessed by motor nerve and cortical stimulation. *Journal of Applied Physiology* **80**, 1351–1356.

Herbert, R.D. & Gandevia, S.C. (1999) Twitch interpolation in human muscles: mechanisms and implications for measurement of voluntary activation. *Journal of Neurophysiology* **82**, 2271–2283.

Herbert, R.D., Gandevia, S.C. & Allen, G.M. (1997) Sensitivity of twitch interpolation. *Muscle and Nerve* **20**, 521–523.

Herbert, R.D., Dean, C. & Gandevia, S.C. (1998) Effects of real and imagined training on voluntary muscle activation during maximal isometric contractions. *Acta Physiologica Scandinavica* **163**, 361–368.

Higbie, E.J., Cureton, K.J., Warren, G.L. III & Prior, B.M. (1996) Effects of concentric and eccentric training on muscle strength, cross-sectional area, and neural activation. *Journal of Applied Physiology* **81**, 2173–2181.

Hisaeda, H., Miyagawa, K., Kuno, S., Fukunaga, T. & Muraoka, I. (1996) Influence of two different modes of resistance training in female subjects. *Ergonomics* **39**, 842–852.

Hortobágyi, T. & DeVita, P. (2000) Favorable neuromuscular and cardiovascular responses to 7 days of exercise with an eccentric overload in elderly women. *Journals of Gerontology Series A: Biological Sciences and Medical Sciences* **55**, B401–B410.

Hortobágyi, T., Barrier, J., Beard, D. *et al.* (1996a) Greater initial adaptations to submaximal muscle lengthening than maximal shortening. *Journal of Applied Physiology* **81**, 1677–1682.

Hortobágyi, T., Hill, J.P., Houmard, J.A., Fraser, D.D., Lambert, N.J. & Israel, R.G. (1996b) Adaptive responses to muscle lengthening and shortening in humans. *Journal of Applied Physiology* **80**, 765–772.

Hortobágyi, T., Lambert, N.J. & Hill, J.P. (1997) Greater cross education following training with muscle lengthening than shortening. *Medicine and Science in Sports and Exercise* **29**, 107–112.

Hortobàgyi, T., Scott, K., Lambert, J., Hamilton, G. & Tracy, J. (1999) Cross-education of muscle strength is greater with stimulated than voluntary contractions. *Motor Control* **3**, 205–219.

Housh, D.J., Housh, T.J., Johnson, G.O. & Chu, W.K. (1992) Hypertrophic response to unilateral concentric resistance isokinetic resistance training. *Journal of Applied Physiology* **73**, 65–70.

Huber, A., Suter, E. & Herzog, W. (1998) Inhibition of the quadriceps muscles in elite male volleyball players. *Journal of Sports Sciences* **16**, 281–289.

Jakobi, J.M. & Chilibeck, P.D. (2001) Bilateral and unilateral contractions: possible differences in maximal voluntary force. *Canadian Journal of Applied Physiology* **26**, 12–33.

Jamison, J.C. & Caldwell, G.E. (1993) Muscle synergies and isometric torque production—influence of supination and pronation level on elbow flexion. *Journal of Neurophysiology* **70**, 947–960.

Jongen, H.A.H., Denier van der Gon, J.J. & Gielen, C.C.A.M. (1989) Inhomogeneous activation of motoneurone pools as revealed by co-contraction of antagonistic human arm muscles. *Experimental Brain Research* **75**, 555–562.

Kamen, G., Taylor, P. & Beehler, P.J. (1984) Ulnar and posterior tibial nerve conduction velocity in athletes. *International Journal of Sports Medicine* **5**, 26–30.

Kamen, G., Knight, C.A., Laroche, D.P. & Asermely, D.G. (1998) Resistance training increases vastus lateralis motor unit firing rates in young and old adults. *Medicine and Science in Sports and Exercise* **30** (Suppl.), S337.

Kanehisa, H. & Miyashita, M. (1983) Effect of isometric and isokinetic muscle training on static strength and dynamic power. *European Journal of Applied Physiology* **50**, 365–371.

Kasprisin, J.E. & Grabiner, M.D. (2000) Joint angle-dependence of elbow flexor activation levels during isometric and isokinetic maximum voluntary contractions. *Clinical Biomechanics* **15**, 743–749.

Kawakami, Y., Abe, T., Kuno, S.Y. & Fukunaga, T. (1995) Training-induced changes in muscle architecture and specific tension. *European Journal of Applied Physiology* **72**, 37–43.

Kawakami, Y., Akima, H., Kubo, K. *et al.* (2001) Changes in muscle size, architecture, and neural activation after 20 days of bed rest with and without resistance exercise. *European Journal of Applied Physiology* **84**, 7–12.

Keen, D.A., Yue, G.H. & Enoka, R.M. (1994) Training-related enhancement in the control of motor output in elderly humans. *Journal of Applied Physiology* **77**, 2648–2658.

Kellis, E. (1998) Quantification of quadriceps and hamstring antagonist activity. *Sports Medicine* **25**, 37–62.

Kellis, E. & Baltzopoulos, V. (1997) The effects of antagonist moment on the resultant knee joint moment during isokinetic testing of the knee extensors. *European Journal of Applied Physiology* **76**, 253–259.

Kellis, E. & Baltzopoulos, V. (1998) Muscle activation differences in eccentric and concentric isokinetic exercise. *Medicine and Science in Sports and Exercise* **30**, 1616–1623.

Kellis, E. & Baltzopoulos, V. (1999) The effects of the antagonist muscle force on intersegmental loading during isokinetic efforts of the knee extensors. *Journal of Biomechanics* **32**, 19–25.

Kent-Braun, J.A. (1999) Central and peripheral contributions to muscle fatigue in humans during sustained maximal effort. *European Journal of Applied Physiology* **80**, 57–63.

Kent-Braun, J.A. & Le Blanc, R. (1996) Quantitation of central activation failure during maximal voluntary contractions in humans. *Muscle and Nerve* **19**, 861–869. 1997 Comment in *Muscle and Nerve* **20**, 521–523.

Koh, T.J. (1995) Do adaptations in serial sarcomere number occur with strength training? *Human Movement Science* **14**, 61–77.

Koh, T.J. & Herzog, W. (1995) Evaluation of voluntary and elicited dorsiflexor torque-angle relationships. *Journal of Applied Physiology* **79**, 2007–2013.

Komi, P.V. (1986) Training of muscle strength and power: interaction of neuromotoric, hypertrophic and mechanical factors. *International Journal of Sports Medicine* **7** (Suppl.), 10–16.

Komi, P.V., Viitasalo, J., Rauramaa, R. & Vihko, V. (1978) Effect of isometric strength training on mechanical, electrical and metabolic aspects of muscle function. *European Journal of Applied Physiology* **40**, 45–55.

Kukulka, C.G. & Clamann, H.P. (1981) Comparison of the recruitment and discharge properties of motor units in human brachial biceps and adductor pollicis during isometric contractions. *Brain Research* **219**, 45–55.

Laidlaw, D.H., Kornatz, K.W., Keen, D.A., Suzuki, S. & Enoka, R.M. (1999) Strength training improves the steadiness of slow lengthening contractions performed by old adults. *Journal of Applied Physiology* **87**, 1786–1795.

Laprade, J., Culham, E. & Brouwer, B. (1998) Comparison of five isometric exercises in the recruitment of the vastus medialis oblique in persons with and without patellofemoral pain syndrome. *Journal of Orthopaedic and Sports Physical Therapy* **27**, 197–204.

Leong, B., Kamen, G., Patten, C. & Burke, J.R. (1999) Maximal motor unit discharge rates in the quadriceps muscles of older weight lifters. *Medicine and Science in Sports and Exercise* **31**, 1638–1644.

Lestienne, F. (1979) Effects of inertial load and velocity on the braking process of voluntary limb movements. *Experimental Brain Research* **35**, 407–418.

Lind, A.R. & Petrofsky, J.S. (1978) Isometric tension from rotary stimulation of fast and slow cat muscle. *Muscle and Nerve* **1**, 213–218.

Lyle, N. & Rutherford, O.M. (1998) A comparison of voluntary versus stimulated strength training of the human adductor pollicis muscle. *Journal of Sports Sciences* **16**, 267–270.

Macaluso, A., De Vito, G., Felici, F. & Nimmo, M.A. (2000) Electromyogram changes during sustained contraction after resistance training in women in their 3rd and 8th decades. *European Journal of Applied Physiology* **82**, 418–424.

McCall, G.E., Byrnes, W.C., Dickinson, A., Pattany, P.M. & Fleck, S.J. (1996) Muscle fiber hypertrophy, hyperplasia, and capillary density in college men after resistance training. *Journal of Applied Physiology* **81**, 2004–2012.

MacDougall, J.D. (1986) Morphological changes in human skeletal muscle following strength training and immobilization. In: *Human Muscle Power* (eds N.L. Jones, N. McCartney & A.J. McComas), pp. 269–288. Human Kinetics, Champaign, IL.

MacDougall, J.D., Sale, D.G., Elder, G.C.B. & Sutton, J.R. (1982) Muscle ultrastructural characteristics of elite powerlifters and bodybuilders. *European Journal of Applied Physiology* **48**, 117–126.

McKenzie, D.K., Bigland-Ritchie, B., Gorman, R.B. & Gandevia, S.C. (1992) Central and peripheral fatigue of human diaphragm and limb muscles assessed by twitch interpolation. *Journal of Physiology* **454**, 643–656.

Marsden, C.D., Obeso, J.A. & Rothwell, J.C. (1983) The function of antagonist muscle during fast limb movement in man. *Journal of Physiology* **335**, 1–13.

Marsh, E., Sale, D., McComas, A.J. & Quinlan, J. (1981) Influence of joint position on ankle dorsiflexion in humans. *Journal of Applied Physiology* **51**, 160–167.

Martin, A., Martin, L. & Morlon, B. (1995) Changes induced by eccentric training on force–velocity relationships of the elbow flexor muscles. *European Journal of Applied Physiology* **72**, 183–185.

Miller, R.G., Mirka, A. & Maxfield, M. (1981) Rate of tension development in isometric contractions of a human hand muscle. *Experimental Neurology* **73**, 267–285.

Milner, T.E., Cloutier, C., Leger, A.B. & Franklin, D.W. (1995) Inability to activate muscles maximally during cocontraction and the effect on joint stiffness. *Experimental Brain Research* **107**, 293–305.

Milner-Brown, H.S., Stein, R.B. & Yemm, R. (1973) The orderly recruitment of human motor units during voluntary isometric contractions. *Journal of Physiology* **230**, 359–370.

Milner-Brown, H.S., Stein, R.B. & Lee, R.G. (1975) Synchronization of human motor units: possible roles of exercise and supraspinal reflexes. *Electroencephalography and Clinical Neurophysiology* **38**, 245–254.

Moritani, T. (1993) Neuromuscular adaptations during the acquisition of muscle strength, power and motor tasks. *Journal of Biomechanics* **26** (Suppl. 1), 95–108.

Moritani, T. & deVries, H.A. (1979) Neural factors vs hypertrophy in time course of muscle strength gain. *American Journal of Physical Medicine and Rehabilitation* **58**, 115–130.

Moritani, T., Oddsson, L. & Thorstensson, A. (1990) Differences in modulation of the gastrocnemius and soleus H-reflexes during hopping in man. *Acta Physiologica Scandinavica* **138**, 575–576.

Morrisey, M.C., Harman, E.A. & Johnson, M.J. (1995) Resistance training modes: specificity and effectiveness. *Medicine and Science in Sports and Exercise* **27**, 648–660.

Nakazawa, K., Kawakami, Y., Fukunaga, T., Yano, H. & Miyashita, M. (1993) Differences in activation patterns in elbow flexor muscles during isometric, concentric and eccentric contractions. *European Journal of Applied Physiology* **66**, 214–220.

Nardone, A. & Schieppati, M. (1988) Shift of activity from slow to fast muscle during voluntary lengthening contractions of the triceps surae muscles in humans. *Journal of Physiology* **395**, 363–381.

Nardone, A., Romano, C. & Schieppati, M. (1989) Selective recruitment of high-threshold human motor units during voluntary isotonic lengthening of active muscles. *Journal of Physiology* **409**, 451–471.

Narici, M.V., Roi, G.S., Landoni, L., Minetti, A.E. & Cerretelli, P. (1989) Changes in force, cross-sectional area and neural activation during strength training and detraining of the human quadriceps. *European Journal of Applied Physiology* **59**, 310–319.

Narici, M.V., Hoppeler, H., Kayser, B. *et al.* (1996) Human quadriceps cross-sectional area, torque and neural activation during 6 months strength training. *Acta Physiologica Scandinavica* **157**, 175–186.

O'Hagan, F.T., Sale, D.G., MacDougall, J.D. & Garner, S.H. (1995) Comparative effectiveness of accommodating and weight resistance training modes. *Medicine and Science in Sports and Exercise* **27**, 1210–1219.

Osternig, L.R., Hamill, J., Lander, J.E. & Robertson, R. (1986) Co-activation of sprinter and distance runner muscles in isokinetic exercise. *Medicine and Science in Sports and Exercise* **18**, 431–435.

Osterning, L.R., Robertson, R.N., Troxel, R.K. & Hansen, P. (1990) Differential responses to proprioceptive neuromuscular facilitation (PNF) stretch techniques. *Medicine and Science in Sports and Exercise* **22**, 106–111.

Osternig, L.R., Caster, B.L. & James, C.R. (1995) Contralateral hamstring (biceps femoris) coactivation patterns and anterior cruciate ligament dysfunction. *Medicine and Science in Sports and Exercise* **27**, 805–808.

Ozmun, J.C., Mikesky, A.E. & Surburg, P.R. (1994) Neuromuscular adaptations following prepubescent strength training. *Medicine and Science in Sports and Exercise* **26**, 510–514.

Patten, C., Kamen, G. & Rowland, D.M. (2001) Adaptations in maximal motor unit discharge rate to strength training in young and older adults. *Muscle and Nerve* **24**, 542–550.

Perot, C., Andre, L., Dupont, L. & Vanhoutte, C. (1996) Relative contribution of the long and short heads of the biceps brachii during single or dual isometric tasks. *Journal of Electromyography and Kinesiology* **6**, 3–11.

Peters, E.J. & Fuglevand, A.J. (1999) Cessation of human motor unit discharge during sustained maximal voluntary contraction. *Neuroscience Letters* **274**, 66–70.

Phillips, S.M. (2000) Short-term training: when do repeated bouts of resistance exercise become training? *Canadian Journal of Applied Physiology* **25**, 185–193.

Ploutz, L.L., Tesch, P.A., Biro, R.L. & Dudley, G.A. (1994) Effect of resistance training on muscle use during exercise. *Journal of Applied Physiology* **76**, 1675–1681.

Rabita, G., Perot, C. & Lensel-Corbeil, G. (2000) Differential effect of knee extension isometric training on the different muscles of the quadriceps femoris in humans. *European Journal of Applied Physiology* **83**, 531–538.

Rack, P.M.H. & Westbury, D.R. (1969) The effects of length and stimulus rate on tension in the isometric cat soleus muscle. *Journal of Physiology* **204**, 443–460.

Rassier, D.E., MacIntosh, B.R. & Herzog, W. (1999) Length dependence of active force production in skeletal muscle. *Journal of Applied Physiology* **86**, 1445–1457.

Rutherford, O.M. (1988) Muscular coordination and strength training. Implications for injury rehabilitation. *Sports Medicine* **5**, 196–202.

Rutherford, O.M. & Jones, D.A. (1986) The role of learning and coordination in strength training. *European Journal of Applied Physiology* **55**, 100–105.

Rutherford, O.M., Greig, C.A., Sargeant, A.J. & Jones, D.A. (1986) Strength training and power output: transference effects in the human quadriceps muscle. *Journal of Sports Sciences* **4**, 101–107.

Rutherford, O.M., Purcell, C. & Newham, D.J. (2001) The human force–velocity relationship; activity in the knee flexor and extensor muscles before and after eccentric practice. *European Journal of Applied Physiology* **84**, 133–140.

Sale, D.G. (1988) Neural adaptation to resistance training. *Medicine and Science in Sports and Exercise* **20** (Suppl.), S135–S145.

Sale, D.G. (1992) Neural adaptation to strength training. In: *Strength and Power in Sport*, 1st edn (ed. P. V. Komi), pp. 249–265. Blackwell Scientific Publications, Oxford.

Sale, D. & MacDougall, D. (1981) Specificity in strength training: a review for the coach and athlete. *Canadian Journal of Applied Sports Science* **6**, 87–92.

Sale, D.G., MacDougall, J.D., Upton, A.R.M. & McComas, A.J. (1983a) Effect of strength training on motoneuron excitability in man. *Medicine and Science in Sports and Exercise* **15**, 57–62.

Sale, D.G., Upton, A.R.M., McComas, A.J. & MacDougall, J.D. (1983b) Neuromuscular function in weight-trainers. *Experimental Neurology* **82**, 521–531.

Sale, D.G., Martin, J.E. & Moroz, D.E. (1992) Hypertrophy without increased isometric strength after weight training. *European Journal of Applied Physiology* **64**, 51–55.

Saplinskas, J.S., Chobotas, M.A. & Yashchaninas, I.I. (1980) The time of completed motor acts and impulse activity of single motor units according to the training level and sport specialization of tested persons. *Electromyography and Clinical Neurophysiology* **20**, 529–539.

Sarti, M.A., Monfort, M., Fuster, M.A. & Villaplana, L.A. (1996) Muscle activity in upper and lower rectus abdominus during abdominal exercises. *Archives of Physical Medicine and Rehabilitation* **77**, 1293–1297.

van Schaik, C.S., Hicks, A.L. & McCartney, N. (1994) An evaluation of the length–tension relationship in elderly human ankle dorsiflexors. *Journals of Gerontology: Biological Sciences* **49**, B121–B127.

Schmidtbleicher, D. & Gollhofer, A. (1982) Neuromuskuläre Untersuchungen zur Bestimmung inviduieller Belastungsgrösen für ein Teifsprung-training. *Leistungssport* **12**, 298–307.

Semmler, J.G. & Nordstrom, M.A. (1998) Motor unit discharge and force tremor in skill- and strength-trained individuals. *Experimental Brain Research* **119**, 27–38.

Sheard, P.W. (2000) Tension delivery from short fibers in long muscles. *Exercise and Sport Sciences Reviews* **28**, 51–56.

Signorile, J.F., Kacsik, D., Perry, A. *et al.* (1995) Effect of foot position on the electromyographical activity of superficial quadriceps muscles during the parallel squat and knee extension. *Journal of Strength and Conditioning Research* **9**, 182–187.

Sleivert, G.G., Backus, R.D. & Wenger, H.A. (1995) The influence of a strength-sprint training sequence on multi-joint power output. *Medicine and Science in Sports and Exercise* **27**, 1655–1665.

Smith, R.C. & Rutherford, O.M. (1995) The role of metabolites in strength training. I. A comparison of eccentric and concentric contractions. *European Journal of Applied Physiology* **71**, 332–336.

Solomonow, M. & Krogsgaard, M. (2001) Sensorimotor control of knee stability. A review. *Scandinavian Journal of Medicine and Science in Sports* **11**, 64–80.

Solomonow, M., Baten, C., Smit, J. *et al.* (1990) Electromyogram power spectra frequencies associated with motor unit recruitment strategies. *Journal of Applied Physiology* **68**, 1177–1185.

Staron, R.S., Karapondo, D.L., Kraemer, W.J. *et al.* (1994) Skeletal muscle adaptations during early phase of heavy-resistance training in men and women. *Journal of Applied Physiology* **76**, 1247–1255.

Stein, R.B. & Parmiggiani, F. (1979) Optimal motor patterns for activating mammalian muscle. *Brain Research* **175**, 372–376.

Strojnik, V. (1995) Muscle activation level during maximal voluntary effort. *European Journal of Applied Physiology* **72**, 144–149.

Strojnik, V. (1998) The effects of superimposed electrical stimulation of the quadriceps muscles on performance in different motor tasks. *Journal of Sports Medicine and Physical Fitness* **38**, 194–200.

Taylor, J.L. & Gandevia, S.C. (2001) Transcranial magnetic stimulation and human muscle fatigue. *Muscle and Nerve* **24**, 18–29.

Taylor, J.L., Allen, G.M., Butler, J.E. & Gandevia, S.C. (2000) Supraspinal fatigue during intermittent maximal voluntary contractions of the human elbow flexors. *Journal of Applied Physiology* **89**, 305–313.

Tesch, P.A. (1999) *Target Bodybuilding*. Human Kinetics, Champaign, IL.

Thépaut-Mathieu, C., Van Hoecke, J. & Maton, B. (1988) Myoelectrical and mechanical changes linked to length specificity during isometric training. *Journal of Applied Physiology* **64**, 1500–1505.

Thorstensson, A., Karlsson, J., Viitasalo, J.H.T., Luhtanen, P. & Komi, P.V. (1976b) Effect of strength training on EMG of human skeletal muscle. *Acta Physiologica Scandinavica* **98**, 232–236.

Trappe, S., Costill, D. & Thomas, R. (2000) Effect of swim taper on whole muscle and single muscle fiber contractile properties. *Medicine and Science in Sports and Exercise* **32**, 48–56.

Tyler, A.E. & Hutton, R.S. (1986) Was Sherrington right about co-contractions? *Brain Research* **370**, 171–175.

Upton, A.R.M. & Radford, P.F. (1975) Motoneuron excitability in elite sprinters. In: *Biomechanics* (ed. P. V. Komi), pp. 82–87. University Park Press, Baltimore.

Van Cutsem, M., Duchateau, J. & Hainaut, K. (1998) Changes in single motor unit behaviour contribute to the increase in contraction speed after dynamic training in humans. *Journal of Physiology* **513**, 295–305.

Van Zuylen, E.J., Gielen, C.C.A.M. & Denier van der Gon, J.J. (1988) Coordination and inhomogeneous activation of human arm muscles during isometric torques. *Journal of Neurophysiology* **60**, 1523–1548.

Weir, J.P., Housh, T.J. & Weir, L.L. (1994) Electromyographic evaluation of joint angle specificity and cross-training after isometric training. *Journal of Applied Physiology* **77**, 197–201.

Weir, J.P., Housh, T.J., Weir, L.L. & Johnson, G.O. (1995) Effects of unilateral isometric strength training on joint angle specificity and cross-training. *European Journal of Applied Physiology* **70**, 337–343.

Westing, S.H., Seger, J.Y. & Thorstensson, A. (1990) Effects of electrical stimulation on eccentric and concentric torque–velocity relationships during knee extension in man. *Acta Physiologica Scandinavica* **140**, 17–22.

Widrick, J.J., Knuth, S.T., Norenberg, K.M. *et al.* (1999) Effect of a 17 day spaceflight on contractile properties of human soleus muscle fibres. *Journal of Physiology* **516**, 915–930.

Wierzbicka, M.M., Wiegner, A.W. & Shahani, B.T. (1986) Role of agonist and antagonist muscles in fast arm movements in man. *Experimental Brain Research* **63**, 331–340.

Wilson, G.J., Murphy, A.J. & Walshe, A. (1996) The specificity of strength training: the effect of posture. *European Journal of Applied Physiology* **73**, 346–352.

Yue, G. & Cole, K.J. (1992) Strength increases from the motor program: comparison of training with maximal voluntary and imagined muscle contractions. *Journal of Neurophysiology* **67**, 1114–1123.

Yue, G., Alexander, A.L., Laidlaw, D.H., Gmitro, A.F., Unger, E.C. & Enoka, R.M. (1994) Sensitivity of muscle proton spin-spin relaxation time as an index of muscle activation. *Journal of Applied Physiology* **77**, 84–92.

Yue, G.H., Xue, M., Ng, T. & Enoka, R.M. (1995) The decision to move may begin in the prefrontal cortex. *Society of Neuroscience Abstracts* **21**, 1421.

Yue, G.H., Ranganathan, V.K., Siemionow, V., Liu, J.Z. & Sahgal, V. (2000) Evidence of inability to fully activate human limb muscle. *Muscle and Nerve* **23**, 376–384.

Zehr, E.P. & Sale, D.G. (1994) Ballistic movement: motor control and muscle activation. *Canadian Journal of Applied Physiology* **19**, 363–378.

Zhou, S. (2000) Chronic neural adaptations to unilateral exercise: mechanisms of cross education. *Exercise and Sport Sciences Reviews* **28**, 177–184.

Chapter 16

Mechanisms of Muscle and Motor Unit Adaptation to Explosive Power Training

JACQUES DUCHATEAU AND KARL HAINAUT

Introduction

In many sports activities, the ability to rapidly develop force is equally important as or even more important than the maximal force itself. Movements that are performed with maximal velocity are usually considered to be ballistic actions (Desmedt & Godaux 1977). Such movements are called 'preprogrammed', which means that the motor command is released as a whole and is not controlled by sensory feedback (Keele 1968). In contrast, slow movements are performed in closed-loop fashion and are continuously controlled by input from the peripheral sensory system (Ghez 1991). This distinction between motor actions is important because it is well known that the neuromuscular system adapts specifically to the modalities of the movements involved during the training programmes. For example, when an individual performs a strength training programme, the increase in strength is greatest for tasks that are similar to the training exercise (see Sale, Chapter 15). The task details that influence this effect include the posture during training, the type of muscle contraction and the load and speed of contraction (Thorstensson *et al.* 1976; Kaneko *et al.* 1983; Duchateau & Hainaut 1984; Häkkinen *et al.* 1985a,b; Thépaut-Mathieu *et al.* 1988; Wilson *et al.* 1996; Pousson *et al.* 1999). These findings clearly indicate that the peak force or power a muscle can achieve during a specific task depends not only on the capability of the muscular system, but also on qualitative features of the motor command (Sale 1988; Enoka 1997; Duchateau & Enoka 2002).

Evidence of muscular and neural adaptations after a strength training programme can be expressed by the comparison between the gain in force recorded during maximal voluntary contraction (MVC) and electrically induced tetanus (Duchateau & Hainaut 1988). Six weeks of training the adductor pollicis with voluntary contractions against a load of 60% of maximum resulted in a greater increase in MVC force compared to tetanic force (22% vs. 15%, respectively). Whereas the increase in tetanic force represents the extent of muscular adaptation, the difference between these two forces indicates the extent of increased activation for this particular muscle. Other studies have also reported evidence of neural adaptation after strength training based on an increase in average electromyographic (EMG) activity (Moritani & de Vries 1979; Häkkinen & Komi 1983; Narici *et al.* 1990) and by an accentuated increase in force compared to the muscle mass (e.g. hypertrophy; Jones & Rutherford 1987; Colliander & Tesch 1990).

Such neural and muscular adaptations can also explain the increase in rate of tension development after training as suggested by some studies (Häkkinen *et al.* 1985a,b; Komi 1986; Schmidtbleicher 1992; Behm & Sale 1993). This chapter focuses on the adaptations and the underlying mechanisms that occur with training that involves dynamic (ballistic) contractions performed against small loads. The adaptation of single motor units in agonist muscles will be emphasized.

Muscular adaptations

Contractile properties

Muscle strength. It has been reported not only that long-lasting heavy-resistance training increases the maximal voluntary strength of muscle (Thorstensson *et al.* 1976; MacDougall *et al.* 1980; McDonagh & Davies 1984), but also that even moderate training programmes induce significant increases in intrinsic force during electrically evoked muscle contraction (Duchateau & Hainaut 1984). In the latter work, the human adductor pollicis was trained by voluntary contractions and the maximal force was tested using supramaximal electrical stimulation (100 Hz) of the motor nerve at the wrist. This was achieved in order to distinguish contractile adaptations from neural ones. The study indicated that voluntary isometric and dynamic exercises have different effects on the muscle maximal force and speed of contraction. During the dynamic training sessions, 10 series of 15 fast contractions were performed, with a counterweight of about 30–40% of the maximal muscle force. In a second group, 10 maximal isometric contractions were developed against a strap and maintained for 5 s. After 3 months of daily training, the maximal muscle strength in subjects who performed isometric contractions increased by 20%, whereas in subjects who trained using dynamic contractions the maximal muscle strength was augmented by only 11% (Fig. 16.1a). This difference is not surprising since it is well known that the gain in force is positively correlated to the intensity of the contraction. In this study, muscle force was nearly maximal throughout the isometric contractions, but not during dynamic ones.

Contraction kinetics and muscle power. In animals, studies have shown that muscle contractile kinetics can specifically adapt to different frequencies of electrical stimulation. It was observed that a slow muscle that was chronically stimulated at high frequency became faster (Gorza *et al.* 1988), whereas a fast muscle stimulated at low frequency became slower (Pette & Vrbova 1992).

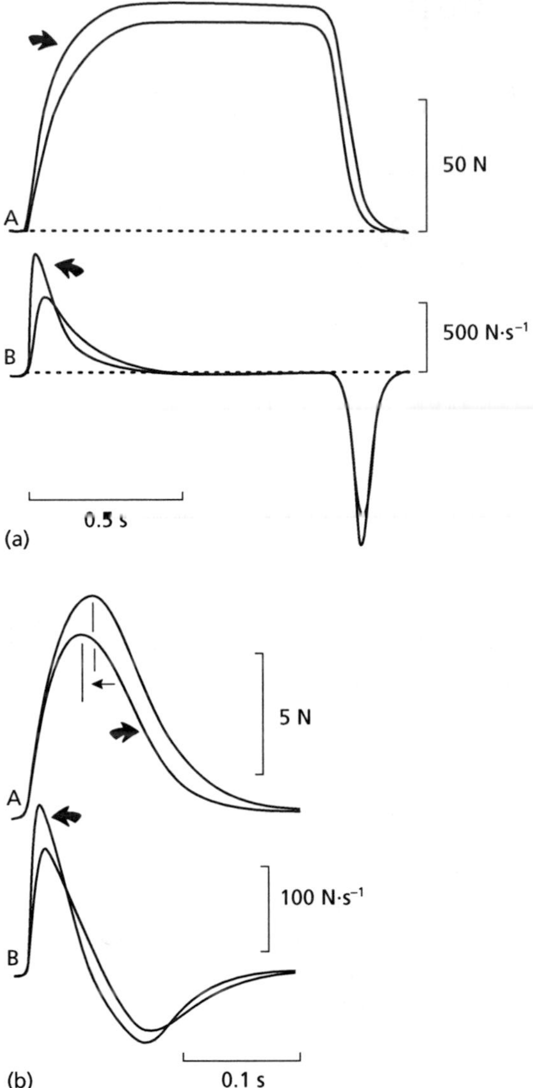

Fig. 16.1 Effects of 3 months of daily dynamic training on the contractile properties of the human adductor pollicis muscle. (a), isometric tetanus (A) recorded at a stimulation frequency of 100 Hz, before and after (arrow) training in one subject. Traces in (B) are the records of corresponding rates of tension development and relaxation given by electronic differentiation of the mechanograms. (b), mechanical twitch obtained in response to a single supramaximal electrical stimulation (A) and corresponding first derivatives (B), before and after (arrow) training. Note that the increase in maximal rate of tension development is associated with a reduced time-to-peak. (Data are from Duchateau & Hainaut 1984.)

These results, which were recorded in rather extreme conditions, are different from those prevailing in sports training. They suggest, however, that muscle contraction kinetics adapt specifically to the frequency of activation, independent of changes in innervation (Buller & Lewis 1965; Barany & Close 1971). In experiments performed in physiological conditions comparable to physical training of athletes (Duchateau & Hainaut 1984), it was observed that dynamic training augmented the rate of rise of tetanic contractions to a greater extent than isometric training (31 vs. 18%). This observation is illustrated in Fig. 16.1(a) by the first derivatives of the tetanus responses, recorded before and after dynamic training. It is interesting that the maximal velocity of muscle shortening, electrically evoked without additional load, increased after dynamic training (21%), but not after isometric exercises.

The analysis of the shape of the force–velocity relationship, illustrated in Fig. 16.2 and the corresponding power curve, before and after training, is of practical importance in sports. In fact, it is not only the maximal muscle force that should be considered, but first of all the optimal force–velocity relationship and thus power, with respect to different sports. The relationship between force and velocity showed that the speed of movement for small loads is essentially related to the maximal speed of tension development, whereas for heavy loads it is more closely related to the muscle maximal strength. The findings that dynamic training increases the velocity of shortening for small loads (Fig. 16.2a) and that isometric exercises augment predominantly this velocity for high mechanical resistances (not illustrated but see Duchateau & Hainaut 1984), were another indication of the specific effects of the two different types of training programmes. This point of view is also supported by the comparison of the force–velocity relations, normalized to the muscle maximal force, before and after dynamic training (Fig. 16.2b). The two curves are only significantly different at forces below 50% of the maximum. Such results suggest moreover that the muscle contractile kinetics were intrinsically modified by dynamic training. The analysis of the muscle power curves (Fig. 16.2c,d) indicates that both types of training augment muscle power for different loads, but the peak power increase is smaller after dynamic training vs. isometric exercises (19 vs. 51%; see Duchateau & Hainaut 1984). However, when expressed in normalized values, only dynamic training shifts the power peak towards smaller loads (Fig. 16.2d). This observation is in line with the viewpoint that the contractile kinetics were intrinsically modified by dynamic exercises.

Excitation–contraction (E–C) coupling

E–C coupling includes the sequence of events which is triggered by the membrane action potential and controls the contractile proteins' interaction (Sandow 1965). The above-documented evidences of the specific adaptation of muscle contractile properties to different training programmes raised the question of their effects on E–C coupling. This coupling can be approached indirectly in intact human muscles by the analysis of the mechanical twitch time course and the corresponding compound action potential or M-wave (cf. Desmedt & Hainaut 1968). In the above-quoted daily training programmes of 3 months' duration, no significant change in M-wave was observed, but the corresponding mechanical activity of the muscle showed a time course acceleration. The maximal speed of contraction was augmented by 20% and 25%, respectively, after isometric training and after dynamic exercises. Maximal speed of twitch relaxation increased by 12% and 16% after isometric and dynamic training, respectively. However, only dynamic exercises reduced twitch time-to-peak (11%), thus reducing time given to the contractile component to stretch the muscle elastic elements which consequently reduced twitch amplitude by 10% (Fig. 16.1b). After isometric training, this amplitude increased (19%) since the time-to-peak did not change, even though there was a faster speed of contraction. The twitch to tetanus ratio (P_t/P_0) was reduced by 18% after dynamic training, an observation which is in line with the characteristics of accelerated

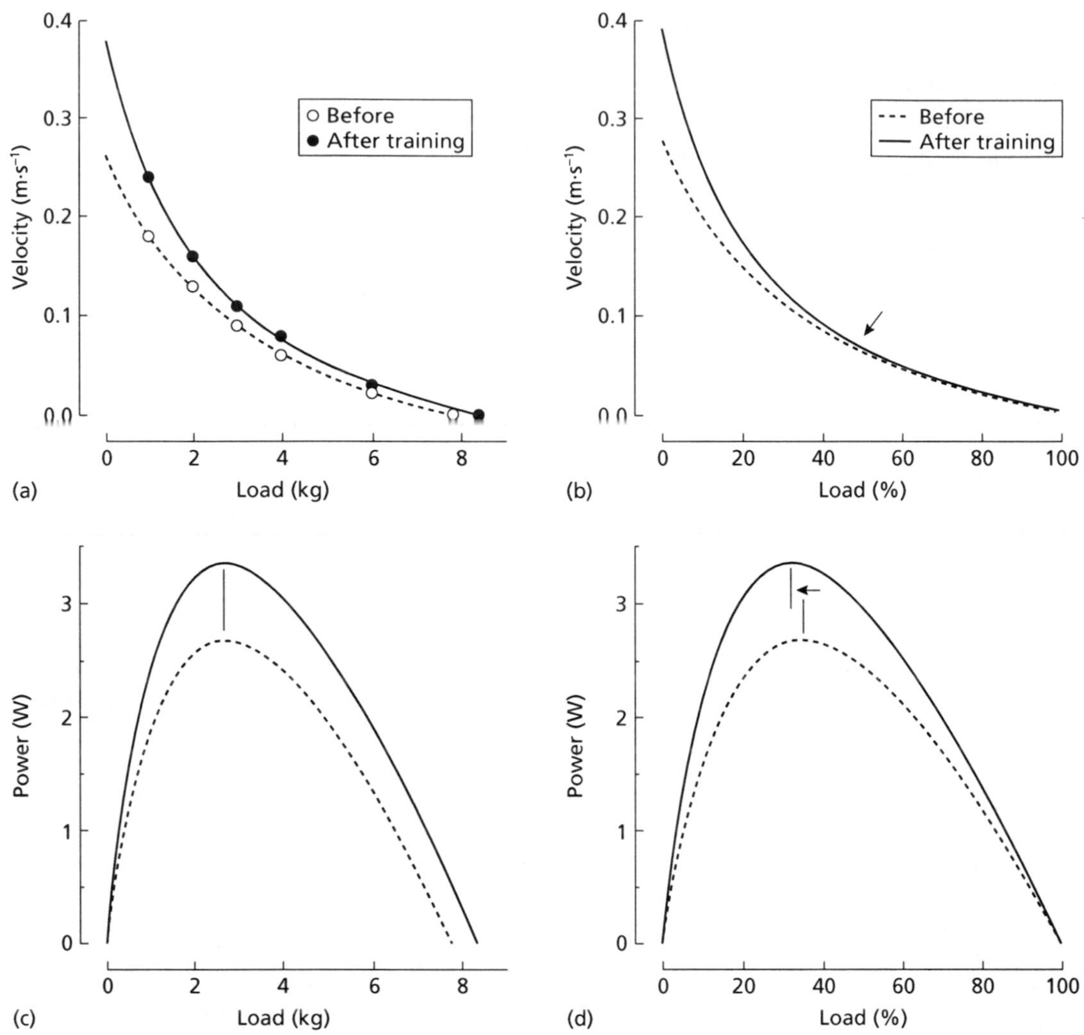

Fig. 16.2 Effects of dynamic training on the force (load)–velocity relationship ((a) and (b)) and power curve ((c) and (d)) of the human adductor pollicis muscle. Muscle contraction was induced by tetanic maximal electrical stimulation at 100 Hz frequency and data plotted by Hill's equation. Loads are expressed in absolute value ((a) and (c)) or as a percentage of the maximal tetanic force ((b) and (d)). (Data are from Duchateau & Hainaut 1984.)

contractile kinetics (Close 1972), or intensification of the muscle E–C coupling (Desmedt & Hainaut 1968).

Mechanical properties of single motor units

Because the muscle contractile kinetics adapt specifically to the type of contraction performed during training, the next question was whether either kind of training programme might influence the contractile capability of the different motor units types (Burke & Edgerton 1975). Since it was obviously impossible to test the same units before and after training, motor units of comparable normalized thresholds (with respect to the muscle maximal force) were compared (Hainaut *et al.* 1981). After isometric training, all motor units showed roughly a proportionally identical force increase without change of twitch time-to-peak and half-relaxation time. After dynamic training, motor units also showed increased force, but the increase was less than that achieved with isometric exercises. In addition, after dynamic exercises, low-threshold motor units presented a larger percentage increase of twitch force than the faster motor units that were recruited at higher force thresholds. Another interesting difference is that the twitch time-to-peak of the whole motor unit population significantly decreased by 9% (Fig. 16.3a) as a result of the dynamic training. This indicated that the twitch time course was accelerated. After training, all motor units showed a decreased recruitment threshold when expressed as a percentage of maximal force. Thus, in order to reach muscle maximal force of contraction, motor unit maximal firing rate should have been increased. There was no evidence of a change in the 'size principle' (Henneman *et al.* 1965) after dynamic training. In fact, a linear relationship was consistently observed between the motor unit size, indicated by its twitch force, and recruitment threshold (Fig. 16.3b).

Mechanisms related to muscular adaptations

Human muscle appears to adapt its contractile properties specifically to the type of exercise training. The augmentation of maximal contraction force should be related to a net increase in contractile proteins and in turn muscle mass (Goldspink 1977; McDonagh & Davies 1984; Narici *et al.* 1996; MacDougall, Chapter 13). The observation that, in training conditions comparable with those prevailing in sports, the M-wave is not changed, suggests that the number of muscle cells is not augmented (Duchateau & Hainaut 1984). It should however, be kept in mind that hyperplasia has been reported after training, but that it is of rather limited significance with respect to the total number of muscle fibres in adults (cf. Fawzi 2000; MacDougall, Chapter 13). The smaller maximal force increase after dynamic exercises is consistent with the fact that the activation duration

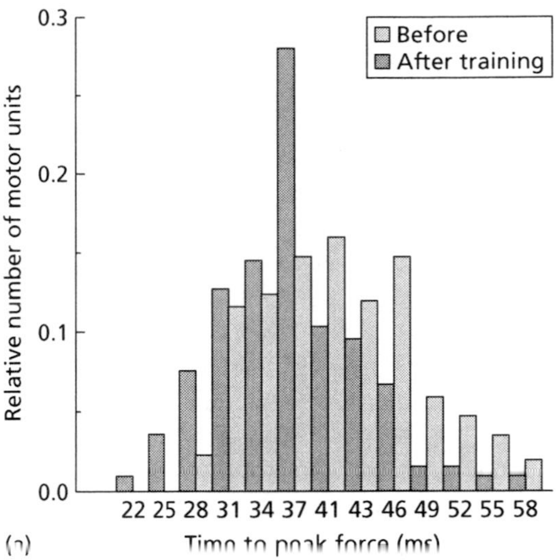

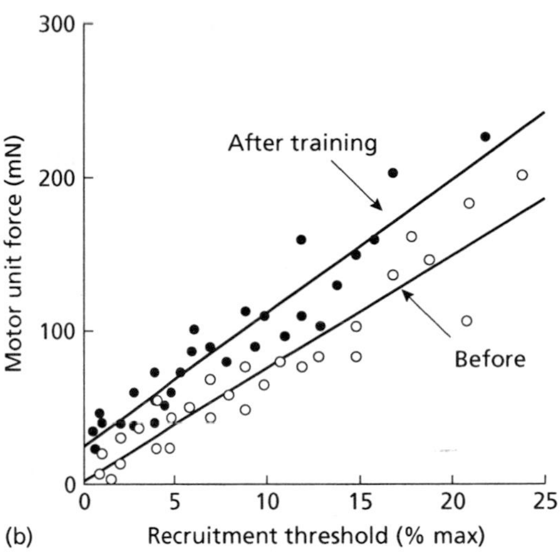

Fig. 16.3 Effects of dynamic training on the mechanical properties of single motor units recorded by spike-triggered averaging method (cf. Milner-Brown *et al.* 1973). (a) Histograms showing the time-to-peak distribution of 112 and 132 motor units before and after training, respectively. Note the shift of the distribution towards shorter time-to-peak values after training. (b) Motor unit force plotted as a function of the recruitment threshold (expressed as a percentage of MVC) during a ramp contraction, before and after dynamic training. The regression lines are statistically different ($P < 0.05$) before and after training.

of different recruitment threshold motor units was not identical. This is because larger motor units are derecruited after the movement onset inertia, and will thus not train throughout the contractions. Such a viewpoint is consistent with the observation that smaller motor units, which are activated until the end of the contractions, show a greater force augmentation compared with larger motor units during dynamic training. This is not the case after isometric training because nearly all motor units are activated throughout the contractions (Hainaut *et al.* 1981).

Increase in maximal rate of tension development and acceleration of twitch time course, which are greater after dynamic training, could be related to an enhanced myosin ATPase activity. It is well known that the maximal speed of shortening is closely related to the myosin ATPase activity (Barany 1967) and that high-velocity (or sprint) training is liable to increase the maximal ATPase activity of the myofibrils (Bell *et al.* 1992) and promote the conversion of muscle myosin from its slower to faster forms (Jansson *et al.* 1990; Andersen *et al.* 1993). An additional mechanism that could explain the increased muscle speed of shortening is enhanced phasic ionized calcium movements. It has been shown in single giant barnacle muscle fibres, using the aequorin technique, that contraction time course changes are closely controlled by changes in calcium movements (Hainaut & Desmedt 1974a,b; Duchateau & Hainaut 1986b). The finding that only dynamic training reduces twitch contraction time suggests that some factors, such as the quantity and/or the quality of sarcoplasmic reticulum, might be specifically enhanced by this type of exercise. The sarcoplasmic reticulum is the organelle which mainly governs phasic ionized calcium movements, and there is experimental evidence that fast muscle fibres contain more sarcoplasmic reticulum than slow ones (Brody 1976). It has also been reported that the sarcoplasmic reticulum can be qualitatively transformed by repetitive electrical activation (Ramirez & Pette 1974). The hypothesis that dynamic training specifically changes calcium movements is consistent with the observation that contraction time may be more dependent on the quality of the reticulum than on the myosin ATPase activity (Brody 1976). It is thus speculative, but nevertheless interesting, to suggest that dynamic training induces larger increases in myosin ATPase activity and phasic calcium movements, compared to isometric exercises.

Adaptation of muscle contractile kinetics to exercise training could also be related to changes in muscle stiffness. In fact decreased series elastic component compliance has been observed after eccentric exercise (Pousson *et al.* 1990). Decreased slope of the stiffness–torque relationship was reported after 'plyometric' training (Cornu *et al.* 1997). It is possible that training would also increase the lateral force transmission to adjacent sarcomeres via the intermediate filament system and the extracellular matrix via lateral connections to the endomysial connective tissue (Patel & Lieber 1997). These changes could facilitate the force transmission to the skeleton. Whatever the underlying mechanisms, the adaptations reported above are the result of muscular changes.

Neural adaptations

In addition to the intrinsic speed-related properties of a muscle, the extent of the neural input to the muscle is of functional importance in the performance of rapid contractions or movements. This association is clear when one compares the rate of EMG, which represents the neural input to the muscle, and the rate of force development during maximum fast isometric contractions. Subjects that present high EMG activity at the beginning of the contraction are also those who show the greatest rate of force development (see fig. 3 in Komi 1986).

A question of importance in sports is related to the capability of an athlete to increase his or her neural input during fast contractions by specific training. A few studies have shown that a training programme with dynamic contractions increases the rate of tension development by an intensification of the neural input to the muscle

(Häkkinen *et al.* 1985b; Behm & Sale 1993; Moritani 1993; Van Cutsem *et al.* 1998). Figure 16.4(a) is an example of such adaptation in one subject, in which force and surface EMG of the tibialis anterior during ballistic isometric contractions of the ankle dorsiflexor muscles are compared before and after 12 weeks of training (Van Cutsem *et al.* 1998). In this study, the training programme consisted of five sessions per week and each session involved 10 sets of 10 contractions against a load that was 30–40% of maximum. When contractions of similar force level (expressed as a percentage of the maximum torque) were compared, it appeared that the rate of torque development and the associated EMG both increased with training (Fig. 16.4a). This increase in rate of torque development was observed at a proportionally comparable extent, whatever the torque level produced during the ballistic contraction (Fig. 16.4b). After training, the average maximal rate of tension development of the five fastest ballistic contractions in all of the five subjects was increased by 82.3% and by 52.9% when expressed as absolute or relative values, respectively. Concomitantly, the time-to-peak tension was shortened by 15.9%. These mechanical adaptations were associated with a mean enhanced EMG activity of 42.7%. This increased EMG activity is particularly evident early in the contraction, since the average time to reach its half-integrated maximal value was shortened by 15.6%. In addition, an earlier activation of the muscle was observed after training (Fig. 16.4a). Because these EMG changes were recorded without any change in the amplitude of the M-wave, they can be interpreted as modifications of the neural command of the contraction. Furthermore, the increase in EMG was truly related to a training adaptation and not a familiarization effect because a control group, tested at 1-, 6-and 12-week intervals, did not show any significant changes.

Various possible neural mechanisms are usually suggested that could explain the increase in neural input to a given muscle. The most frequently proposed mechanisms are: (i) a selective activation of fast high-threshold motor units; (ii) an enhanced synchronization between motor

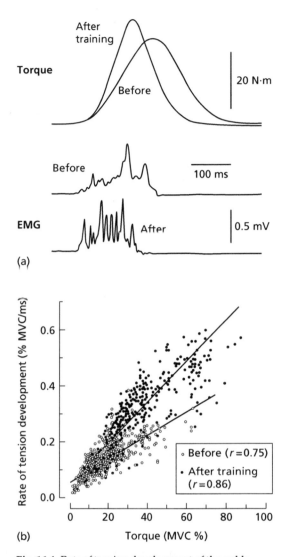

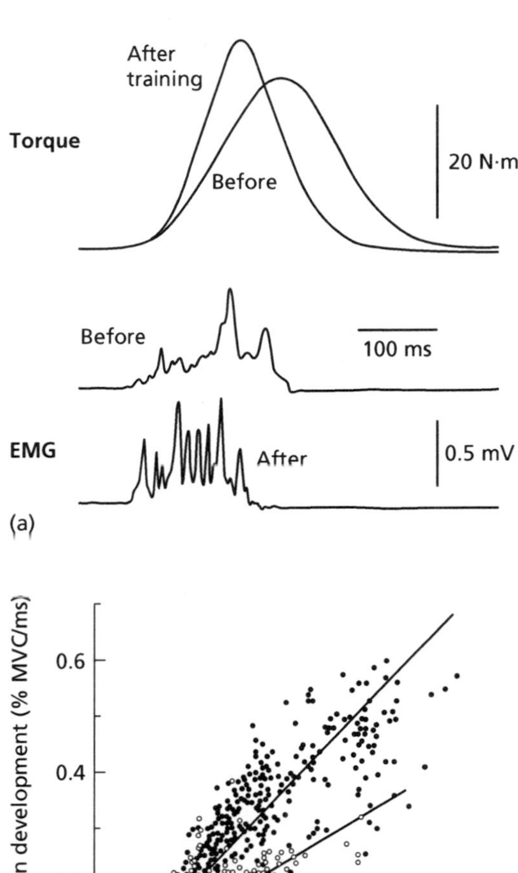

Fig. 16.4 Rate of tension development of the ankle dorsiflexors during ballistic contractions, before and after dynamic training. (a) Comparison of the torque and rectified EMG recorded in the tibialis anterior of one subject during ballistic contractions with a similar MVC percentage (41 vs. 44%), before after training. Note the increased rate of tension development after training and earlier and intensified EMG activity at the onset of the contraction. (b) Relationship for all subjects between the rate of tension development and torque (expressed as a percentage of MVC) during ballistic contractions. The slopes of the relationships before and after training are significantly different ($P < 0.001$). (From Van Cutsem *et al.* 1998, with permission.)

units; and (iii) an increase of motor unit discharge rate.

Selective activation of fast high-threshold motor units

In graded contractions of increasing force, agonist motor units are recruited according to the 'size principle' as documented by Henneman *et al.* in 1965. This principle implies that small (slow) units are activated at a lower force threshold than large (fast) units. This principle, first described in animals, has been found to be valid in human muscles during isometric (Milner-Brown *et al.* 1973) or shortening contractions (Desmedt & Godaux 1979). It has also been shown that the size principle was also the general rule during ballistic contractions (Desmedt & Godaux 1977; Garland *et al.* 1996). However, in the latter conditions, the threshold of motor unit recruitment was lower compared to slow contractions (Desmedt & Godaux 1977). Because during ballistic contractions the strong excitatory drive is able to activate the whole motoneurone pool within a few milliseconds, these small differences in the activation time between motoneurones can sometimes be overridden by the differences in conduction velocity between small and large axons. Indeed, higher conduction velocity was observed in high-threshold units compared to low-threshold units. In spite of this peripheral counteraction, the normal rank order is mostly preserved in a single muscle during ballistic contractions (Büdingen & Freund 1976; Desmedt & Godaux 1977, 1979; Garland *et al.* 1996). To our knowledge, only one study has examined the possibility of a change in the orderly recruitment of motor units after a training programme with dynamic contractions, but no selective recruitment of high-threshold units was observed (Van Cutsem *et al.* 1998). These results, recorded in a single muscle, do not exclude the possibility of changes in the motor unit activation order in synergistic muscles (Duchateau *et al.* 1986; Nardone & Schieppati 1988; Moritani *et al.* 1990). Such exceptions have been reported during very rapid stereotyped movements in the cat (Smith *et al.* 1980), and during eccentric (Nardone *et al.* 1989; Enoka 1996) or electrically induced contractions in humans (Feiereisen *et al.* 1997).

Synchronization between motor units

Motor unit synchronization is another frequently proposed mechanism that explains the increase in the maximal force and rate of tension development (Milner-Brown *et al.* 1975; Komi 1986; Schmidtbleicher 1992). In the study conducted by Milner-Brown *et al.* (1973), synchronization of motor unit impulses was defined as the coincident timing of impulses from two or more motor units. It was observed that weightlifters have a higher synchronization ratio compared to control subjects (Milner-Brown *et al.* 1975; Semmler & Nordstrom 1998) and that strength training increases synchronization between motor units (Milner-Brown *et al.* 1975). Although it is difficult to explain how synchronization would increase the maximal force (see Sale 1988; Yao *et al.* 2000), it is possible that this mechanism could contribute to the increase in the rate of tension development (Semmler & Enoka 2000). The observation of a more segmented aspect of the EMG activity during ballistic contractions after training (Fig. 16.4) could be related either to a greater synchronization between motor units (Komi 1986) or to a tendency of motor units to pulse at a similar frequency (Fuglevand *et al.* 1993). Interestingly, such increased segmentation of the EMG activity was also recorded during stretch–shortening exercises after plyometric training (Schmidtbleicher 1992). Although synchronization among motor units is undoubtedly influenced by changes in the level of chronic physical activity, this has yet to be convincingly demonstrated (Enoka 1997).

Increase of motor unit discharge rate

Increase of motor unit discharge rate has often been proposed as a possible mechanism for

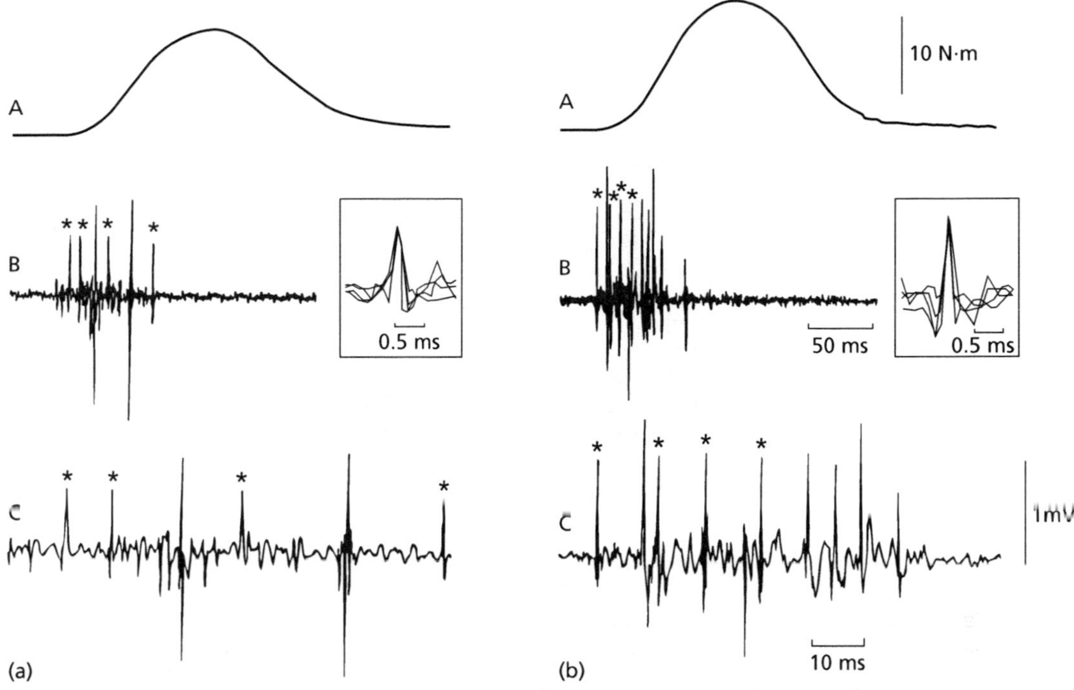

Fig. 16.5 Behaviour of single motor units from the tibialis anterior during ballistic contraction of similar force levels (41 vs. 44% of MVC), before (a) and after (b) dynamic training. The traces correspond to the mechanical force (A) and the intramuscular EMG plotted at slow (B) and fast (C) speeds. (a), typical example of the firing pattern of a single motor unit in untrained muscle showng a short time lapse between the first two spikes followed by longer interspike periods. The first three interspike intervals are 8, 23 and 36 ms, respectively. (b), illustrates the usual motor unit behaviour in trained muscle showing that the high onset of the instantaneous firing rate is maintained during the subsequent spikes. The first three interspike intervals are 11.8, 10 and 11 ms, respectively. The asterisks indicate the discharge of the same motor unit and their traces are superimposed with an extended display (B). (From Van Cutsem *et al.* 1998, with permission.)

enhancing the rate of force development (Cracraft & Petajan 1977; Jansson *et al.* 1990), but this hypothesis has not been experimentally tested until recently. This was done by recording the behaviour of single motor units in the tibialis anterior at the onset of ballistic isometric contractions, by means of an intramuscular wire electrode (Van Cutsem *et al.* 1998). To assess the contribution of motor unit discharge pattern to the increase in the rate of force development, the instantaneous rate for the first four action potentials was determined in single motor units before ($n = 475$) and after ($n = 633$) training. This analysis was limited to the first four action potentials because: (i) few units fired more than four times before training; (ii) at that time the recording was not contaminated by possible electrode movements; and (iii) the maximal rate of tension development was reached.

In the untrained muscle, the discharge rate of single motor units followed the classical behaviour described in the literature during ballistic contractions (Desmedt & Godaux 1977, 1979; Bawa & Calancie 1983). As illustrated by Fig. 16.5(a), the unit started to discharge with a short interspike interval, followed by a progressive interval increase which indicated that the instantaneous discharge rate progressively decreased.

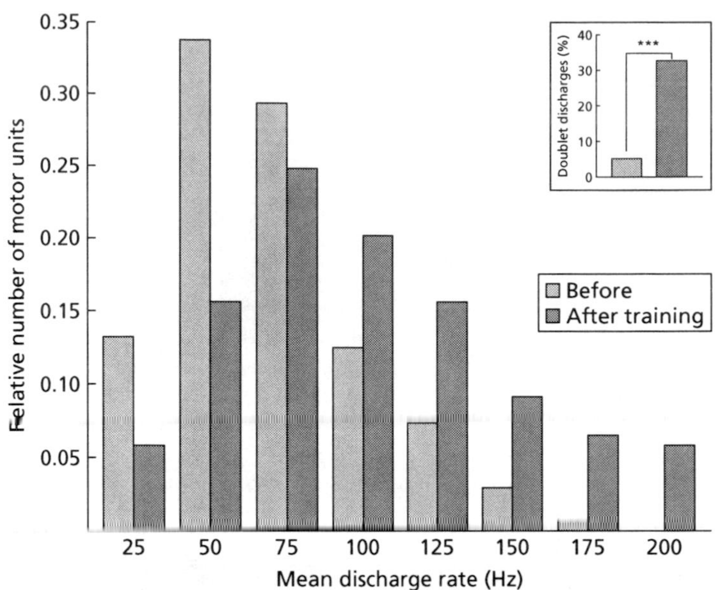

Fig. 16.6 Histograms showing the distribution of the mean discharge rate recorded during the first three interspike intervals of ballistic contractions for the whole motor units population studied before and after dynamic training. Doublet discharges of less than 5 ms intervals are not included in the distribution. The comparison of the distributions, before and after training, are significantly different ($P < 0.001$). In the insert, the histograms illustrate the percentage of doublet discharges of less than 5 ms intervals for the whole motor units population before and after dynamic training. Note that, among the motor units recorded before training, only 5.2% of the tested population showed the presence of doublets at the onset of the EMG burst whereas after training, 32.7% of the units started to fire with interspike intervals between 2 and 5 ms.

It is interesting that after 3 months of dynamic training there was a change in motor unit discharge pattern. As illustrated by Fig. 16.5(b), the decline in the instantaneous discharge frequency of the motor units was no more present in the trained muscle. Without taking into account frequencies above 200 Hz (see the reason below), in the whole population of units the mean discharge frequencies for the first, second and third intervals were 84.6, 64.8 and 59.2 Hz, respectively, before training and 90.2, 89.4 and 89.2 Hz, respectively, after training. The gain in discharge rate was thus larger for the third than for the second and first interspike intervals. Figure 16.6 illustrates the effect of training on the instantaneous discharge rate when the first three interspike intervals are averaged. It is clear from this figure that training increased the discharge rate of the whole motor unit population.

Doublet discharges

In some circumstances, motor unit double discharges (called doublets) are a common observation during intramuscular EMG recordings (Denslow 1948; Bawa & Calancie 1983; Kudina & Churikova 1990; Garland & Griffin 1999). It is generally considered that two consecutive discharges of less than a 20-ms interval are 'doublets' (Simpson 1969). Such double discharges have been observed during graded or sustained submaximal, as well as during fast ramp and ballistic contractions (Bawa & Calancie 1983; Kudina & Churikova 1990; Garland *et al.* 1996; Van Cutsem *et al.* 1998). Because it is impossible to objectively determine the transition between single and double firing, we decided to consider an interval equal to or less than 5 ms as being a doublet. Among the motor units recorded before

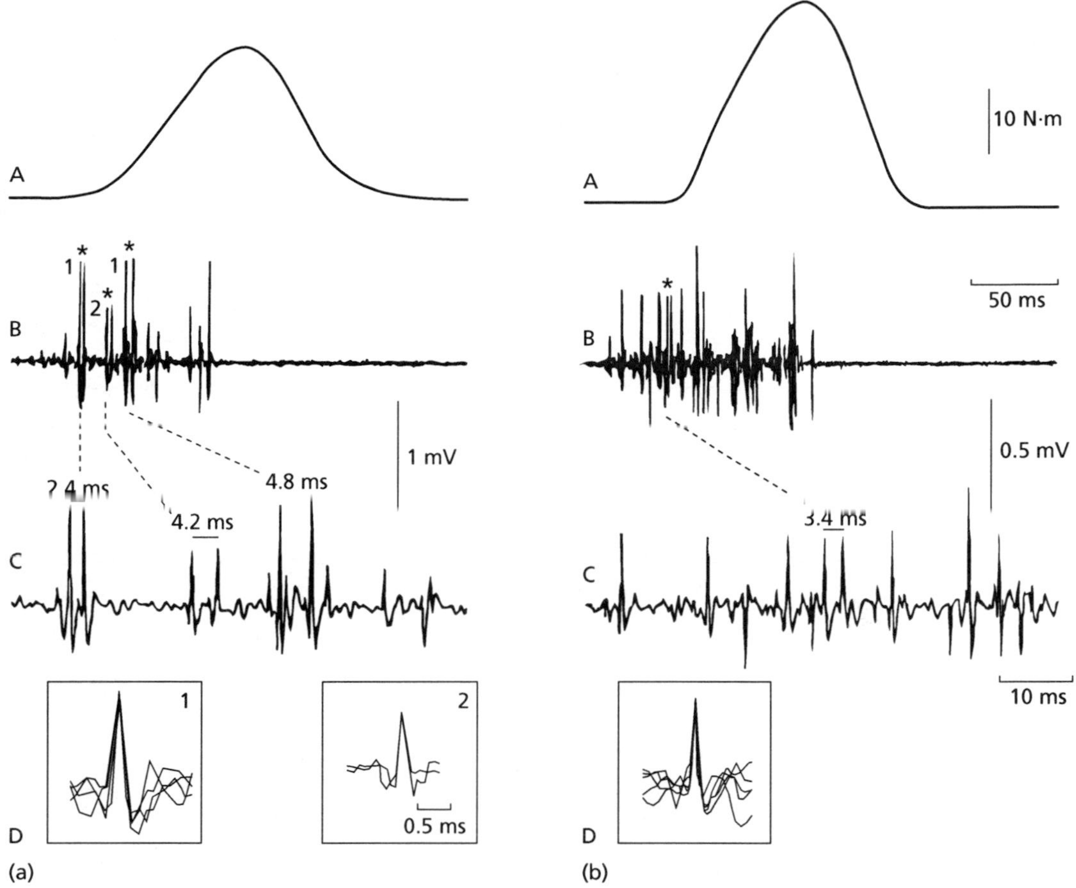

Fig. 16.7 Examples of doublet discharges of single motor units from the tibialis anterior during ballistic contraction after dynamic training. The traces correspond to the mechanical force (A), and the intramuscular EMG plotted at slow (B) and fast (C) speeds. (a) illustrates two different motor units which started to discharge with a doublet. Motor unit 1 fired two doublets (2.4 and 4.8 ms, respectively) while motor unit 2 discharged with a double spike of 4.2 ms interval. (b) illustrates a doublet which appeared later during the contraction. The motor unit illustrated showed three single firings at intervals of, respectively, 14, 12.5 and 6 ms, followed by a 3.4-ms doublet. The asterisks indicate double discharges and their traces are superimposed with an extended display (d). Note that in (b) D, the double discharge has been superimposed on the first three single spikes. (From Van Cutsem *et al.* 1998, with permission.)

training, only 5.2% showed doublets at the onset of the EMG burst (Fig. 16.6). In the trained muscles, 32.7% of the motor units recorded started to fire with interspike intervals between 2 and 5 ms. In some cases, even repetitive doublets of a motor unit occurred as illustrated by Fig. 16.7(a). Under these conditions, the interspike interval of the doublet increased during the discharge sequence. Interestingly, some motor units did not display this doublet firing at the onset of the contraction but did so later during the contraction (Fig. 16.7b).

Mechanisms underlying the increase in firing rate and of doublet discharges

In untrained muscles, motor unit firing rate probably does not reach the optimal level in order to drive the muscle to its maximum rate of tension development. This is supported by the observation that the maximum rate of tension development during tetanic contractions is only reached at an electrical stimulation frequency of 200–250 Hz (Miller *et al.* 1981; Duchateau & Hainaut, unpublished observation). Therefore, the observation of earlier motor unit activation, extra doublets and enhanced maximal firing rate after dynamic training should contribute to the increase in the speed of voluntary ballistic contractions.

High motor unit discharge rates (150–200 Hz) at the onset of sustained contractions (Marsden *et al.* 1971) and the presence of doublet responses of short intervals (3.2–4 ms) during magnetic cortical stimulation (Gandevia & Rothwell 1987; Day *et al.* 1989; Bawa & Lemon 1993) have been reported. These instantaneous high frequencies, which were also observed at the onset of motoneurone firing induced by fast ramp current injection (Baldissera *et al.* 1987), correspond to the 'secondary' range of motoneurone discharges described by Kernell (1965). Since motoneurone firing rate is known to be related to the intensity of the injected current, the increase of short interspike intervals observed after training could be related to an enhanced massive synaptic input. An alternative explanation is that increased motor unit firing rate and doublet discharges are due to changes in intrinsic properties of the motoneurone membrane. It is well known that a motoneurone capable of producing a double discharge may undergo a state of increased depolarization, or delayed depolarization, that occurs during the falling phase of the action potential. The delayed depolarization appears to result from an antidromic invasion of the dendrites following the initial action potential, which causes a small inflection on the falling phase of the initial action potential (Granit *et al.* 1963; Nelson & Burke 1967). During this period, the motoneurone should be more susceptible to increased synaptic input, which may reach the threshold level and produce a second action potential at a very brief interval.

Our observations that the presence of doublets after training is not related to the recruitment threshold of the motor units do not support the idea that increased synaptic input plays a major role in the greater number of recorded doublets. In fact, low-threshold motor units, with larger input resistance, should have shown a greater tendency towards doublet discharges, but this was not the case in the present experiments. The observation, in some units, that doublet discharges do not appear at the onset of firing but later in the discharge sequence is another argument which supports the hypothesis of a change in intrinsic properties of the motoneurone membrane. This is in line with the increase in motoneurone excitability observed after training by Sale and collaborators (1983 and Chapter 15).

Functional significance of doublet discharges

It is concluded from the above discussion that these doublets contribute to the increase in the maximal rate of tension development and/or to the enforcement of submaximal rates, depending on the moment at which they appear in the EMG burst. This is interesting since maximal rate of tension development has been reported as being reached during the second (or third twitch) of a tetanus (see Stein & Parmiggiani 1979; Duchateau & Hainaut 1986a) and to be closely controlled by phasic intracellular ionized calcium movements (Duchateau & Hainaut 1986b). However, it has previously been reported that at very short intervals (roughly 1 ms) the muscle action potential (M-wave) elicited by two pulses was identical to that elicited by a single pulse in the adductor pollicis (Desmedt & Hainaut 1968). Thus, a tendency of the motoneurone to fire doublets at such short intervals during voluntary contractions would be ignored by the membrane because of its refractory state. Since the doublets observed in the present experiments included an interpulse interval greater (ranging from 2 to 5 ms) than the refractory period (roughly 1.5 ms), the functional significance of doublets in the enhanced rate of tension development clearly appears. In addition, a recent computer simulation study (Van Cutsem *et al.*, unpublished data) indicated that such high-frequency double discharges effectively contribute to the increase in the rate of tension development.

Conclusion

Dynamic training using small loads increases the maximal rate of tension development. As for the maximal force, these adaptations are due not only to muscular but also to neural changes and are specific to the type of contraction performed during training. At the muscular level, these adaptations appear to be mainly controlled by intracellular mechanisms (enhanced myosin ATPase activity and/or intensified phasic ionized calcium movements) and changes in muscle compliance. At the neural level, earlier motor unit activation, extra doublets and enhanced maximal firing rate contribute to the increase in the speed of voluntary muscle contraction after dynamic training. The observation that velocity-specific responses to isometric and concentric isokinetic training were the same suggests that it is the intent to contract ballistically, rather than an actual ballistic movement, that mainly determines the adaptation in speed (Behm & Sale 1993). The data from this study emphasize the significance of the neural adaptations in the increase in the rate of tension development.

References

Andersen, J.L., Klitgaard, H. & Saltin, B. (1993) Myosin heavy chain isoforms in single fibres from m. vastus lateralis of sprinters: influence of training intensity. *Acta Physiologica Scandinavica* **151**, 135–142.

Baldissera, P., Campadelli, P. & Piccinelli, L. (1987) The dynamic response of cat gastrocnemius motor units investigated by ramp-current injection into their motoneurones. *Journal of Physiology* **387**, 317–330.

Barany, M. (1967) ATPase activity of myosin correlated with speed of muscle shortening. *Journal of General Physiology* **50**, 197–216.

Barany, M. & Close, R. (1971) The transformation of myosin cross-innervated rat muscles. *Journal of Physiology* **213**, 455–474.

Bawa, P. & Calancie, B. (1983) Repetitive doublets in human flexor carpi radialis muscle. *Journal of Physiology* **339**, 123–132.

Bawa, P. & Lemon, R.N. (1993) Recruitment of motor units in response to transcranial magnetic stimulation in man. *Journal of Physiology* **471**, 445–464.

Behm, D.G. & Sale, D.G. (1993) Intended rather than actual movement velocity determines velocity-specific training response. *Journal of Applied Physiology* **74**, 359–368.

Bell, G.J., Petersen, S.R., Maclean, I., Reid, D.C. & Quinney, H.A. (1992) Effect of high velocity resistance training on peak torque, cross sectional area and myofibrillar ATPase activity. *Journal of Sports Medicine and Physical Fitness* **32**, 10–18.

Brody, I.A. (1976) Regulation of isometric contraction in skeletal muscle. *Experimental Neurology* **50**, 673–683.

Büdingen, H.J. & Freund, H.J. (1976) The relationship between the rate of rise of isometric tension and motor unit recruitment in a human forearm muscle. *Pflügers Archiv* **362**, 61–67.

Buller, A.J. & Lewis, D.M. (1965) The rate of tension development in isometric tetanic contractions of mammalian fast and slow skeletal muscle. *Journal of Physiology* **176**, 337–354.

Burke, R.E. & Edgerton, R.V. (1975) Motor unit properties and selective involvement in movement. *Exercise and Sport Sciences Reviews* **3**, 31–81.

Close, R.I. (1972) Dynamic properties of mammalian skeletal muscles. *Physiological Reviews* **52**, 129–197.

Colliander, E.B. & Tesch, P.A. (1990) Effects of eccentric and concentric muscle actions in resistance training. *Acta Physiologica Scandinavica* **140**, 31–39.

Cornu, C., Almeida Silveira, M.I. & Goubel, F. (1997) Influence of plyometric training on the mechanical impedance of the human ankle joint. *European Journal of Applied Physiology* **76**, 282–288.

Cracraft, J.D. & Petajan, J.H. (1977) Effect of muscle training on the pattern of firing of single motor units. *American Journal of Physical Medicine* **56**, 183–193.

Day, B.L., Dressler, D., Maertens De Noordhout, A. *et al.* (1989) Electric and magnetic stimulation of human motor cortex: surface EMG and single motor unit responses. *Journal of Physiology* **412**, 449–473.

Denslow, J.S. (1948) Double discharges in human motor units. *Journal of Neurophysiology* **11**, 209–215.

Desmedt, J.E. & Godaux, E. (1977) Ballistic contractions in man: characteristic recruitment patterns of single motor units of the tibialis anterior muscle. *Journal of Physiology* **264**, 673–693.

Desmedt, J.E. & Godaux, E. (1979) Voluntary motor commands in human ballistic contractions. *Annals of Neurology* **5**, 415–421.

Desmedt, J.E. & Hainaut, K. (1968) Kinetics of myofilament activation in potentiated contraction: staircase phenomenon in human skeletal muscle. *Nature* **217**, 529–532.

Duchateau, J. & Enoka, R.M. (2002) Neural adaptations with chronic activity patterns in able-bodied humans. *American Journal of Physical Medicine and Rehabilitation* in press.

Duchateau, J. & Hainaut, K. (1984) Isometric or dynamic training: differential effects on mechanical properties of a human muscle. *Journal of Applied Physiology* **56**, 296–301.

Duchateau, J. & Hainaut, K. (1986a) Nonlinear summation of contractions in striated muscle. I. Twitch potentiation in human muscle. *Journal of Muscle Research and Cell Motility* **7**, 11–17.

Duchateau, J. & Hainaut, K. (1986b) Nonlinear summation of contractions in striated muscle. II. Potentiation of intracellular Ca^{2+} movements in single barnacle muscle fibres. *Journal of Muscle Research and Cell Motility* **7**, 18–24.

Duchateau, J. & Hainaut, K. (1988) Training of submaximal electrostimulation in a human muscle. *Medicine and Science in Sports and Exercise* **20**, 99–104.

Duchateau, J., Le Bozec, S. & Hainaut, K. (1986) Contribution of slow and fast muscle to the triceps surae to a cyclic movement. *European Journal of Applied Physiology* **55**, 476–481.

Enoka, R.M. (1996) Eccentric contractions require unique activation strategies by the nervous system. *Journal of Applied Physiology* **81**, 2339–2346.

Enoka, R.M. (1997) Neural adaptations with chronic physical activity. *Journal of Biomechanics* **30**, 447–455.

Fawzi, K. (2000) Adaptation of human skeletal muscle of training and anabolic steroids. *Acta Physiologica Scandinavica* **168**, 1–71.

Feiereisen, P., Duchateau, J. & Hainaut, K. (1997) Motor unit recruitment order during voluntary and electrically induced contractions in the tibialis anterior. *Experimental Brain Research* **114**, 117–123.

Fuglevand, A.J., Winter, D.A. & Patla, A.E. (1993) Models or recuitment and rate coding organization in motor-unit pools. *Journal of Neurophysiology* **70**, 2470–2488.

Gandevia, S.C. & Rothwell, J.C. (1987) Knowledge of motor commands and the recruitment of human motoneurons. *Brain* **110**, 1117–1130.

Garland, S.J. & Griffin, L. (1999) Motor unit double discharges: statistical anomaly or functional entity? *Canadian Journal of Applied Physiology* **24**, 113–130.

Garland, S.J., Cooke, J.D., Miller, K.J., Ohtsuki, T. & Ivanova, T. (1996) Motor unit activity during human single joint movements. *Journal of Neurophysiology* **76**, 1982–1990.

Ghez, C. (1991) The control of movements. In: *Principles of Neural Sciences* (eds E. R. Kandel, J. H. Schwartz & T. M. Jessell), pp. 531–547. Prentice Hall International, London.

Goldspink, D.F. (1977) The influence of activity on muscle size and protein turnover. *Journal of Physiology* **264**, 283–296.

Gorza, L., Gundersen, K., Lomo, T., Schiaffino, S. & Westgaard, R.H. (1988) Slow-to-fast transformation of denervated soleus muscles by chronic high frequency stimulation in the rat. *Journal of Physiology* **402**, 627–649.

Granit, R., Kernell, D. & Smith, R.S. (1963) Delayed depolarization and the repetitive response to intracellular stimulation of mammalian motoneurones. *Journal of Physiology* **168**, 890–910.

Hainaut, K. & Desmedt, J.E. (1974a) Calcium ionophore A23187 potentiates twitch and intracellular calcium release in single muscle fibres. *Nature* **252**, 407–408.

Hainaut, K. & Desmedt, J.E. (1974b) Effect of dantrolene sodium on calcium movements in single muscle fibres. *Nature* **252**, 723–730.

Hainaut, K., Duchateau, J. & Desmedt, J.E. (1981) Differential effects on slow and fast motor units different programs of brief daily training in man. In: *New Developments in Electromyography and Clinical Neurophysiology*, Vol. 9 (ed. J. E. Desmedt), pp. 241–249. Karger, Basel.

Häkkinen, K. & Komi, P.V. (1983) Electromyographic changes during strength training and detraining. *Medicine and Science in Sports and Exercise* **15**, 455–460.

Häkkinen, K.P., Komi, P.V. & Alen, M. (1985a) Changes in isometric force- and relaxation-time, electromyographic and muscle fibre characteristics of human skeletal muscle during strength training and detraining. *Acta Physiologica Scandinavica* **125**, 587–600.

Häkkinen, K.P., Komi, P.V. & Alen, M. (1985b) Effect of explosive type strength training on isometric force- and relaxation-time, electromyographic and muscle fibre characteristics of leg extensor muscles. *Acta Physiologica Scandinavica* **125**, 587–600.

Henneman, E., Somjen, G. & Carpenter, D.O. (1965) Functional significance of cell size in spinal motoneurons. *Journal of Neurophysiology* **28**, 560–580.

Jansson, E., Esbjörnsson, M., Holm, I. & Jacobs, I. (1990) Increase in the proportion of fast-twitch muscle fibres by sprint training in males. *Acta Physiologica Scandinavica* **140**, 359–363.

Jones, D.A. & Rutherford, O.M. (1987) Human muscle strength training: the effects of three different regimes and the nature of the resultant changes. *Journal of Physiology* **391**, 1–11.

Kaneko, M., Fuchimoto, T., Toji, H. & Suei, K. (1983) Training effect of different loads on the force–velocity relationship and mechanical power output in human muscle. *Scandinavian Journal of Sports Sciences* **5**, 50–55.

Keele, S.W. (1968) Movement control in skilled motor performance. *Psychological Bulletin* **70**, 387–403.

Kernell, D. (1965) High repetitive firing of cat lumbosacral motoneurones stimulated by long lasting injected currents. *Acta Physiologica Scandinavica* **65**, 84–86.

Komi, P.V. (1986) Training of muscle strength and power: interaction of neuromotoric, hypertrophic and mechanical factors. *International Journal of Sports Medicine* **7**, 10–15.

Kudina, L.P. & Churikova, L.I. (1990) Testing excitability of human motoneurones capable of firing double discharges. *Electroencephalography and Clinical Neurophysiology* **75**, 334–341.

McDonagh, M.J.N. & Davies, C.T.M. (1984) Adaptive response of mammalian skeletal muscle to exercise with high loads. *European Journal of Applied Physiology* **52**, 139–155.

MacDougall, J.D., Elder, G.C.B., Sale, D.G., Moroz, J.R. & Sutton, J.R. (1980) Effects of strength training and immobilization of human muscle fibres. *European Journal of Applied Physiology* **43**, 25–34.

Marsden, D.C., Meadows, J.C. & Merton, P.A. (1971) Isolated single motor units in human muscle and their rate of discharge during voluntary effort. *Journal of Physiology* **217**, 12–13.

Miller, R.G., Mirka, A. & Maxfield, M. (1981) Rate of tension development in isometric contractions of a human hand muscle. *Experimental Neurology* **73**, 267–285.

Milner-Brown, H.S., Stein, R.B. & Yemm, R. (1973) The contractile properties of human motor units during voluntary isometric contractions. *Journal of Physiology* **228**, 285–306.

Milner-Brown, H.S., Stein, R. & Lee, R.G. (1975) Synchronization of human motor units: possible rôle of exercise and supraspinal reflex. *Electroencephalography and Clinical Neurophysiology* **38**, 245–254.

Moritani, T. (1993) Neuromuscular adaptations during the acquisition of muscle strength, power and motor tasks. *Journal of Biomechanics* **26**, 95–107.

Moritani, T. & De Vries, H.A. (1979) Neural factors vs hypertrophy in time course of muscle strength gain. *American Journal of Physical Medicine and Rehabilitation* **58**, 115–130.

Moritani, T., Oddsson, L. & Thorstensson, A. (1990) Differences in modulation of the gastrocnemius and soleus H-reflexes during hopping in man. *Acta Physiologica Scandinavica* **138**, 575–576.

Nardone, A. & Schieppati, M. (1988) Shift of activity from slow to fast muscle during voluntary lengthening contractions of the triceps surae muscles in humans. *Journal of Physiology* **395**, 363–381.

Nardone, A., Romano, C. & Schieppati, M. (1989) Selective recruitment of high-threshold human motor units during voluntary isotonic lengthening of active muscles. *Journal of Physiology* **409**, 451–471.

Narici, M.V., Roi, G.S., Landoni, L., Minetti, A.E. & Cerretelli, P. (1990) Changes in force, cross-sectional area and neural activation during strength training and detraining of the human quadriceps. *European Journal of Applied Physiology* **59**, 310–319.

Narici, M.V., Hoppeler, H., Kayser, B. *et al.* (1996) Human quadriceps cross-sectional area, torque and neural activation during 6 months strength training. *Acta Physiologica Scandinavica* **157**, 175–186.

Nelson, P.G. & Burke, R.E. (1967) Delayed depolarization in cat spinal motoneurones. *Experimental Neurology* **17**, 16–26.

Patel, T.J. & Lieber, R.L. (1997) Force transmission in skeletal muscle: from actomyosin to external tendons. *Exercise and Sport Sciences Reviews* **25**, 321–363.

Pette, D. & Vrbova, G. (1992) Adaptation of mammalian skeletal muscle fibers to chronic electrical stimulation. *Reviews of Physiology, Biochemistry and Pharmacology* **120**, 115–202.

Pousson, M., Van Hoecke, J. & Goubel, F. (1990) Changes in elastic characteristics of human muscle induced by eccentric exercise. *Journal of Biomechanics* **23**(4), 343–348.

Pousson, M., Amiridis, L.G., Cometti, G. & Van Hoecke, J. (1999) Velocity-specific training in elbow flexors. *European Journal of Applied Physiology* **80**, 367–372.

Ramirez, B.U. & Pette, D. (1974) Effects of long-term electrical stimulation on sarcoplasmic reticulum of fast rabbit muscle. *FEBS Letters* **49**, 180–190.

Sale, D.G. (1988) Neural adaptation to resistance training. *Medicine and Science in Sports and Exercise* **20**(5), 135–145.

Sale, D.G., MacDougall, J.E., Upton, A.R.M. & McComas, A.J. (1983) Effect of strength training upon motoneuron excitability in man. *Medicine and Science in Sports and Exercise* **15**, 57–62.

Sandow, A. (1965) Excitation–contraction coupling in skeletal muscle. *Pharmacological Review* **17**, 265–320.

Schmidtbleicher, D. (1992) Training of power events. In: *Strength and Power in Sport* (ed. P. V. Komi), pp. 381–395. Blackwell Scientific Publications, Oxford.

Semmler, J.G. & Enoka, R.M. (2000) Neural contributions to the changes in muscle strength. In: *Biomechanics in Sport: The Scientific Basis of Performance* (ed. V. M. Zatsiorsky), pp. 3–20. Blackwell Science, Oxford.

Semmler, J.G. & Nordstrom, M.A. (1998) Motor unit discharge and force tremor in skill- and strength-trained individuals. *Experimental Brain Research* **119**, 27–38.

Simpson, J.A. (1969) Terminology of electromyography. *Electroencephalography and Clinical Neurophysiology* **26**, 224–226.

Smith, J.L., Betts, B., Edgerton, V.R. & Zernicke, R.F. (1980) Rapid ankle extension during paw shakes: selective recruitment of fast ankle extensors. *Journal of Neurophysiology* **43**, 612–620.

Stein, R.B. & Parmiggiani, F. (1979) Optimal motor patterns for activation of mammalian muscle. *Brain Research* **175**, 372–376.

Thépaut-Mathieu, C., Van Hoecke, J. & Maton, B. (1988) Myoelectric and mechanical changes are linked to length specificity during isometric training. *Journal of Applied Physiology* **64**, 1500–1505.

Thorstensson, A., Hulten, B., von Döbeln, W. & Karlsson, J. (1976) Effect of strength training on enzyme activities and fibre characteristics in human skeletal muscle. *Acta Physiologica Scandinavica* **96**, 392–398.

Van Cutsem, M., Duchateau, J. & Hainaut, K. (1998) Changes in single motor unit behaviour contribute to the increase in contraction speed after dynamic training in humans. *Journal of Physiology* **513**, 295–305.

Wilson, G.J., Murphy, A.J. & Walshe, A. (1996) The specificity of strength training: the effect of posture. *European Journal of Applied Physiology* **73**, 346–352.

Yao, W., Fuglevand, A.J. & Enoka, R.M. (2000) Motor-unit synchronization increases EMG amplitude and decreases force steadiness of simulated contractions. *Journal of Neurophysiology* **83**, 441–452.

Chapter 17

Proprioceptive Training: Considerations for Strength and Power Production

ALBERT GOLLHOFER

Introduction

The effects of strength and power training have been investigated extensively. Most of the studies concentrate on the mechanisms causing adaptations either reflected in the muscle size or of neuronal activation characteristics. Functional limitations are elaborated that demonstrate the borderlines of the adaptations of muscle areas or volumes as well as of the individual potential of modulation of the muscle fibre type composition. Since most of the current studies have been conducted using classical strength or power training programmes (MacDougall *et al.* 1979; Häkkinen & Komi 1986; MacDougall 1986; Tesch 1987; Sale 1992), the neuromuscular mechanisms that produce adaptive changes in motor systems, and the sensory systems controlling motor systems in sensorimotor training programmes, are poorly understood. The improvement of efferent, voluntarily elicited muscular activation associated with acute or chronic training regimens has been referred either to alterations in the recruitment characteristics or to the frequency pattern of the motoneurones involved. A consensus exists that alterations in maximum strength can be achieved either by enhancement of the muscular protein potential as a consequence of hypertrophy and/or hyperplasia, or by functional adaptations in the neuronal control of the musculature.

Functional adaptations causing changes in basic strength, determined as the improvement in muscle force (maximum voluntary contraction, MVC) after training, are much more frequently investigated than training-induced plasticity of the muscle power, which is commonly assessed by the rate of force development. This is remarkable, as in virtually all situations in sports and in daily activity an efficient means of activating muscles quickly, or of producing high impulses within given time periods is much more desirable.

From a neuromuscular perspective, the actual excitation of the motoneuronal system is determined by both efferent and afferent activation processes. In most of the classical strength training papers, the mechanisms associated with alterations in the efferent, voluntarily generated activation are determined as the factors responsible for neuronal adaptations. The precise role of afferent contributions is not as well understood.

For many years, the fundamental role of sensory feedback in modulating muscular activations has been studied in locomotion and in postural tasks. Questions as to what extent alterations in afferent feedback may also enhance the motor output, understood as a positive feedback mechanism, have not been addressed extensively in the strength training literature. As an exception, the functional importance of active sensory, stretch-related feedback has primarily been investigated only for one specific type of muscular action, the stretch–shortening cycle (Komi 1984; Gollhofer *et al.* 1987). Based on isolated studies the important role of stretch reflexes for regulation of stiffness of the tendomuscular system has been verified. Nichols (1987) demonstrated that an electrically stimulated muscle responds to ramp stretches with linear, spring-like tension increments only if the muscle has remained its intact afferent reflex system. Hoffer and Andreassen (1981) revealed under eccentric conditions that the net contribution of stretch-sensitive activation under eccentric conditions is considerably important amongst a large range of other operating forces.

Despite the apparent importance of afferent neuromuscular activation most of the strength and power training studies do not usually focus on the issue as to whether sensory contributions, provided by proprioceptive mechanisms, may influence the production of force and power itself. Therefore, the major purpose of this chapter is to describe the adaptations of the neuromuscular system after proprioceptive training programmes. Functional considerations will be elaborated in order to reveal relevant mechanisms indicating that improvements in proprioceptive sensitivity apparently can be beneficial for normal muscular activation processes as well.

Proprioception

Human posture and motion are controlled by a complex interaction of centrally and peripherally organized neuronal networks. Task-specific voluntary movement is permanently under the influence of information feedback from various sources of proprioceptive receptors. This control system is highly effective if the feedback is organized 'in real time' and even more effective if feedforward mechanisms are anticipating the motor requirements. From mechanoreceptors in the fingertips it is known that for a precision grip the actual forces are slightly higher than necessary to hold the object (Johansson & Westling 1984, 1987). It is well known (Eliasson *et al.* 1995) that a disturbance of load will result in a compensatory force occurring with a latency of 40 ms. This reaction is thought to be organized by mechanoreceptors and is functionally important for quick adjustments due to external load variations.

In order to differentiate between the various sources of feedback contributions three specific types of 'receptions' are distinguished: exteroception, interoception and proprioception.

The exteroceptive contribution is organized by the receptors that transmit environmental information (visual, auditory, etc.) to the nervous system. Interoception describes the amount of information that is processed within the body. Proprioception allows the perception of position and movement of limbs with reference to both the entire body and single limbs.

Therefore proprioception is a basic information source for the control of body movements basically in the context of balance regulation. With regard to single limbs, proprioception provides most of the required information about the active and passive state of joint complex stabilization. Both components, balance control and joint stabilization, already interact in arguably simple tasks like (for example) securing of the upright stance (Gruber *et al.* 2000).

Proprioception can be subdivided in three submodalities: *the position sense*, a conscious representation of static joint positions, makes it possible to get an impression of three-dimensional space; *the movement sense* (kinaesthesia) organizes the awareness of dynamic changes of joint positions in relation to one and another; and *the force sense* provides information about the current balanced state between internally generated forces and the externally applied moments to the joint systems.

The concept of proprioception merely describes the sensory reception of stimuli as well as the coding of these neurological signals in combination with the afferent feedback to the central nervous system (CNS) (Lephart *et al.* 2000).

Numerous, differently specialized receptors that can be identified in the peripheral limbs guarantee dense networks and high efficiency of this information system. These receptors are connected to the spinal cord via afferent nerve fibres. The interneuronal pool of nerve cells represents the first major control system where all this afferent information converges (Fig. 17.1). As a consequence of central input and peripheral convergence, motoneurones of synergistic or antagonistic muscles may be inhibited or facili-

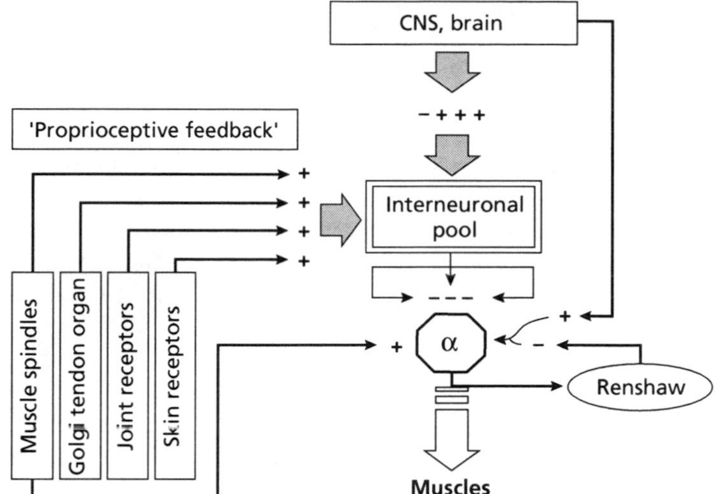

Fig. 17.1 Schematic drawing demonstrating the various efferent and afferent influences on the final pathway of a motoneurone activating skeletal muscles.

tated according to the motor requirements of a distinct movement.

Integration of sensory feedback for movement control, a task-specific modulation

From a biomechanical point of view, gait, for example, is characterized by changes of the centre of pressure (COP) with respect to the actual projection of the centre of mass (COM) to the supporting area during a distinct motor task (Winter 1996). The ability of the nervous system to detect joint positions, movement directions and force applications is mainly processed by sensory afferents. In addition, precise information, already on the joint level already, is necessary to balance gravitational forces as well as any active changes in motor output in order to counteract the gravitational forces and to produce coordinated movements.

The proprioceptive system is part of the entire somatosensory system. On the periphery, for example, the joint systems of arms and legs must be synchronized in order to meet the coordinative demands during distinct tasks. Here, the proprioceptive input is mandatory to align vestibular and visual feedback systems as well, and to continuously modulate the muscular activation of the limb muscles (see Chapter 2). However, control of gravitational load and situational compensation of external load during an ongoing movement or within a given task, is both task and phase dependent. Several authors describe the existence of specifically adapted load receptors (Gollhofer *et al.* 1989; Dietz *et al.* 1992; Prochazka 1996). Not only in rhythmic locomotor activity but also in compensatory activations of mechanically induced joint perturbations, load receptors play an important role in the proprioceptive feedback. From human experiments, it is speculated that especially the Golgi tendon organ with its short latencies is a good candidate to represent these types of load receptors (Dietz *et al.* 1992). However, it has been suggested (Duysens *et al.* 2000) that load is not only sensed by a specific load receptor. A variety of other types of receptors that were previously thought to have other functions may also feedback load. Thus, a new definition of load sensitivity has to be considered.

From single motoneurone recordings it is known that even small variations in the frequency of the excitation drive will result in a largely different motor output. Duchateau *et al.* (1999) (for details see also Chapter 16) have shown that an extra doublet of stimuli, supplied in the activation of the motoneurones, enhances the force output for a considerable time period. This transfer of fast alterations in neuromuscular activation into low-frequency responses of force output may be the major, mechanically important aspect. In situations like stumbling reactions or in tilt movements of the ankle joint complex, the polysynaptically mediated reflexes are superimposed on the basic activation pattern, thus leading to extra stimuli that instantaneously enhance the actual motor frequency (Vallbo 1981; Vallbo & Al-Falahe 1990) and therefore the motor output.

Proprioceptive contribution in stretch–shortening cycle (SSC)

An immediate transfer from the preactivated and eccentrically stretched muscle–tendon complex to the concentric push-off basically determines the efficacy of motor output in the SSC. Detailed analysis of EMG profiles of the leg extensor muscles during hopping, jumping or running revealed that the reflex contribution (Fig. 17.2) interindividually appears to be fairly consistent with a latency of 30–40 ms after touchdown (i.e. landing on force platforms). Moreover, the muscle-specific latencies increase from the most proximal to the most distal muscles, which can be attributed to variations in the length of the reflex loop. On the basis of averaged EMG profiles, these high peak contributions occur intraindividually with a distinct, but constant time delay, related to the instant of ground contact. Although it is not possible to methodologically separate afferent from efferent activation contributions in natural human movement, it has been argued that these peaks, comparable to the short-latency component (SLC) of the monosynaptic stretch reflex, are functionally important in enhancing the efficacy of the motor output in SSC.

On the basis of the background activity which is provided during the preactivation phase (EMG prior to contact), high stretch reflex activities may be expected after a powerful stretch of the muscle–tendon complex (Greenwood & Hopkins 1976; Dietz *et al.* 1984; Gollhofer & Schmidtbleicher 1989). From basic studies (Nichols 1974, 1987; Hufschmidt & Schwaller 1987) it is known that active stretch reflexes are prerequisite mechanisms for an effective enlargement of the short-range elastic stiffness (SRES), thus linearizing the stress–strain characteristics of the entire muscle–tendon complexes.

From a functional point of view, the concept of strain–strain linearization necessitates that the muscle–tendon complex is strained effectively only within the limits of SRES. Strains beyond this 'critical' range lead to a forceful 'yielding' of the cross-links of the actomyosin complexes, concomitant with a potential loss of energy stored in

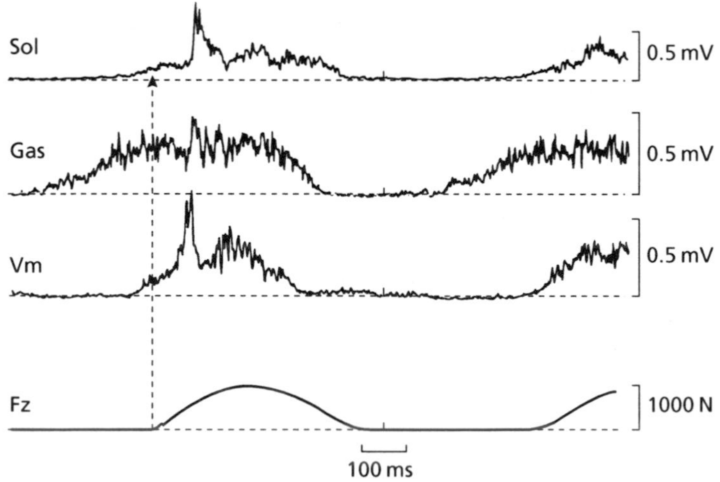

Fig. 17.2 Comparison of the averaged ($n = 12$) EMG profiles of soleus (sol), gastrocnemius (Gas) and vastus medialis (Vm) muscles and vertical ground reaction force. Data are collected from subjects hopping on the spot with one leg.

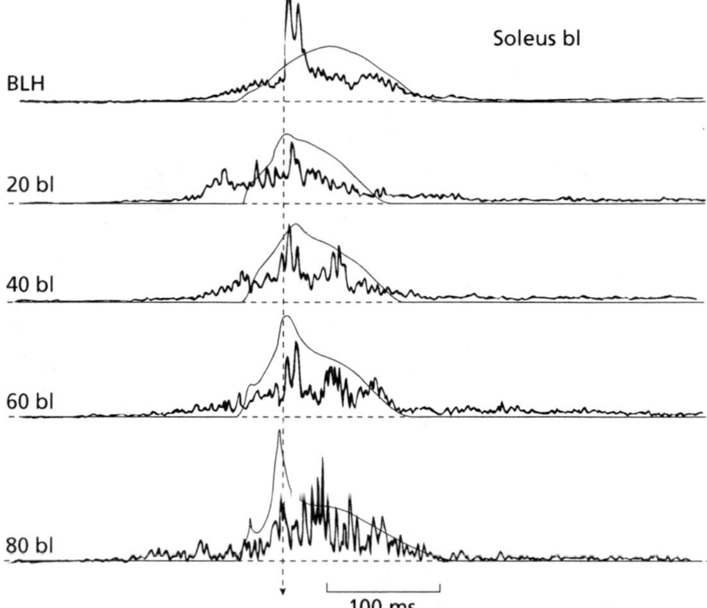

Fig. 17.3 EMG pattern of soleus muscle and vertical ground reaction force in drop jumps with increased stretch load (from top: BLH, both-leg hopping; 20bl–80bl, drop jumps from 20 cm to 80 cm height). The vertical line indicates the first 40 ms after touching the force plates; 40 ms after touch down, basically monosynaptic reflex contribution may be expected.

the lengthened cross-bridges (Flitney & Hirst 1974; Ford *et al.* 1978).

Based on Fig. 17.3, it is noteworthy that stretch-induced reflexes are not necessarily increased if the stretch load, i.e. dropping height, is enlarged. Functionally, it would be most desirable to have activated the high stretch reflexes when the tendomuscular system is mechanically involved. However, the reduced amplitudes of the reflex component observed in drop jumps with high stretch loads suggest diminished reflex facilitation functionally serving as a protection strategy to prevent excessive loading of the tendomuscular complex (for more details the reader is referred to Chapter 10).

In conclusion, the stretch reflex components are likely to contribute to muscle stiffness in reactive movements like stretch–shortening cycles, especially during the eccentric part of the movement.

Proprioceptive training to exercise afferent activation contributions

During rehabilitation of injuries to the locomotor system, proprioceptive training is widely accepted to restore neuromuscular functions. The various receptors in the joint complexes, in the tendons and ligaments, and in the muscular and skin structures are thought to be trained in order to enhance proprioceptive contributions in functional situations. Similarly to the reasoning for reactive movements, proprioceptive training aims to improve the efficacy of the afferent feedback, in order to attain functional limb control and to achieve appropriate neuromuscular access to the muscles encompassing joint complexes. The proprioceptive function of the ankle joint complex was investigated by Konradsen *et al.* (1993) and Tropp (1986). As they compared postural stability of healthy subjects to those with chronic ankle instability. Other approaches have investigated the sensory angular reproduction of different joint dynamics under active or passive conditions (Freeman *et al.* 1965; Glick *et al.* 1976; Tropp 1986; Lövenberg *et al.* 1995). These studies demonstrated a proprioceptive deficit during reproduction of distinct angular dynamics in the case of chronic ankle instability.

Enhancement of proprioceptive-generated muscle activation has been assumed from

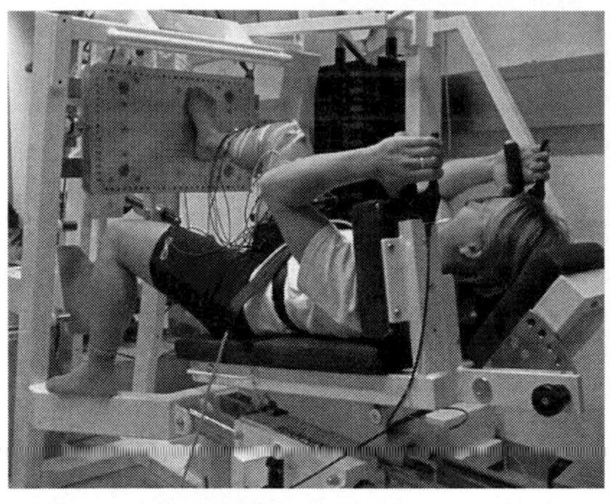

(a)

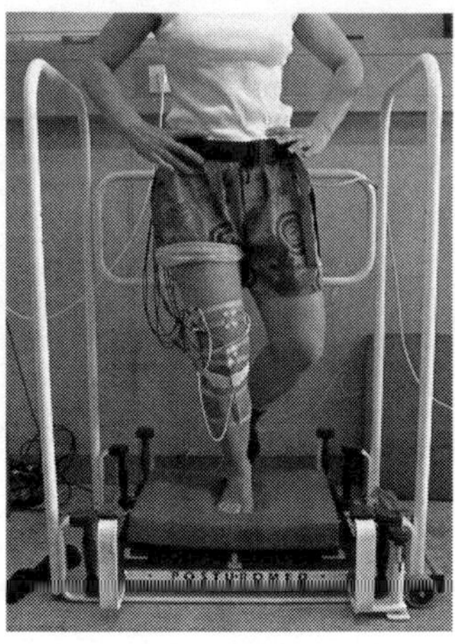

(b)

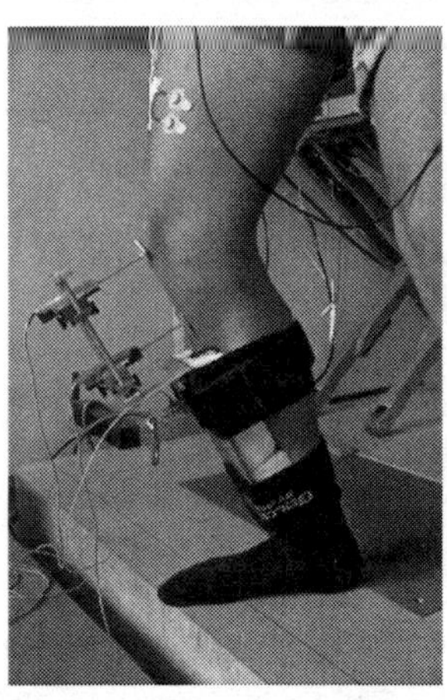

(c)

Fig. 17.4 Experimental conditions. (a) Maximum strength test. Subjects exerted maximal isometric contractions against the force plate. (b) Postural stabilization. Subjects performed postural balance on one leg over a recording period of 40 s. (c) Functional tibia translation. A mechanical stress applied to the tibia produced a short displacement between shank and thigh. By means of linear potentiometers the tibia translation could be determined.

experiments of the knee (Perlau *et al.* 1995) and ankle joint (Jerosch & Bischof 1994). However, only few controlled studies are available that demonstrate at the electromyographical level that proprioceptive training indeed improves the afferent supply in general.

In a series of experiments, Gollhofer (2000) investigated the neuromuscular adaptations following proprioceptive training interventions. Based on longitudinal studies, the author presents experimental data that demonstrate the adaptability of the afferent and efferent contributions.

It was observed that a training designed to improve postural balance over 4 weeks with a frequency of 4 times per week had substantial impact not only on the voluntary activation characteristics, assessed by isometric strength tests (MVC), but also on the proprioceptive activation of the trained muscle groups. Sixty-five volunteers practised postural exercises on unstable platforms, on ankle pads and on uneven surfaces. Classical strength training was not allowed.

Pre- and post measurements comprised (a) force examinations of the leg extension, (b) postural stabilization on a two-dimensional platform (POSTUROMED®) and (c) determination of functional knee joint stiffness (Fig. 17.4). Functional knee joint stiffness was assessed by a specifically designed apparatus that created a mechanical displacement at the tibia relative to

Table 17.1 Pre- and post values, percentage differences and significances of the basic parameters evaluated in the 4-week training programme.

Variable	Pre-	Post-	Difference (Δ %)	Significance ($P < 0.5$)
Maximum strength test				
Rate of force development (RFD, N·m·s^{-1})	7.8	8.5	9	*
Time of RFD (TRFD, ms)	48	44	–8.3	0.21
Postural stabilization				
Postural displacement (m)	1.49	0.72	–48	***
IEMG thigh·displacement (mV·s·m^{-1})	8.5	15.0	76.5	***
IEMG shank·displacement (mV·s·m^{-1})	10.7	15.5	44.9	***
Functional tibia translation				
Tibia translation (mm)	4.6	3.9	–15.2	**
Knee joint stiffness (N·mm^{-1})	37.2	41.8	12.4	0.08
Extensor reflex activity (30–90·ms) (mV·ms)	12.2	9.5	–22.1	***
Flexor reflex activity (30–90·ms) (mV·ms)	5.5	5.1	–7.3	0.53

the thigh. Subjects were in an upright stance and loaded their legs equally. This mechanical stress produced an anterior drawer at the knee joint under functional, i.e. axial-loaded conditions. Quantification of the mechanical parameters of the anterior drawer and determination of the neuronal response allows a comprehensive examination of the functional status of the knee joint complex (Bruhn 1999).

The 4-week training programme produced significant improvements in the maximum rate of force development (RFD) (Table 17.1). Moreover, the absolute times to reach the RFD were reduced. Overall, the subjects could produce their maximum explosive power within shorter time periods after the training. Postural stabilization was drastically reduced, which explains the improved ability of the subjects to control balance. However, calculating the 'proprioception ratio' expressed as the ratio of neuromuscular activity per unit of displacement integrated EMG ((IEMG) activity per displacement), a significant post-training increase could be established both for the thigh as well as for the shank muscles. Biomechanical tests of the tibia translation revealed a significant reduction in the amount of translation and in the overall joint stiffness. Additionally, neuromuscular responses following mechanical translation were enhanced in the post-training examinations.

Our recent data on long-term adaptation to proprioceptive training (Bruhn *et al.* 2001) is in good agreement with the concept that stiffness enhancement of joint complexes after training is basically related to neuromuscular adaptations. The often observed adaptations in isometric, voluntary activations may indicate the improved neuromuscular function through enhanced muscular power.

Active dynamic joint stabilization: a reflex controlled strategy of high-frequency intermuscular coordination

There is an extensive debate in the literature as to whether neuromuscular parameter explains the dysfunction in joint instability. On the one side, the determination of reflex latencies following mechanical perturbation is often used to separate between stable and unstable joint systems. In 1992, Karlsson and Andreasson (1992) observed significantly prolonged reflex latencies in the peroneal muscles of subjects with unilateral instability on the affected side, following a 30° inversion tilt movement. On the other side, several studies report enhanced reflex activation, determined as the integrated EMG activity following a well-defined perturbation in subjects with and without joint protection systems (Lohrer *et al.* 1999). Consistent with the responses

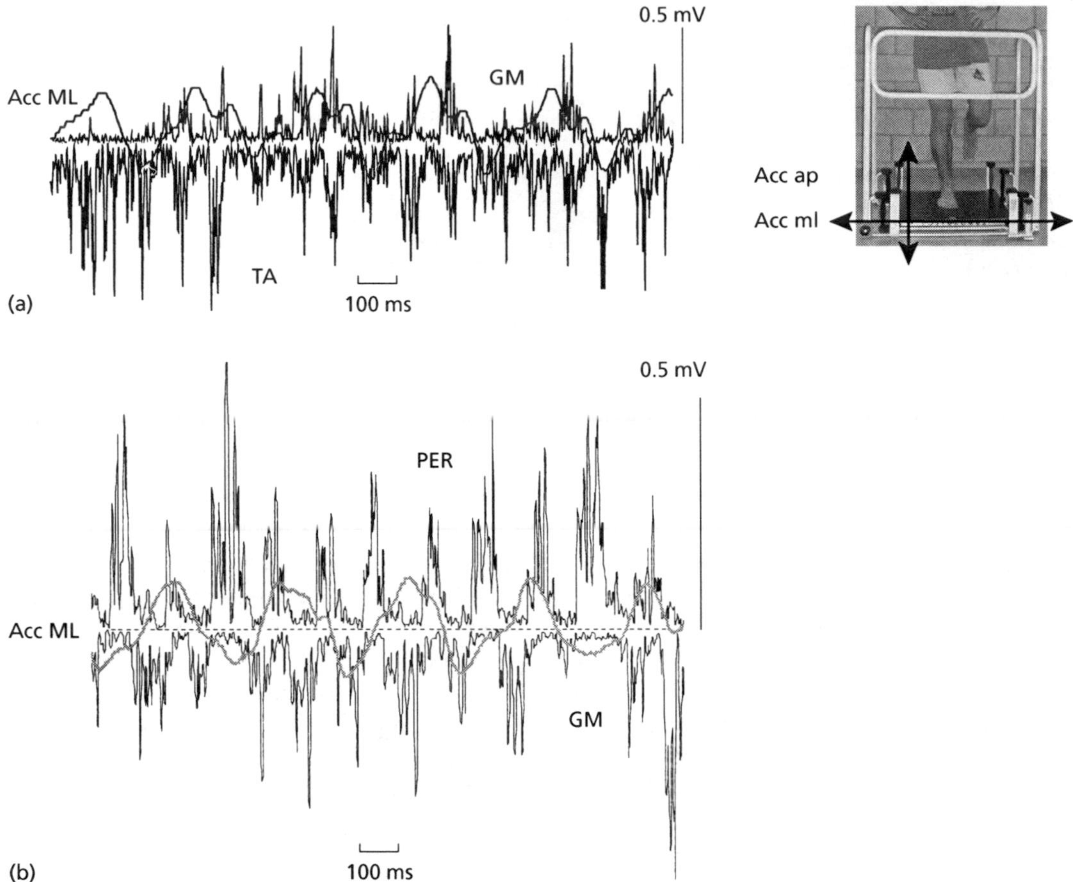

Fig. 17.5 (a) Rectified EMG patterns of gastrocnemius (GM) (up) and tibialis anterior (TA) (down) muscles and acceleration trace in mediolateral (accML) direction during postural stabilization on a two-dimensional unstable platform. The EMG patterns are obviously synchronized on the basis of an interburst frequency of 8 Hz. (b) Rectified EMG patterns of peroneus (PER) and gastrocnemius (GA) (down) muscles and acceleration trace in mediolateral (accML) direction during postural stabilization on a two-dimensional unstable platform. The EMG patterns show an antagonistic activation pattern on the basis of an interburst frequency of 8 Hz.

observed in posture, the reflex latencies of the peroneal muscles are within 60 and 90 ms after mechanical stimulus. There is general agreement that these responses are polysynaptic (Johnson & Johnson 1993; Konradsen *et al.* 1993; Scheuffelen *et al.* 1993). From a functional point of view, prolonged reflex latencies may basically explain that in very fast displacements the reflexive systems may contribute too late to active joint stabilization in very fast displacements. From a physiological point of view, the enhanced reflex latencies in the patients may be ascribed to the failure of the fastest responding structures in the reflex arc. These pathways, however, may not necessarily be the most important ones for an effective joint stabilization function. Thus, reliance on determination of reflex latencies may not cover all aspects of functional joint disposition.

Scheuffelen *et al.* (1993) demonstrated that in situations when large mechanical amplitudes are applied to the ankle joint system, it is functionally most important to have an early and powerful access to the musculature encompassing the stimulated joint. The muscles need to be supplied with an adequate amount of neuromuscular activity, in order to resist the mechanical perturbation and to stiffen the joint complex to avoid ruptures of ligamentous or capsular structures. Consequently, proprioceptive training programmes are employed in rehabilitation to 'teach' the agonist and antagonist muscles to stabilize a joint complex actively.

In order to verify this hypothesis, Gollhofer *et al.* (2000) investigated in a thorough electrophysiological analysis the EMG profiles of dynamic stabilization control. As an illustration, the EMG patterns of one subject are depicted in Fig. 17.5(a,b). Obviously, the dynamic task of postural stabilization requires fast regulation in the activation of the muscles involved. This control is achieved partly by fast neuronal interactions between agonist and antagonist activation with high intermuscular frequency. The pattern of this 'neuronal communication' consists of phasic bursts interacting with a frequency of up to 8.2 Hz. Due to the phasic type of neuronal activation and to the high frequency, it is most likely that these bursts are not organized by central programmes but by spinal circuits processing afferent, proprioceptive feedback onto the α motoneurone system.

Functional role of proprioceptive input on isometric force development

From single motor unit recordings (Macefield *et al.* 1991), it is well known that in isometric conditions the discharge rate is reduced when the afferent contributions are cut off (Fig. 17.6). Based on data from seven motor units, the discharge rate is even more affected by an isometric fatigue contraction over 30 s. On the basis of frequency analysis, the authors concluded that intact afferentation provides for adequate fusimotor drive, thus enhancing the sensitivity of the muscle spindle system. Higher discharge frequencies, however, are responsible for faster rates of force development of the motoneurone (Desmedt & Godaux 1977; Grimby *et al.* 1981). Based on H-reflex data obtained during ramp contraction, several observations favour the

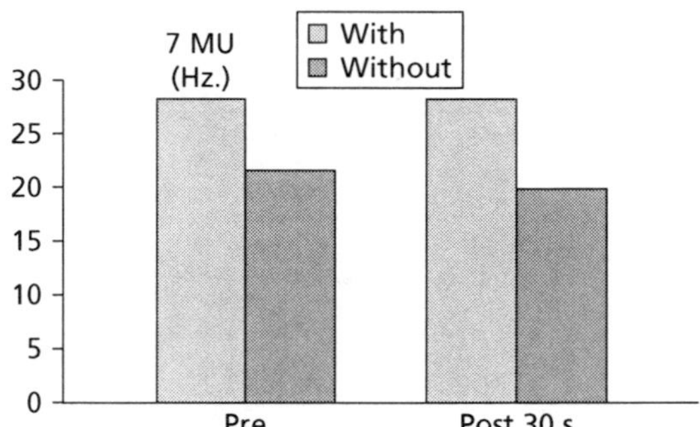

Fig. 17.6 Discharge rate before and after a 30-s contraction of seven motor units. The bars indicate the discharge frequencies with and without afferent feedback. (Modified from Macefield *et al.* 1991.)

hypothesis that afferent reflex contribution also has a gating effect on isometric strength development (Meunier & Pierrot-Deseilligny 1989). The authors compared the extrafascilitatory drive to the motoneurones during ramp-and-hold contractions under different ramp velocities and under various levels of voluntary contraction (MVC) (Fig. 17.7). The data show that the supplementary facilitation of the motoneurone pool is optimal in the early phase of typically fast ramp velocities performed with high MVC percentages. The authors interpret their findings with a tonic presynaptic inhibition on the Ia terminals, basically under centrally programmed control.

In proprioceptive adaptation studies, it is often observed that training-induced, proprioceptive gains in monosynaptic reflex behaviour is correlated with the improvements in the rise of force development: Subjects who performed in a 4-week training programme designed for proprioceptive joint stabilization enhanced their capability for explosive strength significantly compared to subjects who exercised pure isometric and concentric muscular performances (Gollhofer *et al.* 1997). The improvements in muscle activation and in force development within the first 100 ms after activation onset were in line with the adaptations in the monosynaptic stretch reflex sensitivity (Fig. 17.8).

The mechanical importance of these proprioceptive gains seems to reflect the enhanced

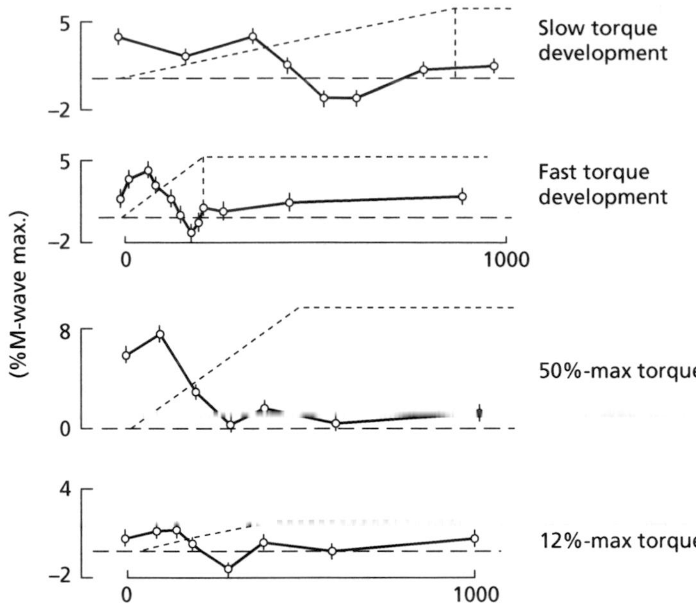

Fig. 17.7 Supplementary facilitation expressed as percentages of the maximum M-wave in four different ramp contraction tasks. (Modified from Meunier & Pierrot-Designy 1989.)

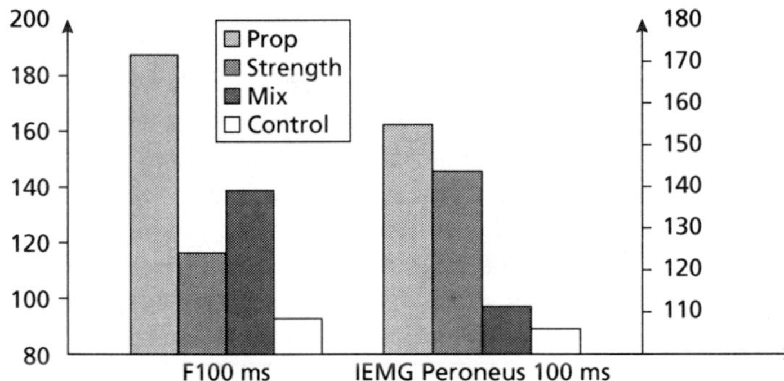

Fig. 17.8 Functional adaptation following a differentially designed training regimen (averages (prevalues = 100%)). The bars indicate the improvements of four different groups exercising either with proprioceptive (Prop), isometric (Strength), combined (Mix (Prop + Strength)) training loads. Control group (Control) was not involved in the training process.

ability of the neuromuscular system to activate the muscles more efficiently at the onset of force development. Functionally, this may be important in order to stiffen joint complexes in disturbance conditions. This control is achieved by fast neuronal interactions between agonist and antagonist activation with high intermuscular frequency (see Fig. 17.5a,b). The pattern of this neuronal communication consists of phasic bursts interacting with high frequencies.

Based on these high frequencies and on the highly specific intermuscular coordination, it is most likely that the neuromuscular activation observed in joint stabilization tasks is generated by reflex activation, controlled at the spinal level. Central or even supraspinal generators are rather unlikely, as the frequency of the observed intermuscular pattern is too high to assume regulation via central pathways. Therefore, the control mechanisms are assumed to be on the spinal level.

Conclusion

The mechanical importance of enhanced afferent gains in the neuromuscular control seems to reflect the changed ability of the neuromuscular system to activate the muscles more efficiently at the onset of force development. Especially in disturbance conditions, quicker access to the muscles may be of vital importance to stiffen joint complexes. Not only in rehabilitation, but to an even greater extent in athletic training like in alpine skiing, proprioceptive training programmes may be an efficient tool to improve the agonist/antagonist intermuscular communication. Furthermore, it may have functional importance in all sport disciplines with explosive power demands.

From a physiological point of view, muscle spindle afferents are not simply stereotyped responses to unexpected stretches. Embedded in the neuromuscular pattern they provide high stiffness in the tendomuscular system, not only in the SSC. Moreover, they are highly efficient in the isometric force development.

References

Bruhn, S. (1999) *Funktionelle Stabilität am Kniegelenk.* Dissertation, University of Stuttgart.

Bruhn, S., Gollhofer, A. & Gruber, M. (2001) Sensorimotor training for prevention and rehabilitation of knee joint injuries. *European Journal of Sport Traumatology* **23**(2). Editrice Kurtis, Milano.

Desmedt, J.E. & Godaux, E. (1977) Fast motor units are not preferentially activated in rapid voluntary contractions in man. *Nature* **267**, 717–719.

Dietz, V., Quintern, J. & Berger, W. (1984) Corrective reactions to stumbling in man. Functional significance of spinal and transcortical reflexes. *Neuroscience Letters* **44**, 131–135.

Dietz, V., Gollhofer, A., Kleiber, M. & Trippel, M. (1992) Regulation of bipedal stance: dependency on 'load' receptors. *Experimental Brain Research* **89**, 229–231.

Duchateau, J., Van Cutsem, M. & Hainaut, K. (1999) Mechanisms underlying neural adaptions following dynamic training. In: *Sport Science 1999 in Europe. Proceedings of the 4th ECSS Congress* (eds P. Parisi, F. Pigozzi & G. Prinzi), p. 182. Rome University of Motor Sciences, Rome.

Duysens, J., Clarac, F. & Cruse, H. (2000) Load-regulating mechanisms in gait and posture. Comparative aspects. *Physiological Reviews* **80**(1), 83–133.

Eliasson, A.C., Forssberg, H., Ikuta, K., Apel, K., Westling, G. & Johannsson, R. (1995) Development of human precision grip. V. Anticipatory and triggered grip actions during sudden loading. *Experimental Brain Research* **106**, 425–433.

Flitney, F.W. & Hirst, D.G. (1974) Cross-bridge detachment and sacromere 'give' during stretch of active frog's muscle. *Journal of Physiology* **276**, 449–465.

Ford, L.E., Huxley, A.F. & Simmons, R.M. (1978) Tension responses to sudden length change in stimulated frog muscle fibres near slack length. *Journal of Physiology* **269**, 441–515.

Freeman, M., Dean, M. & Hanham, I. (1965) The etiology and prevention of functional instability of the foot. *Journal of Bone and Joint Surgery* **47B**, 678–685.

Glick, J.M., Gordon, R.B. & Nishimoto, D. (1976) The prevention and treatment of ankle injuries. *American Journal of Sports Medicine* **4**(4), 136–141.

Gollhofer, A. (2000) Importance of proprioceptive activation on functional neuromuscular properties. In: *Proceedings of the XVIII Symposium on Biomechanics in Sports* (eds Y. Hong & D.P. Johns), pp. 117–125. Department of Sport Science and Physical Education, University of Hong Kong, Hong Kong.

Gollhofer, A. & Schmidtbleicher, D. (1989) Stretch reflex responses of the human m. triceps surae following mechanical stimulation. *Journal of Biomechanics* **22**, 1016.

Gollhofer, A., Komi, P.V., Fujitsuka, N. & Miyashita, M. (1987) Fatigue during stretch–shortening cycle exercises. II. Changes in neuromuscular activation patterns of human skeletal muscle. *International Journal of Sports Medicine* **8**, 38–41.

Gollhofer, A., Horstmann, G.A., Berger, W. & Dietz, V. (1989) Compensation of transitional and rotational perturbations in human posture: stabilization of the centre of gravity. *Neuroscience Letters* **105**, 73–78.

Gollhofer, A., Scheuffelen, C. & Lohrer, H. (1997) Neuromuskuläre Trainingsformen und ihre funktionelle Auswirkung auf die Stabilisierung im Sprunggelenk. *Novartis 7* (eds L. Zichner, M. Engelhardt & J. Freiwald), pp. 109–122. Maurer Verlag, Geislingen, Germany.

Gollhofer, A., Lohrer, H. & Alt, W. (2000) Propriozeption—grundlegende Überlegungen zur sensorimotorischen Steuerung. *Orthopädieschuhtechnik—Sonderheft Propriozeption*, 10–14.

Greenwood, R. & Hopkins, A. (1976) Landing from an unexpected fall and a voluntary step. *Brain Research* **99**, 375–386.

Grimby, L., Hannerz, J. & Hedman, B. (1981) The fatigue and voluntary discharge properties of single motor units in man. *Journal of Physiology (London)* **316**, 545–554.

Gruber, M., Bruhn, S. & Gollhofer, A. (2000) Training induced adaptations of functional stability of the knee joint. In: *Proceedings of 5th Annual Congress of the European College of Sport Science* (eds J. Avela, P.V. Komi & J. Komulainen). Department of Biology of Physical Activity and LIKES Research Centre, Jyväskylä, Finland, p. 296.

Häkkinen, K. & Komi, P.V. (1986) Training-induced changes in neuromuscular performance under voluntary and reflex conditions. *European Journal of Applied Physiology* **55**, 147–155.

Hoffer, J.A. & Andreassen, S. (1981) Regulation of soleus muscle stiffness in premammillary cats: intrinsic and reflex components. *Journal of Neurophysiology* **45**, 267–285.

Hufschmidt, A. & Schwaller, I. (1987) Short-range elasticity and resting tension of relaxed human lower leg muscles. *Journal of Physiology* **393**, 451–465.

Jerosch, J. & Bischof, M. (1994) Der Einfluß der Propriozeptivität auf die funktionelle Stabilität des oberen Sprunggelenkes unter besonderer Berücksichtigung von Stabilisierungshilfen. *Sportverletzung Sportschaden* **8**, 111–121.

Johansson, R.S. & Westling, G. (1984) Roles of glabrous skin receptors and sensimotor memory in automatic control of precision grip when lifting rougher or more slippery objects. *Experimental Brain Research* **56**, 550–564.

Johansson, R.S. & Westling, G. (1987) Signals in tactile afferents from the fingers eliciting adaptive motor responses during precision grip. *Experimental Brain Research* **66**, 141–154.

Johnson, M.B. & Johnson, C.L. (1993) Electromyographic response of peroneal muscles in surgical and nonsurgical injured ankles during sudden inversion. *Journal of Orthopaedic and Sports Physical Therapy* **18**(3), 497–501.

Karlsson, J. & Andeasson, G.O. (1992) The effect of external ankle support in chronic lateral ankle joint stability. An electromyographic study. *American Journal of Sports Medicine* **20**(3), 257–261.

Komi, P.V. (1984) Physiological and biomechanical correlates of muscle function: effects of muscle structure and stretch–shortening cycle on force and speed. *Exercise and Sport Sciences Reviews* **12**, 81–121.

Konradsen, L., Ravn, J.B. & Sorensen, A.I. (1993) Proprioception at the ankle: the effect of anaesthetic blockade of ligament receptors. *Journal of Bone and Joint Surgery (Brit)* **75-B**, 433–436.

Lephart, S.M., Riemann, B.L. & Fu, F.H. (2000) Introduction to sensorimotor system. In: *Proprioception and Neuromuscular Control in Joint Stability Human Kinetics* (eds S. M. Lephart & F. H. Fu), pp. 1–5.

Lohrer, H., Alt, W. & Gollhofer, A. (1999) Neuromuscular properties and functional aspects of taped ankles. *American Journal of Sports Medicine* **27**(1), 69–75.

Lövenberg, R., Kärrholm, J., Sundelin, G. & Ahlgren, O. (1995) Prolonged reaction time in patients with chronic lateral instability of the ankle. *American Journal of Sports Medicine* **23**(4), 414–417.

MacDougall, J.D. (1986) Morphological changes in human skeletal muscle following strength training and immobilization. In: *Human Kinetics* (eds N. L. Jones, N. McCartney & A. J. McComas), pp. 269–288. Champaign, IL.

MacDougall, J.D., Sale, D.G., Moroz, J.R., Elder, G., Sutton, J.R. & Howald, H. (1979) Mitochondrial volume density in human skeletal muscle following heavy resistance training. *Medicine and Science in Sports and Exercise* **11**(2), 164–166.

Macefield, G., Gandevia, S.C., Gorman, R., Bigland-Ritchie, B. & Burke, D. (1991) The discharge rate of human motoneurons innervating ankle dorsiflexors in the absence of afferent feedback. *Journal of Physiology* **438**, 219P.

Meunier, S. & Pierrot-Deseilligny, E. (1989) Gating of the afferent volley of the monosynaptic stretch reflex during movement in man. *Journal of Physiology* **419**, 753–763.

Nichols, T.R. (1974) *Soleus muscle stiffness and its reflex control*. Unpublished doctoral dissertation, Harvard University, Cambridge, MA.

Nichols, T.R. (1987) The regulation of muscle stiffness. *Medicine and Science in Sports and Exercise* **26**, 36–47.

Perlau, R., Frank, C. & Fick, G. (1995) The effect of elastic bandages on human knee proprioception in the uninjured population. *American Journal of Sports Medicine* **23**(2), 251–255.

Prochazka, A. (1996) Proprioceptive feedback and movement regulation. In: *Handbook of Physiology. Exercise: Regulation and Integration of Multiple Systems* (eds L.B. Rowell & J.T. Shepherd), 12(3), pp. 89–127. American Physiological Society, Bethesda, MD.

Sale, D.G. (1992) Neural adaptation to strength training. In: *Strength and Power in Sport* (ed. P. V. Komi), pp. 249–265. Blackwell Scientific Publications, Oxford.

Scheuffelen, Ch, Rapp, W., Gollhofer, A. & Lohrer, H. (1993) Orthotic devices in functional treatment of ankle sprain. *International Journal of Sports Medicine* **14**, 1–9.

Tesch, P.A. (1987) Acute and long term metabolic changes consequent to heavy-resistance training. *Medicine and Sport Science* **26**, 67–89.

Tropp, H. (1986) Pronator muscle weakness in functional instability of the ankle joint. *International Journal of Sports Medicine* **7**, 291–294.

Vallbo, A.B. (1981) Basic patterns of muscle spindle discharge in man. In: *Muscle Receptors and Movement. Proceedings of a Symposium* (eds A. Taylor & A. Prochazka), pp. 263–275. MacMillan, London.

Vallbo, A.B. & Al-Falahe, N.A. (1990) Human muscle spindle response in a motor learning task. *Journal of Physiology (London)* **421**, 553–568.

Winter, D.A. (1996) *Anatomy, Biomechanics and Control of Balance during Standing and Walking*. Waterloo Biomechanics. Waterloo, Ontario, Canada.

Chapter 18

Connective Tissue and Bone Response to Strength Training

MICHAEL H. STONE AND CHRISTINA KARATZAFERI

Introduction

Structurally connective tissue provides our basic framework and supportive structure. Connective tissue also forms the structural foundation of our force-conveying network. Therefore, alterations in connective tissue size and strength resulting from disuse or from chronic exercise can have profound effects on both health and performance capabilities.

Strength training has become a vital part of training programmes, which have varied goals including enhanced physical performance, prevention of injuries, improved general fitness, increased muscle size and use in rehabilitation programmes (Stone & Wilson 1985; Stone 1990; Stone *et al.* 2000). Considering the uses of strength training and its well-documented effects on muscle it is reasonable to believe that strength training can have marked effects on connective tissue. Although a relatively large amount of data is available on the effects of endurance training or passive stretch on connective tissue, less is known about the effects of strength training. It has only been in the last 10–12 years that substantial data have become available as to the effects of strength training on connective tissue.

This chapter deals with the potential effects of strength training on connective tissue. Inferences will be made from studies of endurance training and passive stretch, and implications from strength training studies will be considered.

Anatomical and biochemical characteristics

Connective tissue is made up of collagen, elastin or reticular cells, and fibres. These cells and fibres are embedded in a ground substance containing tissue fluid and various metabolites. The ground substance contains relatively large amounts of aminopolysaccharides or glycoproteins giving it a gelatinous characteristic. Collagen is the major fibre in all types of connective tissue, comprising about 30% of total body protein (Van Pilsum 1982; Viiduk 1986).

Collagen molecules consist of three chains each in a left-handed helix of approximately 100 residues. These three chains are wound around each other in a right-handed helix with glycine residues at crossing points occurring at every third residue. The approximate formula is X-Y-Gly. Most of the amino acid residues are glycine (33%); hydroxyproline makes up about 15% and proline 12%. Collagen molecules form fibrils that are staggered in a parallel manner and range from 10 to 200 nm depending upon the type of collagen. Each molecule is displaced from adjacent molecules by 0, 1, 2, 3 or 4 axial stagger lengths of 234 ± 1 residues (Schultz 1982). The staggered nature of collagen molecules results in banding with electron microscopy (Fig. 18.1).

The cyclic nature of the amino acid residues (X-Y-Gly) results in increased stability by limiting rotation. Additional amino acids may act as hydrophobically charged clusters and occupy

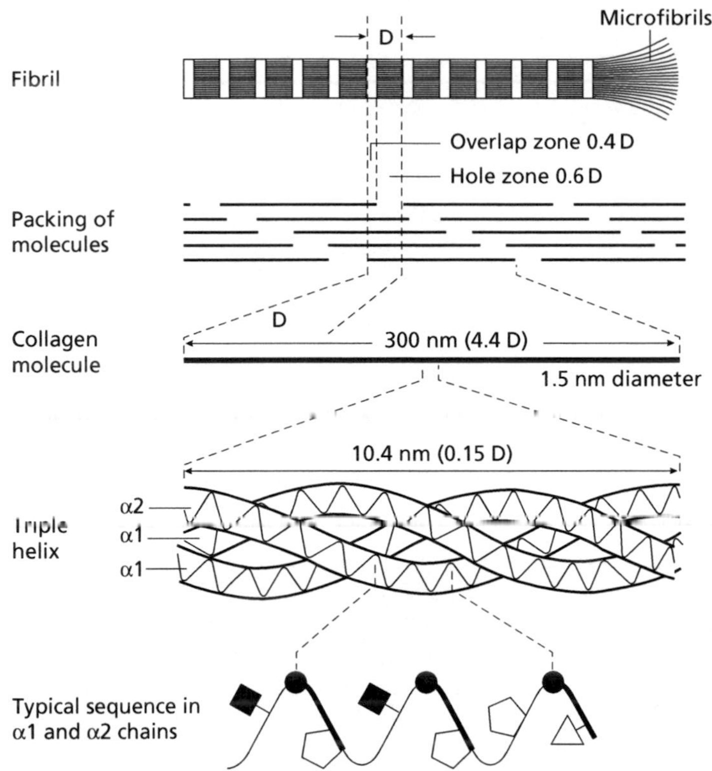

Fig. 18.1 Structure of collagen.

Table 18.1 Primary collagen types.

Type	Distribution	Form	Characteristics
I	Bone, tendon, skin, dentine, ligament, fascia, arteries, uterus	$[a1(I)]_2a2$	Hybrid composed of two chains low in hydroxylysine and glycosylated hydroxylysine
II	Cartilage	$[a1(II)]_3$	High in hydroxylysine
III	Skin, arteries, uterus	$[a1(III)]_3$	High in hydroxylysine, low in hydroxylysine disulphide bonds
IV	Basement membrane	$[a1(IV)]_3$	Large globular regions, high in hydroxylysine, glycosylated hydroxylysine
V	Basement membrane, lens capsule	aA and aB	Similar to IV

the X or Y positions. Specific genes code for the basic structure of collagen chains (Schultz 1982). At least five different types of collagen exist, with different organ distribution (Table 18.1).

Additional stabilization can be achieved by post-translational cross-linking. Cross-links are formed by the oxidation of lysyl side chains to aldehydes and eventual formation of aldol bridges between collagen fibrils (Viidik 1968). Cross-linking increases with age, leading to increased stability and tensile strength (Viidik 1968). This can be considered at least partially responsible for the observed differences in tendon elastic properties *in vivo* with ageing (Shadwick 1990; Kubo *et al.* 2001a). Moreover, total collagen concentration in skeletal muscle is higher in old animals as a result of a decreased rate of degradation. Endurance training has been shown to lower skeletal muscle passive stiffness of old rats by reducing the concentration of mature collagen cross-links (Gosselin *et al.* 1998).

Mechanical properties of connective tissue

The composition and design of collagenous tissues (e.g. tendon, cartilage, human heel pad) is varied according to the function they are to fulfil. Different designs lead to different material properties. In addition, within a type of tissue, for example tendon, the 'fatigue quality' is adjusted to suit its 'stress in life' (Ker 1999).

The development of stress–strain curves has been a valuable tool in studying the mechanical properties of connective tissue. The stress–strain curve can be developed from a load–deformation curve where load is expressed as units of cross-sectional area and deformation is expressed as units of original length (Viiduk 1986). Typically, the point of failure (σ_{max}) or the energy absorbed to the point of failure has been an important variable in comparing tissue strength (Fig. 18.2).

Stress–strain curves can be either passive or active. For example, ligament or tendon strength can be examined passively by simple stretching to failure. Active stress–strain curves can be accomplished using muscle–tendon preparations where the muscle is electrically stimulated at the appropriate time (Garret *et al.* 1987).

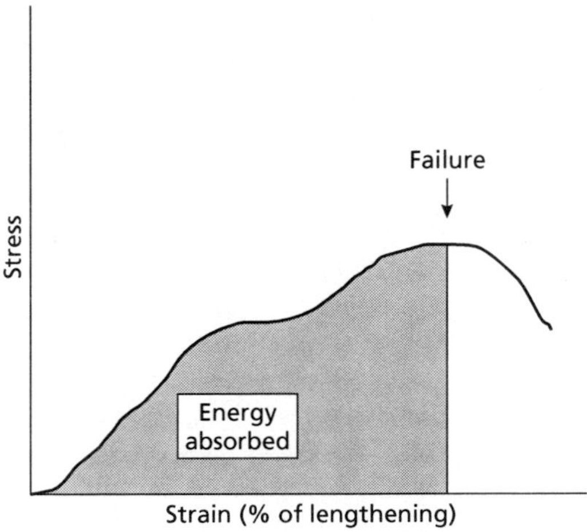

Fig. 18.2 Stress–strain curve for connective tissue.

In the past tendon (and ligament) mechanical properties were largely studied using isolated tissue preparations; recently the use of real-time ultrasonography has allowed for *in vivo* investigations of some of the mechanical properties of human tendon structures (e.g. Maganaris & Paul 1999). These *in vivo* studies indicate that the mechanical properties of intact tendons are similar to those of the isolated preparations.

Effects of physical training on connective tissue

Large amounts of connective tissue exist around and within muscle including the epimysium, perimysium, endomysium (mainly type I and III collagens) and basement membrane of muscle cells (mainly type IV, V and the newly described XV collagens). Connective tissue also makes up tendons and ligaments. This connective tissue is responsible for conveying force from the muscle to the bone lever system and for maintaining the structural form of the muscle organ. Adaptations of connective tissue to exercise and training can include a variety of morphological and biochemical changes.

Biochemical alterations

Exercise, particularly high-force eccentric exercise, places considerable stress on muscle and on connective tissue. Eccentric exercise, which produces delayed muscle soreness, has been associated with increased serum concentrations of hydroxyproline (Abraham 1977). Forced elongation of rat muscle caused considerable structural damage as well as an infiltration of lymphoid cells. Within 5 days proteoglycan localization was apparent, suggesting regeneration of damaged connective tissue (Fritz & Stauber 1988; Stauber *et al.* 1988). Repetitive force production, particularly that associated with stretch–shortening cycles, even at relatively low force levels can also result in markers of damage and regeneration.

For example, prolonged endurance exercise (24-h run) resulted in increased serum concentrations of enzymes associated with synthesis of type III collagen (Takala *et al.* 1976).

Most of the training studies which have been concerned with the effects of training on tendons and ligaments have used endurance exercise and animal models. Endurance training produced increased nuclei number and tendon weights in young mice but no change in tendon weight of adult mice (Ingelmark 1948). Ligament weights have shown increases in male but not in female adult rats (Tipton *et al.* 1975b). Endurance training can also increase the aerobic enzyme activity and rate of collagen synthesis in animal tendons (Tipton *et al.* 1974). Eight weeks of endurance training increased the collagen content (46%) of immature rooster Achilles tendons, but did not affect DNA, dry tendon weight or proteoglycan concentration (Curwin *et al.* 1988). Additionally, fewer (50%) pyridinoline cross-links were present in the trained tendons compared to controls. These results suggest that the training caused a greater matrix–collagen turnover in growing roosters, resulting in reduced maturation of tendon collagen (Curwin *et al.* 1988), and thus reduced stiffness. Hydroxyproline is found as a constant fraction of collagen (Van Pilsum 1982). Because hydroxyproline is found in few other tissues (elastin and complement) which are not associated with tendons or ligaments, its measurement may reflect changes in the collagen content of connective tissue (Viiduk 1986). Hydroxyproline concentration was unchanged in the tendons of young mice (Kiiskinen & Heikkinen 1976) or the ligaments of adult rats (Tipton *et al.* 1970) but was increased in adult dogs (Tipton *et al.* 1975a). Training-induced changes in hydroxyproline concentration should be viewed with caution. Apparent changes in hydroxyproline may be a result of actual hydroxyproline loss or gain within the connective tissue, or it could represent changes (loss or gain) in other tissue components. Therefore, changes in hydroxyproline concentration would represent changes in tissue state but not necessarily the nature of the change (Viiduk 1986). In a study where both passive stiffness and hydroxyproline levels were measured in young and old male rats, 10 weeks of endurance training appeared to attenuate the age-associated increase in passive muscle stiffness (Gosselin *et al.* 1998). This may have implications for the reduction of exercise-induced injuries of ageing muscle, especially during lengthening contractions. Interestingly, static stretching appeared to acutely increase elasticity in medial gastrocnemius human tendon structures (Kubo *et al.* 2001b), which could further contribute to the reduction of connective tissue injury.

Another marker of collagen biosynthesis is the activities of prolyl-4-hydroxylase (PH) and galactosyl-hydroxylsyl glucosyltransferase (GGT), enzymes that catalyse modifications in the collagen polypeptide chains. Endurance training increased PH and GGT activities, indicating an increased collagen synthesis. In streptozotocin-induced diabetes, total PH and GGT activities were reduced and hydroxyproline levels increased in rat vastus lateralis, rectus femoris and gastrocnemius muscle. However, physical training was unable to attenuate the effects of diabetes on collagen synthesis (Han *et al.* 1995).

Compensatory hypertrophy models or chronic stretch do not reflect the same chronic adaptations as resistive training. Differential effects on connective tissue are possible because of differences in the exercise intensity between endurance training and compensatory hypertrophy models of training or chronic stretch. Muscle connective tissue sheaths (epimysium, perimysium, endomysium) are a primary component accounting for muscle tensile strength, the viscoelastic properties of muscle, and the framework for conveying muscle force to the tendons and bone (Fleck & Falkel 1986). Endurance training is associated with increased prolyl-4-hydroxylase activity in skeletal muscle but did not increase total collagen content, suggesting a higher turnover rate (Kovanen *et al.* 1980, 1984; Kovanen & Suominen 1989). However, compensatory rat plantaris hypertrophy (Turto *et al.* 1974) did show increased collagen content as did loading the intact chicken wing (Laurent *et al.* 1978).

Eccentric muscle actions can be an integral part of heavy-resistance training and of explosive sports. A single bout of physical exercise resulting in muscle damage caused an acute increase in prolyl-4-hydroxylation capacity of mice hindlimb muscles (Myllylä *et al.* 1986). These data suggest that strength training may damage connective tissue as well as muscle and that this tissue damage may be important in regeneration (see Chapter 6).

MacDougall *et al.* (1984) estimated the total collagen and other non-contractile protein content of biceps among untrained subjects and two groups of bodybuilders. The proportion of collagen was similar in untrained, novice and elite groups, with collagen representing 69% and 7% being identified as other components. This finding indicates a stable relative collagen content but an increased total collagen content as a result of body building. The increased total collagen content likely represents an increase in muscle sheath strength.

The possibility of a general systemic response of connective tissue is supported by several observations in both animals and humans. Hydroxyproline concentration increased in the skin of immature and adult mice as a result of endurance training (Kiiskinen & Heikkinen 1976; Suominen *et al.* 1978). Skin elasticity was observed to be enhanced following 8 weeks of physical training in 69-year-old men and women (Suominen *et al.* 1977, 1978). Strength training has been shown to stimulate endomysial connective tissue in young men (Brzank & Peiper 1986).

Mechanical alterations

While disuse and inactivity cause atrophy and weakening of connective tissue, physical training can increase maximum tensile strength and the amount of energy absorbed before failure (Stone 1988). Physical activity returns damaged tendons and ligaments to normal tensile strength values faster than complete rest (Tipton *et al.* 1975b). Endurance training causes increased maximum tensile strength in isolated tendons, and in bone–tendon and bone–ligament preparations (Elliot & Crawford 1965; Viiduk 1968; Tipton *et al.* 1974).

Care must be taken in interpreting much of the animal data on connective tissue strength. Trained animals are typically compared to untrained caged animals. Confinement may reduce connective tissue size and maximum tensile strength; therefore, training may simply return tissue properties to unconfined values (Butler *et al.* 1978; Stone 1988). Additionally, the strain rates used in these studies were below normal physiological rates, making generalizations back to intact unconfined animals difficult (Butler *et al.* 1978).

The flexor muscles of most adult animals produce higher maximum force outputs than the extensor muscles (Elliot & Crawford 1965). Flexor tendons of adult pigs have a greater maximum tensile strength and contain more collagen than tendons from extensor muscles, and can store more elastic energy (Woo *et al.* 1982; Shadwick 1990). Developmentally, this suggests that the forces encountered by these tendons at least partially influence the collagen content and maximum tensile strength at maturation. After physical training, extensor muscle tendons increased collagen content and stiffness, reaching values similar to the flexor tendons (Woo *et al.* 1982). This suggests that strengthening of muscle may affect gains in connective tissue maximum tensile strength and elastic energy storage capabilities.

The stress placed on tendons as a result of voluntary muscle contraction has been estimated to be 30% of the maximum tensile strength (Hirsch 1974). This leaves a 200% safety margin. During normal intact functioning in which both concentric and eccentric actions occur, about 50% of the safety margin is used (Alexander 1981). The safety margin may be increased during fast rates of loading as a result of locking the viscous components of tissue (Noyes 1977). The nature of tissue failure is also a function of strain rate (Noyes 1977). At very slow strain rates, failure occurs at the junction of bone–tendon or bone–ligament. At faster strain rates, failure occurs at the tendon or ligament. If the junction fails, the tendon or ligament is not being tested. When muscle–tendon preparations are being tested, failure occurs at the belly of the muscle or most often at the muscle–tendon junction, regardless of strain rates (Garret *et al.* 1987; Safran *et al.* 1988).

Connective tissue subjected to a constant stress elongates with time (stress–relaxation), resulting in a fall in tension below initial values (Laban 1962). Similar phenomena occur in muscle–tendon preparations (Safran *et al.* 1988). Warm-up afforded by isometric action prior to stretching (at physiological strain rates) elongated the muscle–tendon unit to a greater length and required more force at failure than muscles not warmed up (Safran *et al.* 1988). The warm-up stretches the muscle–tendon unit resulting in an increased length at a given load; this places less tension on the muscle–tendon junction and reduces injury potential. Similar increases in stress relaxation have been shown to occur in rabbit tendons as a result of exercise (Viiduk 1968). Essentially, the safety margin is increased by warm-up. However, in 'real life' situations the use of stretching as part of a warm-up procedure may result in a trade-off. While stretching may reduce injuries it may also hinder performance in strength or power performances by reducing compliance or altering muscle stiffness or through a neural inhibitory pathway (Folwes *et al.* 2000; Schilling & Stone 2000).

Sprint training mainly consists of sprint running and resistance training and will probably affect viscoelastic tendon properties. It has been reported that compliance of the tendon structures of the vastus lateralis (VL) can have a direct relationship to 100-m running time (Kubo *et al.* 2000). However, in that study no significant differences in compliance of the VL and medial gastrocnemius were found between sprinters and controls. The authors also suggested that a greater elasticity (longer elongation) of the VL tendon structures among the sprinters could act as a protective adaptation against injury.

Muscle force may also be important in extending the safety margin before failure of the muscle–tendon junction. A greater force at failure and a greater absorbance of energy before failure of the muscle–tendon junction (MTJ) results from both tetanic and wave-summated muscle action in various rabbit muscle tendon preparations (Garret *et al.* 1987). The authors suggest that stored elastic energy and the force of eccentric action were important factors in increasing the amount of energy absorbed prior to failure. It is possible that increased eccentric muscle action force resulting from strength training may further improve energy absorbance and reduce injury potential.

These data suggest that physical training, including strength training, may alter the properties of tendons and ligaments such that they are larger, stronger and more resistant to injury. From this standpoint, strength training exercise could trigger events that both alter force-generating characteristics and enhance protective mechanisms. For example, eccentric contractions have been shown to trigger intense protein synthesis at the MTJ, resulting in MTJ remodelling (Frenette & Côté 2000), which could potentially increase the strength of this area.

It should be noted that certain drugs commonly used in medicine or athletics may have profound effects on tendon and ligament strength. These drugs include certain antibiotics such as fluoroquinolones and corticosteroids. Corticosteroids are used to treat a variety of inflammatory problems such as tendinitis and bursitis. Corticosteroids are catabolic in nature and may cause atrophy, wasting and weakening of connective tissue, especially if injected directly into a tendon or ligament. Tendon rupture may have occurred as a result of the use of these drugs (Chechick *et al.* 1982; Stannard & Bucknell 1993). Anabolic steroids can be used by strength/power athletes to enhance performance. However, some evidence suggests that anabolic steroids (androgens) change the biomechanics of connective tissue such that a tendon or ligament may have a decreased tensile strength (Wood *et al.* 1988) or increased stiffness (Inhofe *et al.* 1995) regardless of training, thus increasing the injury potential. These effects in both animal and human tendons have been noted without any discernible alterations in biochemistry or ultrastructure (Inhofe *et al.* 1995; Evans *et al.* 1998). However, among human males, high doses of androgens have been associated with biochemical alterations in urine and serum which are consistent with increased type I and III synthesis among human (Parssinen *et al.* 2000).

Exercises and training may also affect changes in cartilage strength. For example, the stiffness of articular cartilage of the knee and ankle is apparently related to the degree of functional stress placed upon it during exercise (Yao & Seedhom 1993). While low volumes of exercise, including high-force exercise, may stimulate cartilage growth (van de Lest *et al.* 2000; Lapvetelainen *et al.* 2001) high volumes of very strenuous exercises (high force) may reduce cartilage integrity and increase injury potential leading to mechanical failure (Brama *et al.* 2000; Barneveld & van Weeren 1999). Thus training with different volumes or intensities of exercise may produce different effects, as shown in the following examples.

Positive effects. Some evidence suggests that the observed increased activity of chondrocytes resulting from appropriate volumes of exercise is mediated by increased insulin-like growth factor I (IGF-I) concentrations in the synovial fluid. Thus exercise can alter the synovial fluid in such manner that it produces a 'favourable' effect on cartilage proteoglycan (PG) content by enhancing PG synthesis and reducing its breakdown. (van de Lest *et al.* 2000).

Negative effects. While mechanical failure has a central role in degenerative cartilage disease, the exact cause is difficult to ascertain. In the case of chondromalacia of the patella, the severity of the lesion is probably unrelated to collagen content or cross-linking, but appears to depend on proteoglycan concentration (Väätäinen *et al.* 1998). These differential observations would indicate that there may be an optimum level (volume) of training which can result in cartilage strengthening effects. However, if the volume of exercise is too great then weakening of cartilage can occur.

The exact effects due to the mechanical loading of cartilage by strength training are not clear. For example, it is not uncommon, especially among athletes, to use squatting as a primary component of a strength training programme. Peak compressive forces in the knee during squatting can range from approximately 550 to 8000 N. While it is known that excessive loading of the menisci and articular cartilage can lead to degenerative changes, it is not known at what magnitude compressive forces become injurious to cartilage (Escamilla 2001). It should also be noted that compressive forces have been demonstrated to be important in knee stabilization by resisting shear forces and reducing tibial translation. This enhanced stabilization would offer protection from traumatic tearing of the cartilage as well as protection for the cruciate ligaments.

Although these data from animal and human biomechanical studies suggest that long periods of very heavy strength training may increase the injury potential for cartilage, there is at present little evidence of increased incidence of traumatic injuries or degenerative disease among well-trained strength and power athletes or former athletes. Indeed studies and reviews dealing with injury potential do not show excessive injury rates among highly trained strength athletes, including injuries related to cartilage damage or degeneration (Kuland *et al.* 1978; Fitzgerald & McLatchie 1980; Chandler *et al.* 1989; Hamill 1994; Stone *et al.* 1994).

Bone mineral density and bone mass

Bone acts as structural support and as a lever system in transferring muscle force into locomotion and other physical activities. It is a storage depot for phosphorus and calcium. Bone is a plastic material, changing density, mass and form according to stresses encountered in development (Falch 1982). Bone density and bone mass are related to the strength of the tissue.

WEIGHTLESSNESS AND IMMOBILIZATION

Weightlessness (Vogel & Whittle 1976) and

immobilization (Hanson *et al.* 1975) can cause profound loss of bone density and mass. Immobilization causes a marked increase in urinary calcium excretion, which reflects the loss of bone material (Falch 1982). Low-intensity exercise does not reduce the amount of urinary calcium lost in otherwise immobilized subjects. Standing at attention for 3 h decreased urinary calcium loss but physical activity performed lying down or in a wheelchair did not (Falch 1982). These data suggest that the antigravity muscles must be activated to maintain or enhance bone density and mass. Fleck and Falkel (1986) suggest that resistive training may activate the antigravity muscles. In this context, regular in-flight muscle activation (i.e. resistance training) could reduce the degenerative effects on bone. Among animals in a microgravity environment, housing conditions may exert a profound role, in effect producing a form of resistance training. When they were group housed, even a relatively long spaceflight had minimal effects on bone mass and bone turnover in young rats in contrast to previous work where animals were single housed (Wronski *et al.* 1998). In humans, attempts to obviate the effects of microgravity environments by using various resistance-training protocols have been met with varying degrees of success—more research is necessary (NASA Round Table 1996).

SIGNIFICANCE OF INCREASED BONE MASS

The degree to which physical training can enhance bone mineral deposition and strength is an important consideration. Stronger bones may protect against injury as a result of daily work tasks or athletic competition. The loss of bone tissue (osteoporosis) occurs with the ageing process; if bone density and maximum tensile strength can be enhanced before the osteoporotic process begins then complications can be minimized.

FITNESS LEVEL

The level of athlete and type of physical activity may also influence bone density. Cross-sectional comparisons of physically active men and women generally suggest that a positive relationship exists between physical activity level and bone density and mass. Several studies (Chow *et al.* 1986; Pocock *et al.* 1986; Tsuzuku *et al.* 1998) have related bone density, particularly of the lumbar vertebra, to measures of fitness including maximum muscular strength and aerobic power ($\dot{V}O_{2\,max}$). Additionally, some evidence suggests that childhood physical activity may have a marked subsequent influence on adult bone density (Conroy *et al.* 1990; McCulloch *et al.* 1990). However, not all training programmes necessarily produce the same result (Stone 1988).

BONE MINERAL SITE DEPOSITION

Several cross-sectional studies suggest that physical activity can affect increased bone mineral density (Helela 1969; Dalen & Olsen 1974; Chow *et al.* 1986; Stillman *et al.* 1986). Bone mineral deposition may be expected to be greatest at the site or area subjected to the greatest stress. For example, it may be expected that the dominant limbs of athletes are subjected to higher stress and more total work than non-dominant limbs, and this may be reflected in differences in bone mineral incorporation and bone densities and mass. The humerus of the dominant arm in tennis players has been shown to have a greater mass (Jones *et al.* 1977) and bone width and mineral content (Montoye *et al.* 1980). Similar results have been reported for baseball players (Watson 1974). Among various athletes the femur of the dominant leg also shows higher bone density than the non-dominant leg (Nilsson & Westlin 1971).

AEROBIC TRAINING

Cross-sectional studies of highly trained aerobic athletes have produced somewhat mixed results as to the effects of aerobic activities, particularly jogging, on bone density. Male long-distance runners (> 64 km per week) had similar tibial and radial bone densities, but significantly lower vertebral bone densities compared to sedentary or moderately (< 64 km per week) trained runners (Bilanin *et al.* 1989). Young (13.1 years) male and female distance runners compared to untrained age-, height- and weight-matched controls (Rodgers *et al.* 1990), were shown to have significantly lower mid-ulnar length (15.9 vs. 17.0 cm), bone mineral density (0.67 vs. 0.76 $g \cdot cm^{-1}$) and mineral/width (0.57 vs. 0.62 $g \cdot cm^{-2}$). Bone mineral density was more affected in males than in females. Buchanan *et al.* (1988) studied 30 women aged 18–22 years. The groups examined were sedentary, eumenorrhoeic athletes and amenorrhoeic/oligomenorrhoeic athletes. None of the women used resistance training. No significant differences in lumbar spine densities were found between groups. However, the amenorrhoeic/oligomenorrhoeic group did have the lowest bone density. The authors concluded that hormone profile was an important factor in bone density status. Similar findings have been reported by Moen *et al.* (1990) for lumbar spine bone density among female distance runners (15–18 years). Bone density and bone mass may be adversely affected by amenorrhoea regardless of the volume, intensity or type of exercise (Olsen 1989). One problem with cross-sectional studies of athletes, especially recently (about the last 10–12 years), is the proliferation of strength training programmes into all types of sports which makes data interpretation difficult.

Longitudinal studies generally reflect the results of the cross-sectional studies. Among groups with low bone density, non-resistive training programmes have shown increases toward normal bone density in degenerated bone (Goodship *et al.* 1979; Chien *et al.* 2000). However, Dalen and Olsen (1974) did not find that aerobic training affected bone mineral content in office workers over 3 months. Marguiles *et al.* (1986) examined the effects of military training on tibial bone density in 259 infantry recruits over 14 weeks. The average increase in bone density was 5.2% for the right leg and 11.1% for the left leg. However, 41% of the original 268 recruits did not complete the training course and the increase in bone density was related to the training time completed. Many recruits dropped out because of stress fractures. Williams *et al.* (1984) found that male runners averaging 141 km per week had a greater bone density of the calcaneus compared to runners averaging 65 km or less per week, suggesting a threshold for training volume.

Among postmenopausal women, aerobic dance was more effective in reducing bone loss over a 6-month period than was walking (White *et al.* 1984). Chow *et al.* (1986) divided 58 women into three groups: control, aerobic dance and aerobic dance plus very low intensity strength training with hand-held weights. After 1 year results suggested that bone density had increased in the combined exercise group, showed little change in the aerobic dance group, and showed a small reduction in the controls. This result indicates that combined aerobic and strength training exercise can be more effective in remodelling bone than aerobic training alone, a finding agreeing with that of McDermott *et al.* (2001). Differences in the effect of aerobic training on bone mineral density may be influenced by the degree of weightbearing, strain rate and the volume and intensity of training.

STRENGTH TRAINING

High-force and high-impact activities such as jumping and weight training appear to be associated with modifications in bone geometry at the loaded sites (Notomi *et al.* 2000; Pettersson *et al.* 2000) and can affect changes axially (throughout the length of bone) provided appropriate weightbearing is involved. Therefore athletes engaged in high-impact and high-force sporting and training activities should demonstrate enhanced bone density. Consequently, when examining various sports, bone density has been found to be related to the demands of the required physical activity (Bennell *et al.* 1997; Matsumoto *et al.* 1997; Calbert *et al.* 1999; Pettersson *et al.* 2000).

Nilsson and Westlin (1971) were among the first to examine bone density in relation to sporting demands. They (Nilsson & Westlin 1971) found that the bone densities of the lower limb were greater in international athletes compared to lower-level athletes who possessed greater bone densities than untrained controls. Additionally, it was shown that sports requiring repeatedly high-force movements, such as weightlifting and throwing events, had higher bone densities than distance runners and soccer players. Swimmers (non-weightbearing exercise) had the lowest bone densities (Nilsson & Westlin 1971). Indeed weightlifters have consistently been shown to have higher then normal bone density (Suominen 1993; Klesges *et al.* 1996). This effect of higher bone densities is evident even among young weightlifters. Conroy *et al.* (1990) studying junior elite weightlifters (17.4 years) demonstrated bone mineral density, compared to reference data (20–39 years), to be 113% (spine L2–4) and 134% (proximal femur neck) greater. Additionally, significant relationships were found between bone mineral density at the spine, femur neck, trochanter and Ward's triangle, and maximum lifting ability in the snatch, clean and jerk, and total (snatch plus clean and jerk).

Higher bone mineral densities have also been observed among power lifters. Granhed *et al.* (1987) demonstrated that among eight power lifters the calculated force applied at L3 (3rd lumbar vertebra) and the total load lifted during training over the previous year were related to the bone mineral content of the spine. Compressive forces on L3 ranged from 18 to 36.4 kN. The bone mineral content was highly correlated to training load ($r = 0.82$). Tsuzuku *et al.* (1998) found that young male power lifters had higher bone densities, compared to normal, in the lumbar spine as well as whole-body differences. A recent case study by Dickerman *et al.* (2000) reported the highest bone mineral density values ever recorded in the lumbar spine in the 110-kg class world record holder in the squat lift (average 1.859 $g \cdot cm^{-2}$ compared to a control 1.197 $g \cdot cm^{-2}$). The estimated lumbar critical compressive force during a squat lift of 469 kg was double that of the previously reported critical value of 18 000 N (Dickerman *et al.* 2000). Moreover, these results further emphasize the relationship between maximum muscular strength and bone density (Tsuzuku *et al.* 1998; Rhodes *et al.* 2000).

Among non-athletes resistance training has also been associated with increased bone mineral density. Twelve males who regularly engaged in resistance training for at least 1 year were compared to 50 age-matched controls (19–50 years). Increased density ($g \cdot cm^{-2}$) was found at the lumbar spine (1.35 vs. 1.22), trochanter (0.99 vs. 0.96) and femoral neck (1.18 vs. 1.02), but not at mid-radius (0.77 vs. 0.77), suggesting that resistance training is associated with increased bone density at weightbearing but not non-weightbearing sites (Colletti *et al.* 1989).

Longitudinal studies have also shown that strength training can beneficially alter bone mineral deposition. Of particular interest have been the effects of resistance training among postmenopausal women, due to the associative osteoporosis, particularly as it affects the lumbar spine. For example, over a 5-month period, partner-assisted and body weight training in postmenopausal women caused a 3.8% increase in the distal radius, with the control group decreasing 1.9% (Simkin *et al.* 1987). Two days per week of resistance training has shown a significant increase in lumbar spine bone density over a 1-year period in postmenopausal women (Nelson *et al.* 1994).

Younger women can also show improved bone mineral density (BMD). Twelve months of weight training produced a significant increase in lumbar bone density compared to controls in premenopausal women (Gleeson *et al.* 1990). Lumbar spine bone density (and other sites) was also improved 1.9% in premenopausal women (28–39 years) over 18 months with the use of resistance training (Lohman *et al.* 1995).

Older men have also benefited from resistance training. Sixteen weeks of progressive resistance exercise (75–90% of 1 RM) produced significantly increased BMD at Ward's triangle in elderly men (67 ± 1 years). Increased BMD was observed at several sites compared to controls in younger men (54.6 ± 3.2 years) after 24 weeks of resistance training.

It should be noted that alterations in lean body mass, percentage fat and maximum strength typically accompanied the changes in BMD. These data from studies in older men and women indicate that strength training can improve BMD as well as other physical and performance variables.

INTENSITY AND WEIGHTBEARING CONSIDERATIONS

Lane *et al.* (1988) compared aerobic training (jogging) with weight training over a 5-month period. When programme adherence was taken into account, the weight training produced significantly better increases in lumbar bone density than the aerobic group, a finding supported by animal data (Notomi *et al.* 2000).

The importance of intensity of exercise and weightbearing was pointed out by Martin *et al.* (1981). Beagles were exercised on a treadmill at 3.3 $km \cdot h^{-1}$ for 75 min, 5 days per week for 71 weeks. The dogs wore weighted jackets, the weight of which was increased up to approximately 130% of the dog's body mass by week 23 and was held constant for the remaining 48 weeks. The rate of bone mineral incorporation in the tibia was enhanced compared to sedentary controls. Previous research with no weighted jackets showed no effect on bone density or rate of mineral incorporation (Martin *et al.* 1981). In humans, comparisons of athletes competing in different sports that have different weightbearing and impact characteristics (strain rates) indicate the importance of these two components in optimizing BMD alterations. Athletes involved in high-impact activities such as basketball and volleyball when compared to moderate (track and soccer) and non-impact (swimming) sports tend to show markedly higher BMD values (Creighton *et al.* 2001). Longitudinal studies support the findings among athletes. For example: Maddalozzo and Snow (2000) compared the 24-week effects of a machine-based moderate-intensity programme with a standing free weight training programme (i.e. weightbearing). They concluded that the standing programme was more effective at improving the BMD of the spine in older men (54.6 ± 3.2 years) and women (52.8 ± 3.3 years). These data again indicate that strength training, particularly with higher strain rates and a weightbearing component, can substantially alter BMD.

Mechanisms promoting connective tissue remodelling

Tissue injury

Exercise, especially exercise with a large eccentric action component, can result in muscle damage (Ebbling & Clarkson 1989). Very long term running (24 h) affected changes, likely to be injury to collagen-synthesizing cells, resulting in elevated serum concentrations of galactosylhydroxylysyl glucosyltransferase (S-GGT) and serum type III procollagen amino-terminal propeptide (S-PRO-(III)-N-P) (Takala *et al.* 1976). The change in concentration in neither S-GGT nor S-PRO-(III)-N-P corresponded with changes in serum CPK (creatine phosphokinase) or LDH (lactate dehydrogenase). The S-GGT returned to normal after exercise but the S-PRO-(III)-N-P continued to increase (40%) after exercise. This would likely stimulate type III collagen synthesis.

High forces associated with eccentric actions cause considerable stress to the muscle and connective tissue. Products of collagen injury and damage as a result of exercise may act as chemotactic agents for monocytes to transfer from blood to muscle (Armstrong *et al.* 1983). Upon entering an injured area monocytes transform into macrophages, which have a phagocytic function. The invading cells may be a consequence rather than a cause of damage and are acting to remove damaged cellular components (Jones *et al.* 1986). The invading cells may have myogenic activity (Stauber *et al.* 1988). Proteoglycans, components of connective tissue that are influenced by the muscle damage process, are important in regulating the myogenic process (Fritz & Stauber 1988). Thus, connective tissue may have a regulatory as well as a structural role in the damage and repair process (Ebbling & Clarkson 1989).

Growth-promoting peptides, such as insulin-like growth factor I (IGF-I) and connective tissue growth factor (CTGF) may also play a role in connective tissue regeneration and growth (Parkhouse *et al.* 2000). Many of these growth-promoting factors are activated by autocrine and paracrine responses to tissue damage or repetitive stretching or through hormonal activation (Bishoff 1984; Perrone *et al.* 1995; Yarasheki *et al.* 1997). Resistance training, having a high eccentric component or having a sufficient volume, which causes muscle damage, could promote the production of such growth-promoting factors.

Bone mineral incorporation stimulus

Remodelling is a function of stress and strain encountered by bone. The adaptation of bone is modified by various factors including nutritional, hormonal and functional strain. It has been suggested that a 'minimum effective strain' exists, which is the lowest strain necessary to maintain balanced remodelling and to preserve bone at relatively constant values (Frost 1986). However, magnitude is only one factor contributing to the functional strain that is a stimulus for bone remodelling. Three primary factors that modify bone are (Lanyon 1987):

1 the magnitude of strain;
2 the strain rate; and
3 the distribution of the strain.

Small strains will not contribute to effective bone remodelling regardless of distribution (Lanyon 1987). These factors may explain the relatively small changes in bone associated with typical aerobic training (Notomi *et al.* 2000). Additionally, amenorrhoeic women with low oestrogen concentrations performing aerobic training may experience two problems. First, the aerobic training may not be of sufficient intensity to adequately effect bone remodelling, and the low oestrogen concentrations may reduce calcium reabsorption.

Strength training may more adequately satisfy the criteria for bone remodelling (Notomi *et al.* 2000). Furthermore, the strain rate may be particularly important in bone remodelling. Exercise designed to increase peak bone mass and density or prevent decreases, such as those occurring with age, should involve high strain rates, but need be of relatively short duration. Certain types of strength/power training such as weightlifting training, which includes various fast movements and high rates of force development as well as whole-body exercises, likely provide a high magnitude of strain, varied strain distributions and high strain rates.

Hormonal influences

Exercise and training can cause marked changes in blood hormones (Terjung 1980; Stone 1990). Anabolic hormones including testosterone and growth hormone can increase as a result of exercise (including strength exercises) of appropriate intensity (Terjung 1980; Stone *et al.* 1991; Häkkinen *et al.* 2000). The testosterone/cortisol ratio may reflect the relative anabolic state (Häkkinen *et al.* 1985). Appropriate resistance training may increase this ratio, which may induce increases in lean body mass, including connective tissue (Häkkinen *et al.* 1985).

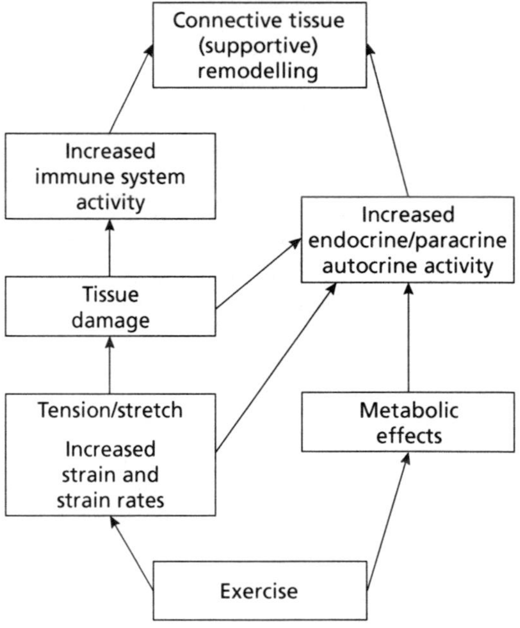

Fig. 18.3 Mechanisms for connective tissue remodelling.

Overtraining may reduce this ratio as well as affect other hormones, e.g. oestrogen, which could adversely affect connective tissue growth and maintenance (Stone 1990; Stone *et al.* 1991). It is of interest that high volumes of endurance training have been associated with decreased bone density in both men and women (Bilanin *et al.* 1989; Michel *et al.* 1989) and alterations in bone density may be associated with lower concentrations of testosterone (Smith & Rutherford 1993).

Testosterone, insulin, other hormones, minerals and vitamins directly related to bone mineral deposition can be stimulated by resistance training. For example, weightlifting training increased the resting concentrations of testosterone in junior weightlifters over a 1-year period (Fry *et al.* 1994). Males weight training for 1 year were found to have increased serum Gla protein and serum vitamin D concentrations, both markers of bone formation, compared to controls (Bell *et al.* 1988). The bioavailability of hormones such as IGF-I may also be increased through resistance training (Parkhouse *et al.* 2000). Other factors affecting connective tissue remodelling could include hormone number and sensitivity as well as paracrine and autocrine activity (Fig. 18.3).

Summary

Evidence suggests that chronic physical activity, particularly resistance training, can modify connective tissue. It appears that to most effectively stimulate connective tissue growth: (i) the intensity of the exercises used must be high; (ii) antigravity muscles should be active, especially for axial bone remodelling; and (iii) load-bearing activities requiring large strains and strain rates may be most effective in stimulating bone formation. Furthermore, overtraining and microgravity environments can adversely affect connective tissue growth (Fig. 18.4).

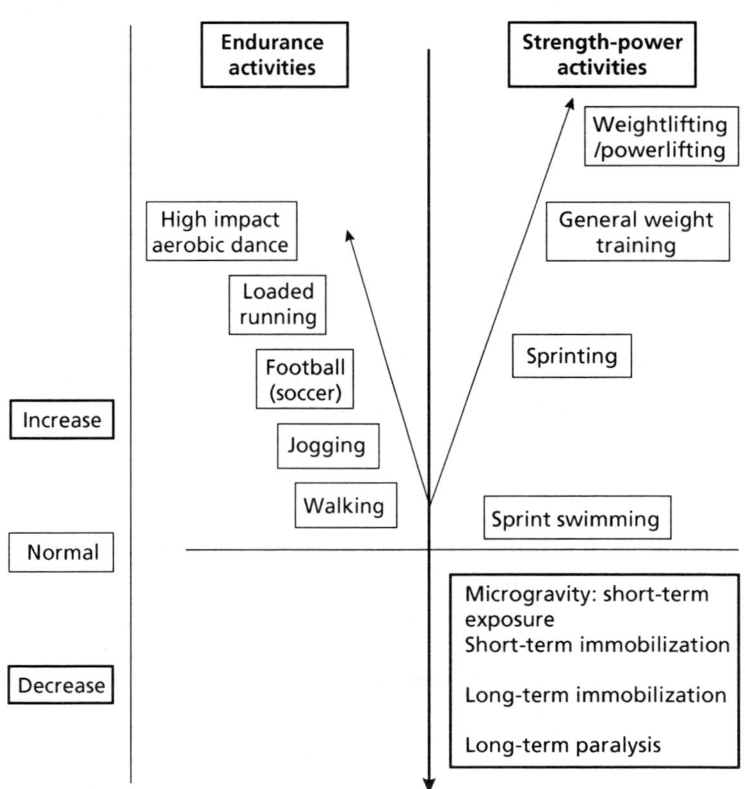

Fig. 18.4 Connective tissue size and strength: theoretical effects of physical activity.

Acknowledgement

The authors are indebted to Frances Welsh for her assistance in preparing this chapter.

References

Abraham, W.M. (1977) Factors in delayed muscle soreness. *Medicine and Science in Sports* **9**, 11–20.

Alexander, R. Mc (1981) Factors of safety in the structure of animals. *Scientific Progress* **67**, 109–130.

Armstrong, R.B., Ogilvie, R.W. & Schwane, J.A. (1983) Eccentric exercise-induced injury to rat skeletal muscle. *Journal of Applied Physiology* **54**, 80–93.

Barneveld, A. & van Weeren, P.R. (1999) Conclusions regarding the influence of exercises on the development of the equine musculoskeletal system with special reference to osteochondrosis. *Equine Veterinary Journal (Suppl.)* **31**, 112–119.

Bell, N.H., Godsen, R.N., Henry, D.P., Shary, J. & Epstein, S. (1988) The effects of muscle-building exercise on vitamin D and mineral metabolism. *Medicine and Science in Sports and Exercise* **21**, 66–70.

Bennell, K.L., Malcolm, S.A., Kahn, K.M. *et al.* (1997) Bone mass and bone turnover in power athletes, endurance athletes and controls: a 12 month longitudinal study. *Bone* **20**, 477–484.

Bilanin, J.O., Blanchard, M.S. & Russek-Cohen, E. (1989) Lower vertebral bone density in male long distance runners. *Medicine and Science in Sports and Exercise* **21**, 66–70.

Bishoff, R. (1986) A satellite cell mitogen from crushed adult muscle. *Developmental Biology* **15**, 140–147.

Brama, P.A., Tekoppele, J.M., Basnk, R.A., Barneveld, A., Firth, E.C. & van Weeren, P.R. (2000) The influence of strenous exercises on collagen characteristics of articular cartilage in thoroughbreds age 2 years. *Equine Veterinary Journal* **32**, 551–554.

Brzank, K.D. & Peiper, K.S. (1986) Effect of intensive strength building exercise training on the fine structure of human skeletal muscle capillaries. *Anatomischer Anzeiger* **161**, 243–248.

Buchanan, J.R., Myers, C., Lloyd, T., Leuenberger, P. & Demers, L.M. (1988) Determinants of trabecular bone density in women: the role of androgens, estrogens and exercise. *Journal of Bone and Mineral Research* **3**, 673–680.

Butler, D.L., Grood, E.S., Noyes, F.R. & Zernicke, R.F. (1978) Biomechanics of ligaments and tendons. *Exercise and Sport Sciences Reviews* **6**, 125–181.

Calbert, J.A., Diaz Herrera, P. & Rodriguez, L.P. (1999) High bone mineral density in male elite professional volleyball players. *Osteoporosis International* **10**, 468–474.

Chandler, T.J., Wilson, G.D. & Stone, M.H. (1989) The effect of the squat exercise on knee stability. *Medicine and Science in Sports and Exercise* **21**, 299–303.

Chechick, A., Amit, Y., Israeli, A. & Horozowski, H. (1982) Recurrent rupture of the achilles tendon induced by corticosteroid injection. *British Journal of Sports Medicine* **16**, 89–90.

Chien, M.Y., Wu, Y.T., Hsu, A.T., Ynag, R.S. & Lai, J.S. (2000) Efficacy of a 24-week aerobic exercise program for osteopenic postmenopausal women. *Calcified Tissue International* **67**, 443–448.

Chow, R.K., Harrison, J.E., Brown, C.F. & Hajek, V. (1986) Physical fitness effect on bone mass in postmenopausal women. *Archives of Physical Medicine and Rehabilitation* **67**, 231–234.

Colletti, L.A., Edwards, J., Gordon, L., Shary, J. & Bell, N.H. (1989) The effects of muscle building exercise on bone mineral density of the radius, spine and hip in young men. *Calcified Tissue International* **45**, 12–14.

Conroy, B.P., Kraemer, W.J., Dalsky, G.P. *et al.* (1990) Bone mineral density in elite junior weightlifters. *Medicine and Science in Sports and Exercise* **22**, S77.

Creighton, D.L., Morgan, A.L., Boardley, D. & Brolinsson, P.G. (2001) Weight-bearing exercise markers of bone turnover in female athletes. *Journal of Applied Physiology* **90**, 565–570.

Curwin, S.L., Vailas, A.C. & Wood, J. (1988) Immature tendon adaptation to strenuous exercise. *Journal of Applied Physiology* **65**, 2297–2301.

Dalen, N. & Olsen, K.E. (1974) Bone mineral content and physical activity. *Acta Orthopaedica Scandinavica* **45**, 170–174.

Dickerman, R.D., Pertus, R.M. & Smith, G.H. (2000) The upper range of lumbar spine bone mineral density? An examination of the current world record holder in the squat lift. *International Journal of Sports Medicine* **21**, 469–470.

Ebbling, C.B. & Clarkson, P.M. (1989) Exercise-induced muscle damage and adaptation. *Sports Science* **7**, 207–234.

Elliot, D.H. & Crawford, G.N.C. (1965) The thickness and collagen content of tendon relative to strength and cross-sectional area of muscle. *Proceedings of the Royal Society of London Series B* **162**, 137–146.

Escamilla, R.F. (2001) Knee biomechanics of the squat exercise. *Medicine and Science in Sports and Exercise* **33**, 127–141.

Evans, N.A., Bowrey, D.J. & Newman, G.R. (1998) Ultrastructural analysis of ruptured tendon from anabolic steroid users. *Injury* **29**, 769–773.

Falch, J.A. (1982) The effects of physical activity on the skeleton. *Scandinavian Journal of Social Medicine (Suppl.)* **29**, 55–58.

Fitzgerald, B. & McLatchie, G.R. (1980) Degenerative joint disease in weightlifters. *British Journal of Sports Medicine* **14**, 97–101.

Fleck, S.J. & Falkel, J.E. (1986) Value of resistance training for the reduction of sports injuries. *Sports Medicine* **3**, 61–68.

Folwes, J.R., Sale, D.G. & MacDougall, J.D. (2000) Reduced strength after passive stretch of the human plantarflexors. *Journal of Applied Physiology* **89**, 1179–1188.

Frenette, J. & Côté, C.H. (2000) Modulation of structural protein content of the myotendinous junction following eccentric contractions. *International Journal of Sports Medicine* **21**, 313–320.

Fritz, V.K. & Stauber, W.T. (1988) Characterisation of muscles injured by forced lengthening. II. Proteoglycans. *Medicine and Science in Sports and Exercise* **20**, 354–361.

Frost, H.M. (1986) *The Intermediate Organisation of the Skeleton*. CRC Press, Boca Raton.

Fry, A.C., Kraemer, W.J., Stone, M.H. *et al.* (1994) Endo- [illegible] before and after one year of weightlifting training. *Canadian Journal of Applied Physiology* **19**, 400–410.

Garret, W.E., Safran, M.R., Seaber, A.V., Glisson, R.R. & Ribbeck, B.M. (1987) Biomechanical comparison of stimulated and non-stimulated skeletal muscle pulled to failure. *American Journal of Sports Medicine* **15**, 448–454.

Gleeson, P.G., Protas, E.J., Leblanc, A.D., Schneider, V.S. & Evans, H.J. (1990) Effects of weight lifting on bone mineral density in premenopausal women. *Journal of Bone and Mineral Research* **5**, 153–158.

Goodship, A.E., Lanyon, L.E. & McFie, H. (1979) Functional adaptations of bone to increased stress. *Journal of Bone and Joint Surgery* **61A**, 539–546.

Gosselin, L.E., Adams, C., Cotter, T., McCormick, R.A. & Thomas, D.P. (1998) Effect of exercise training on passive stiffness in locomotor skeletal muscle: role of extracellular matrix. *Journal of Applied Physiology* **85**, 1011–1016.

Granhed, H., Jonson, R. & Hansson, T. (1987) The loads on the spine during extreme weightlifting. *Spine* **12**, 146–149.

Häkkinen, K., Pakarinen, A., Kraemer, W.J., Newton, R.U. & Alen, M. (2000) Basal concentrations and acute responses of serum hormones and strength development during heavy resistance training in middle-aged and elderly men and women. *Journal of Gerontology* **55**, B95–B105.

Häkkinen, K., Pakarinen, A., Markku, A. & Komi, P.V. (1985) Serum hormones during prolonged training of neuromuscular performance. *European Journal of Applied Physiology* **53**, 287–293.

Hamill, B.P. (1994) Relative safety of weightlifting and weight training. *Journal of Strength and Conditioning Research* **8**(1), 53–57.

Han, X., Karpakka, J., Kainulainen, H. & Takala, T.E.S. (1995) Effects of streptozotocin-induced diabetes, physical training and their combination on collagen biosynthesis in rat skeletal muscle. *Acta Physiologica Scandinavica* **155**, 9–16.

Hanson, T.H., Roos, B.O. & Nachemson, A. (1975) Development of osteopenia in the fourth lumbar vertebrae during prolonged bedrest after operation for scoliosis. *Acta Orthopaedica Scandinavica* **46**, 621–630.

Helela, T. (1969) Variations of thickness of cortical bone in two populations. *Annals of Clinical Research* **1**, 227–231.

Hirsch, G. (1974) Tensile properties during tendon healing. *Acta Orthopaedica Scandinavica Supplement* **153**.

Ingelmark, B.E. (1948) Der Bau der sehnen wahrend Verschiederaltersperioden und unter wechselendes funktionellen Bedigngungen. I. *Acta Anatomica* **6**, 113–140.

Inhofe, P.D., Grana, W.A., Egle, D., Min, K.W. & Tomanek, J. (1995) The effects of anabolic steroids on rat tendon, an ultrastructural, biomechanical and biochemical analysis. *American Journal of Sports Medicine* **23**, 227–232.

Jones, H.H., Priest, J.D., Hayes, W.C., Tichnor, C.C. & Nagel, D.A. (1977) Humeral hypertrophy in response to exercise. *Journal of Bone and Joint Surgery* **59A**, 204–208.

Jones, D.A., Newham, D.J., Round, J.M. & Tolfree, S.E.J. (1986) Experimental human muscle damage: morphological changes in relation to other indices of damage. *Journal of Physiology* **375**, 435–448.

Ker, R.F. (1999) The design of soft collagenous load-bearing tissues. *Journal of Experimental Biology* **202**, 3315–3324.

Kiiskinen, A. & Heikkinen, H. (1976) Physical training and connective tissue in young mice. *British Journal of Dermatology* **95**, 525–529.

Klesges, R.C., Ward, K.D. & Davis, J. (1996) Changes in bone mineral content in male athletes: mechanisms of action and intervention effects. *Journal of the American Medical Association* **276**, 226–230.

Kovanen, V. & Suominen, H. (1989) Age- and training-related changes in the collagen metabolism of rat skeletal muscle. *European Journal of Applied Physiology* **58**, 765–771.

Kovanen, V., Suominen, H. & Heikkenen, E. (1980) Connective tissue of fast and slow skeletal muscle in rats—effects of endurance training. *Acta Physiologica Scandinavica* **108**, 173–180.

Kovanen, V., Suominen, H. & Heikkenen, E. (1984) Collagen of fast twitch and slow twitch muscle fibers in different types of rat skeletal muscle. *European Journal of Applied Physiology* **52**, 235–242.

Kubo, K., Kanehisa, H., Kawakami, Y. & Fukunaga (2000) Elasticity of tendon structures of the lower limbs in sprinters. *Acta Physiologica Scandinavica* **168**, 327–335.

Kubo, K., Kanehisa, H., Kawakami, Y. & Fukunaga (2001a) Growth changes in the elastic properties of human tendon structures. *International Journal of Sports Medicine* **22**, 138–143.

Kubo, K., Kanehisa, H., Kawakami, Y. & Fukunaga (2001b) Influence of static stretching on viscoelastic properties of human tendon structures in vivo. *Journal of Applied Physiology* **90**, 520–527.

Kuland, D.N., Dewy, J.B. & Brubaker, C.E. (1978) Olympic weightlifting injuries. *The Physician and Sports Medicine* **6**, 111–119.

Laban, M.M. (1962) Collagen tissue: implications of its response to stress in vitro. *Archives of Physical Medicine and Rehabilitation* **43**, 461–466.

Lane, N., Bevier, W., Bouxsein, M., Wiswell, R., Carter, D. & Marcus, R. (1988) Effect of exercise intensity on bone mineral. *Medicine and Science in Sports and Exercise* **20**, S51.

Lanyon, L.E. (1987) Functional strain in bone tissue as an objective and controlling stimulus for adaptive bone remodelling. *Journal of Biomechanics* **2**, 1083–1093.

Lapvetelainen, T., Hyttinen, M., Lindblom, J. *et al.* (2001) More knee joint osteoarthritis (OA) in mice after inactivation of one allele of type LL procollagen but less OA after lifelong voluntary wheel running exercise. *Osteoarthritis and Cartilage* **9**, 152–160.

Laurent, G.J., Sparrow, M.P., Bates, P.C. & Millward, D.J. (1978) Collagen content and turnover in cardiac and skeletal muscles of the adult fowl and the changes during stretch induced growth. *Biochemistry Journal* **176**, 419–427.

Lohman, T., Going, S., Pamenter, R. *et al.* (1995) Effects of resistance training on regional and total bone mineral density in premenopausal women: a randomized prospective study. *Journal of Bone and Mineral Research* **10**, 1015–1024.

McCulloch, R.G., Baily, D.A., Houston, C.S. & Dodd, B.L. (1990) Effects of physical activity, dietary calcium intake, and selected lifestyle factors on bone density in young women. *Canadian Medical Association Journal* **142**, 221–232.

McDermott, M.T., Christensen, R.S. & Lattimer, J. (2001) The effects of regio-specific resistance and aerobic exercises on bone mineral density in premenopausal women. *Military Medicine* **166**, 318–121.

MacDougall, J.D., Sale, D.G., Always, S.E. & Sutton, J.R. (1984) Muscle fibre number in biceps brachii in body builders and control subjects. *Journal of Applied Physiology* **57**, 1399–1403.

Maddalozzo, G.F. & Snow, C.M. (2000) High intensity resistance training: effects on bone in older men and women. *Calcified Tissue International* **66**, 399–404.

Maganaris, C.N. & Paul, J.P. (1999) In vivo human tendon mechanical properties. *Journal of Physiology (London)* **521**, 307–313.

Marguiles, J.K., Simkin, A., Leichtor, A. *et al.* (1986) Effects of intense physical activity on the bone mineral content in the lower limbs of young adults. *Journal of Bone and Joint Surgery* **68A**, 1090–1093.

Martin, R.K., Albright, J.P., Clark, W.R. & Niffnegger, J.A. (1981) Load-carrying effects on the adult beagle tibia. *Medicine and Science in Sports and Exercise* **13**, 343–349.

Matsumoto, T., Nakagawa, S., Nishida, S. & Hirota, R. (1997) Bone density and bone metabolic markers in active collegiate athletes: findings in long distance runners, judoists and swimmers. *International Journal of Sports Medicine* **18**, 408–412.

Michel, B.A., Bloch, D.A. & Fries, J.F. (1989) Weight-bearing exercise, overexercise, and lumbar bone density over age 50 years. *Archives of Internal Medicine* **149**, 2325–2329.

Moen, S., Sanborn, C., Bonnick, S. *et al.* (1990) Lumbar bone density in female distance runners. *Medicine and Science in Sports and Exercise* **22**, 377.

Montoye, H.J., Smith, E.L., Fardon, D.F. & Howley, E.T. (1980) Bone mineral in senior tennis players. *Scandinavian Journal of Sports Science* **2**, 26–32.

Myllylä, R., Salminen, A., Peltonen, L., Takala, T.E.S. & Vihko, V. (1986) Collagen metabolism of mouse skeletal muscle during repair of exercise injuries. *Pflügers Archiv* **407**, 64–70.

NASA Round Table, Baldwin, K.M., White, T.P., Arnaud, S.B. *et al.* (1996) Musculoskeletal adaptations to weightlessness and development of effective counter measures. *Medicine and Science in Sports and Exercise* **10**, 1247–1253.

Nelson, M.E., Fiatarone, M.A., Morganti, C.M., Trice, I., Greenberg, R.A. & Evans, W.J. (1994) Effects of high-intensity strength training on multiple risk factors for osteoporotic fractures. *Journal of the American Medical Association* **272**, 1909–1914.

Nilsson, B.E. & Westlin, N.E. (1971) Bone density in athletes. *Clinical Orthopaedics* **77**, 179–182.

Notomi, T., Okazaki, Y., Okimoto, N., Saitoh, S., Nakamura, T. & Suzuki, M. (2000) A comparison of resistance and aerobic training for mass, strength and turnover of bone in growing rats. *European Journal of Applied Physiology* **83**, 469–474.

Noyes, F.R. (1977) Functional properties of knee ligaments and alterations induced by immobilisation: a correlative biomechanical and histological study in primates. *Clinical Orthopaedics* **123**, 210–242.

Olsen, B.R. (1989) Exercise induced amenorrhea. *American Family Physician* **39**, 213–221.

Parkhouse, W.S., Coupland, D.C., Li, C. & Vanderhoek, K.J. (2000) IGF-1 bioavailability is increased by resistance training in older women with low bone mineral density. *Mechanics of Ageing Development* **113**, 75–83.

Parssinen, M., Karila, T., Kovanen, V. & Seppala, T. (2000) The effect of supraphysiological doses of anabolic androgenic steroids on collagen metabolism. *International Journal of Sports Medicine* **21**, 406–411.

Perrone, C.E., Fenwick-Smith, D. & Vandenbourgh, H.H. (1995) Collagen and stretch modulate autocrine secretion of insulin-like growth factor-1 and insulin-like growth factor binding proteins from differentiated skeletal muscle cells. *Journal of Biological Chemistry* **270**, 20099–20106.

Pettersson, U., Nordström, P., Alfredson, H., Henriksson-Larsen, K. & Lorentzon, P. (2000) Effect of high impact activity on bone mass and size in adolescent females: a comparative study between two different types of sports. *Calcified Tissue International* **67**, 207–214.

Pocock, N.A., Eisman, J.A., Yeates, M.G., Sambrook, F.N. & Eberl, S. (1986) Physical fitness is a major determinant of femoral neck and lumbar spine bone mineral density. *Journal of Clinical Investigation* **78**, 618–621.

Rhodes, E.C., Martin, A.D., Taunton, J.E., Donnelly, M., Warren, J. & Elliot, J. (2000) Effects of one year resistance training on the relation between muscular strength and bone density in elderly women. *British Journal of Sports Medicine* **34**, 18–22.

Rodgers, C.D., Vanheest, J.L., Nowak, J.L., Van Huss, W.D., Heusner, W.W. & Seefeldt, V.D. (1990) Bone mineral content in young endurance-trained male and female runners. *Medicine and Science in Sports and Exercise* **22**, 576.

Safran, M.R., Garret, W.E., Seaber, A.V., Glisson, R.R. & Ribbeck, B.M. (1988) The role of warmup in muscular injury prevention. *American Journal of Sports Medicine* **16**, 123–129.

Schilling, B. & Stone, M.H. (2000) Stretching: acute effects on strength and power performance. *Strength and Conditioning* **22**(1), 44–50.

Schultz, R.M. (1982) Proteins II. In: *Biochemistry with Clinical Correlations* (ed. T. M. Devlin), pp. 124–132. John Wiley & Sons, New York.

Shadwick, R.E. (1990) Elastic energy storage in tendons: mechanical differences related to function and age. *Journal of Applied Physiology* **68**, 1033–1040.

Simkin, A., Ayalon, J. & Leichter, I. (1987) Increased trabecular bone density due to bone loading exercises in postmenopausal women. *Calcified Tissue International* **40**, 59–63.

Smith, R. & Rutherford, O.M. (1993) Spine and total body mineral density and serum testosterone levels in male athletes. *European Journal of Applied Physiology* **674**, 330–334.

Stannard, J.P. & Bucknell, A.L. (1993) Rupture of the triceps tendon associated with steroid injections. *American Journal of Sports Medicine* **21**, 482–485.

Stauber, W.T., Fritz, B.K., Vogelbach, D.W. & Dahlmann, B. (1988) Characterisation of muscles injured by forced lengthening. I. Cellular infiltrates. *Medicine and Science in Sports and Exercise* **20**, 345–353.

Stillman, R.J., Lohman, T.G., Slaughter, M.H. & Massey, B.H. (1986) Physical activity and bone mineral incorporation content in women aged 30–85 years. *Medicine and Science in Sports and Exercise* **18**, 576–580.

Stone, M.H. (1988) Implications for connective tissue and bone alterations resulting from resistance exercise training. *Medicine and Science in Sports and Exercise* **20**, S162–S168.

Stone, M.H. (1990) Muscle conditioning and muscle injuries. *Medicine and Science in Sports and Exercise* **22**, 457–462.

Stone, M.H. & Wilson, G.D. (1985) Selected physiological effects of weight-training. *Medical Clinics of North America* **69**(1), 109–122.

Stone, M.H., Keith, R.E., Kearney, J.T., Fleck, S.J., Wilson, G.D. & Triplett, N.T. (1991) Overtraining: a review of the signs, symptoms and possible causes. *Journal of Applied Sports Science Research* **5**(1), 35–50.

Stone, M.H., Fry, A.C., Ritchie, M., Stoessel-Ross, L. & Marsit, J.L. (1994) Injury potential and safety aspects of weightlifting movements. *Strength and Conditioning* **16**(3), 15–24.

Stone, M.H., Collins, D., Plisk, S., Haff, G. & Stone, M.E. (2000) Training principles: evaluation of modes and methods of resistance training. *Strength and Conditioning* **22**(3), 65–76.

Suominen, H. (1993) Bone mineral density and long-term exercise: an overview of cross-sectional athlete studies. *Sports Medicine* **16**, 316–330.

Suominen, W.T., Heikkinen, E. & Parkatti, T. (1977) Effect of eight weeks physical training on muscle and connective tissue of the m. vastus lateralis in 69-year old men and women. *Journal of Gerontology* **32**, 33–37.

Suominen, H., Heikkinen, E., Moiso, H. & Viljama, K. (1978) Physical and chemical properties of skin in habitual trained and sedentary 31–70 year old men. *British Journal of Dermatology* **99**, 147–154.

Takala, T.E., Vuori, J., Antinen, H., Vaanen, K. & Myllyla, R. (1976) Prolonged exercise causes an increase in the activity of galactosyl hydroxylysyl glucosyl-transferase and in the concentration of type III procollagen amino propeptide in human serum. *Pflügers Archiv* **407**, 500–503.

Terjung, R. (1980) Endocrine response to exercise. *Exercise and Sport Sciences Reviews* **7**, 153–180.

Tipton, C.M., James, S.L., Merger, J.W. & Tcheng, T.K. (1970) Influence of exercise on strength of medial collateral knee ligaments of dogs. *American Journal of Physiology* **218**, 894–902.

Tipton, C.M., Matthes, R.D. & Sandage, D.S. (1974) In situ measurements of junction strength and ligament elongation in rats. *Journal of Applied Physiology* **37**, 758–762.

Tipton, C.M., Martin, R.K., Matthes, R.D. & Carey, R.A. (1975a) Hydroxyproline concentrations in ligaments from trained and non-trained dogs. In: *Metabolic Adaptations to Prolonged Physical Training* (eds H. Howald & J. R. Purtmans), pp. 262–267. Birkhauser-Verlag, Basel.

Tipton, C.M., Matthes, R.D., Maynard, J.A. & Carey, R.A. (1975b) The influence of physical activity on ligaments and tendons. *Medicine and Science in Sports* **7**, 165–175.

Tsuzuku, S., Ikegami, Y. & Yabe, K. (1998) Effects of high-intensity resistance training on bone mineral density in young powerlifters. *Calcified Tissue International* **63**, 283–286.

Turto, H., Lindy, S. & Holme, J. (1974) Protocollagen proline hydroxylase activity in work-induced hypertrophy of rat muscle. *American Journal of Physiology* **226**, 63–65.

Väätäinen, U., Kiviranta, I., Jaroma, H., Arokosi, J., Tammi, M. & Kovanen, V. (1998) Collagen crosslinks in chondromalacia of the patella. *International Journal of Sports Medicine* **19**, 144–148.

Van de Lest, C.H., van de Hoogen, B.M. & van Weeren, P.R. (2000) Loading-induced changes in synovial fluid affect cartilage metabolism. *Biorheology* **37**, 45–55.

Van Pilsum, J.F. (1982) Metabolism of individual tissues. In: *Biochemistry with Clinical Correlations* (ed. T. M. Devlin), pp. 1050–1052. John Wiley & Sons, New York.

Viiduk, A. (1968) Elasticity and tensile strength of the anterior cruciate ligament in rabbits as influenced by training. *Acta Physiologica Scandinavica* **74**, 372–380.

Viiduk, A. (1986) Adaptability of connective tissue. In: *Biochemistry of Exercise* VI (ed. B. Stalin), pp. 545–562. Academic Press, London.

Vogel, J.M. & Whittle, M.W. (1976) Bone mineral content changes in the skylab astronauts. *American Journal of Roentgenology* **126**, 1296.

Watson, R.C. (1974) Bone growth and physical activity in young males. In: *International Conference on Bone Mineral Measurements*, pp. 380–385. US Department of Health, Education, and Welfare Publications, NIH 75–683.

White, M.K., Martin, R.B., Yeater, R.A., Butcher, R.L. & Radin, E.L. (1984) The effects of exercise on post-menopausal women. *International Orthopaedics* **7**, 209–214.

Williams, J.A., Wagner, J., Wasnich, R. & Heilburn, L. (1984) The effects of long distance running upon appendicular bone mineral content. *Medicine and Science in Sports and Exercise* **16**, 223–227.

Woo, S.L.Y., Gomex, M.A., Woo, Y.K. & Akeson, W.H. (1982) Mechanical properties of tendons and ligaments. II. The relationship between immobilisation and exercise on tissue remodelling. *Biorheology* **19**, 397–408.

Wood, T.O., Cooke, P.H. & Goodship, A.E. (1988) The effect of exercise and anabolic steroids on the mechanical properties and crimp morphology of the rat tendon. *American Journal of Sports Medicine* **16**, 153–158.

Wronski, T.J., Li, M., Shen, Y. *et al.* (1998) Lack of effect of spaceflight on bone mass and bone formation in group-housed rats. *Journal of Applied Physiology* **85**, 279–285.

Yao, J.Q. & Seedhom, B.B. (1993) Mechanical conditioning of articular cartilage to prevalent stresses. *British Journal of Rheumatology* **32**, 956–965.

Yarasheki, K.E., Campbell, J.A. & Korht, W.M. (1997) Effect of resistance exercise and growth hormone on bone density in older men. *Clinical Endocrinology* **47**, 223–229.

Chapter 19

Endocrine Responses and Adaptations to Strength and Power Training

WILLIAM J. KRAEMER AND NICHOLAS A. RATAMESS

Introduction

Strength and power training present a potent stimulus to the musculoskeletal system. This type of stress elicits a wide variety of physiological responses and subsequent adaptations instrumental to the increases in muscular strength, power, hypertrophy and local muscular endurance observed during resistance training (Kraemer & Ratamess 2000). One such physiological system vital to acute resistance exercise performance and tissue remodelling is the neuroendocrine system (Kraemer 2000). Furthermore, chronic adaptations in the neuroendocrine system have been related to force production (Häkkinen 1989).

Hormonal increases in response to resistance exercise take place in a physiological environment that is quite unique. More specifically, tissue repair mechanisms are activated as part of the remodelling process during the recovery period from the mechanical and chemical stresses of exercise. A variety of hormonal mechanisms influence tissue growth and remodelling (e.g. muscle, bone and other connective tissue) which are critical to strength and power performance.

Several hormones are discussed in this chapter. Emphasis is placed upon those anabolic and catabolic hormones most relevant to skeletal muscle tissue remodelling. Adaptations to resistance training entail three general classifications: (i) acute changes during and after resistance exercise; (ii) chronic changes in resting concentrations; and (iii) chronic changes in the acute response to a resistance exercise stimulus. Other factors such as nutritional intake, training experience, gender, age and/or maturity, interaction with other modalities of exercise and diurnal variations, as well as the resistance training programme, affect the endocrine responses and adaptations to resistance training and are discussed in this chapter.

The resistance exercise stimulus

The resistance exercise stimulus is the primary factor determining both the acute and chronic hormonal responses and adaptations. The acute programme variables associated with resistance training have been described in detail (Kraemer & Fleck 1988; Fleck & Kraemer 1997; Kraemer & Ratamess 2000; Kraemer *et al.* 2000). These variables include:

- Exercise selection and order.
- Mode of muscle action.
- Intensity.
- Volume (e.g. number of exercises, sets and total repetitions).
- Repetition velocity.
- Rest periods between sets and exercises.
- Frequency.
- Muscle groups trained (e.g. total body, upper/lower body split, muscle group split routine).

All of these training programme variables affect the acute metabolic, neural, muscular and cardiovascular responses to resistance exercise. Such systems interact with the endocrine system in the acute expression of muscular strength,

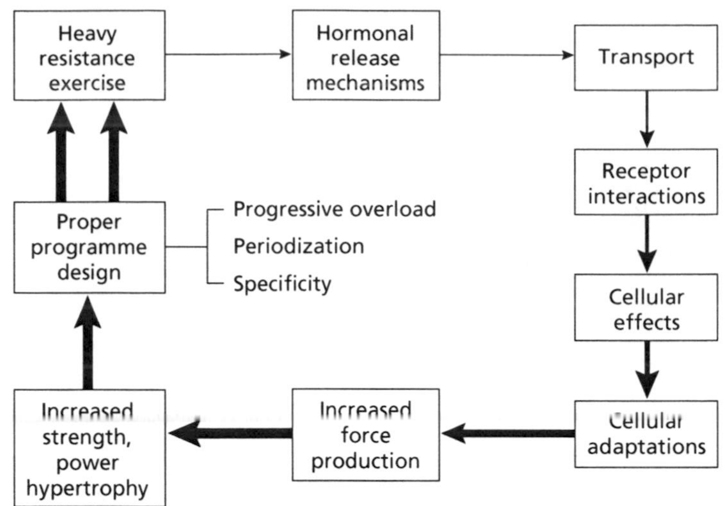

Fig. 19.1 Theoretical sequence of events demonstrating the influence of resistance exercise on hormonal effects leading to increased strength and power performances.

power and endurance and in the subsequent chronic adaptations. A general schematic sequence of events is presented in Fig. 19.1.

Proper resistance training programme design will incorporate three fundamental concepts of progression, i.e. progressive overload, variation and specificity, which attempt to maximize adaptations of the neuromuscular system (Kraemer & Ratamess 2000). For example, with progressive overload motor unit recruitment will increase (Sale 1988). Recruitment of a greater number of muscle fibres enables hormone–tissue interaction with a larger percentage of the total muscle mass. Thus, the potential for improvement significantly increases.

The mechanisms of hormonal interaction with muscle tissue are based on several factors (see Chapter 5). Acute increases in circulating blood hormone concentrations observed during and immediately following a resistance exercise protocol present a greater probability of interaction with receptors. Coinciding with blood hormonal concentrations is the number of receptors available for binding and subsequent cellular changes. Secondly, considering that adaptations to heavy-resistance exercise are 'anabolic' in nature, the recovery mechanisms involved are related to tissue remodelling and repair. Lastly, improper resistance training programme design (e.g. detraining and/or overtraining) may limit the potential benefit and optimal physiological adaptations. Accordingly, hormonal mechanisms will either adversely affect tissue development or minimally activate mechanisms that augment the adaptational processes. Thus, the training programme as well as genetic predisposition, gender, fitness level and the potential for adaptation all play significant roles in the hormonal responses to resistance exercise.

Acute increases in circulating concentrations of hormones in the blood result via several mechanisms. These include shifts in fluid volume, changes in extrahepatic clearance rates, changes in hepatic clearance rates secondary to hepatic blood flow, hormonal degradation, venous pooling of blood and receptor interactions (Jezova & Vigas 1981; Kraemer *et al.* 1992; Schwab *et al.* 1993). One or more of these may be involved in exposing cellular receptors to a greater magnitude of hormones, thereby increasing the likelihood of receptor interactions leading to tissue remodelling. In addition, the interaction of these hormones (e.g. stimulatory, inhibitory or permissive actions) is of great importance during resistance training as both metabolic and force production demands must be met in addition to tissue repair. The time course of blood sampling during resistance exercise is also very important as it provides a physiological window for viewing the effects of the exercise stress. Because resistance exercise is intermittent in nature, samples are typically obtained immediately following the exercise stress. When examining longer recovery periods, diurnal hormonal variations must be controlled for. Lastly, the pre-exercise concentrations will ultimately affect the acute resistance exercise response of the hormone and determine the magnitude of change. Thus, training effects on the basal concentrations, timing of blood samples due to diurnal variations, and other induced effects on the pre-exercise concentrations must be accounted for when evaluating exercise-induced responses.

Hormonal changes in peripheral blood

In a study by Kraemer *et al.* (1998b) the consistency of response of various hormones in the blood on 3 consecutive days of exercise demonstrated the reproducibility of the hormone response (a response fingerprint, so to speak) to a given resistance training workout protocol (see Fig. 19.2) can be replicated with great consistency. Such data indicate that hormones are tightly linked to the characteristics of the resistance exercise protocol and can be replicated day to day.

Blood can be drawn from athletes at various stages of training and hormone concentrations in the blood samples determined. While interpretation of blood concentrations of hormones can be 'tricky', as it is only one part of the whole hormonal response puzzle, such data do provide an indication of the status or responses of the glands or functional status of the mechanisms controlled by the hormone. It should be noted that peripheral concentrations of hormones in the blood do not indicate the status of the various receptor populations, the non-receptor effects or the effects of a hormone within the cell. It is typically assumed, however, that if large increases in hormone concentration are observed, higher probabilities for interactions with receptors or target cells exist. Decreases in hormonal concentrations indicate several possible fates for the hormone including higher uptake into the target tissue receptors and/or greater degradation of the hormone and/or decreased secretion of the hormone. Many different physiological mechanisms may contribute in varying degrees to the observed changes in peripheral blood concentrations of hormones. Figure 19.3 shows a sequence of mechanisms that may affect the concentration of the hormone. A few of the major ones are the following.

• *Synthesis and degradation rates*. Each hormone has its own synthesis rates (e.g. steroidogenesis 35 min) and half-life for degradation depending upon whether it is free or bound.

• *Interactions with binding proteins in the blood.* Hormones bind with specialized proteins in the blood that help with transport. Free hormones

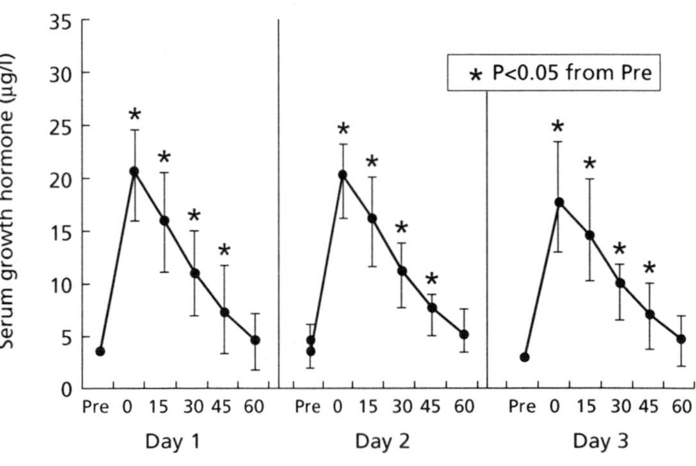

Fig. 19.2 Responses of growth hormone to repeated days of the same resistance exercise protocol, showing the remarkable reproducibility of hormonal changes in the circulation in response to resistance exercise stress. (Adapted from Kraemer *et al.* 1998b.)

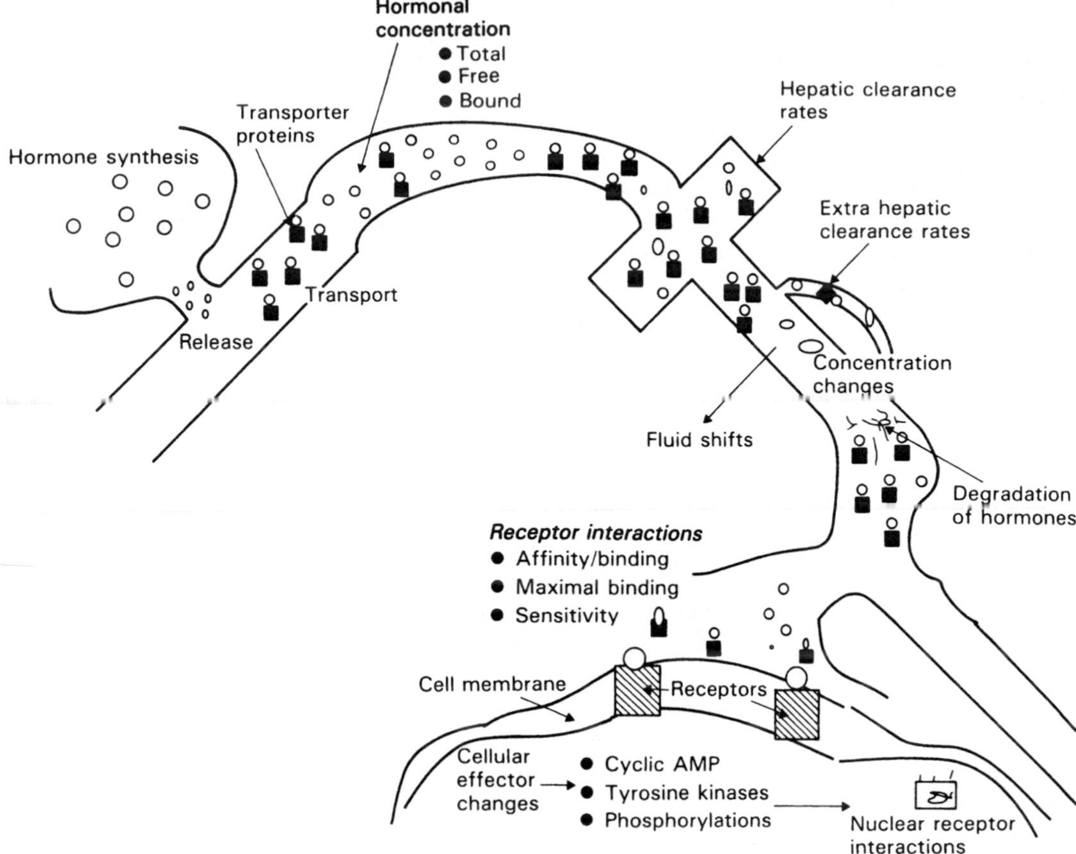

Fig. 19.3 Circulatory fates of hormone transport from synthesis and secretion to target receptor interactions with the cell.

and bound hormones all interact differently with tissue; ultimately, it is the free hormone that interacts with the membrane or other cellular receptors.

• *Fluid volume shifts.* Body fluid tends to shift from the blood to the cells as a result of exercise. This shift can increase hormone concentrations in the blood without any changes of secretion from endocrine glands. It has been hypothesized that regardless of the mechanism of increase, such concentration changes increase receptor interaction probabilities.

• *Clearance rates.* Tissue (especially liver) clearance rates of a hormone; that is, the time it takes a hormone to go through the circulation of the tissue. Hormones circulate through various tissues and organs, the liver being one of the major processing organs in the body. Time delays are seen as the hormone goes through the circulation in the liver and other tissues (e.g. lungs). The clearance time of a tissue keeps the hormone out of the circulation and away from contact with target receptors in other parts of the body, or can degrade it and make it non-functional.

• *Venous pooling of blood.* Blood flow back to the heart is slowed by pooling of blood in veins; the blood is delayed in the peripheral circulation by intense muscle activity (muscle actions greater than 45% of maximal). Thus, blood flow must recover during intervals when muscle activity is reduced. The pooling of the blood can increase the concentrations of hormones in the venous blood and also increase time of exposure to target tissues.

• *Receptor interactions.* All these mechanisms interact to produce a certain concentration of a hormone in the blood, which influences the potential for interaction with the receptors in target tissue and their subsequent secondary effects, leading to the final effect of the hormone on a cell.

While organs such as muscle and connective tissue are the ultimate targets of most resistance training programmes, many adaptations occur within the endocrine system as well. These changes are temporally related to changes in the target organs and the toleration of exercise stress. The potential for adaptation in the endocrine system is great with so many different sites and mechanisms that can be affected. The following are examples of the potential types of adaptations that are possible.

• Amount of synthesis and storage of hormones.
• Transport of hormones via binding proteins.
• Time needed for the clearance of hormones through hepatic and extrahepatic tissues.
• Amount of hormonal degradation that takes place over a given period of time.
• How much of a blood to tissue fluid shift occurs with exercise stress.
• How tightly the hormone binds to its receptor (receptor affinity), which does not occur with exercise training.
• How many receptors are in the tissue.
• The magnitude of the signal sent to the cell nucleus by the hormone–receptor complex or second messenger.
• The degree of interaction with the cell nucleus (which would dictate how much muscle protein is to be produced).

Testosterone

Acute responses to a resistance exercise protocol

Resistance training has been shown to acutely increase peripheral blood concentrations of total testosterone in most studies in men (Weiss *et al.* 1983; Chandler *et al.* 1994; Hickson *et al.* 1994; Häkkinen & Pakarinen 1995; Kraemer *et al.* 1998b, 1999) while in young women no change (Häkkinen & Pakarinen 1995) or an increase (Cumming *et al.* 1987; Nindl *et al.* 2001d) may take place. A wide variety of responses to various resistance exercise protocols have been observed and some of the variations are shown in Fig. 19.4. In addition, testosterone increases observed during resistance exercise have also been attributed to adrenergic stimulation (Jezova & Vigas 1981) and lactate-stimulated secretion (Lu *et al.* 1997). The possible actions of testosterone have been previously reviewed (see Chapter 5). It has been suggested that adaptations in testosterone synthesis and/or secretory capacity of the Leydig cells in the testes may be an important cause of the elevation (Fry & Kraemer 1997). Its role in augmentation of other hormonal anabolic mechanisms appears to be of primary interest. In addition, the effects of testosterone on peripheral neuronal tissue are beginning to be appreciated (Nagaya & Herrera 1995). Since testosterone increases have been observed during endurance exercise, variations in its actions may be due to differences in the cellular environment consequent to resistance training.

It is the free, or unbound, fraction of testosterone that is biologically active such that changes in the pool of free testosterone play a critical role in receptor binding and subsequent increases in protein synthesis. In this manner, the lack of change in total testosterone concentration may not always be reflective of the bioavailability of this hormone. Thus, a decrease in sex hormone binding globulin (SHBG) coupled with no change in total testosterone concentrations indicates a potential beneficial adaptation to resistance training.

Scant data are available concerning the acute free testosterone resistance exercise response. Häkkinen *et al.* (1987, 1988a,b) have observed that free testosterone remains unaltered or decreases after resistance exercise workouts. Recently, Kraemer *et al.* (1999b) reported significant elevations in serum free testosterone during an acute bout of resistance exercise in both young and

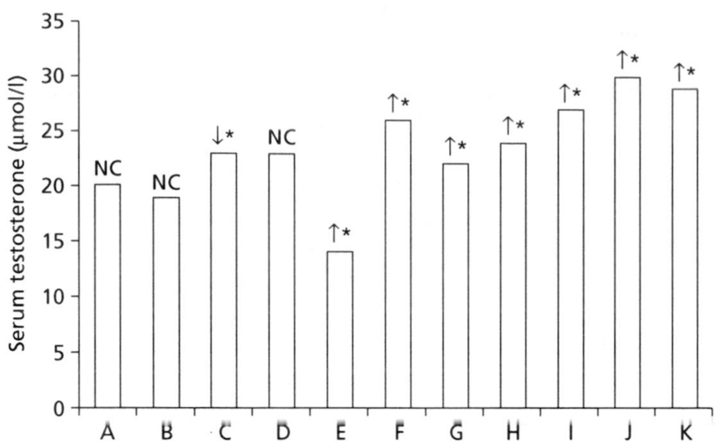

Fig. 19.4 Acute testosterone responses to various resistance exercise protocols in men. *, $P < 0.05$ from corresponding resting or pre-exercise value; ↑ or ↓ signify direction of change; NC signifies no change from rest. A, 1 set of bench presses, maximal number at 70% of 1 RM (1 repetition maximum) (Guezennec *et al.* 1986); B, 6 sets of 8 repetitions of bench press-ups at 70% of 1 RM (Guezennec *et al.* 1986); C, full Olympic exercise workout (second day) (Häkkinen *et al.* 1988a); D, full Olympic exercise workout (first workout) (Häkkinen *et al.* 1988a); E, 3 sets of 4 exercises at 80% of 1 RM (Weiss *et al.* 1983); F, 5 sets of deadlifts at 5 RM—unskilled participants (Fahey *et al.* 1976); G, 5 sets of deadlifts at 5 RM—skilled participants (Fahey *et al.* 1976); H, 4 sets of squats for 6 repetitions at 90–95% of 6 RM (Schwab *et al.* 1993); I & J, 8 exercises performed for 3 sets of 10 RM with 1-min rest intervals (Kraemer *et al.* 1990, 1991); K, bench press, sit-up, leg press for 5 sets of 10 RM with 3-min rest intervals (Häkkinen & Pakarinen 1995).

elderly men. Interestingly, the magnitude of increase was slightly greater after 10 weeks of periodized strength training compared to the pretraining response. In addition, a significant increase in resting serum free testosterone was observed in the young men. Positive correlations have been reported between the serum testosterone/SHBG ratio and changes in muscular strength during long-term resistance training (Häkkinen *et al.* 1985), suggesting that the level of biologically active unbound testosterone may be of great importance for trainability during prolonged resistance training (Häkkinen 1989). However, further research is warranted in this area as it appears that the bound hormone could significantly influence the rate of hormone delivery (Elkins 1990).

In men several factors appear to influence the acute serum concentrations of total testosterone. The magnitude of increase during resistance exercise has been shown to be affected by the muscle mass involved (Volek *et al.* 1997), exercise selection (Volek *et al.* 1997), intensity and volume (Kraemer *et al.* 1990, 1991; Häkkinen & Pakarinen 1993; Schwab *et al.* 1993; Bosco *et al.* 2000; Raastad *et al.* 2000), nutrition intake (Kraemer *et al.* 1998b) and training experience (Kraemer *et al.* 1998a), but is independent of the individual's absolute level of muscular strength (Kraemer & Fleck 1988).

The exercises selected and amount of muscle mass involved may affect the acute response of total testosterone to resistance exercise. Large muscle mass exercises such as the Olympic lifts (Kraemer *et al.* 1992) and deadlift (Fahey *et al.* 1976) have been shown to produce significant elevations in testosterone. Volek *et al.* (1997) reported an approximate 15% acute increase in testosterone concentration following a protocol consisting of jump squats as opposed to a 7% increase in testosterone following a protocol consisting entirely of the bench press. These large muscle mass exercises have been shown to be potent metabolic stressors (Ballor *et al.* 1987); thus a strong metabolic component has been suggested as a stimulus for testosterone release (Lu *et al.* 1997). Based on the limited data it does appear that programmes designed to stimulate testosterone secretion should consist of large muscle mass exercises. In addition, the sequencing of exercises has not received attention in the literature concerning the acute testosterone response. It has been suggested for strength training that large muscle mass exercises be performed before small muscle mass exercises (Kraemer & Ratamess 2000). In light of this information, it has been suggested that performance of large muscle mass exercises (i.e. squat, deadlift, power clean) early in the workout may produce significant elevations in testosterone which may potentially expose smaller muscles to a greater response than that resulting from performance of small muscle mass exercises only. However, further research is warranted examining this exercise order hypothesis.

The interaction of intensity and volume of the resistance training programme affects the acute testosterone responses. Gotshalk *et al.* (1997) showed that 3 sets of 10 RM with 1-min rest periods produced higher concentrations than 1 set of 10 RM. Weiss *et al.* (1983) reported a significant increase in serum testosterone following 3 sets of 4 exercises performed to failure using 80% of 1 RM with 2-min rest intervals. Raastad *et al.* (2000) used two similar protocols, with the exception that one group used 70% of 3–6 RM and the second group used 100% of 3–6 RM and reported significantly greater testosterone and cortisol response following the high-intensity protocol up to 1 h post exercise. Schwab *et al.* (1993) compared a protocol of 4 × 6 (90–95% of 6 RM) to 4 × 9–10 (60–65% of load used for high intensity) for the squat and reported similar increases in testosterone following both protocols (31 and 27% increase, respectively, for the high- and moderate-intensity protocols). However, testosterone did not significantly increase until after the fourth set. The authors concluded that a threshold of volume may be needed to elicit significant increases in testosterone. A similar observation was made by Bosco *et al.* (2000) who reported significant increases in testosterone with high-volume resistance training with no change during lower-volume resistance training (20 sets of 2–4 repetitions of half squats vs. 10 sets of 2–3 repetitions) in weightlifters. However, in this study testosterone concentrations decreased in a group of bodybuilders who performed a low-intensity protocol with higher volume than the weightlifters, thus demonstrating the interaction between volume and intensity of resistance exercise for stimulating testosterone secretion. Häkkinen and Pakarinen (1993) compared two squat training programmes: (i) 20 sets of 1 RM; and (ii) 10 sets of 10 repetitions with 70% of 1 RM, and reported that significant increases in total and free testosterone occurred only in the higher-volume workout. Guezennec *et al.* (1986) reported only minor increases in testosterone during conventional strength training (i.e. 3–4 sets of 3–10 repetitions at 70–95% of 1 RM, 2.5-min rest periods). However, when load was increased further and repetitions decreased to 3, a limited testosterone response was observed. These results also demonstrate a possible glycolytic component for stimulating testosterone release. These results were further supported by a series of studies by Kraemer *et al.* (1990, 1991) in which a body building programme (moderate load, high volume) with short rest periods produced greater testosterone responses than high-load, low-volume training with long (i.e. 3-min) rest periods and by Bosco *et al.* (2000) who reported a decrease in testosterone concentrations with a low volume (6 sets of 16 repetitions total) programme with 8-min rest intervals.

Nutritional supplementation appears to affect the acute testosterone response to resistance exercise. Kraemer *et al.* (1998b) compared the hormonal response to 3 consecutive days of lifting with either a placebo or a carbohydrate/protein supplement, and reported higher testosterone concentrations during the placebo treatment than with a carbohydrate/protein supplement. The additional caloric intake appeared to attenuate circulating testosterone. The rationale for this occurrence is unclear but it may be due to the increased utilization by the androgen receptor. A previous study reported decreased circulating concentrations of testosterone in response to low dietary fat intake and a diet with a high protein/carbohydrate ratio (Volek *et al.* 1997). The mechanism(s) of such a response is unclear and remains to be elucidated. In addition, elevations in insulin concentrations have coincided with decreased testosterone in another study examining protein/carbohydrate supplementation where a similar decreased testosterone response was observed (Chandler *et al.* 1994). Thus, a possible interaction between insulin and testosterone may also contribute to this as one of the mediating mechanisms.

The age and training experience of the individuals play a critical role when examining the acute response of testosterone. Fahey *et al.* (1976) were unable to demonstrate significant increases in males of high school age during resistance exercise whereas college-aged men showed a greater response. Kraemer *et al.* (1992) reported a greater acute increase in junior weightlifters with more than 2 years of lifting experience compared to junior weightlifters with less than 2 years of experience and suggested that increases may occur if the strength training experience is 2 years or more in young men of 14–18 years of age. Kraemer *et al.* (1998a) were unable to demonstrate an acute increase during resistance exercise until previously untrained men had completed at least 6 weeks of an 8-week resistance training programme. However, Craig *et al.* (1989) reported that 12 weeks of resistance training did not alter the acute response to a workout. Older individuals have been shown to produce significant elevations of testosterone during an acute bout of resistance exercise; however, the absolute concentrations are significantly lower than that of younger individuals (Kraemer *et al.* 1999b).

The acute testosterone response in women appears to be very limited (Stoessel *et al.* 1991; Kraemer *et al.* 1993b; Häkkinen & Pakarinen 1995; Bosco *et al.* 2000) as only few studies have shown any change (Cumming *et al.* 1987; Nindl *et al.*, 2001d). Nindl *et al.* (in press) found significant increases in total testosterone (1.24 vs. 1.55 $nmol{\cdot}l^{-1}$; ~25% increase), free testosterone (7.18 vs. 9.0 $pg{\cdot}ml^{-1}$; ~25% increase) and SHGB (145.4 vs. 150.9 $nmol{\cdot}l^{-1}$; ~4% increase) in women in response to 6 sets of a 10-RM squat exercise routine. With the small increases, *n* sizes and individual variations among women play a vital role in detecting the small treatment effects. In addition, variations in adrenal androgen content may play a significant role and be related to differences in women's trainability with resistance exercise. Absolute changes in testosterone concentrations in women are less responsive to resistance exercise than in men (Stoessel *et al.* 1991), especially when the volume is low and rest intervals are high (Bosco *et al.* 2000). In direct comparison of the same protocol (3 exercises, 5 × 10 RM; and 4 exercises, 3 × failure × 80% of 1 RM, respectively) in men and women, Häkkinen and Pakarinen (1995) and Weiss *et al.* (1983) reported significant increases in young men but not in young women. Rather, it appears other anabolic hormones (e.g. growth hormone; insulin-like growth factor I, IGF-I) may be more influential for promoting muscle hypertrophy in women. Nevertheless, small increases appear to be possible with acute resistance exercise in women and the effects of this response over time need to be studied.

The effect of training frequency on the acute testosterone response has not been addressed. Häkkinen *et al.* (1988b) reported a greater testosterone response during afternoon sessions compared to morning sessions in elite weight lifters during multiple training sessions per day. Multiple training sessions per day are common in these athletes in order to maximize performance. However, it is difficult to interpret hormonal data at different training times as diurnal variations are very influential; so also is total training volume, as serum testosterone concentrations increased to normal when training frequency was reduced to one workout per day (Häkkinen *et al.* 1987).

Chronic changes in resting concentrations of testosterone

Changes in resting testosterone concentrations during resistance training have been inconsistent.

There does not appear to be a gradual increase or consistent pattern in resting testosterone concentrations with resistance training in men and women (Alen *et al.* 1988; Potteiger *et al.* 1995), although significant elevations have been reported in both prepubertal and pubertal boys (Tsolakis *et al.* 2000). Rather, it appears that resting concentrations reflect the state of muscle tissue such that increases or decreases may occur at various stages depending on the volume and intensity of the training stimulus (Häkkinen *et al.* 1987), as well as the resistance training experience of the individual (Kraemer *et al.* 1992). These data demonstrate the constantly changing state of muscle tissue and demonstrate the importance of training variation in programme design.

Increased resting concentrations have been reported in some studies (Häkkinen *et al.* 1988c; Staron *et al.* 1994; Kraemer *et al.* 1999b; Marx *et al.* 2001) whereas several studies have shown no differences (Häkkinen *et al.* 1985, 1987; Alen *et al.* 1988; Reaburn *et al.* 1997). Interestingly, the mean concentrations of free and total testosterone have been highly correlated ($r = 0.81–0.83$) to force production (Häkkinen *et al.* 1990). However, following 16 days of overload in rats, testosterone concentrations did not correlate highly with changes in muscle mass (Crowley & Matt 1996). McCall *et al.* (1999) and Hickson *et al.* (1994) reported no change in resting concentrations of testosterone during 9–12 weeks of resistance training. Staron *et al.* (1994) reported significant elevations of resting testosterone concentrations following 4 weeks of an 8-week resistance training programme, and changes in Type II fibres were related to changes in resting testosterone. Häkkinen *et al.* (1988c) reported an increase in resting testosterone in elite weightlifters over a 2-year period ($19.8 \pm 5.3 - 25.1 \pm 5.2$ nmol·l^{-1}), but not, however, during 1 year (Häkkinen *et al.* 1987). Reaburn *et al.* (1997) reported no change in testosterone following 8 weeks of resistance training in veteran sprinters. Potteiger *et al.* (1995) reported no significant changes in resting serum testosterone concentrations over 24 weeks of periodized training in male and female strength athletes. In women, no changes have been observed during 3 and 16 weeks of strength and power training (Häkkinen *et al.* 1990, 1992). However, a recent study by Marx *et al.* (2001) reported significant elevations in resting serum testosterone with the response greater with higher-volume, periodized multiple-set training compared to a single-set programme during 6 months of training.

Perhaps more significant for long-term endocrine adaptations to resistance training is the number of androgen receptors (e.g. via up-regulation or down-regulation) potentially interacting with the biologically active free testosterone. Very few studies have examined changes at the receptor level. Resistance training has been shown to up-regulate androgen receptors in rats (Inoue *et al.* 1993). In addition, Deschenes *et al.* (1994) have shown that the receptor response is different in Type I and Type II muscle in response to resistance vs. endurance exercise in rats. Recently, Bamman *et al.* (2001) compared concentric and eccentric loading (8 sets of squats) and reported that androgen receptor mRNA increased 63% following the eccentric loading and 102% following the concentric loading without concomitant increases in serum testosterone concentrations. These results indicate a positive adaptation at the cellular level without significant changes in circulating hormones. It appears that muscle contractility and/ or mechanical damage has a potent effect in regulating androgen receptor number, thereby increasing the likelihood of hormonal interaction and subsequent protein synthesis.

Androgen precursors

The biosynthetic pathway of testosterone contains many steps. Some of these precursor molecules have been investigated during resistance training. The rationale is that a change in precursors may ultimately affect circulating testosterone concentrations and potentially the anabolic state of muscle tissue. Androstenedione and dehydroepiandrosterone (DHEA) are adrenal androgens which are testosterone precursors (Longcope 1996). These two compounds have received much attention in the literature recently due to their popularity as nutritional supplements and their use in athletics (Pecci & Lombardo 2000). Studies have shown that recommended doses (100–300 mg·day^{-1}) of these compounds do not increase circulating testosterone concentrations in healthy men (King *et al.* 1999; Wallace *et al.* 1999; Ballantyne *et al.* 2000) although the concentrations of DHEA, androstenedione and luteinizing hormone (LH) were significantly elevated. Therefore, the potential ergogenic effects of precursor hormones as they relate to muscle hypertrophy and associated strength and power performances remain to be seen and require further examination, particularly since many individuals consume higher than the recommended dose. The method of administration (oral vs. sublingual vs. injection) may also play a role in such intakes of precursor hormones of testosterone.

Adrenal androgens may play a greater role in women considering the low levels of testosterone present. Additionally, variations in the concentrations of adrenal androgens among women may affect the trainability of women. At rest, women typically have higher concentrations of androstenedione than men (Weiss *et al.* 1983). However, androstenedione is significantly less potent than testosterone. Few studies have examined the acute response to resistance exercise. Using a programme consisting of 4 exercises for 3 sets to failure with 80% of 1 RM and 2-min rest intervals, Weiss *et al.* (1983) reported increases in circulating androstenedione of 8–11% in both men and women in response to an acute bout of resistance exercise. However, little is known concerning the impact of acute increases in androstenedione on muscle strength and hypertrophy increases.

Chronic resistance training (e.g. 24 weeks of strength and power training) has been shown to decrease serum concentrations of the testosterone precursors 17-OH-progesterone, androstenedione and DHEA (Alen *et al.* 1988). The impact of these findings is unclear but may suggest a greater potential rate of androgen turnover in response to resistance training. Thus, the influence of these precursors during long-term resistance training also warrants further investigation.

Responses of luteinizing hormone

Luteinizing hormone (LH) is a pulsatile protein hormone secreted from the basophilic cells of the anterior pituitary, which is the primary regulator of testosterone secretion from the Leydig cells of the testes (Fry & Kraemer 1997). LH concentrations are positively related to the intensity and volume of resistance training (Häkkinen *et al.* 1987; Busso *et al.* 1992). Resting concentrations of LH may not change significantly in men and women during strength and power training within 16–24 weeks (Häkkinen *et al.* 1985, 1990), but slight increases have been shown in strength athletes during intense training periods (Häkkinen *et al.* 1988c; Häkkinen & Pakarinen 1991) with concentrations of LH returning to basal values during normal training (Häkkinen & Pakarinen 1991). It appears that the interaction of intensity and volume are important stimulators. Busso *et al.* (1992) compared a 4-week intensive training programme in elite weightlifters with a 2-week reduced training period and reported a decrease in serum testosterone concentrations with an increase in serum LH during the intense training phase. It was hypothesized that the decrease in testosterone contributed to the increase in LH in which testosterone concentrations did not return to normal until the reduced training phase. Interestingly, serum LH correlated highly with fitness level. In addition, an acute bout of resistance exercise does not induce LH secretion (Häkkinen *et al.* 1988a), therefore suggesting that acute increases in serum testosterone concentrations are due to other regulatory mechanisms. Nindl *et al.* (2001b) found after examining 10 men for 13 h after a resistance exercise protocol that there was a decline in overnight testosterone. These data demonstrate that the decline in overnight testosterone concentrations after acute heavy-resistance exercise is accompanied by elevated cortisol concentrations and a blunted LH production rate. These changes in the pituitary–adrenal–testicular axis are centrally mediated and presumably reflect the myriad of metabolic processes.

Sex hormone binding globulin

Circulating testosterone is predominantly bound to the transport protein SHBG which preserves the integrity of the hormone. A change in SHBG concentrations may influence the binding capacity of testosterone and the magnitude of free testosterone available for diffusion across the cell membrane to interact with membrane-bound steroid receptors. Differential responses have been observed during resistance training. No changes in resting or acute SHBG concentrations have been reported following 12 and 24 weeks of resistance training (Häkkinen *et al.* 1985; McCall *et al.* 1999), following 1 week of intensive Olympic weightlifting (Häkkinen *et al.* 1988a), over a 2-year period in elite Olympic weightlifters (Häkkinen *et al.* 1988c) in men, and following 3 and 16 weeks of strength and power training in women (Häkkinen *et al.* 1990, 1992). However, one study reported an acute increase following 8 weeks of resistance training in previously untrained women (Kraemer *et al.* 1998). Long-term resistance training may result in reduced serum concentrations of SHBG (Häkkinen *et al.* 1987). Häkkinen *et al.* (1988b) reported no acute increases in SHBG during an early morning workout in elite Olympic weightlifters, but reported increases during an afternoon workout on the same day (i.e. two workouts in one day).

Growth hormone

Acute response to resistance exercise

Human growth hormone (GH) is a peptide hormone (22-kDa single-chain polypeptide with 191 amino acids and two disulphide cross-linkages) secreted from the acidophilic cells of the anterior pituitary (Fry & Kraemer 1997). Recent evidence has shown that GH has several different molecular weight variants of the 22-kDa form, many with potential biological activity (McCall *et al.* 1999). Yet a diversity in post-transcriptional and post-translational events as well as the somatotroph types results in a much more complicated picture. The result is a wide array of monomeric variants and higher-level polymers. The majority of these plasma GH variants can be summarized best by dividing them into three broad categories based upon molecular weight. Approximately 31.5% are unbound monomeric forms of GH (22 kDa, 20 kDa and acidic). Various covalently and non-covalently linked homo- and heterodimers of the three monomeric forms account for 29% (40–50 kDa). Higher molecular weight (tri- to pentameric) polymeric aggregates (14%) and binding protein–monomer complexes (24.5%) are all greater than 60 kDa. The small remaining percentage is comprised of varying amounts of GH peptide fragments believed to originate from the pituitary as well as to result from partial degradation in peripheral tissues and subsequent recirculation or smaller novel peptides yet undetermined. Investigators have characterized three distinct molecular weight ranges to generally characterize GH variants as 'little' (20–22 kDa), 'big' (40–50 kDa) and 'big big' (> 60 kDa). The gene-based molecular weight of the typical GH monomer is the 22-kDa GH molecule.

Although net uptake of GH has been observed during dynamic exercise in humans (Brahm *et al.* 1997), some of the effects of GH are mediated through insulin-like growth factors (IGFs), primarily IGF-I (see Chapter 5). Little is known concerning the acute and chronic response of different molecular weight variants of the GH molecule to resistance training since the immunoreactive methodologies used were not sensitive to all forms of GH. Thus, the remainder of this section (and all subsequent responses and adaptations) typically refers to the well-known 22-kDa form of GH (see Chapter 5 for an overview of other GH responses).

The variety of exercise responses of the 22-kDa GH in the blood to resistance exercise can be variable depending upon the programme used (see Fig. 19.5). Human GH has been shown to increase during resistance exercise and 30 min

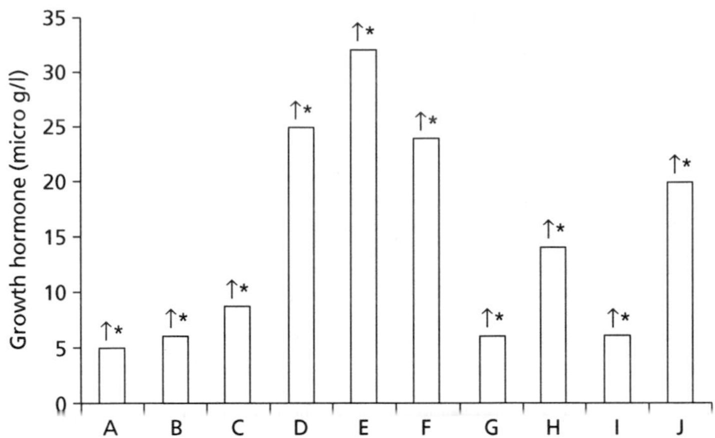

Fig. 19.5 Acute growth hormone responses to various resistance exercise protocols in men. *, $P < 0.05$ from corresponding resting or pre-exercise value; ↑ or ↓ signify direction of change. A, 7 sets of 7 repetitions at 85% of 7 RM (Van Helder *et al.* 1984); B, Olympic lifting training session (first day) at 70–100% of 1 RM (Häkkinen *et al.* 1988c); C, 8 exercises for 3 sets of 10 RM with 1-min rest intervals (McCall *et al.* 1999); D, 4 exercises for 2 sets of 8–10 repetitions with 75% of 1 RM with 90-s rest intervals (Chandler *et al.* 1994); E, Olympic weightlifting session (Kraemer *et al.* 1992); F & H, 8 exercises for 3 sets of 10 RM with 1-min rest intervals (Kraemer *et al.* 1990, 1991); G & I, 8 exercises for 3–5 sets of 5 RM with 3-min rest intervals (Kraemer *et al.* 1990, 1991); J, bench press, sit-up, leg press for 5 sets of 10 RM with 3-min rest intervals (Häkkinen & Pakarinen 1995).

post exercise with the magnitude dependent upon exercise selection (Häkkinen *et al.* 1988a,b; Kraemer *et al.* 1992), intensity (Van Helder *et al.* 1984; Pyka *et al.* 1992), volume (Häkkinen *et al.* 1988a,b; Häkkinen & Pakarinen 1993; Bosco *et al.* 2000; Williams *et al.* 2002), rest periods between sets (Kraemer *et al.* 1990, 1991, 1995a) and carbohydrate/protein supplementation (Chandler *et al.* 1994); independent of muscular strength (Kraemer 1988), training experience in men (Kraemer *et al.* 1992) but not women (Taylor *et al.* 2000), and may be somewhat attenuated with short-term detraining (Kraemer *et al.*, 2002). By measuring arterial and venous concentrations of GH during and following an acute bout of resistance exercise, it was shown that GH uptake in skeletal muscle (quadriceps) increases significantly (Brahm *et al.* 1997). These data show that GH may act directly or through the IGF system. In addition, high correlations have been reported between blood lactate and serum GH concentrations (Häkkinen & Pakarinen 1993). It has been proposed that H^+ accumulation produced by lactic acidosis may be the primary factor influencing GH release (Kraemer *et al.* 1993). This finding was supported by an attenuated GH response following induced alkalosis during high-intensity cycling (Gordon *et al.* 1994). Hypoxia, breath holding, acid–base shifts and protein catabolism have been reported to influence GH release (Kraemer *et al.* 1993b). Thus, the metabolic demands of resistance exercise play a significant role in GH concentrations.

Not all resistance training programmes will produce a significant elevation in serum GH concentrations; thus a threshold volume and intensity (i.e. level of exertion) may be needed. Van Helder *et al.* (1984) did not report a significant increase in GH using very light loads for high repetitions. Taylor *et al.* (2000) reported a greater acute increase in resistance-trained women than in non-trained women to the same glycolytic protocol. However, the trained women were capable of lifting greater loads and perhaps this affected the overall magnitude of exertion. It has been shown that the acute GH response is somewhat limited in older individuals (Craig *et al.* 1989; Pyka *et al.* 1992; Kraemer *et al.* 1999b).

However, it has been suggested that a major factor contributing to this limited GH response may be the magnitude of exertion displayed. Pyka *et al.* (1992) also reported lower lactates in the elderly subjects, thereby supporting the hypothesis that maximal effort is necessary for optimizing the exercise-induced secretion of GH. However, resistance training over 12 weeks in the elderly has been shown to promote a greater acute GH response to a resistance exercise protocol (Craig *et al.* 1989), possibly suggesting the greater response was due to an increased ability to exert oneself.

Resistance training programmes may span a wide continuum of loads and repetition numbers for various exercises, lifting velocities, and rest intervals depending on the goals of the individual (Fleck & Kraemer 1997). Moderate-to-high intensity, high-volume programmes using short rest periods have shown the greatest acute GH response compared to conventional strength or power training using high loads, low repetitions and long rest intervals in men (Kraemer *et al.* 1990, 1991). Similar results have been reported in women, although the resting concentrations of GH are significantly higher in women during the early follicular phase of the menstrual cycle (Kraemer *et al.* 1993b). Häkkinen and Pakarinen (1993) reported that 20 sets of 1 RM in the squat only produced a slight increase in GH, whereas a substantial increase in GH was observed following 10 sets of 10 repetitions with 70% of 1 RM. Multiple-set protocols have elicited greater GH response than single-set protocols (Craig & Kang 1994; Mulligan *et al.* 1996; Gotshalk *et al.* 1997), thus showing the importance of training volume. These data indicate that programmes moderate in intensity but high in total work or volume using short rest intervals (e.g. body building or programmes targeting local muscular endurance) may elicit the greatest increases in GH concentrations, this probably being due to high metabolic demands.

Recently, it has been shown that the muscle action may affect the acute GH response to resistance exercise. Kraemer *et al.* (2001b) had subjects train for 19 weeks performing either all concentric repetitions, concentric repetitions with double the volume, or concentric and eccentric repetitions, and the acute response to a resistance exercise protocol consisting of either concentric or eccentric muscle actions was measured before and afterwards. The GH response was high for the concentric training groups for the concentric protocol; however, the acute response was greater for the eccentric protocol for the concentric/eccentric training group. The data indicate that GH is sensitive to the muscle actions used during resistance training. It has been shown that the anterior pituitary may be directly innervated by nerve fibres mostly with synapses on corticotroph and somatotroph cells (Ju 1999). It has also been suggested that 'neural–humoral' regulation of GH secretion may take place such that a rapid neural response is observed during the initial stress with the humoral phase subsequently occurring (Ju 1999). If such is the case then it may be possible for higher brain centres (e.g. the motor cortex), to play an active role in regulating GH secretion during stress, and this regulatory mechanism appears to be sensitive to the specific muscle actions used during resistance training.

In a rare look at the effects of resistance exercise on GH and some of the molecular variants over the course of a night, Nindl *et al.* (2001c) examined the hypothesis that acute heavy-resistance exercise would increase overnight concentrations of circulating GH. Ten young men underwent two overnight serial blood draws sampled every 10 min from 1700 h to 0600 h: a control and a resistance exercise condition. The high-volume heavy-resistance exercise protocol (i.e. high-volume, multiset exercise bout 50 sets total: squat, bench press, leg press, latissimus pulldown that alternated between 10 and 5 repetition maximum sets with 90-s rest periods between sets) was conducted from 1500 h to 1700 h. Three different immunoassays were used to measure GH concentrations including polyclonal, monoclonal and immunofunctional assays each describing a different aspect of the GH molecule (e.g. immunofunctional assay measures those molecules that have both epitopes available for dimerization and signal transduction). In general, GH was lower over time compared to the non-exercise control condition. It was revealed that there was a lower mean pulse amplitude for the exercise vs. control when assessed using the assays, as well as a differential temporal pattern of release (i.e. lower GH from 2100 h to 0300 h, but higher GH from 0300 h to 0600 h for the exercise vs. control). The lower responses following exercise may implicate greater uptake by the receptors or alternate use of other forms of the GH molecule. Assay effects were observed showing that what happens to GH is a function of the assay detection system that is used. It might be concluded that daytime resistance exercise can influence the temporal pattern of overnight GH pulsatility and there may be biological relevance as different types of GH molecules were also differentially affected.

Chronic changes in resting GH concentrations

Resistance training does not appear to affect resting concentrations of GH. No changes in resting GH concentrations have been observed in several studies (Kraemer *et al.* 1999b; McCall *et al.* 1999; Marx *et al.* 2001). This contention is also supported by data demonstrating normal resting concentrations of GH in elite Olympic weightlifters (Häkkinen *et al.* 1988a,b). These data are consistent with dynamic feedback mechanisms GH is involved with and its roles in the homeostatic control of several variables, e.g. glucose. This may be due to the interactive effects of different GH molecules, aggregates and variants with training. In addition, these data suggest that the acute responses of GH to resistance exercise may be the most prominent mechanism for interacting acutely with tissue target receptors leading to remodelling. The exercise-induced increase has been significantly correlated with the magnitude of Type I and Type II muscle fibre hypertrophy ($r = 0.62 - 0.74$) (McCall *et al.* 1999). These relationships could be indicative of a role for repeated acute resistance exercise-induced GH elevations on cellular adaptations in trained muscle. Changes in receptor sensitivity, other molecular size GH molecules playing a role, differences in feedback mechanisms, IGF-I potentiation, and diurnal variations may also play significant roles with resistance training.

Cortisol

Acute response to resistance exercise

Glucocorticoids are released from the adrenal cortex in response to exercise. Of these, cortisol accounts for approximately 95% of all glucocorticoid activity (Guyton 1991). Cortisol has catabolic functions which have greater effects in Type II muscle fibres (Kraemer 2000). Studies have shown significant elevations in cortisol and adrenocorticotrophic hormone (ACTH) during an acute bout of resistance exercise (Guezennec *et al.* 1986; Kraemer *et al.* 1987, 1992, 1993b, 1996, 1999b; Häkkinen *et al.* 1988), with the response similar between men and women (Kraemer *et al.* 1993b), although one study has reported an increase in cortisol in men but not women who performed the same protocol (Häkkinen & Pakarinen 1995). The acute cortisol response appears to be independent of training status at least in adolescent weightlifters (Kraemer *et al.* 1992). It has been reported that the acute increase in cortisol secretion during resistance exercise may be attenuated in anabolic steroid users (Boone *et al.* 1990). Although it has been suggested by one investigator that elevations in cortisol may attenuate the effects of testosterone (Cumming *et al.* 1989), no such relationships have been reported for resistance exercise-induced elevations.

Interestingly, programmes that elicit the greatest cortisol response also elicit the greatest acute GH and lactate response. Significant correlations between blood lactate and serum cortisol ($r = 0.64$) have been reported (Kraemer *et al.* 1989). In addition, acute elevations in serum cortisol have been highly correlated ($r = 0.84$) to 24-h post-exercise serum creatine kinase concentrations (Kraemer *et al.* 1993b). Metabolically demanding protocols (i.e. high volume, moderate to high intensity with short rest periods, have shown the greatest acute cortisol responses (Kraemer *et al.* 1987, 1993b; Häkkinen & Pakarinen 1993) with little change during conventional strength/power training. It appears that rest period length is an important variable for eliciting a significant cortisol response (Kraemer *et al.* 1987, 1993b). This may be due to the greater reliance on glycolytic sources and impact on glucose metabolism. Kraemer *et al.* (1996) reported that performing 8 sets of 10 RM leg press exercise with 1-min rest periods between sets elicited a significantly greater acute cortisol response than the same protocol using 3-min rest periods. Therefore, while chronic high levels of cortisol may have adverse effects on some systems and inhibit some cellular processes (e.g. inhibiting activation of T cells), acute increases may be part of a larger acute set of signalling mechanisms and a remodelling process in muscle tissue.

Chronic adaptations in resting cortisol concentrations

Cortisol concentrations have been generally thought to reflect the long-term training stress. Chronic resistance training does not appear to produce consistent patterns of cortisol secretion as no change (Häkkinen *et al.* 1987, 1988c, 1990, 1992; Fry *et al.* 1994; Potteiger *et al.* 1995), decreases (Häkkinen *et al.* 1985; Alen *et al.* 1988; Kraemer *et al.* 1998a; McCall *et al.* 1999; Marx *et al.* 2001) and increases (Häkkinen & Pakarinen 1991) have been reported during normal strength and power training in men and women and during overreaching-type training. Häkkinen *et al.* (1985) reported greater reductions in resting serum cortisol after 24 weeks of strength training compared to power training. Marx *et al.* (2001) compared periodized multiple-set resistance training to single-set training over 6 months and reported that only the higher-volume group experienced a significant reduction in resting serum cortisol. Recently, Kraemer *et al.* (1999b) reported that resting concentrations of serum cortisol decreased by the 3rd week of a 10-week programme in elderly individuals. A recent animal study has shown that cortisol concentrations may explain most of the variance (~ 60%) in muscle mass changes (Crowley & Matt 1996). Thus it appears that the acute cortisol responses may reflect metabolic stress whereas the chronic adaptation may be involved with tissue homeostasis involving protein metabolism (Florini 1987). Again, as pointed out in the earlier chapter on hormonal mechanisms, there is the finding that with resistance training, testosterone receptors may become adapted to the higher levels of cortisol (i.e. corticosterone in rats) produced with acute exercise stress and become 'disinhibited' whereby the cortisol molecules do not affect the testosterone production or binding characteristics at the level of the testes (unpublished observations). Here again, an increase in cortisol alone may not reflect the adaptive nature of the muscle itself but other cellular targets may still be negatively affected by the acute increases in cortisol (immune cells). Such differential effects related to cell targets require further examination within the context of acute resistance exercise and chronic training.

Testosterone/cortisol ratio

The testosterone/cortisol ratio (T/C ratio) and/or free testosterone/cortisol ratio have been suggested to be indicators of the anabolic/catabolic status during resistance training (Häkkinen 1989). Thus, either an increase in testosterone, a decrease in cortisol, or both would indicate tissue anabolism. However, this appears to be an oversimplification and is at best only a gross indirect measure of the anabolic/catabolic properties of skeletal muscle (Fry & Kraemer 1997). Several studies have shown changes in the T/C ratio during strength and power training and this ratio has been positively related to performance (Häkkinen *et al.* 1985; Alen *et al.* 1988). Stressful training (overreaching) in elite weightlifters has been shown to decrease the T/C ratio (Häkkinen *et al.* 1987). Periodized, higher-volume programmes have been shown to produce a significantly greater increase in the T/C ratio than a low-volume single-set programme (Marx *et al.* 2001). However, in an animal study where the T/C ratio was manipulated to investigate muscle hypertrophy, it was reported that the T/C ratio was not a useful indicator of tissue anabolism (Crowley & Matt 1996). Thus, the popular use of the T/C ratio in monitoring overall anabolic and catabolic status of the human body has been shown to reflect some biological status with training. However, it remains unclear as to what system it is actually reflecting as its underlying biological basis as this may not be muscle *per se*.

Insulin-like growth factors

Acute response to resistance exercise

Many of the actions of GH are regulated by the small polypeptides insulin-like growth factors I and II (IGF-I and IGF-II). IGFs are secreted by the liver in response to GH-stimulated DNA synthesis. The acute response of IGF-I to resistance exercise remains unclear. Most studies have shown no change in IGF-I during or immediately following an acute bout of resistance exercise (Chandler *et al.* 1994; Kraemer *et al.* 1995a, 1998b), whereas a few studies have shown acute increases during and after resistance exercise (Kraemer *et al.* 1990, 1991). The lack of change has been attributed to delayed secretion of IGF-I, i.e. 3–9 h, following GH-stimulated messenger RNA synthesis (Kraemer *et al.* 1993b), as peak values may not be reached until 16–28 h post stimulated GH release (Chandler *et al.* 1994). Thus, the majority of research indicates that the response of IGF-I is delayed. In addition, it has been shown that an acute bout of resistance exercise did not influence IGF-I specifically but significantly affected the manner in which IGF-I was partitioned among its family of binding proteins (Nindl *et al.* 2001). Therefore, an acute bout of resistance may or may not increase circulating IGF-I concentrations but appears to affect its activity by modifying its affinity for binding proteins.

IGF-I has been shown to have autocrine/paracrine functions within muscle cells (Adams 1998; Goldspink 1999). This isoform of IGF-I in muscle has been called mechanogrowth factor (MGF) (Goldspink 1999). It appears to be produced by overloaded muscle and subsequent mechanical damage, e.g. resistance training, and is a prominent regulator of tissue repair (Goldspink 1999; Bamman *et al.* 2001). Bamman *et al.* (2001) reported significant elevations in muscle IGF-I mRNA following resistance exercise, particularly during eccentric resistance exercise. Brahm *et al.* (1997) have shown that during intensive exercise, arterial concentrations of IGF-I remained constant. However, venous concentrations of IGF-I increased which may indicate that the increase may be accounted for by greater release from the muscles. It has been suggested by some investigators that these serum increases in IGF-I during an acute bout of resistance exercise are the result of cell disruption and greater blood flow (Brahm *et al.* 1997; Kraemer 2000), thus causing IGF-I release from storage sites. Although further research is warranted, it does appear that the muscle isoform of IGF-I may play a prominent role during tissue remodelling. Furthermore, the absolute concentration pre-exercise of IGF-I may influence the responsiveness to exercise stress, with few changes taking place in subjects with higher concentrations at rest.

Chronic adaptations to resistance training

No change in resting concentrations of IGF-I has been reported during short-term resistance training (Kraemer *et al.* 1999b; McCall *et al.* 1999) unless concurrent with carbohydrate/protein supplementation (Kraemer *et al.* 1998b). However, long-term studies in women have shown elevations in resting IGF-I, particularly during high-volume training (Koziris *et al.* 1999; Marx *et al.* 2001). Recently, Borst *et al.* (2001) reported significant elevations in resting serum IGF-I following only 13 weeks of a 25-week training programme. The increases reported by Borst *et al.* (2001) were similar in single-set and multiple-set training groups despite a significantly greater strength increase observed in the 3-set group. In addition, a significant decrease in IGF binding protein 3 (IGFBP-3) was observed between weeks 13 and 25 which the authors suggested may be a positive adaptation for the strength increase by increasing the concentration of free IGF-I. Marx *et al.* (2001) reported significant increases in resting serum IGF-I concentrations in previously untrained women following 6 months of training. In addition, the magnitude was greater when a high-volume, multiple-set programme was used vs. the 1-set circuit. Thus, it appears that the volume and intensity of training are important for chronic IGF-I adaptations.

Insulin

Insulin has been shown to significantly affect muscle protein synthesis when adequate amino acid concentrations are available (Wolfe 2000). Serum insulin concentrations parallel changes in blood glucose (Chandler *et al.* 1994). Serum insulin concentrations have been shown to decrease during an acute bout of resistance exercise (Raastad *et al.* 2000), possibly due to α-adrenergic inhibition of insulin secretion (Galbo *et al.* 1977). In addition, a resistance exercise workout does not appear to directly affect insulin secretion independently of blood glucose concentrations unless carbohydrate, protein or a combination of carbohydrate/protein supplements are taken during the workout in which significant elevations have been reported (Chandler *et al.* 1994; Kraemer *et al.* 1998b). In addition, resistance training does not appear to significantly affect insulin sensitivity. Power lifters have shown comparable rates of insulin-stimulated whole-body and femoral muscle glucose uptake to those of sedentary men but far lower than those of endurance-trained athletes (Takala *et al.* 1999). Although a potent anabolic hormone, insulin appears to be most affected by blood glucose concentrations and/or dietary intake.

Catecholamines

Catecholamines appear to reflect the acute demands and physical stress of the resistance exercise protocol. Catecholamines are important for increasing force production, muscle action rate and energy availability, as well as having several other functions including the augmentation of hormones such as testosterone (Kraemer 2000). An acute bout of resistance exercise has been shown to increase plasma concentrations of epinephrine (Guezennec *et al.* 1986; Kraemer *et al.* 1987, 1999a), norepinephrine (Guezennec *et al.* 1986; Kraemer *et al.* 1987, 1999a) and dopamine (Kraemer *et al.* 1987, 1999a). The magnitude may be dependent upon the force of muscle action, amount of muscle stimulated, volume of resistance exercise and rest intervals (Kraemer *et al.* 1987). In a study by Bush *et al.* (1999), it was shown that power and force production significantly affect the responses of norepinephrine and epinephrine, with higher force production producing greater elevations even when work is corrected for in the compared protocols. In addition, the more intense the protocol (intensity or short rest periods) the longer the elevations in epinephrine and norepinephrine that can be observed up to 5 min post exercise (Kraemer *et al.* 1987; Bush *et al.* 1999). A high-intensity, short rest period (10–60 s) heavy-resistance exercise protocol (10 exercises, 3 sets, 10 RM) frequently used in body building training sessions increased plasma epinephrine, norepinephrine and dopamine through 5 min of recovery (Kraemer *et al.* 1987).

An interesting observation prior to resistance exercise has been the 'anticipatory rise' in catecholamine concentrations (Kraemer *et al.* 1991, 1999a). Prior to intense exercise a significant elevation in plasma epinephrine and norepinephrine have been observed (Kraemer *et al.* 1991, 1999a). This anticipatory rise may be part of the body's psychophysiological adjustment for performance of a maximal effort exercise stress.

Chronic adaptations to resistance training remain unclear. It has been suggested that training reduces the catecholamine response to resistance exercise (Guezennec *et al.* 1986). However, alterations in the acute response may reflect the demands of the programme such that systematic variation and progressive overload may obviate any subsequent decrease. Nevertheless, this system appears to be a very dynamic system subject to a host of physical and psychological influences of stress.

β-Endorphins

Less is known concerning the role of β-endorphins during resistance exercise and training. Increases have been reported during resistance exercise (Eliot *et al.* 1984). Kraemer *et al.* (1992) reported significant elevations in plasma β-endorphin concentration at 5 and 15 min post exercise following a weightlifting workout in elite junior weightlifters. The acute increase has been attributed to the magnitude of muscle mass used (multiple-joint exercises), rest interval length and intensity and volume of the resistance exercise programme (Kraemer *et al.* 1992, 1993a), and has been correlated highly (e.g. $r = 0.72 - 0.82$) to blood lactate concentrations (Kraemer *et al.* 1989, 1993a). Kraemer *et al.* (1993a) reported that body building type workouts (high volume, moderate load, short rest periods) produce the most substantial increases in plasma β-endorphin concentrations compared to traditional strength training (high load, low repetitions, long rest periods). The β-endorphin changes along with cortisol and growth hormone suggest that the hypopituitary–adrenal–cortical axis is significantly stimulated during resistance exercise yet is not affected by training experience or muscle strength (Kraemer *et al.* 1992). The role of β-endorphins during resistance training remains unclear but may involve some beneficial adaptations conducive to the enhancement of strenuous training sessions or adherence to exercise training.

Thyroid hormones

The role of thyroid hormones during resistance training remains unclear but may be permissive in its interaction with other hormones. In moderately trained individuals over 24 weeks of strength training only significant decreases were reported for serum thyroxine (T4) and free T4 whereas no changes were observed in thyroid-stimulating hormone (TSH) or triiodothyronine (T3) (Pakarinen *et al.* 1988). Pakarinen *et al.* (1991) reported significant decreases in TSH, T3 and T4 during 1 intensive week of resistance training (two workouts per day) in elite weightlifters. However, over the course of 1 year of training in elite weightlifters no changes were observed for any thyroid hormone until the precompetition period (i.e. lower volume of training) where significant increases in free T4 and T3 were reported (Alen *et al.* 1993). These thyroid hormone changes returned to baseline when the intensity increased in the next training phase. It appears that resistance training may alter thyroid function potentially through inhibition at the hypothalamic–pituitary axis, decreasing the release of TSH and subsequent T3 and T4 concentrations. However, the impact of these alterations remains speculative at the present time. Due to the tight homeostatic control of thyroid hormones, resting circulating increases during chronic resistance training are not expected to be observed (Kraemer 2000).

Leptin

Leptin, a product of the *ob* gene, is a protein hormone thought to relay a satiety signal to the hypothalamus to regulate energy balance and appetite (Kalra *et al.* 1999). Serum leptin concentrations appear to be in proportion to the amount of adipose tissue in the human body, and may be influenced by gender, metabolic hormones (e.g. stimulated by insulin and cortisol and inhibited by β-adrenergic agonists), and current energy requirements (Considine 1997). Most studies have shown no direct impact of exercise on leptin concentrations independent of its effect on adipose tissue (Considine 1997). Similar findings have been reported with resistance training. Gippini *et al.* (1999) reported that leptin did not correlate with body mass index (BMI) in bodybuilders and that resistance training does not influence leptin production independently of changes in body composition. Nindl *et al.* (2002) has shown that leptin can be reduced with an acute high-volume resistance training workout in the late phases of an overnight response curve. This was the first study to show that leptin is responsive to acute resistance exercise stress but one has to examine a very extended recovery curve.

Fluid regulatory hormones

Fluid homeostasis is critical to acute exercise performance in general, although the majority of the literature has examined aerobic modalities of exercises. Fluid regulatory hormones such as arginine vasopressin, atrial peptide, renin, aldosterone and angiotensin II have been shown to increase in response to exercise, with the magnitude dependent on exercise intensity, duration and hydration status (Convertino *et al.* 1981; Mannix *et al.* 1990; Mandroukas *et al.* 1995; Grant *et al.* 1996). Resistance exercise has been shown to reduce plasma volume (Gordon *et al.* 1985) comparable to changes elicited by running and/or cycling at 80–95% of $\dot{V}O_{2max}$ (Collins *et al.* 1986). Kraemer *et al.* (1999a) recently examined the fluid regulatory hormonal responses to resistance exercise. Competitive power lifters performed 1 set of the leg press exercise to exhaustion using 80% of their respective 1 RM. Immediately post exercise into 5 min of recovery, plasma osmolality, atrial peptide, renin activity and angiotensin II were elevated (with the elevations in plasma renin activity and angiotensin II greater in power lifters than in controls). Plasma arginine vasopressin concentration was also elevated but was not statistically significant. These data were the first to demonstrate that fluid balance and the subsequent hormonal response may be affected by as little as the first set of a resistance training workout.

Peptide F

Peptide F is a proenkephalin fragment secreted from chromaffin cells of the adrenal medulla along with epinephrine (Fry & Kraemer 1997). Although the physiological function of peptide is not entirely known, it has been shown that it improves the activation and B cell helper function of T lymphocytes (Triplett-McBride *et al.* 1998). Exercise has been shown to increase concentrations of peptide F (Kraemer *et al.* 1985). Bush *et al.* (1999) showed that peptide F interacted with epinephrine responses during acute and chronic recovery of 240 min suggesting a coregulatory effect. Very little is known about resistance training. Maximal intensity resistance exercise-induced overtraining does not change circulating peptide F concentrations at rest or after exercise (Fry *et al.* 1998). Interestingly, changes in the ratio of peptide F to epinephrine were observed, suggesting that overtraining may alter the secretory patterns of chromaffin cells.

Overtraining

Overtraining is defined as any increase in training volume and/or intensity resulting in long-term performance decrements (Fry & Kraemer 1997). In contrast, overreaching is a short-term increase in volume and/or intensity which is often planned in resistance training programmes and is thought to increase performance when used correctly (Fry & Kraemer 1997). Repeated overreaching may lead to overtraining and subsequent performance decrements in addition to neuroendocrine changes. Two weeks of overreaching has been shown to decrease resting concentrations of testosterone and IGF-I (Raastad *et al.* 2001). These decreases were significantly correlated ($r = 0.69$) to strength decrements (Raastad *et al.* 2001). Decreases in resting concentrations of testosterone have been reported during acute overreaching (Häkkinen *et al.* 1988a). However, short-term overreaching may not result in performance decrements or elevated resting cortisol, and may augment the acute testosterone response to resistance exercise when the individual has had at least 1 year of weightlifting training and previous exposure to the overreaching stimulus (Fry *et al.* 1994).

Volume-related overtraining has been shown to increase cortisol and decrease resting LH and total and free testosterone concentrations, with the free pool of testosterone most sensitive to the overtraining stimuli (Häkkinen & Pakarinen 1991; Fry & Kraemer 1997). In addition, the exercise-induced increase in total testosterone is attenuated during volume-related overtraining (Häkkinen *et al.* 1987). However, intensity-related overtraining does not appear to alter resting concentrations of hormones, thus demonstrating a differential response in comparison to large increases in training volume (Fry & Kraemer 1997). Fry *et al.* (1998) reported no changes in circulating testosterone, free testosterone, cortisol, GH or peptide F concentrations during high-intensity overtraining, e.g. 10 1-RM sets of the squat every day for 2 weeks. Therefore, it appears that intensity-related overtraining does not alter resting hormonal concentrations significantly with a corresponding decrease in performance whereas volume-related overtraining does appear to significantly alter circulating hormone concentrations.

Detraining

Detraining is the cessation of resistance training or significant reduction of training volume, intensity or frequency resulting in reduced performance, e.g. reduced muscle strength, power, hypertrophy and local muscle endurance (Fleck & Kraemer 1997). Alterations in hormonal activity may occur in addition to changes in neural and muscle function. It appears that the duration of the detraining period is important for the magnitude of change as well as the training status and history of the individual (Fleck & Kraemer 1997). Hortobágyi *et al.* (1993) reported significant increases in resting concentrations of GH, testosterone and the T/C ratio, with a significant decrease in cortisol following 2 weeks of detraining in highly trained power lifters and football players. The authors hypothesized that this increase in anabolic hormone concentrations was related to the body's ability to combat the catabolic processes associated with detraining and suggested that short-term detraining may represent an augmented stimulus for tissue remodelling and repair. However, these increases have only been shown during short-term detraining. Kraemer *et al.* 2002) reported no significant changes in testosterone, GH, LH, SHBG, cortisol or ACTH following 6 weeks of detraining. No changes were observed for cortisol, SHBG and LH following 8 weeks of detraining in women (Häkkinen *et al.* 1990). However, detraining periods longer than 8 weeks have shown significant changes. Häkkinen *et al.* (1985) and Alen *et al.* (1988) trained subjects for 24 weeks followed by 12 weeks of detraining and reported a decrease in the T/C ratio which correlated highly to strength decrements. Increases in T4 concentrations have been reported (Pakarinen *et al.* 1988). These hormonal changes coincide with periods of muscle atrophy (Hortobágyi *et al.* 1993) and indicate that hormonal changes play a role in muscle size and strength reductions observed during periods of detraining.

Circadian patterns

Several hormones are secreted in various concentrations throughout the day in a circadian pattern. Salivary testosterone secretion has been shown to be secreted in a circadian manner with the greatest increases observed early in the morning with less throughout the rest of the waking day (Kraemer *et al.* 2001a). Considering that resistance exercise stimulates acute increases in testosterone concentrations, it is of interest to examine whether or not resistance exercise alters circadian patterns. Recently, Kraemer *et al.* (2001a) examined the effect of resistance exercise on normal circadian patterns of salivary testosterone and reported that resistance exercise did not affect circadian patterns of testosterone secretion over a 16-h waking period in resistance-trained men. It has been shown that afternoon resistance exercise-induced increases in serum testosterone are sometimes greater than those observed in the morning (Häkkinen & Pakarinen 1991), thus reflective of diurnal variations. It appears that regulatory mechanisms are quickly re-engaged after a resistance exercise workout such that homeostasis is maintained within 1 h post exercise. This may indicate that the acute cellular interactions in the immediate recovery period following a resistance training session may be of greater importance than previously thought due to the inability to affect waking circadian patterns during the day.

The nocturnal hormonal response has been investigated. McMurray *et al.* (1995) had trained lifters perform 3 sets of 6 exercises to exhaustion at 1900 h–2000 h and sampled blood beforehand and at 20-min intervals afterwards, from 2100 h to 0700 h. Resistance exercise did not alter nocturnal patterns of GH and cortisol secretion. However, testosterone secretion was greater between 0500 h and 0700 h in the resistance exercise group and nocturnal secretion of T4 decreased. It was suggested that the nocturnal changes in these hormones may have implications for tissue anabolism. Studies by Nindl *et al.* (2001a,b,c, 2002) have shown that acute higher-volume resistance exercise performed in trained men during the day will suppress several of the hormonal response patterns at night (i.e. testosterone, GH, IGF-I, cortisol, leptin). How these influence the target tissues remains to be examined. In addition, what happens at the level of the receptor and subsequent molecular effects on the target cells will be of greater interest as changes in circulating concentrations may indicate a number of different outcomes for the hormones.

Compatibility of strength and endurance training

Several studies have indicated that there is an incompatibility between simultaneous high-intensity strength and endurance training such that maximal strength and power appear to be limited (Kraemer *et al.* 1995b; Bell *et al.* 2000). It appears that possible reasons may be related to differences in neural recruitment patterns and/or an attenuation of muscle hypertrophy (Kraemer *et al.* 1995b). In addition, the neuroendocrine system may or may not be altered. Bell *et al.* (2000) reported no changes in resting concentrations of testosterone, GH or SHBG following 12 weeks of combined strength and endurance training. However, greater urinary cortisol was observed in women. Kraemer *et al.* (1995b) had subjects perform a total-body, high-volume resistance training programme 4 days per week along with 4 days per week of endurance training for 12 weeks and reported a substantial increase in exercise-induced cortisol concentrations. These data indicate that the incompatibility may also be the result of overtraining which in itself may produce a catabolic hormonal environment.

Summary

It is evident that hormonal mechanisms are responsive to resistance training. The specific neuroendocrine mechanisms that mediate physiological adaptations in the development of muscle strength, power and hypertrophy remain unclear. It is evident that homeostatic and regulatory mechanisms appear to be intimately involved with both the acute response to resistance exercise and chronic training adaptations. The changes in circulating concentrations provide a brief window of observation to the potential plasticity of the neuroendocrine system and its responsiveness to resistance exercise directed at strength and power development.

References

Adams, G.R. (1998) Role of insulin-like growth factor-I in the regulation of skeletal muscle adaptation to increased loading. *Exercise and Sport Sciences Reviews* **26**, 31–60.

Alen, M., Pakarinen, A., Häkkinen, K. & Komi, P.V. (1988) Responses of serum androgenic-anabolic and catabolic hormones to prolonged strength training. *International Journal of Sports Medicine* **9**, 229–233.

Alen, M., Pakarinen, A. & Häkkinen, K. (1993) Effects of prolonged training on serum thyrotropin and thyroid hormones in elite strength athletes. *Journal of Sport Science* **11**, 493–497.

Ballantyne, C.S., Phillips, S.M., MacDonald, J.R., Tarnopolsky, M.A. & MacDougall, J.D. (2000) The acute effects of androstenedione supplementation in healthy young males. *Canadian Journal of Applied Physiology* **25**, 68–78.

Ballor, D.L., Becque, M.D. & Katch, V.L. (1987) Metabolic responses during hydraulic resistance exercise. *Medicine and Science in Sports and Exercise* **19**, 363–367.

Bamman, M.M., Shipp, J.R., Jiang, J. *et al.* (2001) Mechanical load increases muscle IGF-1 and androgen receptor mRNA concentrations in humans. *American Journal of Physiology* **280**, E383–E390.

Bell, G.J., Syrotuik, D., Martin, T.P., Burnham, R. & Quinney, H.A. (2000) Effect of concurrent strength and endurance training on skeletal muscle properties and hormone concentrations in humans. *European Journal of Applied Physiology* **81**, 418–427.

Boone, J.B., Lambert, C.P., Flynn, M.G., Michaud, T.J., Rodriguez-Zayas, J.A. & Andres, F.F. (1990) Resistance exercise effects on plasma cortisol, testosterone and creatine kinase activity in anabolic-androgenic steroid users. *International Journal of Sports Medicine* **11**, 293–297.

Borst, S.E., De Hoyos, D.V., Garzarella, L. *et al.* (2001) Effects of resistance training on insulin-like growth factor-I and IGF binding proteins. *Medicine and Science in Sports and Exercise* **33**, 648–653.

Bosco, C., Colli, R., Bonomi, R., von Duvillard, S.P. & Viru, A. (2000) Monitoring strength training: neuromuscular and hormonal profile. *Medicine and Science in Sports and Exercise* **32**, 202–208.

Brahm, H., Piehl-Aulin, K., Saltin, B. & Ljunghall, S. (1997) Net fluxes over working thigh of hormones, growth factors and biomarkers of bone metabolism during short lasting dynamic exercise. *Calcified Tissue International* **60**, 175–180.

Bush, J.A., Kraemer, W.J., Mastro, A.M. *et al.* (1999) Exercise and recovery responses of adrenal medullary neurohormones to heavy resistance exercise. *Medicine and Science in Sports and Exercise* **31**(4), 554–559.

Busso, T., Häkkinen, K., Pakarinen, A., Kauhanen, H., Komi, P.V. & Lacour, J. (1992) Hormonal adaptations and modeled responses in elite weightlifters during 6 weeks of training. *European Journal of Applied Physiology* **64**, 381–386.

Chandler, R.M., Byrne, H.K., Patterson, J.G. & Ivy, J.L. (1994) Dietary supplements affect the anabolic hormones after weight-training exercise. *Journal of Applied Physiology* **76**, 839–845.

Collins, M.A., Hill, D.W., Cureton, K.J. & DeMello, J.J. (1986) Plasma volume change during heavy-resistance weight lifting. *European Journal of Applied Physiology* **55**, 44–48.

Considine, R.V. (1997) Weight regulation, leptin and growth hormone. *Hormone Research* **48** (Suppl. 5), 116–121.

Convertino, V.A., Keil, L.C., Bernauer, E.M. & Greenleaf, J.E. (1981) Plasma volume, osmolality, vasopressin, and renin activity during graded exercise in man. *Journal of Applied Physiology* **50**, 123–128.

Craig, B.W. & Kang, H. (1994) Growth hormone release following single versus multiple sets of back squats: total work versus power. *Journal of Strength and Conditioning Research* **8**, 270–275.

Craig, B.W., Brown, R. & Everhart, J. (1989) Effects of progressive resistance training on growth hormone and testosterone levels in young and elderly subjects. *Mechanisms of Ageing and Development* **49**, 159–169.

Crowley, M.A. & Matt, K.S. (1996) Hormonal regulation of skeletal muscle hypertrophy in rats: the testosterone to cortisol ratio. *European Journal of Applied Physiology* **73**, 66–72.

Cumming, D.C., Wall, S.R., Galbraith, M.A. & Belcastro, A.N. (1987) Reproductive hormone responses to resistance exercise. *Medicine and Science in Sports and Exercise* **19**, 234–238.

Cumming, D.C., Wheeler, G.D. & McColl, E.M. (1989) The effect of exercise on reproductive function in men. *Sports Medicine* **7**, 1–17.

Deschenes, M.R., Maresh, C.M., Armstrong, L.E., Covault, J., Kraemer, W.J. & Crivello, J.F. (1994) Endurance and resistance exercise induce muscle fiber type specific responses in androgen binding capacity. *Journal of Steroid Biochemistry and Molecular Biology* **50**, 175–179.

Eliot, D.L., Goldberg, L., Watts, W.J. & Orwoll, E. (1984) Resistance exercise and plasma beta-endorphin/beta-lipotrophin immunoreactivity. *Life Sciences* **34**, 515–518.

Elkins, R. (1990) Measurement of free hormones in blood. *Endocrine Reviews* **11**, 5–45.

Fahey, T.D., Rolph, R., Moungmee, P., Nagel, J. & Mortar, S. (1976) Serum testosterone, body composition, and strength of young adults. *Medicine and Science in Sports and Exercise* **8**, 31–34.

Fleck, S.J. & Kraemer, W.J. (1997) *Designing Resistance Training Programs*, 2nd edn. Human Kinetics, Champaign, IL.

Florini, J.R. (1987) Hormonal control of muscle growth. *Muscle and Nerve* **10**, 577–598.

Fry, A.C. & Kraemer, W.J. (1997) Resistance exercise overtraining and overreaching. Neuroendocrine responses. *Sports Medicine* **23**, 106–129.

Fry, A.C., Kraemer, W.J., Stone, M.H. *et al.* (1994) Endocrine responses to overreaching before and after 1 year of weightlifting. *Canadian Journal of Applied Physiology* **19**, 400–410.

Fry, A.C., Kraemer, W.J. & Ramsey, L.T. (1998) Pituitary–adrenal–gonadal responses to high-intensity resistance exercise overtraining. *Journal of Applied Physiology* **85**, 2352–2359.

Galbo, H., Christensen, N.J. & Holst, J.J. (1977) Catecholamines and pancreatic hormones during autonomic blockade in exercising man. *Acta Physiologica Scandinavica* **101**, 428–437.

Gippini, A., Mato, A., Peino, R., Lage, M., Dieguez, C. & Casanueva, F.F. (1999) Effect of resistance exercise (body building) training on serum leptin levels in young men. Implications for relationship between body mass index and serum leptin. *Journal of Endocrinological Investigation* **22**, 824–828.

Goldspink, G. (1999) Changes in muscle mass and phenotype and the expression of autocrine and systemic growth factors by muscle in response to stretch and overload. *Journal of Anatomy* **194**, 323–334.

Gordon, N.F., Russell, H.M.S., Krüger, P.E. & Cilliers, J.F. (1985) Thermoregulatory responses to weight training. *International Journal of Sports Medicine* **6**, 145–150.

Gordon, S.E., Kraemer, W.J., Vos, N.H., Lynch, J.M. & Knuttgen, H.G. (1994) Effect of acid-base balance on the growth hormone response to acute high-intensity cycle exercise. *Journal of Applied Physiology* **76**, 821–829.

Gotshalk, L.A., Loebel, C.C., Nindl, B.C. *et al.* (1997) Hormonal responses to multiset versus single-set heavy-resistance exercise protocols. *Canadian Journal of Applied Physiology* **22**, 244–255.

Grant, S.M., Green, H.J., Phillips, S.M., Enns, D.L. & Sutton, J.R. (1996) Fluid and electrolyte hormonal responses to exercise and acute plasma volume expansion. *Journal of Applied Physiology* **81**, 2386–2392.

Guezennec, Y., Leger, L., Lhoste, F., Aymonod, M. & Pesquies, P.C. (1986) Hormone and metabolite response to weight-lifting training sessions. *International Journal of Sports Medicine* **7**, 100–105.

Guyton, A.C. (1991) *Textbook of Medical Physiology*, 8th edn. W.B. Saunders, Philadelphia, PA.

Häkkinen, K. (1989) Neuromuscular and hormonal adaptations during strength and power training. A review. *Journal of Sports Medicine and Physical Fitness* **29**, 9–26.

Häkkinen, K. & Pakarinen, A. (1991) Serum hormones in male strength athletes during intensive short term strength training. *European Journal of Applied Physiology* **63**, 191–199.

Häkkinen, K. & Pakarinen, A. (1993) Acute hormonal responses to two different fatiguing heavy-resistance protocols in male athletes. *Journal of Applied Physiology* **74**, 882–887.

Häkkinen, K. & Pakarinen, A. (1995) Acute hormonal responses to heavy resistance exercise in men and women at different ages. *International Journal of Sports Medicine* **16**, 507–513.

Häkkinen, K., Pakarinen, A., Alen, M. & Komi, P.V. (1985) Serum hormones during prolonged training of neuromuscular performance. *European Journal of Applied Physiology* **53**, 287–293.

Häkkinen, K., Pakarinen, A., Alen, M., Kauhanen, H. & Komi, P.V. (1987) Relationships between training volume, physical performance capacity, and serum hormone concentrations during prolonged training in elite weight lifters. *International Journal of Sports Medicine* **8** (Suppl.), 61–65.

Häkkinen, K., Pakarinen, A., Alen, M., Kauhanen, H. & Komi, P.V. (1988a) Daily hormonal and neuromuscular responses to intensive strength training in 1 week. *International Journal of Sports Medicine* **9**, 422–428.

Häkkinen, K., Pakarinen, A., Alen, M., Kauhanen, H. & Komi, P.V. (1988b) Neuromuscular and hormonal responses in elite athletes to two successive strength training sessions in one day. *European Journal of Applied Physiology* **57**, 133–139.

Häkkinen, K., Pakarinen, A., Alen, M., Kauhanen, H. & Komi, P.V. (1988c) Neuromuscular and hormonal adaptations in athletes to strength training in two years. *Journal of Applied Physiology* **65**, 2406–2412.

Häkkinen, K., Pakarinen, A., Kyrolainen, H., Cheng, S., Kim, D.H. & Komi, P.V. (1990) Neuromuscular adaptations and serum hormones in females during prolonged power training. *International Journal of Sports Medicine* **11**, 91–98.

Häkkinen, K., Pakarinen, A. & Kallinen, M. (1992) Neuromuscular adaptations and serum hormones in women during short-term intensive strength training. *European Journal of Applied Physiology* **64**, 106–111.

Hickson, R.C., Hidaka, K., Foster, C., Falduto, M.T. & Chatterton, R.T. (1994) Successive time courses of strength development and steroid hormone responses to heavy-resistance training. *Journal of Applied Physiology* **76**, 663–670.

Hortobágyi, T., Houmard, J.A., Stevenson, J.R., Fraser, D.D., Johns, R.A. & Israel, R.G. (1993) The effects of detraining on power athletes. *Medicine and Science in Sports and Exercise* **25**, 929–935.

Inoue, K., Yamasaki, S., Fushiki, T. *et al.* (1993) Rapid increases in the number of androgen receptors following electrical stimulation of the rat muscle. *European Journal of Applied Physiology* **66**, 134–140.

Jezova, D. & Vigas, M. (1981) Testosterone response to exercise during blockade and stimulation of adrenergic receptors in man. *Hormone Research* **15**, 141–147.

Ju, G. (1999) Evidence for direct neural regulation of the mammalian anterior pituitary. *Clinical and Experimental Pharmacology and Physiology* **26**, 757–759.

Kalra, S.P., Dube, M.G., Pu, S., Xu, B., Horvath, T.L. & Kalra, P.S. (1999) Interacting appetite-regulating pathways in the hypothalamic regulation of body weight. *Endocrine Reviews* **20**, 68–100.

King, D.S., Sharp, R.L., Vukovich, M.D. *et al.* (1999) Effect of oral androstenedione on serum testosterone and adaptations to resistance training in young men: a randomized controlled trial. *Journal of the American Medical Association* **281**, 2020–2028.

Koziris, L.P., Hickson, R.C., Chatterton, R.T. *et al.* (1999) Serum levels of total and free IGF-1 and IGFBP-3 are increased and maintained in long-term training. *Journal of Applied Physiology* **86**, 1436–1442.

Kraemer, W.J. (1988) Endocrine responses to resistance exercise. *Medicine and Science in Sports and Exercise* **20** (Suppl.), S152–S157.

Kraemer, W.J. (2000) Neuroendocrine responses to resistance exercise. In: *Essentials of Strength Training and Conditioning* (ed. T. Baechle), 2nd edn, pp. 91–114. Human Kinetics, Champaign, IL.

Kraemer, W.J. & Fleck, S.J. (1988) Resistance training: exercise prescription. *Physician and Sports Medicine* **16**, 69–81.

Kraemer, W.J. & Ratamess, N.A. (2000) Physiology of resistance training: current issues. In: *Orthopaedic Physical Therapy Clinics of North America: Exercise Technologies* (ed. C. Hughes) 9: 4, pp. 467–513. W.B. Saunders, Philadelphia, PA.

Kraemer, W.J., Noble, B., Culver, B. & Lewis, R.V. (1985) Changes in plasma proenkephalin peptide F and catecholamine levels during graded exercise in men. *Proceedings of the National Academy of Sciences of the United States of America* **82**, 6349–6351.

Kraemer, W.J., Noble, B.J., Clark, M.J. & Culver, B.W. (1987) Physiologic responses to heavy-resistance exercise with very short rest periods. *International Journal of Sports Medicine* **8**, 247–252.

Kraemer, W.J., Fleck, S.J., Callister, R. *et al.* (1989) Training responses of plasma beta-endorphin, adrenocorticotropin, and cortisol. *Medicine and Science in Sports and Exercise* **21**, 146–153.

Kraemer, W.J., Marchitelli, L., Gordon, S.E. *et al.* (1990) Hormonal and growth factor responses to heavy resistance exercise protocols. *Journal of Applied Physiology* **69**, 1442–1450.

Kraemer, W.J., Gordon, S.E., Fleck, S.J. *et al.* (1991) Endogenous anabolic hormonal and growth factor responses to heavy resistance exercise in males and females. *International Journal of Sports Medicine* **12**, 228–235.

Kraemer, W.J., Fry, A.C., Warren, B.J. *et al.* (1992) Acute hormonal responses in elite junior weightlifters. *International Journal of Sports Medicine* **13**, 103–109.

Kraemer, W.J., Dziados, J.E., Marchitelli, L.J. *et al.* (1993a) Effects of different heavy-resistance exercise protocols on plasma β-endorphin concentrations. *Journal of Applied Physiology* **74**, 450–459.

Kraemer, W.J., Fleck, S.J., Dziados, J.E. *et al.* (1993b) Changes in hormonal concentrations after different heavy-resistance exercise protocols in women. *Journal of Applied Physiology* **75**, 594–604.

Kraemer, W.J., Aguilera, B.A., Terada, M. *et al.* (1995a) Responses of IGF-1 to endogenous increases in growth hormone after heavy-resistance exercise. *Journal of Applied Physiology* **79**, 1310–1315.

Kraemer, W.J., Patton, J.F., Gordon, S.E. *et al.* (1995b) Compatibility of high-intensity strength and endurance training on hormonal and skeletal muscle adaptations. *Journal of Applied Physiology* **78**, 976–989.

Kraemer, W.J., Clemson, A., Triplett, N.T., Bush, J.A., Newton, R.U. & Lynch, J.M. (1996) The effects of plasma cortisol elevation on total and differential leukocyte counts in response to heavy-resistance exercise. *European Journal of Applied Physiology* **73**, 93–97.

Kraemer, W.J., Staron, R.S., Hagerman, F.C. *et al.* (1998a) The effects of short-term resistance training on endocrine function in men and women. *European Journal of Applied Physiology* **78**, 69–76.

Kraemer, W.J., Volek, J.S., Bush, J.A., Putukian, M. & Sebastianelli, W.J. (1998b) Hormonal responses to consecutive days of heavy-resistance exercise with or without nutritional supplementation. *Journal of Applied Physiology* **85**, 1544–1555.

Kraemer, W.J., Fleck, S.J., Maresh, C.M. *et al.* (1999a) Acute hormonal responses to a single bout of heavy resistance exercise in trained power lifters and untrained men. *Canadian Journal of Applied Physiology* **24**, 524–537.

Kraemer, W.J., Häkkinen, K., Newton, R.U. *et al.* (1999b) Effects of heavy-resistance training on hormonal response patterns in younger vs. older men. *Journal of Applied Physiology* **87**, 982–992.

Kraemer, W.J., Ratamess, N.A. & Rubin, M.R. (2000) Basic principles of resistance exercise. In: *Nutrition and the Strength Athlete* (ed. C.R. Jackson), pp. 1–328. CRC Press, Boca Raton, Florida.

Kraemer, W.J., Loebel, C.C., Volek, J.S. *et al.* (2001a) The effect of heavy resistance exercise on the circadian rhythm of salivary testosterone in men. *European Journal of Applied Physiology* **84**, 13–18.

Kraemer, W.J., Dudley, G.A., Tesch, P.A. *et al.* (2001b) The influence of muscle action on the acute growth hormone response to resistance exercise and short-term detraining. *Growth Hormone and IGF Research* in press.

Kraemer, W.J., Koziris, L.P., Ratamess, N.A. *et al.* (2002) Muscular performance and hormonal changes during six weeks of detraining in resistance-trained men. *Journal of Strength and Conditioning Research* in press.

Longcope, C. (1996) Dehydroepiandrosterone metabolism. *Journal of Endocrinology* **150** (Suppl.), S125–S127.

Lu, S.S., Lau, C.P., Tung, Y.F. *et al.* (1997) Lactate and the effect of exercise on testosterone secretion: evidence for the involvement of a cAMP-mediated mechanism. *Medicine and Science in Sports and Exercise* **29**, 1048–1054.

McCall, G.E., Goulet, C., Grindeland, R.E., Hodgson, J.A., Bigbee, A.J. & Edgerton, V.R. (1997) Bed rest suppresses bioassayable growth hormone release in response to muscle activity. *Journal of Applied Physiology* **83**, 2086–2090.

McCall, G.E., Byrnes, W.C., Fleck, S.J., Dickinson, A. & Kraemer, W.J. (1999) Acute and chronic hormonal responses to resistance training designed to promote muscle hypertrophy. *Canadian Journal of Applied Physiology* **24**, 96–107.

McMurray, R.G., Eubank, T.K. & Hackney, A.C. (1995) Nocturnal hormonal responses to resistance exercise. *European Journal of Applied Physiology* **72**, 121–126.

Mandroukas, K., Zakas, A., Aggelopoulou, N., Christoulas, K., Abatzides, G. & Karamouzis, M. (1995) Atrial natriuretic factor responses to submaximal and maximal exercise. *British Journal of Sports Medicine* **29**, 248–251.

Mannix, E.T., Palange, P., Aronoff, G.R., Manfredi, F. & Farber, M.O. (1990) Atrial natriuretic peptide and the renin–aldosterone axis during exercise in man. *Medicine and Science in Sports and Exercise* **22**, 785–789.

Marx, J.O., Ratamess, N.A., Nindl, B.C. *et al.* (2001) Low-volume circuit versus high-volume periodized resistance training in women. *Medicine and Science in Sports and Exercise* **33**, 635–643.

Mulligan, S.E., Fleck, S.J., Gordon, S.E., Koziris, L.P., Triplett-McBride, N.T. & Kraemer, W.J. (1996) Influence of resistance exercise volume on serum growth hormone and cortisol concentrations in women. *Journal of Strength and Conditioning Research* **10**, 256–262.

Nagaya, N. & Herrera, A.A. (1995) Effects of testosterone on synaptic efficacy at neuromuscular junctions in asexually dimorphic muscle of male frogs. *Journal of Physiology* **483**, 141–153.

Nindl, B.C., Kraemer, W.J., Marx, J.O. *et al.* (2001a) Overnight responses of the circulating IGF-1 system after acute heavy-resistance exercise. *Journal of Applied Physiology* **90**, 1319–1326.

Nindl, B.C., Kraemer, W.J., Deaver, D.R., Peters, J.L., Marx, J.O. & Loomis, G.A. (2001b) Luteinizing hormone secretion and testosterone concentrations are blunted after acute heavy resistance exercise in men. *Journal of Applied Physiology* **91**, 1251–1258.

Nindl, B.C., Hymer, W.C., Deaver, D.R. & Kraemer, W.J. (2001c) Growth hormone pulsatility profile characteristics following acute heavy resistance exercise. *Journal of Applied Physiology* **91**, 163–172.

Nindl, B.C., Kraemer, W.J., Gotshalk, L.A. *et al.* (2001d) Testosterone responses after acute resistance exercise in women: effects of regional fat distribution. *International Journal of Sports Nutrition and Metabolism* **11**, 451–465.

Nindl, B.C., Kraemer, W.J. & Arciero, P.J. *et al.* (2002) Leptin concentrations experience a delayed reduction after resistance exercise in men. *Medicine and Science in Sports and Exercise* **34**, 608–613.

Pakarinen, A., Alen, M., Häkkinen, K. & Komi, P. (1988) Serum thyroid hormones, thyrotropin and thyroxine binding globulin during prolonged strength training. *European Journal of Applied Physiology* **57**, 394–398.

Pakarinen, A., Häkkinen, K. & Alen, M. (1991) Serum thyroid hormones, thyrotropin, and thyroxine binding globulin in elite athletes during very intense strength training of one week. *Journal of Sports Medicine and Physical Fitness* **31**, 142–146.

Pecci, M.A. & Lombardo, J.A. (2000) Performance-enhancing supplements. *Physical Medicine and Rehabilitation Clinics of North America* **11**, 949–960.

Potteiger, J.A., Judge, L.W., Cerny, J.A. & Potteiger, V.M. (1995) Effects of altering training volume and intensity on body mass, performance, and hormonal concentrations in weight-event athletes. *Journal of Strength and Conditioning Research* **9**, 55–58.

Pyka, G., Wiswell, R.A. & Marcus, R. (1992) Age-dependent effect of resistance exercise on growth hormone secretion in people. *Journal of Clinical Endocrinology and Metabolism* **75**, 404–407.

Raastad, T., Bjoro, T. & Hallen, J. (2000) Hormonal responses to high- and moderate-intensity strength exercise. *European Journal of Applied Physiology* **82**, 121–128.

Raastad, T., Glomsheller, T., Bjoro, T. & Hallen, J. (2001) Changes in human skeletal muscle contractility and hormone status during 2 weeks of heavy strength training. *European Journal of Applied Physiology* **84**, 54–63.

Reaburn, P., Logan, P. & Mackinnon, L. (1997) Serum testosterone response to high-intensity resistance training in male veteran sprint runners. *Journal of Strength and Conditioning Research* **11**, 256–260.

Sale, D.G. (1988) Neural adaptations to resistance training. *Medicine and Science in Sports and Exercise* **20** (Suppl.), S135–S145.

Schwab, R., Johnson, G.O., Housh, T.J., Kinder, J.E. & Weir, J.P. (1993) Acute effects of different intensities of weight lifting on serum testosterone. *Medicine and Science in Sports and Exercise* **25**, 1381–1385.

Staron, R.S., Karapondo, D.L., Kraemer, W.J. *et al.* (1994) Skeletal muscle adaptations during early phase of heavy-resistance training in men and women. *Journal of Applied Physiology* **76**, 1247–1255.

Stoessel, L., Stone, M.H., Keith, R., Marple, D. & Johnson, R. (1991) Selected physiological, psychological and performance characteristics of national-caliber United States women weightlifters. *Journal of Applied Sports Science Research* **5**, 87–95.

Takala, T.O., Nuutila, P., Knuuti, J., Luotolahti, M. & Yki-Jarvinen, H. (1999) Insulin action on heart and skeletal muscle glucose uptake in weight lifters and endurance athletes. *American Journal of Physiology* **276**, E706–E711.

Taylor, J.M., Thompson, H.S., Clarkson, P.M., Miles, M.P. & DeSouza, M.J. (2000) Growth hormone response to an acute bout of resistance exercise in weight-trained and non-weight-trained women. *Journal of Strength and Conditioning Research* **14**, 220–227.

Triplett-McBride, N.T., Mastro, A.M., McBride, J.M. *et al.* (1998) Plasma proenkephalin peptide F and human B cell responses to exercise stress in fit and unfit women. *Peptides* **19**, 731–738.

Tsolakis, C., Messinis, D., Stergioulas, A. & Dessypris, A. (2000) Hormonal responses after strength training and detraining in prepubertal and pubertal boys. *Journal of Strength and Conditioning Research* **14**, 399–404.

Van Helder, W.P., Radomski, M.W. & Goode, R.C. (1984) Growth hormone responses during intermittent weight lifting exercise in men. *European Journal of Applied Physiology* **53**, 31–34.

Volek, J.S., Kraemer, W.J., Bush, J.A., Incledon, T. & Boetes, M. (1997) Testosterone and cortisol in relationship to dietary nutrients and resistance exercise. *Journal of Applied Physiology* **82**, 49–54.

Wallace, M.B., Lim, J., Cutler, A. & Bucci, L. (1999) Effects of dehydroepiandrosterone vs androstenedione supplementation in men. *Medicine and Science in Sports and Exercise* **31**, 1788–1792.

Weiss, L.W., Cureton, K.J. & Thompson, F.N. (1983) Comparison of serum testosterone and androstenedione responses to weight lifting in men and women. *European Journal of Applied Physiology* **50**, 413–419.

Williams, A.G., Ismail, A.N., Sharma, A. & Jones, D.A. (2002) Effects of resistance exercise volume and nutritional supplementation on anabolic and catabolic hormones. *European Journal of Applied Physiology* **86**, 315–321.

Wolfe, R.R. (2000) Effects of insulin on muscle tissue. *Current Opinion in Clinical Nutrition and Metabolic Care* **3**, 67–71.

Chapter 20

Cardiovascular Responses to Strength Training

STEVEN J. FLECK

This chapter focuses on the cardiovascular responses and adaptations to resistance training exercise. Cardiovascular adaptations at rest and during resistance training exercise are of interest because of their relationship to cardiovascular health. Limited data are available on some of the topics discussed in this chapter, especially in the area of the acute responses and chronic adaptations to resistance training during activity. This is in part related to difficulties associated with accurate determination of variables such as blood pressure and cardiac output during activity. Accurate blood pressure determination during activity requires intra-arterial cannulation, although more recently the non-invasive photoplethysmographic technique has been used to determine blood pressure during activity and echocardiographic and cardiac impedance techniques have been used to determine central measures, such as stroke volume, during activity. All of these techniques have some limitations, thus the data must be viewed with some caution. Physiological responses and adaptations may be affected by training volume and intensity. Therefore, conclusions concerning the physiological response and chronic adaptations to weight training in general must be viewed considering the possible effect of training volume and intensity.

Chronic adaptations at rest

Decreased resting heart rate, decreased resting blood pressure and changes in the blood lipid profile are normally associated with decreased cardiovascular risk, while changes in cardiac morphology, stroke volume and cardiac output at rest may indicate normal or abnormal cardiac function and are also indicators of cardiovascular risk. Cardiovascular changes at rest due to weight training (Table 20.1) have been investigated using cross-sectional as well as longitudinal study designs.

Heart rate

Resting heart rates of junior and senior competitive bodybuilders, power lifters and Olympic lifters range from 60 to 78 beats per minute (Colan *et al.* 1985; Smith & Raven 1986; Fleck & Dean 1987; George *et al.* 1995; Haykowsky *et al.* 2000). The vast majority of cross-sectional data indicates that resting heart rates of highly strength-trained athletes are not significantly different from sedentary individuals (Longhurst *et al.* 1980a,b; Snoecky *et al.* 1982; Colan *et al.* 1985; Menapace *et al.* 1982; Spataro *et al.* 1985; Pearson *et al.* 1986; Smith & Raven 1986; Fleck & Dean 1987), although lower than average resting heart rates in highly resistance-trained athletes have also been reported (Saltin & Astrand 1967; Scala *et al.* 1987). Resting heart rate of master-level power lifters has been reported to be 87 beats per minute, which was significantly higher than age-matched control subjects (Haykowsky *et al.* 2000).

Short-term (up to 20 weeks) longitudinal studies report significant decreases of approximately

4–13% in resting heart rate (Kanakis & Hickson 1980; Stone *et al.* 1983b, 1987; Haennel *et al.* 1989; Goldberg *et al.* 1994), and small non-significant decreases (Ricci *et al.* 1982; Stone *et al.* 1983a; Lusiani *et al.* 1986; Blumenthal *et al.* 1990; Goldberg *et al.* 1994). In some longitudinal studies changes in resting heart rate are non-significant; however, in the majority of studies a significant or non-significant decrease in resting heart rate is reported. The mechanism causing a decrease in resting heart rate due to weight training is not clearly elucidated. However, decreased heart rate is typically associated with a combination of increased parasympathetic and decreased sympathetic cardiac tone. Some cardiovascular responses to isometric actions resemble typical weight training activity, and some data indicate that during low-level isometric actions (30% of maximal voluntary contraction) both autonomic branches show increased activity (Gonzalez-Camarena *et al.* 2000) rather than the typical parasympathetic withdrawal and sympathetic augmentation observed during dynamic exercise, such as cycle ergometry, giving rise to the possibility that a decrease in resting heart rate due to weight training may not be due to increased parasympathetic and decreased sympathetic cardiac tone, but to increased activity of both autonomic branches.

Blood pressure

The majority of cross-sectional data clearly show highly strength-trained athletes to have average resting systolic and diastolic blood pressures (Longhurst *et al.* 1980a,b; Menapace *et al.* 1982; Pearson *et al.* 1986; Fleck & Dean 1987; Fleck *et al.* 1989b; Goldberg 1989; Byrne & Wilmore 2000), although significantly above average (Snoecky *et al.* 1982) and less than average (Smith & Raven 1986) resting blood pressures have also been reported in weightlifters. Short-term training studies have reported non-significant changes in resting systolic and diastolic pressures in normotensive individuals (Lusiani *et al.* 1986; Goldberg *et al.* 1988, 1994; Byrne & Wilmore 2000). A significant decrease in resting systolic pressure (3.7%), but no significant change in resting diastolic pressure (Stone *et al.* 1983b) and a significant decrease in diastolic pressure only (Hurley *et al.* 1988) have also been reported in normotensive individuals. In borderline hypertensive individuals significant decreases in both systolic and diastolic resting blood pressure have been reported due to weight training (Hagberg *et al.* 1984; Harris & Holly 1987).

Decreased resting blood pressure when it does occur due to strength training is probably related to decreased body fat and changes in the sympathoadrenal drive (Goldberg *et al.* 1989), whereas explanations of hypertension when observed in highly strength-trained athletes are essential hypertension, chronic overtraining, use of androgens and/or large gains in muscle mass. Although body mass has been positively correlated to systolic blood pressure (Viitasalo *et al.* 1979), beneficial effects on blood pressure have been shown with concomitant increases in lean body mass (Stone *et al.* 1983b; Goldberg *et al.* 1988) indicating that gains in lean body mass can occur without increases in resting blood pressure. Although significant increases and decreases in resting blood pressure have been reported, the majority of both longitudinal and cross-sectional data indicates weight training to result in either no change in or a small decrease in resting blood pressure.

Rate pressure product

The rate pressure product (heart rate × systolic blood pressure) is an estimate of myocardial work and is proportional to myocardial oxygen consumption. Resting rate pressure product has shown decreases after 8 weeks of an Olympic-style weight training programme (Stone *et al.* 1983b). Although rate pressure product is not reported in many studies any study showing a decrease in resting heart rate or systolic blood pressure would result in a decrease in rate pressure product. Thus weight training can decrease rate pressure product suggesting the left ventricle is performing less work and has a lower oxygen consumption at rest.

Table 20.1 Adaptations at rest.

Heart rate	No change or small ↓
Blood pressure	
Systolic	No change or small ↓
Diastolic	No change or small ↓
Rate pressure product	No change or small ↓
Stroke volume	
Absolute	Small ↑ or no change
Relative to BSA	No change
Relative to LBM	No change
Cardiac function	
Systolic	No change
Diastolic	No change
Lipid profile	
Total cholesterol	No change or small ↓
HDL-C	No change or small ↑
LDL-C	No change or small ↓
Total cholesterol/HDL-C	No change or small ↑

Stroke volume

Comparisons of absolute resting stroke volume of highly strength-trained males to normals are equivocal. No difference between (Dickhuth *et al.* 1979; Brown *et al.* 1983) these two groups in absolute stroke volume and a greater value (Pearson *et al.* 1986; Fleck *et al.* 1989a) in the highly strength-trained individuals have been reported. Increased absolute stroke volume when present appears to be due to a significantly greater end-diastolic left ventricular internal dimension and a normal ejection fraction (Fleck 1988). A meta-analysis indicates that calibre of athlete may influence absolute stroke volume with national/international-calibre athletes having a greater absolute stroke volume than lesser-calibre athletes (Fleck 1988). Relative to body surface area only one (Fleck *et al.* 1989a) comparison between highly strength-trained individuals and normals shows a significantly greater value in the strength-trained individuals, while five comparisons show no difference between these two groups (Longhurst *et al.* 1980a; Pearson *et al.* 1986). The study showing stroke volume relative to body surface area to be greater in highly strength-trained individuals does report this difference to be non-significant when stroke volume is expressed relative to lean body mass (Fleck *et al.* 1989a). Meta-analysis of stroke volume relative to body surface area demonstrates no difference by calibre of athlete (Fleck 1988). Thus the greater absolute stroke volume in some national/international-calibre highly strength-trained athletes may be explained in part by body size.

No change in absolute resting stroke volume has been reported due to a short-term weight training programme (Lusiani *et al.* 1986). The preponderance of evidence indicates weight training to have no or little effect upon absolute stroke volume, or stroke volume relative to body surface area or lean body mass.

Lipid profile

Cross-sectional and longitudinal studies examining the effect of resistance training on the blood lipid profile are inconclusive. Literature reviews report male strength-trained athletes to have normal, higher, and lower than normal HDL-C (high-density lipoprotein cholesterol) concentrations, LDL-C (low-density lipoprotein cholesterol) concentrations, total cholesterol concentrations and total cholesterol to HDL-C ratios (Kraemer *et al.* 1988; Hurley 1989; Stone *et al.* 1991). It has also been reported that highly weight-trained females demonstrate some positive changes (Elliot *et al.* 1987; Moffatt *et al.* 1990) and show no difference from control subjects (Morgan *et al.* 1986) in the lipid profile. Cross-sectional data on strength/power athletes have also shown lipid profiles indicative of an increased cardiovascular risk (Berg *et al.* 1980). Longitudinal training studies using males and females as subjects also show inconclusive results. Increases in HDL-C of approximately 10–15% and decreases in LDL-C of approximately 5–39% and decreases in total cholesterol of 3–16% as a result of short-term resistance training in normolipidaemic individuals have been demonstrated (Hurley 1989). However, other longitudinal studies show no significant change in the lipid profile due to short-term resistance training programmes (Kraemer *et al.* 1988; Hurley 1989;

Stone *et al.* 1991; LeMura *et al.* 2000; Staron *et al.* 2000).

All of the cross-sectional and longitudinal study designs used to examine the effect of weight training on the lipid profile can be criticized. Limitations of the studies include: inadequate control of age, diet and training programme and possible androgen use by the subjects; use of only one blood sample in determining the lipid profile; lack of control group; failure to control for changes in body composition; and short duration of longitudinal studies. Additionally, it has been demonstrated that an acute increase in HDL-C and decrease in total cholesterol occurs 24 h after a 90-min resistance exercise session that does not return to baseline values by 48 h after the exercise session (Wallace *et al.* 1991). Some studies did not rule out this possible acute effect of the last training session. Thus conclusions from these studies must be viewed with some caution.

Weight training volume may have some impact on the lipid profile. Bodybuilders have been reported to have lipid profiles similar to runners, whereas power lifters have lower HDL-C and higher LDL-C concentrations than runners when body fat, age and androgen use (which has been shown to depress HDL-C concentrations) are controlled for (Hurley *et al.* 1984, 1987). It has also been reported in middle-aged men that positive changes in the lipid profile do occur over 12 weeks of resistance training (Johnson *et al.* 1982; Blessing *et al.* 1987) with the greatest change occurring during the highest training volume phase of the programme.

Why resistance training might positively affect the lipid profile has not been completely elucidated. A decrease in percentage of body fat has been reported to positively influence the lipid profile (Williams *et al.* 1994; Twisk *et al.* 2000) and resistance training programmes have been reported to decrease percentage body fat. Resistance training may improve oxidative capacity of skeletal muscle due to an increase in the activity of specific aerobic oxidative enzymes (Wang *et al.* 1993). Such a change might occur due to fibre type conversion from Type IIB to the more oxidative Type IIA fibre type (Staron *et al.* 1994) and an increase in capillaries per muscle fibre (McCall *et al.* 1996). There are also possible negative effects of weight training on the lipid profile. Individuals with a higher percentage of Type I muscle fibres have been reported to have a higher HDL-C concentration (Tikkanen *et al.* 1996). Some resistance training programmes have a greater hypertrophic effect on Type II fibres (Tesch 1987). The resulting decrease in the percentage area of Type I fibres may unfavourably affect the lipid profile. For a positive effect on the lipid profile to occur the factors that may potentially favourably affect the lipid profile would have to counteract any factors that may have a deleterious effect on the lipid profile.

Strength training may have a positive effect on the lipid profile. However, further research is needed before this conclusion can be viewed without caution. Programmes with a high total training volume may offer the best possibility for a positive effect on the profile. It has been reported that an aptitude for power/speed athletic events, including weightlifting, does not offer protection from cardiovascular risk in former athletes, whereas an aptitude for endurance athletic events and continuing vigorous physical activity after retirement does offer protection against cardiovascular risk (Kujala *et al.* 2000). Therefore a prudent conclusion might be to encourage strength/power athletes to perform some endurance training and follow dietary practices appropriate to bring about a positive influence on the lipid profile after retirement from competition.

Left ventricular wall thickness

Cardiac morphology, such as ventricular wall thickness (Table 20.2), is most frequently determined using echocardiographic techniques. However, magnetic resonance imaging (MRI) has also been used to examine cardiac morphology (Fleck *et al.* 1989b). Literature reviews conclude that highly strength-trained individuals can have greater than average absolute diastolic posterior left ventricular wall thickness (PWTd) (Fleck

1988; Urhausen & Kindermann 1992) and diastolic intraventricular septum wall thickness (IVSd) (Wolfe *et al.* 1986; Fleck 1988; Urhausen & Kindermann 1992; Perrault & Turcotte 1994). However, wall thickness in highly strength-trained individuals rarely exceeds the upper limits of normal (Wolfe *et al.* 1986; Urhausen & Kindermann 1992) and is normally significantly lower than in disease states such as aortic stenosis, obstructive cardiomyopathy and extreme hypertension (Wolfe *et al.* 1986). It is also important to note that increased ventricular wall thickness is apparent in other types of athletes. A study examining nationally ranked athletes in 27 different sports ranks weightlifting as number eight in terms of impact on left ventricular wall thickness (Spataro *et al.* 1994). The increase in wall thickness, when apparent in weightlifters, is normally attributed to the intermittent elevated blood pressure encountered during strength training exercise (Effron 1989).

When PWTd and IVSd of highly strength-trained individuals are expressed relative to body surface area or to lean body mass rarely is there a difference from normal (Fleck 1988; Fleck *et al.* 1989a; Urhausen & Kindermann 1992; Perrault & Turcotte 1994) which indicates a physiological adaptation rather than an adaptation to a pathological disease state. This is of interest because some studies have found a disproportionate thickening of the IVSd in comparison to the PWTd, possibly indicating a deleterious adaptation, while other studies have found this ratio to be within normal limits (Urhausen & Kindermann 1992). Interestingly a meta-analysis concluded that IVSd thickness and not PWTd were affected by athlete calibre, with national/international- and regional-calibre athletes having a greater IVSd thickness than recreational strength trainers (Fleck 1988). More research is needed to elucidate whether there is disproportionate thickening of the ventricular walls and if it does occur what are the effects on cardiac function.

Short-term longitudinal training studies support the concept that strength training can increase PWTd and IVSd, but that it is not a necessary outcome of all weight training programmes (Fleck 1988; Effron 1989; Perrault & Turcotte 1994). The conclusion that strength training does not have to result in increased PWTd and IVSd is supported by cross-sectional studies showing no significant difference from controls in ventricular wall thickness in female collegiate strength/power-trained athletes (George *et al.* 1995) and junior and master national-calibre power lifters (Haykowsky *et al.* 2000). Whether or not increased ventricular wall thickness does occur with strength training is probably due to differences in the training programmes utilized. The highest blood pressures during a set to concentric failure occur during the last few repetitions of a set (MacDougall *et al.* 1985; Fleck & Dean 1987; Sale *et al.* 1994). Exercises involving large muscle mass, such as leg presses, have been reported to result in higher blood pressures than small muscle mass exercises (MacDougall *et al.* 1985). Therefore whether or not sets are carried to concentric failure and the exercises performed may affect whether or not increases in ventricular wall thickness occur. Other factors that may affect whether or not changes in ventricular wall thickness occur include training intensity, training volume, duration of training, and rest periods between sets.

Right ventricular wall thickness has received considerably less attention than left ventricular wall thickness. However, an MRI study did report no difference in systolic and diastolic right ventricular wall thickness between male junior elite Olympic weightlifters and age- and weight-matched controls (Fleck *et al.* 1989b). The same study did find the weightlifters to have significantly greater left ventricular wall thickness. Thus these results indicate that the right ventricle is not exposed to sufficiently elevated blood pressures to cause hypertrophy of the right ventricular walls during strength training.

Strength training can cause increased absolute left ventricular wall thickness, but it is not a necessary consequence of all strength training programmes. Increased left ventricular wall thickness when apparent is caused by the intermittent elevated blood pressures encountered during strength training. When expressed relative to body surface area or lean body mass generally no increase in left ventricular wall thickness is demonstrated. Additionally, increased left ventricular wall thickness rarely exceeds the upper limits of normal and is significantly below wall thickness increases due to pathological conditions.

Chamber size

Left ventricular internal dimension has most frequently been determined using echocardiography; however, it has also been determined using MRI (Fleck *et al.* 1989b). Highly strength-trained individuals can have a normal or significantly greater absolute diastolic left ventricular internal dimension (LVIDd) than normal (Fleck 1988; Fleck *et al.* 1989b; Urhausen & Kindermann 1992; Perrault & Turcotte 1994; George *et al.* 1995). Similar to left ventricular wall thickness, LVIDd in highly strength-trained individuals normally does not exceed the upper limits of normal (Wolfe *et al.* 1986; Fleck 1988; Urhausen & Kindermann 1992; Perrault & Turcotte 1994) and in most cases is not significantly different from normal when expressed relative to body surface area or lean body mass (Wolfe *et al.* 1986; Fleck 1988; Urhausen & Kindermann 1992). However, absolute and relative to body surface area LVIDd in highly strength-trained individuals can also be slightly but significantly greater than normal when expressed relative to body surface area (Perrault & Turcotte 1994). Short-term longitudinal training studies support the conclusion that the effect of weight training on LVIDd is minimal (Wolfe *et al.* 1986; Fleck 1988; Perrault & Turcotte 1994).

A comparison of nationally ranked athletes in 27 different sports showed weightlifters to be ranked number 22 in terms of effect on LVIDd (Spataro *et al.* 1994). Although weight training may have a minimal effect on LVIDd it is important that this variable is not decreased due to weight training as is the case in pathological pressure overload caused by hypertension or due to various forms of cardiomyopathy (Urhausen & Kindermann 1992). The slight increase or no change in LVIDd coupled with no change or slight increase in left ventricular wall thickness is an important difference between weight training and pathological cardiac hypertrophy, where a large increase in wall thickness is not accompanied by an increase in LVIDd (Urhausen & Kindermann 1992).

Meta-analysis indicates that athlete calibre does not influence whether or not LVIDd is significantly different from normal (Fleck 1988). This conclusion is supported by reports of nationally ranked junior and senior power lifters having normal LVIDd (Haykowsky *et al.* 2000) and by other reports of national-calibre strength-trained athletes having a LVIDd not significantly different from normal (Dickhuth *et al.* 1979; Fleck *et al.* 1989a). Changes in ventricular volume are normally associated with a volume overload; it might therefore be hypothesized that the type of weight training programme performed would affect LVIDd. This is supported by a report of bodybuilders, but not weightlifters, having a greater absolute LVIDd at rest (Deligiannis *et al.* 1988). However, if expressed relative to body surface area or lean body mass neither the bodybuilders or the weightlifters demonstrated LVIDd significantly different from normal.

Right ventricular and atrial internal dimensions have also been examined in highly strength-trained individuals. Bodybuilders typically train with greater numbers of repetitions per set (6–12 repetitions per set), compared to weightlifters who typically perform smaller numbers of repetitions per set (3 or less) for a good portion of their training programme. Thus bodybuilders typically perform a higher-volume training programme compared to weightlifters and it has been reported that bodybuilders but not weightlifters have greater diastolic and systolic right ventricular internal dimensions at rest in absolute and relative to body surface area and lean body mass terms (Deligiannis *et al.* 1988). A cross-sectional study on junior elite Olympic-style weightlifters reports them not to have an absolute, relative to body surface area or relative to lean body mass diastolic or systolic right ventricular internal dimension significantly different from normal (Fleck *et al.* 1989b). Similar to right ventricular internal dimension, left atrial internal dimension of both bodybuilders and weightlifters has been reported to be greater than normal in absolute and relative to body surface area and lean body mass terms, with the bodybuilders having a significantly greater left atrial internal dimension than the weightlifters (Deligiannis *et al.* 1988). This again indicates the type of weight training programme may affect cardiac chamber size.

Generally, weight training has a slight or no significant effect upon LVIDd. This is true when LVIDd is expressed in absolute, relative to body surface area or relative to lean body mass terms. Higher volume weight training programmes may have the greatest potential to affect cardiac chamber sizes.

Left ventricular mass

Left ventricular mass (LVM) can increase due to an increase in either ventricular wall thickness or internal dimensions. Due to the assumptions used to calculate LVM the calculation must be viewed with some caution. For example, a change of 1 mm in left ventricular wall thickness can result in a significant increase of 15% in estimated LVM (Perrault & Turcotte 1994). Both cross-sectional data on highly strength-trained individuals (Fleck 1988; Effron 1989; George *et al.* 1995; Haykowsky *et al.* 2000) and short-term longitudinal (Wolfe *et al.* 1986; Fleck 1988; Effron 1989) studies indicate that absolute LVM can significantly increase due to weight training, but is not a necessary outcome of all weight training programmes. Any difference from control values in cross-sectional studies or increase in longitudinal studies, however, is greatly reduced or non-existent when LVM is expressed relative to body surface area or lean body mass.

The type of training programme performed may influence how LVM is increased. Both bodybuilders and weightlifters have a significantly greater than normal absolute LVM, with LVM not being different between these two groups of athletes (Deligiannis *et al.* 1988). Both bodybuilders and weightlifters in this study had a significantly greater than normal left ventricular wall thickness. However, only the bodybuilders had a significantly greater than normal left ventricular end-diastolic dimension. Thus in the bodybuilders the LVM is increased due to both a greater left ventricular wall thickness and increased chamber size, whereas in the weightlifters the increase is caused primarily by an increase in left ventricular wall thickness. It could be hypothesized that a weight training programme that increases both left ventricular wall thickness and left ventricular internal dimensions would result in the greatest increase in estimated left ventricular mass. Such a programme may be a higher volume weight training programme.

Absolute LVM can be increased due to resistance training; however, such an increase does not occur with all weight training programmes. The type of training programme performed may influence the magnitude of increase in LVM and the means by which an increase in LVM occurs, with higher-volume programmes resulting in an increase in both left ventricular wall thickness and chamber size; and lower-volume programmes resulting in an increase in left ventricular mass primarily due to an increase in wall thickness.

Cardiac function

Abnormalities in systolic and diastolic function are associated with cardiac hypertrophy caused by pathological conditions, such as hypertension and valvular heart disease. Thus there has been concern that cardiac hypertrophy caused by weight training might impair cardiac function. However, the majority of cross-sectional studies demonstrate that the common measures of systolic function, percentage of fractional shortening, ejection fraction and velocity of circumferential shortening, are not altered in resistance-trained individuals (Fleck 1988; Effron 1989; Ellias *et al.* 1991; Urhausen & Kindermann 1992; George *et al.* 1995; Haykowsky *et al.* 2000). In only one cross-sectional study (Colan *et al.* 1987) was a measure of systolic function, percentage of

Table 20.2 Cardiac morphology adaptations at rest.

		Relative to	
	Absolute	BSA	LMB
Wall thickness		↑↑	
Left ventricle	↑ or no change	No change	No change
Septal	↑ or no change	No change	No change
Right ventricle	No change	No change	No change
Chamber volume			
Left ventricle	No change or slight ↑	No change or slight ↑	No change or slight ↑
Right ventricle	No change or slight ↑(?)	No change or slight ↑(?)	No change or slight ↑(?)
Left ventricular mass	↑ or no change	No change	No change

BSA, body surface area (m^2); LBM, lean body mass (kg); ?, minimal data.

fractional shortening, found to be significantly greater (32 vs. 37%) than a control group. Short-term longitudinal training studies are equivocal with no change (Lusiani *et al.* 1986) and a significant increase in percentage fractional shortening shown (Kanakis & Hickson 1980). The majority of evidence indicates weight training has no effect on systolic function, with minimal evidence indicating enhanced systolic function.

Diastolic function has received considerably less attention than systolic function. However, the majority of cross-sectional studies report no significant change from normal in diastolic function of highly weight-trained individuals (Urhausen & Kindermann 1992). However, power lifters with significantly greater absolute and relative to body surface area left ventricular mass have been shown to demonstrate some indication of enhanced diastolic function. Power lifters competing at the national level have been shown to have a significantly enhanced left ventricular peak rate of chamber enlargement and peak rate of wall thinning compared to a control group (Colan *et al.* 1985). Atrial peak filling rate has also been shown to be greater in power lifters than in normal individuals (Pearson *et al.* 1986). This information indicates that diastolic function is not affected, or perhaps slightly enhanced, despite an increase in absolute and relative to body surface area left ventricular mass in highly weight-trained individuals.

Acute response

Acute response refers to the cardiovascular response during one or several sets of a strength training exercise. The acute response has received considerably less attention from the sports science community than the response to chronic long-term training. This may be in part because of the need to use intra-arterial lines to determine blood pressure during resistance exercise as auscultatory sphygmomanometry has limitations, such as not being able to accurately determine blood pressures during the concentric and eccentric phases of repetitions. More recently finger plesmography has been used to determine blood pressure continuously during weight training exercise. It is also difficult to accurately determine cardiac output, stroke volume, and left ventricular end-diastolic and systolic volumes using cardiac impedance or echocardiographic techniques during weight training. Therefore, in some instances, conclusions drawn concerning the acute cardiovascular response to weight training exercise must be viewed with caution (Table 20.3).

Heart rate and blood pressure

Heart rate and both systolic and diastolic blood pressures increase substantially during the performance of dynamic heavy-resistance exercise (Fleck 1988; Hill & Butler 1991). Mean peak

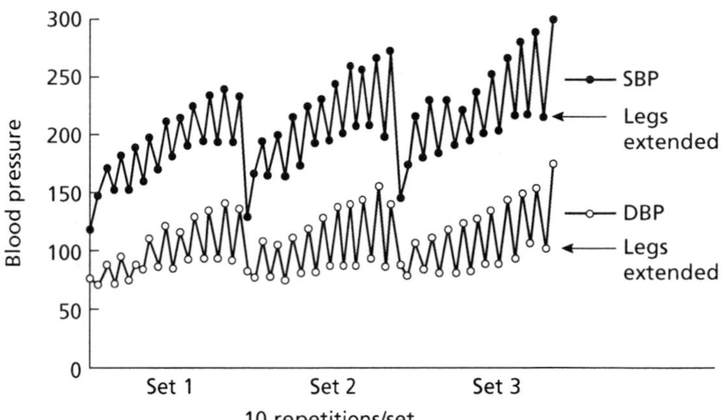

Fig. 20.1 Blood pressure response during 3 successive sets of 10 repetitions at a 10-repetition maximal weight in a two-legged leg press exercise. sbd, systolic blood pressure; dbp, diastolic blood pressure. (From Gotshall *et al.* 1999.)

systolic and diastolic blood pressures as high as 320/250 mmHg and a peak heart rate of 170 beats per minute have been reported during performance of a two-legged leg press set to failure at 95% of 1 RM, in which a Valsalva manoeuvre was allowed (MacDougall *et al.* 1985). Other representative mean peak values include 198/160 mmHg and 135 beats per minute in a single-legged knee extension performed to failure at 80% of 1 RM when a Valsalva manoeuvre was discouraged (Fleck & Dean 1987) and 230/170 mmHg when a Valsalva manoeuvre was allowed during a one-arm arm curl to failure using 95% of 1 RM (MacDougall *et al.* 1985). Blood pressure (Fig. 20.1) and heart rate will increase as the set progresses so the highest blood pressure and heart rate occur during the last several repetitions of a set to volitional fatigue whether or not a Valsalva manoeuvre is allowed (MacDougall *et al.* 1985; Fleck & Dean 1987). Using finger plesmography it has been shown that during three successive sets to failure peak heart rate and blood pressure increase during each successive set (Gotshall *et al.* 1999). Both the heart rate and blood pressure response increase with increased active muscle mass; however, the response is not linear (MacDougall *et al.* 1985; Fleck 1988; Falkel *et al.* 1992).

The increase in blood pressure and heart rate are apparent during machine, free-weight and isokinetic exercise (MacDougall *et al.* 1985; Fleck & Dean 1987; Sale *et al.* 1993; Sale *et al.* 1994; Scharf *et al.* 1994; Kleiner *et al.* 1996; Iellamo *et al.* 1997). Unfortunately due to differences in experimental design, such as whether sets were carried to volitional fatigue, velocity of the movement and length of a set across different exercise modes, few conclusions concerning possible differences between exercise modes can be reached. For example, a comparison of one set of isokinetic, variable resistance and fixed resistance knee extension exercise reported significantly greater peak systolic blood pressure during the isokinetic exercise (Kleiner *et al.* 1996). No difference between resistance training modes was reported for peak diastolic blood pressure or heart rate. All exercises were performed to volitional fatigue at $60°\cdot s^{-1}$. However, duration of the isokinetic set (118 s) was significantly longer than the variable resistance (48 s) or fixed resistance (67 s) sets. Thus the greater systolic blood pressure response during the isokinetic exercise may be due to the longer duration of the set.

Substantial increases in peak intra-arterial blood pressure (348/157 mmHg) and heart rate (157 beats per minute) are apparent during sets of isokinetic exercise to volitional fatigue at $50°\cdot s^{-1}$ (Kleiner *et al.* 1999). However, comparisons of isokinetic action velocity from 30 to $200°\cdot s^{-1}$ show little change with velocity in the peak heart rate and blood pressure response (Haennel *et al.* 1989; Kleiner *et al.* 1999).

The blood pressure response is higher during sets performed to volitional fatigue at 95% of

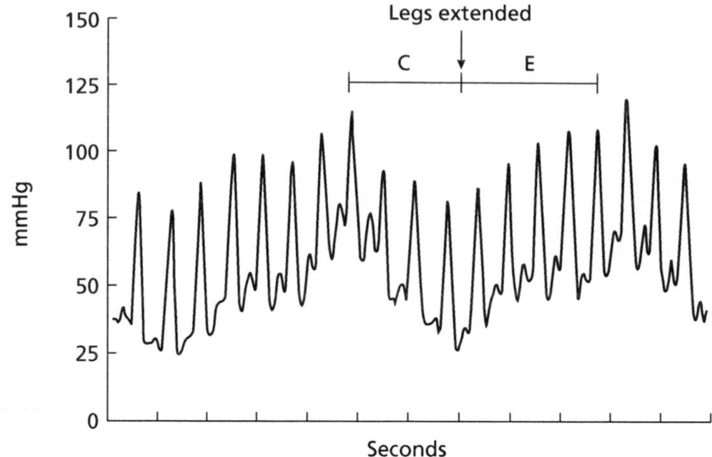

Fig. 20.2 Blood pressure response during one complete repetition of a two-legged leg press exercise. (From Gotshall *et al.* 1999.)

1 RM compared to 100% of 1 RM when a Valsalva manoeuvre is allowed (MacDougall *et al.* 1985). Both the peak heart rate and blood pressure responses during sets at 50, 70, 80, 85 and 87.5% of 1 RM have been shown to increase as the percentage of repetition maximum increases when a Valsalva manoeuvre is allowed (Sale *et al.* 1994). When a Valsalva manoeuvre is discouraged the blood pressure response is higher, but not significantly so, during sets at 90, 80 and 70% of 1 RM compared to sets at 100 and 50% of 1 RM to volitional fatigue (Fleck & Dean 1987), while peak heart rate response during sets to volitional fatigue at 90, 80, 70, and 50% of 1 RM are significantly higher than peak heart rate at 100% of 1 RM with slightly higher heart rates during sets at lower percentages of 1 RM (Fleck *et al.* 1987; Falkel *et al.* 1992). Thus the blood pressure and heart rate response is lower during a repetition at 100% of 1 RM compared to sets performed to volitional fatigue at lower percentages of 1 RM. The blood pressure and heart rate response during dynamic weight training appears to be similar to the response during isometric actions —as the duration of the activity increases so does the heart rate and blood pressure response (Ludbrook *et al.* 1978; Kahn *et al.* 1985), whereas during a repetition at 100% of 1 RM the duration of the activity is not sufficient to result in a maximal blood pressure and heart rate response.

During dynamic resistance exercise, higher systolic and diastolic blood pressures, but not heart rates, have been reported to occur during the concentric compared to the eccentric portion of repetitions (MacDougall *et al.* 1985; Miles *et al.* 1987; Falkel *et al.* 1992). However, blood pressure changes during the concentric and eccentric phases of a repetition. Therefore the point in the range of motion in the eccentric or concentric portion of a repetition at which blood pressure is determined will affect the value. More recently, using finger plesmography (Fig. 20.2) it has been reported that the highest systolic and diastolic blood pressures occur at the start of the concentric portion of the leg press with blood pressure decreasing as the concentric portion of the repetition progresses, and reaching its lowest point when the legs are extended (Gotshall *et al.* 1999). Blood pressure then increases as the legs bend during the eccentric portion of a repetition and again reaches its highest point when the legs are bent as far as possible. This indicates that the blood pressure response is highest at the sticking point of an exercise when the muscular contraction is nearest its maximal force.

Stroke volume and cardiac output

Stroke volume and cardiac output have been determined during resistance training exercise using electrical impedance techniques. Stroke volume and cardiac output are not elevated significantly above resting values during the concentric phase of knee extension exercise during 12 repetitions using a 12-RM resistance when attempts are made to limit the performance of a Valsalva manoeuvre (Miles *et al.* 1987). However, during the eccentric phase of knee extension exercise stroke volume and cardiac output are significantly increased above resting values and significantly greater than during the concentric phase. During knee extension exercise to volitional fatigue at 50, 80 and 100% of 1 RM stroke volume and cardiac output show different patterns of change when a Valsalva manoeuvre is allowed (Falkel *et al.* 1992). Stroke volume during the eccentric phase is significantly above resting values or not significantly different from resting values, while during the concentric phase stroke volume is either significantly below resting values or not significantly different from resting values. Cardiac output during the eccentric phase of knee extension exercise during all sets was significantly above resting values, while cardiac output during the concentric phase during all sets was above resting values but not always significantly so. During squat exercise to volitional failure at 50, 80 and 100% of 1 RM stroke volume and cardiac output have also been shown to vary between the eccentric and concentric phases of a repetition (Falkel *et al.* 1992). During the eccentric phase stroke volume was above resting values, but not always significantly so, during 50 and 100% of 1-RM sets, while stroke volume during the eccentric phase at 80% of 1 RM was significantly below resting values. Concentric stroke volume during the concentric phase was significantly below resting values during all sets. Cardiac output during the eccentric phase of squat exercise was significantly above resting values during all sets, while concentric cardiac output was always above resting values, but not always significantly so. During both the knee extension and squat exercise stroke volume and cardiac output were significantly greater during the eccentric compared to the concentric phases during all sets. A general pattern for both large and small muscle mass exercises is that stroke volume and cardiac output are higher during the eccentric compared to the concentric phase of repetition, while stroke volume during both large and small muscle mass exercises is generally below resting values during the concentric phase and generally above resting values, but not always to a statistically significant level, during the eccentric phase. Cardiac output during the eccentric phase of both large and small muscle mass exercises is generally above resting values. During large muscle group exercises cardiac output is also above resting values during the concentric phase, but during the concentric phase of small muscle mass exercises may show cardiac outputs that are above or below resting values.

Heart rate is not significantly different between the concentric and eccentric phases of a repetition (MacDougall *et al.* 1985; Miles *et al.* 1987; Falkel *et al.* 1992), whereas as discussed above stroke volume is significantly greater during the eccentric compared to the concentric phase of repetition. Thus the greater cardiac output during the eccentric compared to the concentric phase of a repetition is due solely to a greater stroke volume during the eccentric phase.

Stroke volume and cardiac output during both the eccentric and concentric phases of knee extension and squat exercise performed to volitional fatigue at 50, 80 and 100% of 1 RM have been compared (Falkel *et al.* 1992). Generally both stroke volume and cardiac output during both the eccentric and concentric phase at the same percentage of 1 RM are higher during knee extension exercise compared to squat exercise. The greater cardiac output during the knee extension exercise is due to a higher stroke volume, because generally heart rate during squat exercise is significantly higher than during knee extension exercise at the same percentage of 1 RM (Falkel *et al.* 1992).

Mechanisms of the pressor response

Several hypotheses can be advanced concerning possible mechanisms of the pressor response during weight training. An increase in cardiac output can result in an increase in blood pressure. Mean cardiac output may not be elevated during resistance training exercise (Miles *et al.* 1987). However, it has also been reported that cardiac output during both the eccentric and concentric phases of resistance training exercise is significantly elevated above resting values (Falkel *et al.* 1992). Thus increased cardiac output may contribute to the increase in blood pressure during weight training.

Increased intrathoracic or intra-abdominal pressures may have an impact upon the blood pressure response during strength training exercise (Fleck 1988). Intrathoracic pressure increases while performing strength training exercise (MacDougall *et al.* 1985; Falkel *et al.* 1992; Sale *et al.* 1994), especially if a Valsalva manoeuvre is performed. Classically, increased intrathoracic pressures are thought to eventually decrease venous return to the heart and so decrease cardiac output. Mouth pressure, an indirect measure of a Valsalva manoeuvre, or intrathoracic pressure have been shown to indicate greater intrathoracic pressure in individuals showing a reduced cardiac output and stroke volume in resistance training exercise than individuals showing indications of less intrathoracic pressure (Falkel *et al.* 1992). Thus an increase in intrathoracic pressure may limit venous return and so cardiac output, but at the same time this may cause a build-up of blood in the systemic circulation causing an increase in blood pressure. Performance of a Valsalva manoeuvre, which elevates intrathoracic pressure, would therefore lead to a greater blood pressure response than performance of the exercise without a Valsalva manoeuvre. Cardiac output and stroke volume can be above resting values during resistance training exercise. Therefore it can be speculated that the increase in blood pressure during weight training in conjunction with the powerful muscle pump overcomes the decrease in venous return due to an increase in intrathoracic pressure, and helps to maintain stroke volume and cardiac output.

The increase in intrathoracic pressure may have a protective function for the cerebral blood vessels (MacDougall *et al.* 1985). Any increase in intrathoracic pressure is transmitted to the cerebral spinal fluid due to the cerebral spinal fluid bearing on the intervertebral foramina. This reduces the transmural pressure of the cerebral blood vessels, protecting them from damage caused by the increase in blood pressure. This mechanism is similar to that thought to be active during a cough or strain (Hamilton *et al.* 1943).

Increased intramuscular pressure during weight training exercise would increase total peripheral resistance and so decrease blood pressure. For blood to flow through a vessel intraluminal pressure must exceed extravascular pressure. Quite high intramuscular pressures (92 kPa) have been measured during static human muscular actions (Edwards *et al.* 1972). Although there is considerable intramuscular variability, static actions of 40–60% of maximum can occlude blood flow (Bonde-Petersen *et al.* 1975; Sadamoto *et al.* 1983). A decrease in perfusion has been shown to follow an increase in intramuscular pressure (Sejersted *et al.* 1984; Sjogaard *et al.* 1986). Increased intramuscular pressure due to muscular actions are the most probable reason for blood pressures being reportedly higher during the concentric compared to the eccentric portion of a repetition (Miles *et al.* 1987) and are probably responsible for blood pressures being the highest at the sticking point of a repetition (Gotshall *et al.* 1999).

Increased blood pressure during weight training has been hypothesized to help maintain perfusion pressure in relation to the increased intramuscular pressure (MacDougall *et al.* 1985). This appears to be true at least for small human muscles (Wright *et al.* 2000). After fatiguing the adductor pollicis muscle by performing rhythmic isometric actions blood pressure was increased by contracting the knee extensors. Eighteen per cent of the isometric force lost due to fatigue of the adductor pollicis was recovered for each 10% increase in blood pressure. The recovery of contractile force is probably related to an increase in perfusion pressure to the muscle. The applicability to or magnitude of this mechanism in relation to larger muscle groups is unclear.

Table 20.3 Acute response of resistance exercise relative to rest.

	Portion of repetition	
	Concentric	Eccentric
Heart rate, no difference between concentric and eccentric	↑	↑
Stroke volume (?), eccentric value higher than concentric	No difference or ↓	No difference or ↑
Cardiac output (?), eccentric value higher than concentric	No difference or ↑	↑
Blood pressure		
Systolic ↑, highest at exercise sticking point	↑	↑
Diastolic ↑, highest at exercise sticking point	↑	↑
Intrathoracic pressure, highest when a Valsalva manoeuvre is performed	↑	↑

?, minimal data.

Chronic adaptations during activity

Classical cardiovascular training adaptations are reductions in heart rate and blood pressure at a specified submaximal workload. Relatively few studies have examined the effect of chronic weight training on cardiovascular changes during physical activity.

Heart rate, blood pressure and rate pressure product

Cross-sectional studies of highly weight-trained individuals indicate resistance training can reduce cardiovascular stress during weight training and other exercise tasks (Table 20.4). When not encouraged to perform a Valsalva manoeuvre bodybuilders demonstrate lower maximal intra-arterial systolic and diastolic blood pressures and maximal heart rates during sets to volitional fatigue at 50, 70, 80, 90 and 100% of 1 RM than novice weight-trained subjects with 6–9 months of training experience and sedentary subjects. (Fleck & Dean 1987). The bodybuilders were stronger than the other subjects; thus they demonstrated a lower blood pressure and heart rate response at the same relative workload (percentage of 1 RM), but also at higher absolute weight training workloads. Bodybuilders have also been shown to have lower heart rates and rate pressure products, but not blood pressures, during arm ergometry at the same absolute workload compared to normal subjects (Colliander & Tesch 1988). Bodybuilders have also demonstrated lower heart rates at the same relative workload during weight training than power lifters (Falkel *et al.* 1992). These cross-sectional studies indicate that weight training can result in a lower pressor response during physical work including weight training. The lower pressor response shown by bodybuilders may in part be due to a smaller-magnitude Valsalva manoeuvre during resistance exercise in bodybuilders compared to power lifters (Falkel *et al.* 1992).

Short-term longitudinal studies also indicate weight training can bring about a lower pressor response during physical activity. Heart rate, blood pressure and rate pressure product have all been shown to decrease after 12–16 weeks of weight training during treadmill walking, treadmill walking holding light hand weights, and bicycle ergometry (Blessing *et al.* 1987; Goldberg *et al.* 1988, 1994). Short-term training studies also show significant decreases in the heart rate and blood pressure responses during isometric actions (Goldberg *et al.* 1994) and in both senior (66-year-old) adults (McCartney *et al.* 1993) and young adults (Sale *et al.* 1993) during dynamic weight training at the same absolute workload. This longitudinal information clearly indicates that weight training can reduce the pressor response during a variety of physical activities.

However, the blood pressure response at the same relative weight training workload may be unchanged or even increased due to a short-term weight training programme (Sale *et al.* 1994). It is important to note that the same relative workload (percentage of 1 RM) after training is a greater absolute workload. After 19 weeks of weight training peak systolic pressure increases during a set to concentric failure at 85% of 1 RM, but is unchanged during sets at 50, 70, 80 and 87.5% of 1 RM. Peak diastolic pressure attained significantly increased during sets at 50, 70 and 80% of 1 RM, but was unchanged during a set at 87.5% of 1 RM. Peak oesophageal pressure increased significantly during the set at 80% of 1 RM, but was unchanged during the other sets. This indicates a more forceful Valsalva manoeuvre during the set at 80% of 1 RM, while heart rate during all sets at the same relative workload tended to be higher and tended to be lower at the same absolute workload, but not significantly so, after the 19 weeks of training. The information from this longitudinal study is not consistent with the lower blood pressor response shown by bodybuilders during sets to volitional fatigue when a Valsalva manoeuvre is not encouraged (Fleck & Dean 1987). The difference between these two studies may in part be related to whether a not a Valsalva manoeuvre is discouraged or allowed during the weight training exercise.

Myocardial oxygen consumption

A decrease in the rate pressure product indicates a decrease in myocardial work and oxygen consumption. A reduction in total peripheral resistance at rest and during exercise may explain the results of some of the above studies. A decrease in total peripheral resistance during exercise at the same absolute workload could in part explain a decrease in the rate pressure product during exercise. After a weight training programme a submaximal absolute workload would be performed at a lower relative maximum voluntary contraction. This would be possible after a weight training programme because of an increase in maximal strength; thus a smaller percentage of the maximum voluntary contraction would be necessary to develop a submaximal absolute force. This would result in less occlusion and therefore a decrease in total peripheral resistance. This mechanism may be in large part responsible for increases in time to exhaustion during cycling, without an increase in maximal oxygen consumption, after a weight training programme because it allows more blood flow to a working muscle (Marcinik *et al.* 1991).

Laplace's law also offers a possible explanation for a reduction in rate pressure product. Laplace's law can be represented by the formula $T = P \times R / Wt$ where T is myocardial wall tension, P is pressure, R is chamber radius and Wt is wall thickness. Resistance training in many instances increases left ventricular wall thickness with little or no change in left ventricular chamber size. These changes would result in a reduction in myocardial wall tension according to Laplace's law. A reduction in wall tension may simultaneously result in a decrease in myocardial oxygen consumption. Although the mechanisms are not completely elucidated it does appear that weight training may result in a decrease in rate pressure product and so myocardial oxygen consumption.

Stroke volume and cardiac output

The peak stroke volume and cardiac output of bodybuilders is greater than power lifters during sets of the back squat and knee extension exercises to volitional fatigue at 50, 80 and 100% of 1 RM when a Valsalva manoeuvre is allowed (Falkel *et al.* 1992). The higher stroke volume and cardiac output of the bodybuilders were evident during both the concentric and eccentric phases of repetitions. The bodybuilders also demonstrated an indication (mouth pressure) of a lesser-magnitude Valsalva manoeuvre. Thus the difference in stroke volume and cardiac output shown between the bodybuilders and power lifters may be due to the magnitude of the Valsalva manoeuvre performed and so differences in the effect of intrathoracic pressure on venous return and blood pressure. During most of the squat and knee extension exercise sets the bodybuilders demonstrated a higher maximal heart rate than the power lifters, indicating cardiac output is increased in the bodybuilders due to an increase in stroke volume and heart rate. The power lifters had a significantly greater 1 RM than the bodybuilders in both the squat and knee extension exercise, indicating that lifting a greater absolute load may result in a lower stroke volume and cardiac output. The differences between the bodybuilders and power lifters indicates that the type of training programme may affect stroke volume and cardiac output during weight training exercise.

A short-term longitudinal study indicates that training may affect the magnitude of the Valsalva manoeuvre (Sale *et al.* 1994). After 19 weeks of weight training oesophageal pressures during a set at the same relative resistance (percentage of 1 RM) are unchanged. However, at the same absolute resistance, which is now a lower percentage of 1 RM after training, oesophageal pressures during the first several repetitions of a set can be reduced. This indicates a less forceful Valsalva manoeuvre during the first several repetitions of a set at the same absolute resistance after weight training. A reduction in the forcefulness of the Valsalva manoeuvre may allow stroke volume and cardiac output to increase compared to pretraining. Oesophageal pressure during the last repetitions of the set is unaffected by training, and therefore would not alter stroke volume or cardiac output compared to pretraining values.

Immediately after weight training exercise the cardiac output ($30\ l \cdot min^{-1}$) and stroke volume (150–200 ml) of weightlifters are significantly elevated above resting values (Vorobyev 1988), whereas the stroke volume and cardiac output of untrained individuals changes insignificantly immediately after weight training exercises. These studies indicate that stroke volume and cardiac output may be increased during weight training in strength-trained individuals compared to untrained individuals. Any changes in stroke volume and cardiac output brought about by chronic weight training may be related to a reduction in the forcefulness of a Valsalva manoeuvre after training and the type of training performed.

Peak oxygen consumption

Peak oxygen consumption ($\dot{V}O_{2\,peak}$) on a treadmill or bicycle ergometer is considered a marker of cardiovascular fitness. $\dot{V}O_{2\,peak}$ is minimally affected by heavy-resistance training. Cross-sectional data demonstrates that relative $\dot{V}O_{2\,peak}$ of competitive Olympic weightlifters, power lifters and bodybuilders ranges from 41 to $55\ ml \cdot kg^{-1} \cdot min^{-1}$ (Saltin & Astrand 1967; Kraemer *et al.* 1988; Stone *et al.* 1991; George *et al.* 1995). These are average to moderately above average relative $\dot{V}O_{2\,peak}$ values. The wide range indicates that weight training may increase $\dot{V}O_{2\,peak}$, but not all programmes may bring about an increase in relative $\dot{V}O_{2\,peak}$.

Longitudinal data show that heavy-resistance training, using a few repetitions per set with heavy resistances and long rest periods between sets, results in small increases or no change in relative $\dot{V}O_{2\,peak}$ (Fahey & Brown 1973; Hickson *et al.* 1980; Gettman & Pollock 1981; Lee *et al.* 1990). Seven weeks of an Olympic-style weightlifting programme can result in moderate gains in absolute $\dot{V}O_{2\,peak}$ (9%) and relative $\dot{V}O_{2\,peak}$ (8%) (Stone *et al.* 1983b). The first 5 weeks of training in this study consisted of 3–5 sets of 10 repetitions per set of each exercise, 3.5–4.0 min of rest between sets and exercises, and two sessions per day 3 days per week. Vertical jump training was performed 3 days per week during the initial 5 weeks of training. Training during the next 2 weeks was identical to the first 5 weeks, except 3 sets of 5 repetitions per set were performed and vertical jump training performed only 1 day per week. The majority of the gain in $\dot{V}O_{2\,peak}$ occurred during the initial 5 weeks of training, with no further significant gain during the last 2 weeks of training. The results indicate that higher-volume weight training may be necessary to bring about significant gains in $\dot{V}O_{2\,peak}$. However, this conclusion must be viewed with caution because of the inclusion of vertical jump training in the total training programme.

Table 20.4 Adaptations during exercise due to resistance training.

	Absolute workload*	Relative workload*
Heart rate	↓	No change
Blood pressure		
Systolic	↓	No change or ↓ or ↑
Diastolic	↓	No change or ↓ or ↑
Rate pressure product	↓	No change or ↓↑
Stroke volume	↑	?
Cardiac output	↑	?
$V\text{O}_{2\ peak}$	↑	?

*, minimal data and contradictory data; ?, unknown.

Circuit weight training consists of 12–15 repetitions per set using 40–60% of 1 RM with short rest periods of 15–30 s between sets and exercises. With this type of training relative $V\text{O}_{2\ peak}$ increases approximately 4% in men and 8% in women during 8–20 weeks of training (Gettman & Pollock 1981).

Heart rate during physical conditioning must be maintained at 60% of maximum for a minimum of 20 min to elicit significant gains in $V\text{O}_{2\ peak}$ (American College of Sports Medicine 1990). Exercising heart rate and total metabolic cost during a circuit weight training session is significantly higher than during a more traditional heavy weight training session (Pichon *et al.* 1996). This may be in part why circuit weight training elicits a significant increase in $V\text{O}_{2\ peak}$ while little or no change is brought about by a more traditional heavy weight training programme. The relatively long rest periods utilized in a traditional heavy weight training programme allow heart rate to decrease below the recommended 60% of maximum level needed to bring about a significant increase in $V\text{O}_{2\ peak}$. Thus weight training programmes intended to increase $V\text{O}_{2\ peak}$ should utilize short rest periods between sets and exercises.

Even when an increase in $V\text{O}_{2\ peak}$ is elicited by weight training the increase is substantially lower than the 15–25% increases associated with traditional cycling, running and swimming endurance training programmes. Therefore, if a major goal of a training programme is to significantly increase $V\text{O}_{2\ peak}$ some form of aerobic training needs to be included in the programme. The volume of aerobic training necessary to maintain or significantly increase $V\text{O}_{2\ peak}$ when performing weight training can be minimal (Nakao *et al.* 1995). Moderately trained subjects minimally, but significantly, increased relative $V\text{O}_{2\ peak}$ (3–4 $ml \cdot kg^{-1} \cdot min^{-1}$) over 1–2 years of weight training when performing only one aerobic training session per week of running 3.2 km per session. Individuals who only performed weight training during the same time frame demonstrated a small but significant decrease in relative $V\text{O}_{2\ peak}$. No difference in maximal strength gains between the runners and nonrunners was demonstrated.

In conclusion, performance of resistance training exercise does result in a pressor response that affects the cardiovascular system. Information to date indicates that chronic performance of resistance training can result in positive adaptations of the cardiovascular system at rest and during physical activity. Factors such as the volume and intensity of the weight training programme may influence to what extent any adaptation occurs. Further research is definitely needed concerning the cardiovascular response and adaptations to resistance training. In particular, research is needed concerning the effect of training intensity and volume on the acute cardiovascular response and the effects of long-term resistance training on the cardiovascular response at rest and during physical activity.

References

American College of Sports Medicine (1990) The recommended quantity and quality of exercise for developing and maintaining cardiorespiratory and muscular fitness in healthy adults. *Medicine and Science in Sports and Exercise* **22**, 265–274.

Berg, A., Ringwald, G. & Keul, J. (1980) Lipoprotein-cholesterol in well-trained athletes. A preliminary communication: reduced HDL-cholesterol in power athletes. *International Journal of Sports Medicine* **1**, 137–138.

Blessing, D., Stone, M., Byrd, R. *et al.* (1987) Blood lipid and hormonal changes from jogging and weight training in middle-aged men. *Journal of Applied Sports Science Research* **1**, 25–29.

Blumenthal, J.A., Fredrikson, M., Khun, C.M., Ulmer, R.L., Walsh Riddle, M. & Appelbaum, M. (1990) Aerobic exercise reduces level of cardiovascular and sympathoadrenal responses to mental stress in subjects without prior evidence of myocardial ischemia. *American Journal of Cardiology* **65**, 93–98.

Bonde-Petersen, F., Mork, A.L. & Nielsen, E. (1975) Local muscle blood flow and sustained contractions of human arms and back muscles. *European Journal of Applied Physiology and Occupational Physiology* **34**, 43–50.

Brown, S., Byrd, R., Jayasinghe, M.D. & Jones, D. (1983) Echocardiographic characteristics of competitive and recreational weight lifters. *Journal of Cardiovascular Ultrasonography* **2**, 163–165.

Byrne, H.K. & Wilmore, J.H. (2000) The effects of resistance training on resting blood pressure in women. *Journal of Strength and Conditioning Research* **14**, 411–418.

Colan, S., Sanders, S.P., McPherson, D. & Borrow, K.M. (1985) Left ventricular diastolic function in elite athletes with physiologic cardiac hypertrophy. *Journal of the American College of Cardiology* **6**, 545–549.

Colan, S., Sanders, S.P. & Borrow, K.M. (1987) Physiologic hypertrophy: effects on left ventricular systolic mechanisms in athletes. *Journal of the American College of Cardiology* **9**, 776–783.

Colliander, E.B. & Tesch, P. (1988) Blood pressure in resistance-trained athletes. *Canadian Journal of Sports Science* **13**, 31–34.

Deligiannis, A., Zahopoulou, E. & Mandroukas, K. (1988) Echocardiographic study of cardiac dimensions and function in weight lifters and body builders. *International Journal of Sports Cardiology* **5**, 24–32.

Dickhuth, H.H., Simon, G., Kindermann, W., Wildberg, A. & Keul, J. (1979) Echocardiographic studies on athletes of various sport-types and non-athletic persons. *Zeitschrift fur Kardiologie* **68**, 449–453.

Edwards, R.H.T., Hill, D.K. & McDonnell, M.N. (1972) Monothermal and intramuscular pressure measurements during isometric contractions of the human quadriceps muscle. *Journal of Physiology* **224**, 58–59.

Effron, M.B. (1989) Effects of resistance training on left ventricular function. *Medicine and Science in Sports and Exercise* **21**, 694–697.

Ellias, B.A., Berg, K.E., Latin, R.W., Mellion, M.B. & Hofschire, P.J. (1991) Cardiac structure and function in weight trainers, runners, and runner/weight trainers. *Research Quarterly for Exercise and Sport* **62**, 326–332.

Elliot, D.L., Goldberg, L., Kuehl, K.S. & Katlin, D.H. (1987) Characteristics of anabolic-androgenic steroid-free, competitive male and female body builders. *Physician and Sportsmedicine* **15**, 169–179.

Fahey, T.D. & Brown, H. (1973) The effects of an anabolic steroid on the strength, body composition, and endurance of college males when accompanied by a weight training program. *Medicine and Science in Sports* **5**, 272–276.

Falkel, J.E., Fleck, S.J. & Murray, T.F. (1992) Comparison of central hemodynamics between powerlifters and body builders during exercise. *Journal of Applied Sports Science Research* **6**, 24–35.

Fleck, S.J. (1988) Cardiovascular adaptations to resistance training. *Medicine and Science in Sports and Exercise* **20**, S146–S151.

Fleck, S.J. & Dean, L.S. (1987) Resistance-training experience and the pressor response during resistance exercise. *Journal of Applied Physiology* **63**, 116–120.

Fleck, S.J., Bennett, J.B. III, Kraemer, W.J. & Baechle, T.R. (1989a) Left ventricular hypertrophy in highly strength trained males. In: *Sports Cardiology 2nd International Conference* (eds T. Lukich, A. Venerando, P. Zeppilli & A. Gaggi), Vol. 2, pp. 303–311.

Fleck, S.J., Henke, C. & Wilson, W. (1989b) Cardiac MRI of elite junior Olympic weight lifters. *International Journal of Sports Medicine* **10**, 329–333.

George, K.P., Wolfe, L.A., Burggraf, G.W. & Normna, R. (1995) Electrocardiographic and echocardiographic characteristics of female athletes. *Medicine and Science in Sports and Exercise* **27**, 1362–1370.

Gettman, L.R. & Pollock, M.I. (1981) Circuit weight training: a critical review of its physiological benefits. *Physician and Sportsmedicine* **9**, 44–60.

Goldberg, A.P. (1989) Aerobic and resistance exercise modify risk factors for coronary heart disease. *Medicine and Science in Sports and Exercise* **21**, 669–674.

Goldberg, L., Elliot, D.L. & Kuehl, K.S. (1988) Cardiovascular changes at rest and during mixed static and dynamic exercise after weight training. *Journal of Applied Sports Science Research* **2**, 42–45.

Goldberg, L., Elliot, D.L. & Kuehl, K.S. (1994) A comparison of the cardiovascular effects of running and weight training. *Journal of Strength and Conditioning Research* **8**, 219–224.

Gonzalez-Camarena, R., Carrasco-Sosa, S., Roman-Ramos, R., Gaitan-Gonzalez, M.J., Medina-Banuelos, V. & Azpiroz-Leehan, J. (2000) Effect of static and dynamic exercise on heart rate and blood pressure variabilities. *Medicine and Science in Sports and Exercise* **32**, 1719–1728.

Gotshall, R.W., Gootman, J., Byrnes, W.C., Fleck, S.J. & Volovich, T.C. (1999) Noninvasive characterization of the blood pressure response to the double-leg press exercise. *Journal of Exercise Physiology* online **2**, www.css.edu/users/tboone2.

Haennel, R., Teo, K.K., Quinney, A. & Kappagoda, T. (1989) Effects of hydraulic circuit training on cardiovascular function. *Medicine and Science in Sports and Exercise* **21**, 605–612.

Hagberg, J.M., Ehsoni, A.A., Goldring, D., Hernandez, A., Sincore, D.R. & Holloszy, J.O. (1984) Effect of weight training on blood pressure and hemodynamics in hypertensive adolescents. *Journal of Pediatrics* **104**, 147–151.

Hamilton, W.F., Woodbury, R.A. & Harper, H.T. (1943) Arterial, cerebrospinal, and venous pressures in man during cough and strain. *American Journal of Physiology* **141**, 42–50.

Harris, K.A. & Holly, R.G. (1987) Physiological responses to circuit weight training in borderline hypertensive subjects. *Medicine and Science in Sports and Exercise* **19**, 246–252.

Haykowsky, M.J., Quinney, H.A., Gillis, R. & Thompson, C.R. (2000) Left ventricular morphology in junior and master resistance trained athletes. *Medicine and Science in Sports and Exercise* **32**, 349–352.

Hickson, R.C., Rosenkoetter, M.A. & Brown, M.M. (1980) Strength training effects on aerobic power and short-term endurance. *Medicine and Science in Sports and Exercise* **12**, 336–339.

Hill, D.W. & Butler, S.D. (1991) Hemodynamic responses to weightlifting exercise. *Sports Medicine* **12**, 1–7.

Hurley, B.F. (1989) Effects of resistance training on lipoprotein-lipid profiles: a comparison to aerobic exercise training. *Medicine and Science in Sports and Exercise* **21**, 689–693.

Hurley, B.F., Seals, D.R., Hagberg, J.M. *et al.* (1984) High-density-lipoprotein cholesterol in bodybuilders vs powerlifters. *Journal of the American Medical Association* **252**, 507–513.

Hurley, B.F., Hagberg, J.M., Seals, D.R., Ehsani, A.A., Goldberg, A.P. & Holloszy, J.O. (1987) Glucose tolerance and lipid-lipoprotein levels in middle-age powerlifters. *Clinical Physiology* **7**, 11–19.

Hurley, B.F., Hagberg, J.M., Goldberg, A.P. *et al.* (1988) Resistive training can reduce coronary risk factors without altering $Vo_{2\,max}$ or percent body fat. *Medicine and Science in Sports and Exercise* **20**, 150–154.

Iellamo, F., Legramante, J.M., Raimondi, G. *et al.* (1997) Effects of isokinetic, isotonic and isometric submaximal exercise on heart rate and blood pressure. *European Journal of Applied Physiology* **75**, 89–96.

Johnson, C.C., Stone, M.H., Lopez, S.A., Hebert, J.A., Kilgore, L.T. & Byrd, R.J. (1982) Diet and exercise in middle-age men. *Journal of the American Dietic Association* **81**, 695–701.

Kahn, J.F., Kapitaniak, B. & Monod, H. (1985) Comparisons of two modalities when exerting isometric contractions. *European Journal of Applied Physiology* **54**, 331–335.

Kanakis, C. & Hickson, C. (1980) Left ventricular responses to a program of lower-limb strength training. *Chest* **78**, 618–621.

Kleiner, D.M., Blessing, D.L., Davis, W.R. & Mitchell, J.W. (1996) Acute cardiovascular responses to various forms of resistance exercise. *Journal of Strength and Conditioning Research* **10**, 56–61.

Kleiner, D.M., Blessing, D.L., Mitchell, J.W. & Davis, W.R. (1999) A description of the acute cardiovascular responses to isokinetic resistance at three different speeds. *Journal of Strength and Conditioning Research* **13**, 360–366.

Kraemer, W.J., Deschenes, M.R. & Fleck, S.J. (1988) Physiological adaptations to resistance exercise implications for athletic conditioning. *Sports Medicine* **6**, 246–256.

Kujala, U.M., Sarna, S., Kaprio, J., Tikkanen, H.O. & Koskenvuo, M. (2000) Natural selection to sports, later physical activity habits, and coronary heart disease. *British Journal of Sports Medicine* **34**, 445–449.

Lee, A., Craig, B.W., Lucas, J., Pohlman, R. & Stelling, H. (1990) The effect of endurance training, weight training and a combination of endurance and weight training upon the blood lipid profile of young male subjects. *Journal of Applied Sports Science Research* **4**, 68–75.

LeMura, L.M., von Duvillard, S.P., Andreacci, J., Klebez, J.M., Chelland, S.A. & Russo, J. (2000) Lipid and lipoprotein profiles, cardiovascular fitness, body composition and diet during and after resistance, aerobic and combination training in young women. *European Journal of Applied Physiology* **82**, 451–458.

Longhurst, J.C., Kelly, A.R., Gonuea, W.J. & Mitchell, J.H. (1980a) Echocardiographic left ventricular masses in distance runners and weight lifters. *Journal of Applied Physiology: Respiration, Environmental and Exercise Physiology* **48**, 154–162.

Longhurst, J.C., Kelly, A.R., Gonuea, W.J. & Mitchell, J.H. (1980b) Cardiovascular responses to static exercise in distance runners and weight lifters. *Journal of Applied Physiology: Respiration, Environmental and Exercise Physiology* **49**, 676–683.

Ludbrook, J., Faris, I.B., Iannos, J., Jamieson, G.G. & Russel, W.J. (1978) Lack of effect of isometric handgrip exercise on the responses of the carotid sinus baroreceptor reflex in man. *Clinical Science and Molecular Medicine* **55**, 189–194.

Lusiani, L., Ronsisvalle, G., Bonanome, A., Castellani, V., Macchia, C. & Pagan, A. (1986) Echocardiographic evaluation of the dimensions and systolic properties of the left ventricle in freshman athletes during physical training. *European Heart Journal* **7**, 196–203.

McCall, G.E., Byrnes, W.C., Dickinson, A., Pattany, P.M. & Fleck, S.J. (1996) Muscle fiber hypertrophy, hyperplasia, and capillary density in college men after resistance training. *Journal of Applied Physiology* **81**, 2004–2012.

McCartney, N., McKelvie, R.S., Martin, J., Sale, D.G. & MacDougall, J.D. (1993) Weight-training induced attenuation of the circulatory response of older males to weight lifting. *Journal of Applied Physiology* **74**, 1056–1060.

MacDougall, J.D., Tuxen, D., Sale, D.G., Moroz, J.R. & Sutton, J.R. (1985) Arterial blood pressure response to heavy resistance exercise. *Journal of Applied Physiology* **58**, 785–790.

Marcinik, E.J., Potts, J., Schlabach, G., Will, S., Dawson, P. & Hurley, B.F. (1991) Effects of strength training on lactate threshold and endurance performance. *Medicine and Science in Sports and Exercise* **23**, 739–743.

Menapace, F.J., Hammer, W.J., Ritzer, T.F. *et al.* (1982) Left ventricular size in competitive weight lifters: and echocardiographic study. *Medicine and Science in Sports and Exercise* **14**, 72–75.

Miles, D.S., Owens, J.J., Golden, J.C. & Gotshall, R.W. (1987) Central and peripheral hemodynamics during maximal leg extension exercise. *European Journal of Applied Physiology* **56**, 12–17.

Moffatt, R.J., Wallace, M.B. & Sady, S.P. (1990) Effect of anabolic steroids on lipoprotein profiles of female weight lifters. *Physician and Sportsmedicine* **18**, 106–115.

Morgan, D.W., Cruise, R.J., Girardin, B.W., Lutz-Schneider, V., Morgan, D.H. & Qi, W.M. (1986) Hdl-c concentrations in weight-trained, endurance trained, and sedentary females. *Physician and Sportsmedicine* **14**, 166–181.

Nakao, M., Inoue, Y. & Murakami, H. (1995) Longitudinal study of the effect of high-intensity weight training on aerobic capacity. *European Journal of Applied Physiology* **70**, 20–25.

Pearson, A.C., Schiff, M., Mrosek, D., Labovitz, A.J. & Williams, G.A. (1986) Left ventricular diastolic function in weight lifters. *American Journal of Cardiology* **58**, 1254–1259.

Perrault, H. & Turcotte, R.A. (1994) Exercise-induced cardiac hypertrophy fact or fallacy? *Sports Medicine* **17**, 288–308.

Pichon, C.E., Hunter, G.R., Morris, M., Bond, R.L. & Metz, J. (1996) Blood pressure and heart rate response and metabolic cost of circuit versus traditional weight training. *Journal of Strength and Conditioning Research* **10**, 153–156.

Ricci, G., Lajoie, D., Petticlerc, R. *et al.* (1982) Left ventricular size following endurance, sprint, and strength training. *Medicine and Science in Sports and Exercise* **14**, 344–347.

Sadamoto, T., Bonde-Petersen, F. & Suzuki, Y. (1983) Skeletal muscle tension, flow pressure and EMG during sustained isometric contractions in humans. *European Journal of Applied Physiology* **51**, 395–408.

Sale, D.G., Moroz, D.E., McKelvie, R.S., MacDougall, J.D. & McCartney, N. (1993) Comparison of blood pressure response to isokinetic and weight-lifting exercise. *European Journal of Applied Physiology* **67**, 115–120.

Sale, D.G., Moroz, D.E., McKelvie, R.S., MacDougall, J.D. & McCartney, N. (1994) Effect of training on the blood pressure response to weight lifting. *Canadian Journal of Applied Physiology* **19**, 60–74.

Saltin, B. & Astrand, P.O. (1967) Maximal oxygen uptake in athletes. *Journal of Applied Physiology* **23**, 353–358.

Scala, D., McMillian, J., Blessing, D., Rozenek, R. & Stone, M. (1987) Metabolic cost of a preparatory phase of training in weightlifting: a practical observation. *Journal of Applied Sports Science Research* **1**, 48–52.

Scharf, H.-P., Eckhardt, R., Maurus, M. & Puhl, W. (1994) Metabolic and hemodynamic changes during isokinetic muscle training. *International Journal of Sports Medicine* **15**, S56–S59.

Sejersted, O.M., Hargens, A.R., Kardel, K.R., Blom, P., Jensen, O. & Hermansen, L. (1984) Intramuscular fluid pressure during isometric contractions of human skeletal muscle. *Journal of Applied Physiology* **56**, 287–295.

Sjogaard, G., Kiens, B., Jorgensen, K. & Saltin, B. (1986) Intramuscular pressure, EMG and blood flow during low-level prolonged static contraction in man. *Acta Physiologica Scandinavica* **128**, 475–484.

Smith, M.L. & Raven, B.P. (1986) Cardiovascular responses to lower body negative pressure in endurance and static exercise trained men. *Medicine and Science in Sports and Exercise* **18**, 545–550.

Snoecky, L.H.E.H., Abeling, H.F.M., Lambrets, J.A.C., Schmitz, J.J.F., Verstappen, F.T.J. & Reneman, R.S. (1982) Echocardiographic dimensions in athletes in relation to their training programs. *Medicine and Science in Sports and Exercise* **14**, 32–34.

Spataro, A., Pelliccia, A., Caselli, G., Amici, E. & Vernerando, A. (1985) Echocardiographic standards in top-class athletes. *Journal of Sports Cardiology* **2**, 17–27.

Spataro, A., Pellicca, A., Proschan, M.A. *et al.* (1994) Morphology of the 'athlete's heart' assessed by echocardiography in 947 elite athletes representing 27 sports. *American Journal of Cardiology* **74**, 802–806.

Staron, R.S., Karapondo, D.L., Kraemer, W.J. *et al.* (1994) Skeletal muscle adaptations during the early phase of heavy-resistance training in men and women. *Journal of Applied Physiology* **76**, 1247–1255.

Staron, R.S., Murray, T.E., Gilders, R.M., Hagerman, F.C., Hikida, R.S. & Ragg, K.E. (2000) Influence of resistance training on serum lipid and lipoprotein concentrations in young men and women. *Journal of Strength and Conditioning Research* **14**, 37–44.

Stone, M.H., Nelson, J.K., Nader, S. & Carter, D. (1983a) Short-term weight training effects on resting and recovery heart rates. *Athletic Training* **18**, 69–71.

Stone, M.H., Wilson, G.D., Blessing, D. & Rozenek, R. (1983b) Cardiovascular responses to short-term Olympic style weight-training in young man. *Canadian Journal of Applied Sports Science* **8**, 134–139.

Stone, M.H., Pierce, K., Godsen, R. *et al.* (1987) Heart rate and lactate levels during weight-training exercises in trained and untrained men. *Physician and Sportsmedicine* **15**, 97–105.

Stone, M.H., Fleck, S.J., Triplett, N.R. & Kraemer, W.J. (1991) Physiological adaptations to resistance training exercise. *Sports Medicine* **11**, 210–231.

Tesch, P.A. (1987) Acute and long-term metabolic changes consequent to heavy-resistance exercise. *Medicine and Science in Sports and Exercise* **26**, 67–89.

Tikkanen, H.O., Naveri, H. & Harkonen, M. (1996) Skeletal muscle fiber distribution influences serum high-density lipoprotein cholesterol level. *Atherosclerosis* **120**, 1–5.

Twisk, J.W.R., Kemper, H.C.G. & van Mechelen, W. (2000) Tracking of activity and fitness and the relationship with cardiovascular disease risk factors. *Medicine and Science in Sports and Exercise* **32**, 1455–1461.

Urhausen, A. & Kindermann, W. (1992) Echocardiographic findings in strength- and endurance-trained athletes. *Sports Medicine* **13**, 270–284.

Viitasalo, J.T., Komi, P.V. & Karovonen, M.J. (1979) Muscle strength and body composition as determinants of blood pressure in young men. *European Journal of Applied Physiology* **42**, 165–173.

Vorobyev, A.N. (1988) Part 12: Musculo-skeletal and circulatory effects of weightlifting. *Soviet Sports Review* **23**, 144–148.

Wallace, M.B., Moffatt, R.J., Haymes, E.M. & Green, N.R. (1991) Acute effects of resistance exercise on parameters of lipoprotein metabolism. *Medicine and Science in Sports and Exercise* **23**, 199–204.

Wang, N., Hikida, R.S., Staron, R.S. & Simoneau, J.-A. (1993) Muscle fiber types of women after resistance training—quantitative ultrastructure and enzyme activity. *Pflügers Archiv* **424**, 494–502.

Williams, P.T., Stefanick, M.L., Vranizan, K.M. & Wood, P.D. (1994) The effects of weight loss of exercise or by dieting on plasma high-density lipoprotein (hdl) levels in man with low, intermediate, and normal-to-high hdl at baseline. *Metabolism* **43**, 917–924.

Wolfe, L.A., Cunningham, D.A. & Boughner, D.R. (1986) Physical conditioning effects on cardiac dimensions: a review of echocardiographic studies. *Canadian Journal of Applied Sports Science* **11**, 66–79.

Wright, J.R., McCloskey, D.I. & Fitzpatrick, R.C. (2000) Effects of systemic arterial blood pressure on the contractile force of a human hand muscle. *Journal of Applied Physiology* **88**, 1390–1396.

PART 4

SPECIAL PROBLEMS IN STRENGTH AND POWER TRAINING

Chapter 21

Ageing and Neuromuscular Adaptation to Strength Training

KEIJO HÄKKINEN

Ageing, muscle atrophy, activation and decrease in strength and power

Human muscle strength reaches its peak between the ages of 20–30 years, after which time it remains unchanged or decreases only slightly for more than 20 years. However, with increasing age, especially at the onset of the sixth decade, a steeper decline in maximal strength begins in both genders (e.g. Viitasalo *et al.* 1985; Frontera *et al.* 1991; Häkkinen & Häkkinen 1991; Narici *et al.* 1991; Porter *et al.* 1995; Häkkinen *et al.* 1996b, 1998a). The decrease in maximal strength from the age of 30 to the age of 80 can be as large as 30–40%. The age-related decrease in maximal strength may also vary slightly between different muscle groups of the body (Fig. 21.1). The loss of muscle strength in the proximal muscles of the lower extremities seems to be greater than that of the upper extremities, presumably due to a decreasing use of lower compared with upper limb muscles in older groups (e.g. Frontera *et al.* 1991).

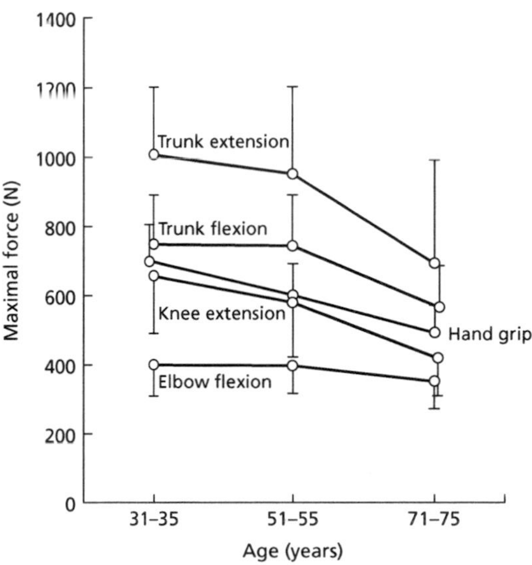

Fig. 21.1 Mean (± SE) maximal isometric strength of various muscle groups in men of three different age groups. (From Viitasalo *et al.* 1985.)

The age-related decrease in muscle strength is related to several factors as summarized in Fig. 21.2 (e.g. Porter *et al.* 1995). Nevertheless, the decrease in maximal strength is related to a great extent to the reduction in muscle mass in both men and women, since ageing is associated with alterations in hormone balance, especially with decreased androgen levels (e.g. Vermulen *et al.* 1972; Chakravati *et al.* 1976; Hammond *et al.* 1978; Häkkinen & Pakarinen 1993), and often also with a decline in the volume of normal physical activities and/or with a decrease in the loads (loading intensity) of these activities. It has been shown that the decline in muscle mass is due to both a reduction in the size of individual muscle fibres, especially of Type II (fast-twitch) fibres, and a loss of individual fibres (Larsson *et al.* 1978; Essen-Gustavsson & Borges 1986; Lexell *et al.* 1988). The data presented in Fig. 21.3 indicate age-related muscle atrophy with preferential atrophy of Type II muscle fibres in the 70-year age group in comparison to the 50-year age group in both men and women. Lexell *et al.* (1988) have demonstrated that ageing atrophy of muscles, at least in

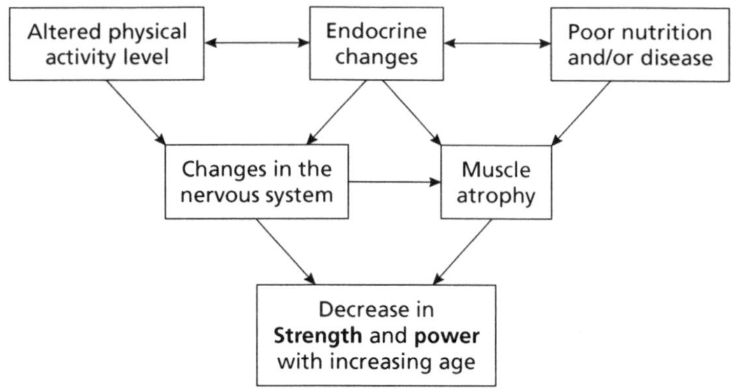

Fig. 21.2 Proposed mechanisms leading to the decreases in muscle strength and power with increasing age. (Modified from Porter *et al.* 1995.)

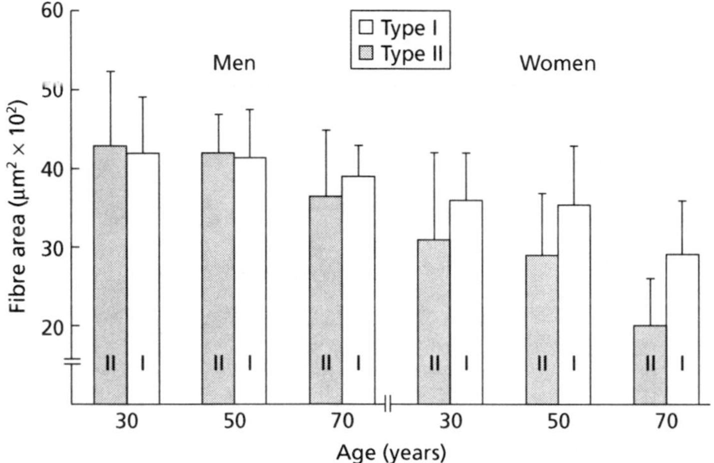

Fig. 21.3 Mean areas of Type I and II muscle fibres of the vastus lateralis in men and women of three different age groups (Essen-Gustavsson & Borges 1986).

the vastus lateralis muscle, is caused mainly by a loss of fibres and to a lesser extent by a reduction in fibre size, mostly in Type II fibres. The reduction in fibre number can be caused either by an irreparable damage of the fibres or by a permanent loss of the contact between the nerves of the muscle fibres. Part of the fibre population seems to undergo a denervation process, although a reinnervation process is also possible with increasing age. Nevertheless, when some muscle fibres are permanently denervated and lost, a subsequent replacement of fat and fibrous tissue follows, leading to a smaller proportion of muscle tissue in ageing men and women. Both a denervation process and inactivity seem to underlie the change in fibre size with increasing age (Lexell *et al.* 1988). Whether the fibre type proportion of the muscle is altered during ageing is a very difficult question to answer. According to Lexell *et al.* (1988) there may be several processes affecting the properties of individual fibres, and alterations due to a specific loss of a motor unit type may be undetected.

Because the proportion of muscle tissue decreases with increasing age, it is clear that age-related decline in the whole cross-sectional area (CSA) of muscle can also be 'easily' demonstrated as shown in Fig. 21.4 for the quadriceps femoris (QF) muscle in men and women of two different age groups. The results indicate that age-related declines in the CSA and in maximal strength of this muscle group seem to take place in parallel. When the individual values in maximal force are related to the individual values

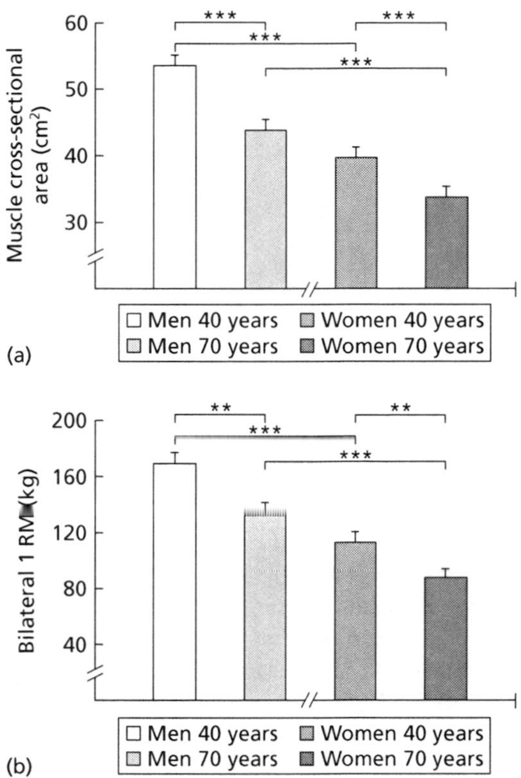

Fig. 21.4 Means (± SE) for cross-sectional area of the quadriceps femoris and 1-RM bilateral leg extension in middle-aged and older men and women (Häkkinen *et al.* 1998a).

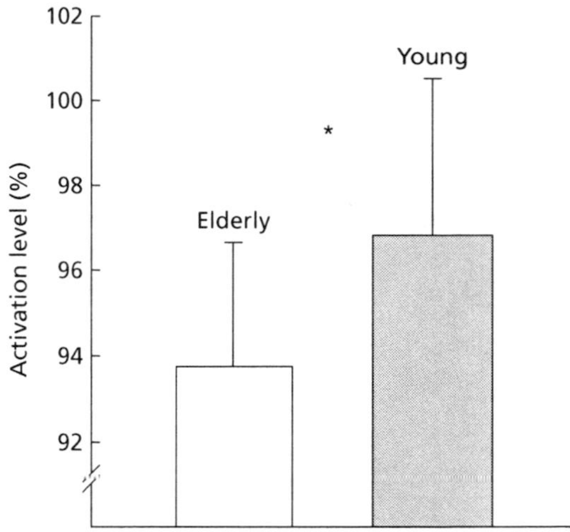

Fig. 21.5 Activation level (%) during maximal voluntary contraction in elderly and young groups (Yue *et al.* 1999).

in the CSA of the muscle, no or only slight differences are usually observed between different age groups. This does support the concept that decrease in strength with increasing age is related to a great extent to the reduction in muscle mass (Frontera *et al.* 1991). However, in the older age group, the interindividual variations in the force values per CSA may be somewhat greater than in the younger groups (Häkkinen & Häkkinen 1991). This indicates that in addition to decrease in muscle mass, decrease in maximal strength, especially at older ages, might also be in part due to a decrease in maximal voluntary neural input to the muscles and/or changes in 'qualitative' characteristics of the muscle tissue.

Actually, age-related declines in strength have been shown to be in part due to decreased maximal voluntary activation of the agonists. This was indicated by an incomplete muscle activation during maximal voluntary efforts performed with the addition of supramaximal single pulses in the case of both the quadriceps femoris (Harridge *et al.* 1999) and the biceps brachii (Yue *et al.* 1999). The incomplete muscle activation (Fig. 21.5) may in part be explained by an age-related decrease observed in the firing rate of motor units (Kamen *et al.* 1995) (Fig. 21.6). In addition to changes in maximal voluntary neural drive to the agonists, there appears to be an age-related increase in antagonist coactivation, especially during dynamic actions (Fig. 21.7). Nevertheless, one could conclude that it seems clear that the extent to which voluntary neural drive would decrease with increasing age is probably much smaller than peripheral neuromuscular ageing changes. Since some data also indicate that age would not necessarily impair voluntary ability to maximally activate some muscles, for example, the first dorsal interosseus of the hand (Enoka *et al.* 1992), the decrease in this activation ability in ageing people may vary between the different muscles and muscle groups in relation to their decreased use in normal daily physical activities.

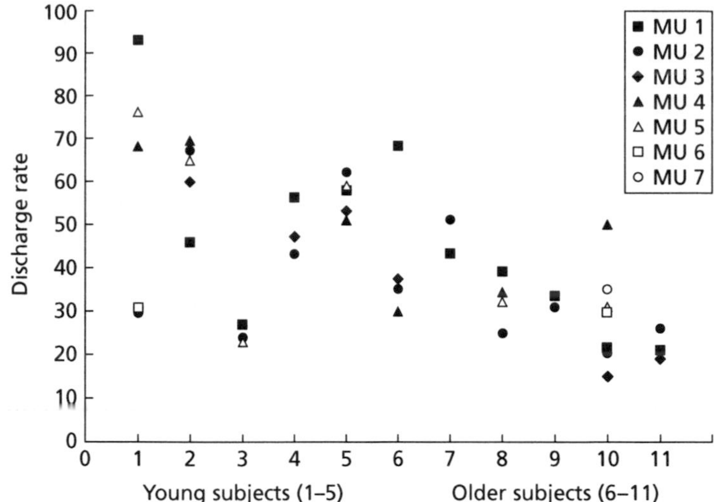

Fig. 21.6 Discharge rate of motor units in young and older subjects (Kamen *et al.* 1995).

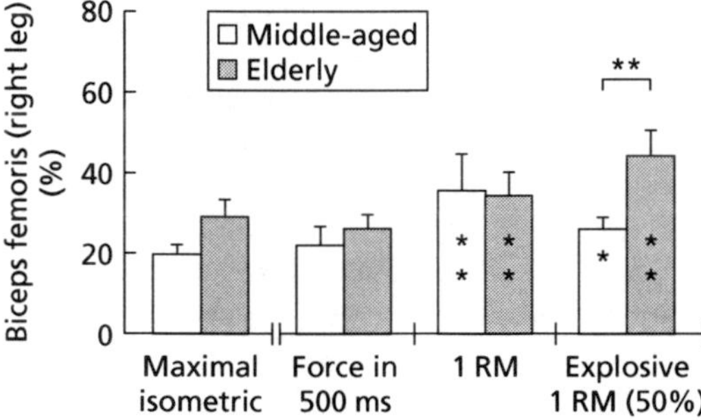

Fig. 21.7 Mean (± SE) IEMG (in relative (%) values) for the biceps femoris during the maximal isometric and the initial (500-ms) (rapidly produced) phases, concentric 1 RM and explosive actions (with a load of 50% of 1 RM) of the leg extensors in middle-aged and elderly subjects. (Modified from Häkkinen *et al.* 1998a.)

Nevertheless, the information available suggests that in order to minimize age-related muscle atrophy and decrease in muscle strength, strength training should be a part of an overall physical training programme in ageing men and women. This should deserve more attention, since older people may usually be involved primarily in endurance, aerobic or stretching types of physical activities performed with low loads.

In normal human movement the time taken to produce a certain submaximal force level may sometimes be as important as the absolute force level itself. Ageing leads to declines in muscle mass and in maximal strength of the muscles, but it has been shown to lead to even greater worsening in explosive force production (e.g. Bosco & Komi 1980; Clarkson *et al.* 1981; Häkkinen & Häkkinen 1991; Häkkinen *et al.* 1998a; Izquierdo *et al.* 1999). The results presented in Fig. 21.8 demonstrate this by showing that the maximal vertical jumping ability decreases largely with increasing age, in both men and women. However, it must be pointed out that vertical jumping ability, especially at older ages, is influenced not only by the level of explosive force production, but also by the level of absolute maximal strength of the muscles which contribute to this neuromuscular performance capacity. Nevertheless, the decrease in explosive strength can also be observed by the drastic differences in the shapes of the force–time curves among younger, middle-aged and older subjects of both genders (Häkkinen & Häkkinen 1991; Häkkinen *et al.* 1995, 1996b, 1998a) as shown in Fig. 21.9 for the leg extensor muscles of men of three different age groups.

The shape of the isometric force–time curve can also be analysed on a relative scale—with

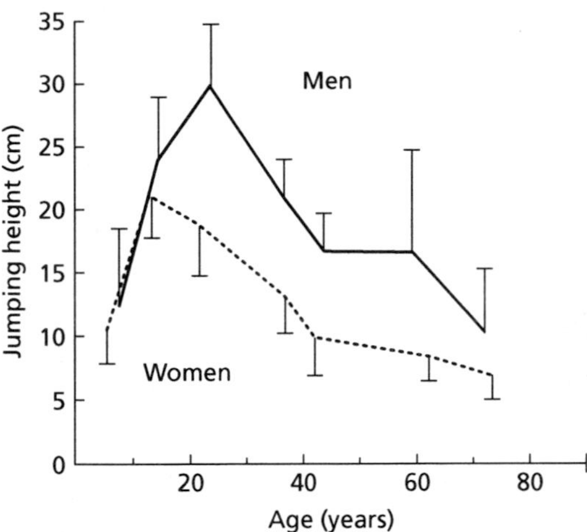

Fig. 21.8 Mean (± SD) heights of rise in the squat jump in men and women of different age groups (Bosco & Komi 1980).

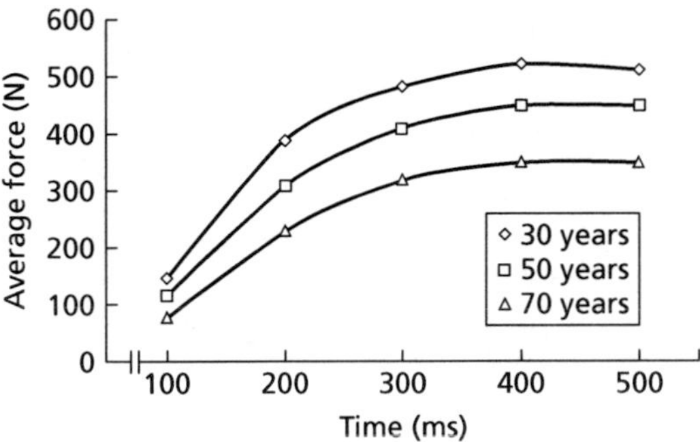

Fig. 21.9 Average force–time curves of isometric bilateral leg extension action in men of three different age groups. (Modified from Häkkinen *et al.* 1995.)

respect to percentage of the maximal force of each individual. It has been shown that the shape of the (relative) isometric force–time curves also changes markedly in ageing people, especially women (Häkkinen & Häkkinen 1991) at the onset of the sixth decade. The force–time curves of the leg extension action presented in Fig. 21.10 for women of three different age groups indicate that explosive force production capacity of muscles decreases in ageing people. These findings also support the concept that atrophying effects of increasing age may be greater on Type II than on Type I fibres and/or that there is a loss of Type II fibres and that the maximal rate of voluntary neural activation of the muscles might also be influenced by ageing. The occurrence of the age-related decrease in the maximal rate of voluntary neural activation is further supported by some recent data (Häkkinen *et al.* 1998a; Kent-Braun & Ng 1999). All of these observations may also have some practical relevance. In order to minimize the effects of ageing on the neuromuscular system, strength training combined with modified power type of exercises could also be useful as a part of an overall physical training for older people. This would also contribute positively to attempts to maintain the daily functional capacity of older people at as high a level as possible, for as long as possible.

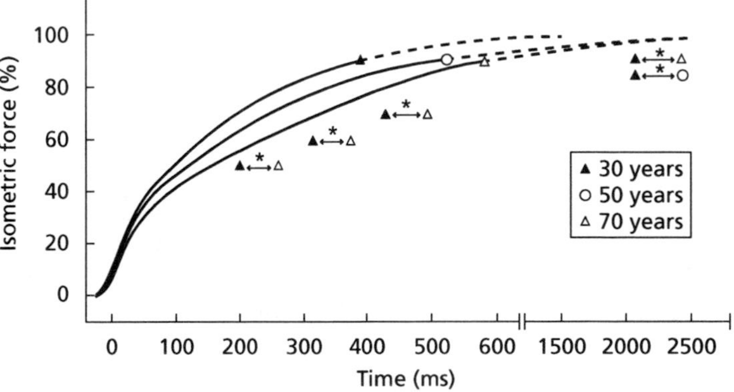

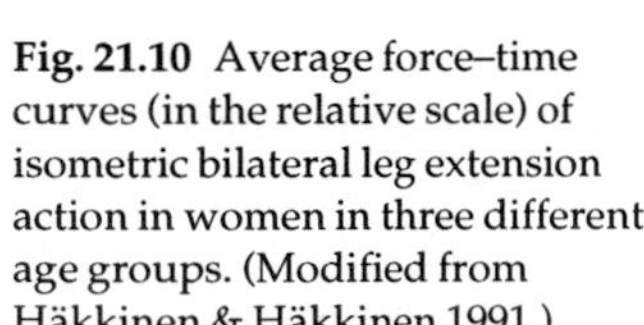
Fig. 21.10 Average force–time curves (in the relative scale) of isometric bilateral leg extension action in women in three different age groups. (Modified from Häkkinen & Häkkinen 1991.)

Table 21.1 Strength gains due to strength training in older men and women.

Authors	Gender	Age (years)	*n*	Action	Duration (weeks)	Strength gain (%)
Frontera *et al.* (1988)	M	60–72	12	Knee extension	12	1 RM (107)
Hagberg *et al.* (1989)	M/F	70–79	23	Chest press	26	1 RM (18)
Brown *et al.* (1990)	M	60–70	14	Elbow flexion	12	1 RM (48)
Fiatarone *et al.* (1990)	M/F	86–96	10	Knee extension	8	1 RM (174)
Charette *et al.* (1991)	F	64–86	13	Leg press	12	1 RM (28)
Hicks *et al.* (1991)	M/F	66.3	11	Dorsiflexion	12	1 RM (48)
Judge *et al.* (1993)	M/F	71–97	18	Knee flexion	12	1 RM (32)
Nichols *et al.* (1993)	F	67.8	18	Upper/lower	24	1 RM (18–71)
Rice *et al.* (1993)	M	65–78	10	Elbow extension	26	1 RM (30)
Pyka *et al.* (1994)	M/F	61–78	25	Upper/lower	30	1 RM 23–62
Fiatarone *et al.* (1994)	M/F	72–98	100	Hip/knee extension	10	1 RM (113)
Häkkinen *et al.* (1994)	M/F	64–73	11	Leg extension	12	MVC (20–37)
Häkkinen *et al.* (1996a)	M/F	60–75	12	Knee extension	12	1 RM (18–21)
Häkkinen *et al.* (1998)	M/F	62–78	11	Leg extension	24	MVC (36–57)
Harridge *et al.* (1999)	M/F	85–97	11	Knee extension	12	MVT (37)
Tracy *et al.* (1999)	M/F	65–75	12	Knee extension	9	1 RM (27–29)
Hagerman *et al.* (2000)	M	60–75	10	Leg press	16	1 RM (72)
Häkkinen *et al.* (2000)	M/F	62–78	11	Knee extension	24	1 RM (16–24)
Roth *et al.* (2000)	F	65–75	6	Knee extension	9	1 RM (25)
Häkkinen *et al.* (2001)	F	60–68	10	Leg extension	21	MVC (37)

Strength gains in middle-aged and older men and women during strength training

Moritani and DeVries (1980) had already demonstrated over 20 years ago that muscle strength in older people could be increased during systematic resistance training. Actually, muscle strength of the elbow flexion improved in a group of older men (70 years) to about the same extent (about 20%) as in another group of young men (22 years) after 8 weeks of strength training. Effects of strength training in older people were examined extensively in the late 1980s and especially in the 1990s. Table 21.1 shows clearly that large strength gains have taken place due to strength training in older men and women at ages ranging from 60 to even 98 years. It can be concluded that systematic strength training can lead to considerable improvements of strength of all muscle groups examined, independent of age and gender, when the loads (loading intensity), the frequency of training sessions per week, and duration of the resistance training period are all sufficient. The results presented in Fig. 21.11 also show that the initial increases in maximal strength are very large during the first 2–4 months of strength training in both middle-aged and older subjects of both genders. Thereafter, strength development may take place at a diminished rate during more prolonged training periods, depending also on the loads, frequency and type of training. Nevertheless, older men and women are able to increase their strength over prolonged resistance training periods lasting for 1 year (Fig. 21.12) or even longer (Morganti *et al.* 1995; McCartney *et al.* 1996; Häkkinen *et al.* 2000a). Thus, an important conclusion from the practical standpoint is the fact that the frequency of strength training in previously untrained middle-aged and older subjects of both genders can be as low as twice a week, when the loads and volume of each training session are sufficient and/or increased progressively (i.e. periodized) throughout the training period.

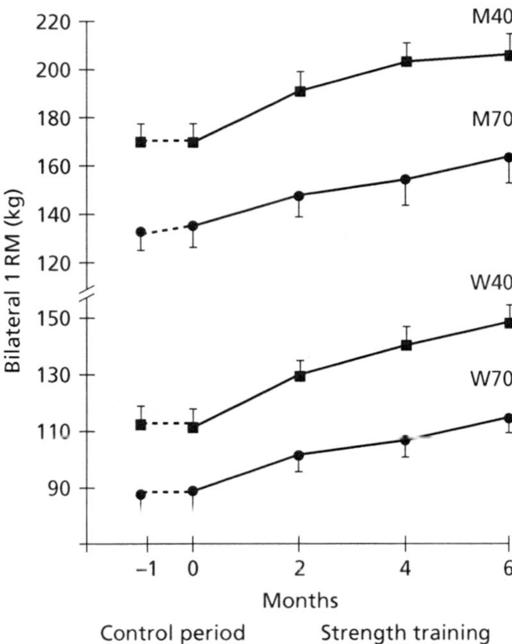

Fig. 21.11 Mean (± SE) maximal bilateral concentric 1 RM of the leg extensor muscles in middle-aged and older men and women during the control and strength training periods (Häkkinen *et al.* 1998b).

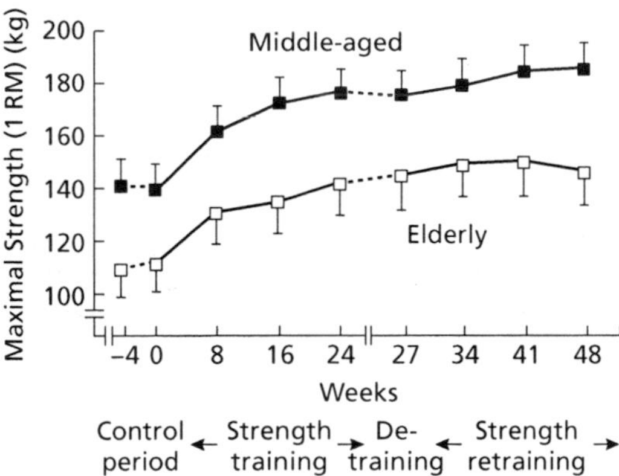

Fig. 21.12 Mean (± SE) maximal bilateral concentric 1 RM of the leg extensor muscles in middle-aged and elderly subjects during the control, strength training, detraining and strength retraining periods (Häkkinen *et al.* 2000a).

Neural adaptations during strength training in middle-aged and older people

In previously untrained young men and women, large initial increases in maximal strength during strength training result primarily from increased motor unit activation of trained muscles, while gradually increasing muscle hypertrophy contributes to strength development during the later phases of training. A widely held view up to the end of the 1980s was that strength gains in older subjects might be due to improved neural recruitment patterns rather than hypertrophy of muscle fibres. The large increases observed in maximal IEMGs of trained muscles, especially during the earlier weeks of strength training, both in middle-aged and older men and women, indicate that considerable training-induced adaptation takes place in the nervous system (Moritani & DeVries 1980; Häkkinen & Häkkinen 1995; Häkkinen *et al.* 1998b, 2000a, 2001a). The data recorded in both middle-aged and older subjects of both genders during the strength training period shown in Fig. 21.13 support this well (Häkkinen *et al.* 1998b). Although the EMG is a complicated signal and represents only an average of the maximal neural activation of the muscle, strength training-induced increases in the magnitude of EMG could result from the increased number of active motor units and/or increase in their firing frequency in younger adults and middle-aged and older subjects of both genders. The actual nature of adaptations in the nervous system is difficult to determine but strength training seems to lead to changes in the facilitatory and/or inhibitory pathways so that: (i) activation of the prime movers is increased; (ii) there is an improved coactivation of the synergists; and (iii) there is reduced coactivation of the antagonist muscles (Komi 1986; Enoka 1988; Sale 1992; Häkkinen 1994). These suggestions are strongly supported by some recent data (Harridge *et al.* 1999) shown in Fig. 21.14 including more direct evidence for neural adaptations due to strength training. The data indicate that an older man did demonstrate an incomplete

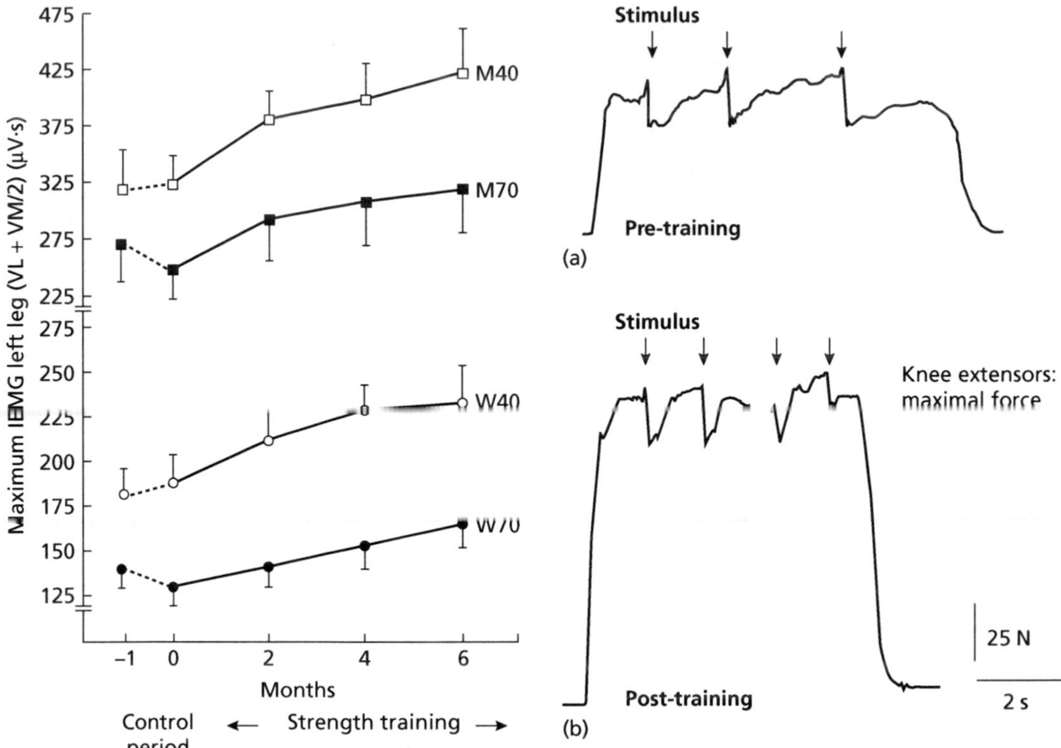

Fig. 21.13 Mean (± SE) maximum IEMGs of the vastus lateralis and vastus medialis in isometric knee extension action in middle-aged and older men and women during the control and strength training periods (Häkkinen *et al.* 2000b).

Fig. 21.14 Original recordings of voluntary force production with a superimposed stimulus of an older man (a) before and (b) after strength training. (From Harridge *et al.* 1999.)

muscle activation of the knee extensors before training, but increased activation by 44% such that he was able, for at least part of a maximal effort, to obtain full activation after 12 weeks of heavy-resistance training. However, older men and women seem to demonstrate large interindividual variation in neural adaptations during strength training (Häkkinen *et al.* 1996a, 1998b, 2000a,b; Harridge *et al.* 1999).

In addition to the increase in the activation of the prime movers a unique feature in strength training in older people is the observation as to considerable decreases in the coactivation of the antagonists in both genders. This has been recorded during both maximal isometric and 1-RM dynamic leg extension actions as shown in Fig. 21.15 for older women in the isometric

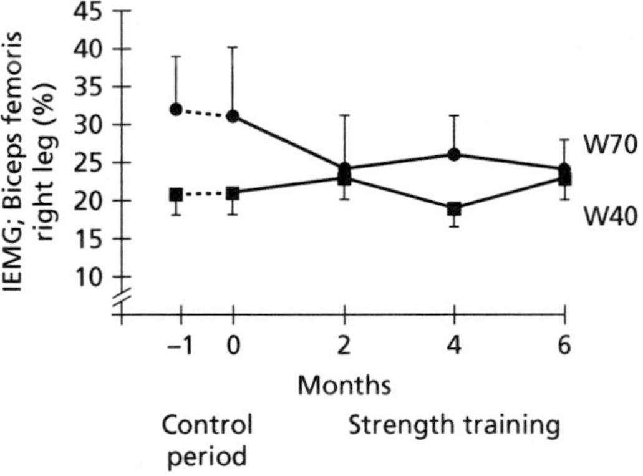

Fig. 21.15 Mean (± SE) integrated electromyographic activity (IEMG in relative to agonist values (%)) for the biceps femoris during maximal voluntary isometric action of the leg extensors in middle-aged and older women during the control and strength training periods. (Modified from Häkkinen *et al.* 1998b.)

action. The change in antagonist coactivation in these older women took place during the initial phases of the training so that the coactivation at the end of the training period was at about the same level in comparison to that recorded for the middle-aged subjects. The results obtained in older subjects of both genders support strongly the concept not only that strength training can lead to the increased activation of the agonist muscles but also that training-induced learning effects in terms of reduced coactivation of the antagonist muscles may also play an important role enhancing the net strength production of the agonist muscles. To what extent this kind of reduced coactivation of the antagonists is mediated by mechanisms in the central nervous system or associated also with peripheral neural control, especially during various dynamic actions, is difficult to interpret. It is also possible that the magnitude and the time course of the changes in antagonist coactivation may be related to the action used in the measurements, to the exercises utilized in the training, and to the initial physical status of the subjects in terms of experience and skill in strength training.

Table 21.2 Increases in muscle fibre size during strength training (12–30 weeks) in older people (60–84 training years).

		Muscle fibre size increase (%)	
Authors	Gender	Type I	Type II
Frontera *et al.* (1988)	M	34	28
Brown *et al.* (1990)	M	14	30
Charette *et al.* (1991)	F	7	20
Grimby *et al.* (1992)	M	8	5
Roman *et al.* (1993)	M	24	37
Pyka *et al.* (1994)			
(a) 15 weeks	M/F	25	20
(b) 30 weeks	M/F	48	62
Häkkinen *et al.* (1998)	M	31	42
Hikida *et al.* (2000)	M	46	43
Häkkinen *et al.* (2001)	F	22	36

Muscle hypertrophy during strength training in middle-aged and older people

Although strength gains in older subjects do take place to a great extent due to improved neural recruitment patterns, it has been shown with sensitive techniques such as fibre area determination by muscle biopsy, or muscle CSA determination by ultrasound, CT and especially MRI scan, that muscle hypertrophy has also accounted to a considerable extent for strength gains in the elderly of both genders. Some recent research results on strength training-induced large increases in the sizes of both Type I and Type II muscle fibres presented in Table 21.2 demonstrate this well. Strength training-induced muscle hypertrophy in older men and women seems to take place in both subtype IIa and IIb fibres (Häkkinen *et al.* 1998c, 2001b). Skeletal muscles of older people of both genders retain the capacity to undergo training-induced hypertrophy when the overall volume, loads, frequency of training and duration of the training period are sufficient. In addition, Type II subtype transformation going from Type IIb to IIab to IIa has been previously observed in younger (Staron *et al.* 1991, 1994; Adams *et al.* 1993; Kraemer *et al.* 1995) and older men (Häkkinen *et al.* 1998c) but not necessarily in older women (Häkkinen *et al.* 2001a). The roles of duration and mode of resistance training as well as that of age in muscle fibre transformation in the Type IIb fibre population need further examination. Although considerable training-induced muscle hypertrophy does occur in older people, the magnitude of the increases in the sizes of individual muscle fibres does not necessarily correspond to the enlargements recorded in the total CSA of trained muscles. Nevertheless, average enlargements in the total muscle CSA may be as large as 10% during a 3-month heavy-resistance strength training period in both middle-aged and older men and women (Häkkinen & Häkkinen 1995). The MRI data presented in Fig. 21.16 further show that strength training-induced muscle hypertrophy in young and older men took place to about the same degree and was also rather similar in all of the four individual muscles of the QF muscle group.

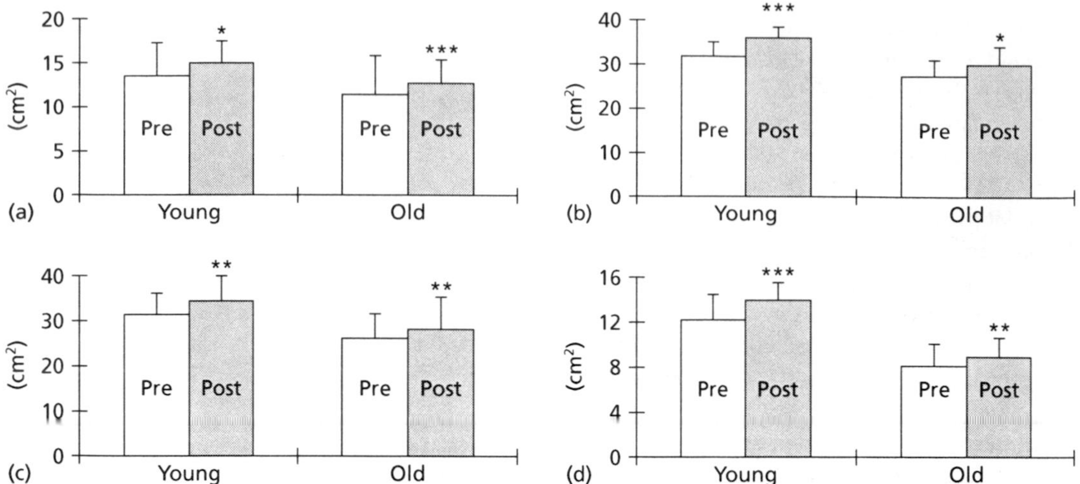

Fig. 21.16 Mean (± SD) cross-sectional areas of the individual muscles of the quadriceps femoris before and after the 10-week strength training period in young and older men. (a) vastus medialis; (b) vastus lateralis; (c) vastus intermedius; (d) rectus femoris. (Modified from Häkkinen *et al.* 1998c.)

However, caution should be exercised when interpreting muscle CSA data obtained only at one particular portion of the limb, since training-induced muscle hypertrophy can be non-uniform along the belly of the muscle in both younger adults (Narici *et al.* 1996) and older people (e.g. Tracy *et al.* 1999; Häkkinen *et al.* 2001b). Tracy *et al.* (1999) examined the phenomenon of selective hypertrophy of the QF in older women and men and showed that strength training-induced muscle hypertrophy was greatest in the region of the largest CSA (at midthigh) and the increases in the CSA became progressively smaller toward the proximal and distal regions of the QF. The authors concluded that the single-slice method may overestimate the true muscle CSA changes in other regions of the QF and may be prone to error. However, the individual muscles of the QF are known to differ, with regard not only to the average CSA of each muscle, but largely to the cross-sectional areas along the belly of these muscles. Interestingly, our recent data (Häkkinen *et al.* 2001b) showed that the increases in the CSA of the total QF took place throughout the length of the femur (Fig. 21.17), while the magnitudes of the CSA increases along the length of the femur did differ specifically between the individual muscles of the QF. Thus, the increases in CSA during the 21-week training were greater in the regions of the largest CSAs, at proximal portions for the vastus lateralis (VL), and at distal portions for the vastus medialis (VM) (Fig. 21.18). Interestingly, this was not the case for the increases recorded in the vastus intermedius or rectus femoris muscles. Although the large training-induced increases observed in the maximal global IEMG of the VL and VM muscles did not differ from each other, the differences in the degree of hypertrophy between the two muscles could be explained by specific differences in muscle activation (and tension) and/or differences in contractile protein synthesis along the belly of the individual muscles (e.g. Narici *et al.* 1996). It should also be pointed out that our study (Häkkinen *et al.* 2001b) used a typical training programme with two common exercises (leg press and knee extension) for the thigh musculature and that the choice of the exercises might contribute to the degree of the selective hypertrophy of the muscles trained. It is also possible that in addition to increased voluntary muscle activation, architectural changes, e.g. changes in pennation angle of the muscle fibres, may have taken place during strength training

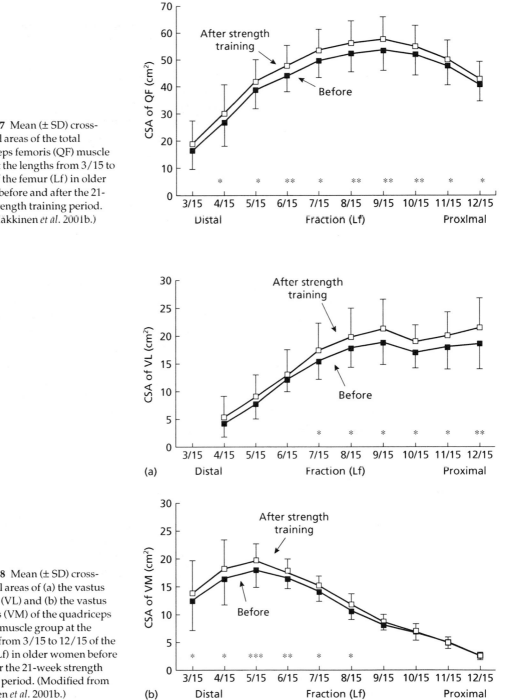

Fig. 21.17 Mean (± SD) cross-sectional areas of the total quadriceps femoris (QF) muscle group at the lengths from 3/15 to 12/15 of the femur (Lf) in older women before and after the 21-week strength training period. (From Häkkinen *et al.* 2001b.)

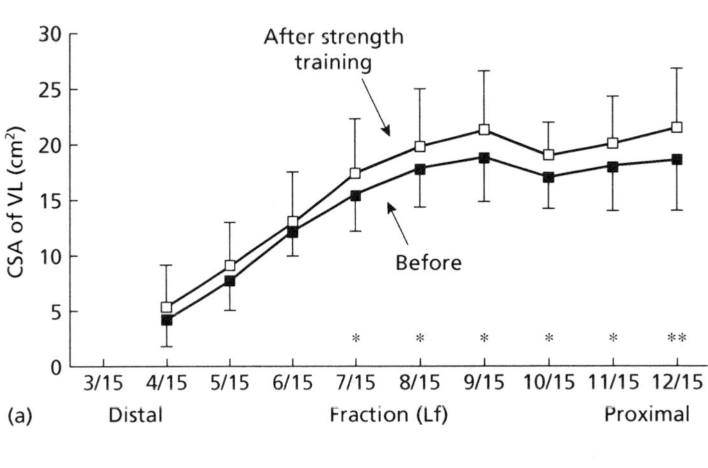

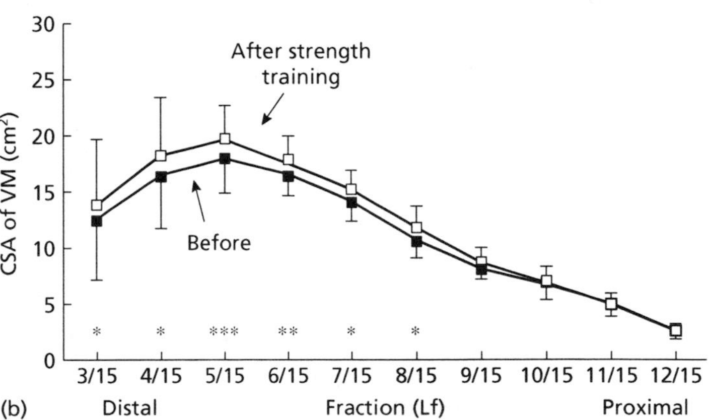

Fig. 21.18 Mean (± SD) cross-sectional areas of (a) the vastus lateralis (VL) and (b) the vastus medialis (VM) of the quadriceps femoris muscle group at the lengths from 3/15 to 12/15 of the femur (Lf) in older women before and after the 21-week strength training period. (Modified from Häkkinen *et al.* 2001b.)

(e.g. Kawakami *et al.* 1993) contributing to strength development. Our data in older women further showed that the increases in CSA of the muscles measured at the length of the muscle biopsy site were significant for the VL and VM and for the whole QF. Thus, the present biopsy site (at the lower third portion of the thigh) for the VL, as commonly used, to determine the degree of hypertrophy of individual muscle fibres, may actually be a reasonable one. In conclusion, the enlargements of the muscle CSA may differ largely between the individual muscles of the QF muscle group, when measured at the same femur length, suggesting the advantages of the multiple-slice method to indicate the 'true' growth of the muscle tissue taking place during strength training.

The possible role of muscle fibre distribution (percentage Type II fibres) on increased strength or the magnitude of muscle hypertrophy during strength training has not been conclusively determined. The recent findings obtained in a group of young and older men indicated that the subjects with a higher relative proportion of Type II fibres demonstrated greater increases in the CSA of the trained muscle than those subjects possessing a lower proportion of Type II in their muscles (Häkkinen *et al.* 1998c). If confirmed, this may be of some importance, especially in older subjects, since ageing is known to be associated with not only muscle atrophy but also a loss of muscle fibres, especially of Type II fibres. However, further research work has to be conducted using experimental designs with longer durations of training, a larger number of subjects, and a larger variability in the age of subjects under investigation, before it can be said that the ultimate degree of muscle hypertrophy and/or strength development in older people would be dependent upon the fibre distribution of trained muscles.

Hormonal factors related to gains in muscle mass and strength

To what extent the degree of training-induced hypertrophy and strength development might be limited in magnitude due to hormonal factors, such as serum levels of anabolic hormones and growth factors, during strength training in older and/or middle-aged men and women needs to be examined in more detail in the future (e.g. Kraemer *et al.* 1998; Häkkinen *et al.* 2001b). However, it seems that when the overall volume/loading of the strength training (such as two or three sessions a week) remains within normal physiological ranges maximal strength can be increased gradually, e.g. throughout the entire 6-month training period with no systematic changes occurring in the serum concentrations of anabolic and catabolic hormones (Häkkinen *et al.* 2000b, 2001b). Second, the data available indicate that although a basal level of the anabolic hormone testosterone is lowered in older women, they seem to be able to gain in strength to about the same extent as middle-aged or young women or men when utilizing a similar type of low-volume total body strength training protocol over the 6-month period. However, in those older women who have demonstrated very low basal testosterone levels, the individual gains in maximal strength and the individual gains in the CSA of the trained muscles during strength training may be minor in comparison to those with higher testosterone concentrations (Häkkinen *et al.* 2000b, 2001b). Therefore, it has been suggested that basal concentrations of blood testosterone may be of great importance, even to the extent that a low level of testosterone may be a limiting factor in older women, for both strength development and overall training-induced muscle hypertrophy, when typical total body heavy-resistance training programmes are utilized. However, it is possible that, even though the blood testosterone levels would remain unaltered, strength training could induce changes e.g. at the receptor level (e.g. Kraemer *et al.* 1999).

Another unique feature is the finding that the acute response of GH to heavy-resistance loading is known to decrease due to ageing in both men and especially older women at the age of about 70 years (Häkkinen & Pakarinen 1995). However, after the 21-week training period the increase in serum GH concentrations in older women at the age of 64 years became significant, not only immediately at postloading but also remaining so up to 30 min postloading (Häkkinen *et al.* 2001b). Due to the pulsatile nature of GH secretion the interpretation of single measures must be done cautiously. However, the observation can be considered as an indication of the training-induced adaptation of the endocrine system showing that the acute GH hormone response may become more systematic after strength training even in older women. It is possible that the magnitude of the acute GH hormone response and the time duration of the response are both important physiological indicators of anabolic adaptations taking place during prolonged strength training even in older women.

Specificity of heavy vs. explosive resistance training

It is well documented that typical heavy-resistance strength training programmes (with high loads and slow movement/action velocities) in young men and women lead to greater increases in maximal force, while the changes in the earlier force portions of the isometric force–time or in the higher velocity portions of the force–velocity curves usually remain considerably minor. This principle of the specificity of the training seems to hold true also during heavy-resistance training in older people (e.g. Frontera *et al.* 1988). The explosive type of strength training, which utilizes exercises performed with slightly lower loads but with much higher movement velocities, usually leads in younger men and women to improvements primarily in the earlier force portions of the force–time or higher velocity portions of the force–velocity curves (e.g. Häkkinen 1994). It has been shown not only that a strength training programme composed of both heavy-resistance and explosive types of exercises for the leg extensor muscles in middle-aged and older men and women led to great increases in maximal force, but also that considerable increases in explosive strength characteristics of the trained muscles were recorded in both isometric (Fig. 21.19) and dynamic actions (Häkkinen *et al.* 1998b). The significant increases observed in the IEMGs of the agonists during the early phase of the isometric knee extension action indicate that the increases in explosive force of the trained muscles might have been explained largely by training-induced increases in the rapid neural activation of the motor units (Van Cutsem *et al.* 1998) and/or that selective hypertrophy of Type II muscle fibres may have also occurred to some degree not only in middle-aged but also in older subjects of both genders. The observation that explosive force production capacity of the neuromuscular system remains trainable even in older subjects should also be of practical value, for example, in primary and secondary prevention of frailty and in physical rehabilitation programmes for ageing men and women.

Since muscle strength and the ability of the leg extensor muscles to develop force rapidly are important performance characteristics contributing to several tasks of daily life such as climbing stairs and walking, or even prevention of falls and trips (Bassey *et al.* 1992; Izquierdo *et al.* 1999), this should be taken into consideration when constructing strength training programmes for both middle-aged and older men and women. Actually, strength training can lead to improvements in these types of functional tasks such as walking speed due to increased strength and power of the trained muscles (e.g. Häkkinen *et al.* 2000a). The results presented in Fig. 21.20 show that, although the change may not be very large, strength training can lead to an increase in the walking speed to some extent throughout the entire training period of 48 weeks in both middle-aged and older persons. The significant correlation observed between the changes in the 1-RM strength and in the walking speed during the second training period in the elderly indicates the importance of muscle strength for walking performance, especially in those older people who possess very low initial levels of strength and power in their muscles. It seems obvious that both middle-aged and older people can carry out successful strength training for prolonged periods and also attain considerable functional adaptations in the neuromuscular system.

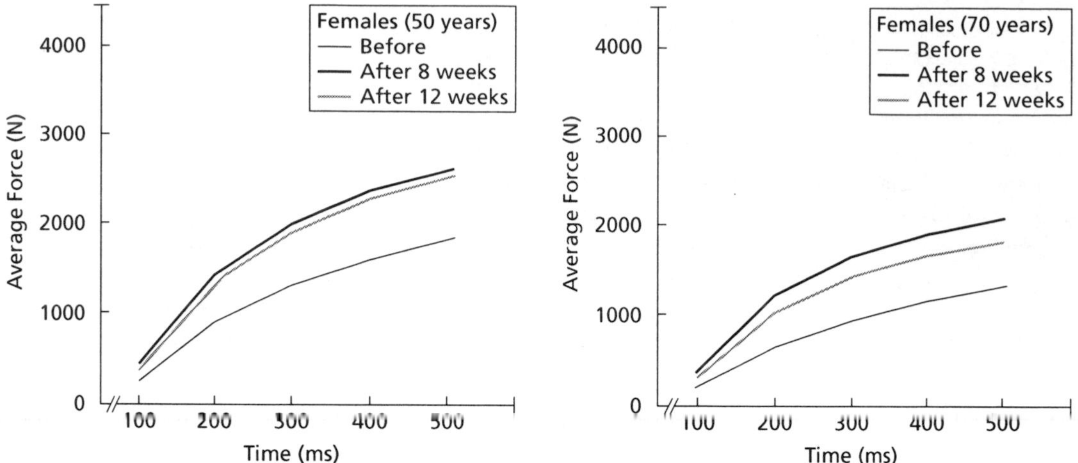

Fig. 21.19 Average force–time curves of isometric bilateral leg extension action in middle-aged and older females before and after heavy-resistance strength training combined with explosive types of exercises. (Modified from Häkkinen & Häkkinen 1995.)

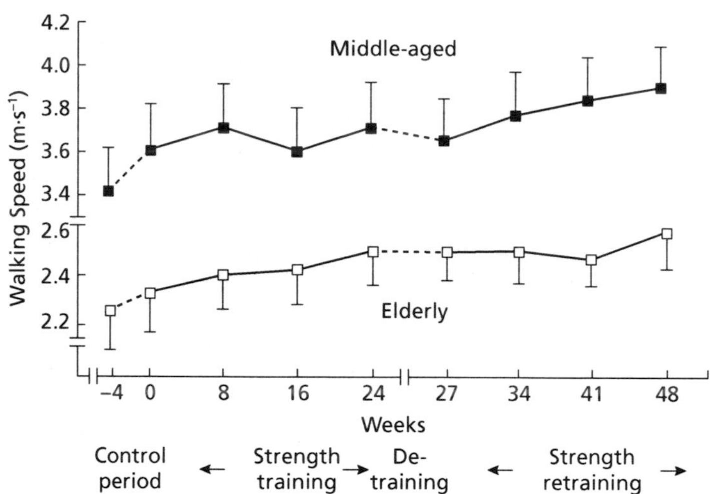

Fig. 21.20 Mean (± SE) maximal walking speed in middle-aged and elderly subjects during the control, strength training, detraining and strength retraining periods. (From Häkkinen *et al.* 2000a.)

Practical conclusions

It has been quite common worldwide for older people to be involved fairly often in endurance-type activities which is no doubt beneficial for cardiorespiratory fitness. However, one can suggest that to minimize the effects of ageing on the neuromuscular system, strength training (combined with some explosive types of exercises) could be recommended as an important part of an overall physical training programme to maintain the functional capacity of middle-aged and especially older people at as high a level as possible for as long as possible. The benefits of maintaining or improving strength and/or explosive strength production of the neuromuscular system in ageing people include correction of gait disturbances, prevention of falls, improved stair climbing and walking, increased mobility, improved performance of activities of daily living and increased capacity for independent living, as well as delayed threshold of dependency. It is justifiable to conclude that proper strength training of ageing people can be utilized as a preventive, therapeutic and rehabilitative tool to optimize neuromuscular function and enhance performance.

References

Adams, G.R., Hather, B.M., Baldwin, K.M. & Dudley, G.A. (1993) Skeletal muscle myosin heavy chain composition and resistance training. *Journal of Applied Physiology* **74**, 911–915.

Bassey, E.J., Fiatarone, M.A., O'Neill, E.F., Kelly, M., Evans, W.J. & Lipsitz, L.A. (1992) Leg extensor power and functional performance in very old men and women. *Clinical Science* **82**, 321–327.

Bosco, C. & Komi, P.V. (1980) Influence of aging on the mechanical behavior of leg extensor muscles. *European Journal of Applied Physiology* **45**, 209–215.

Brown, A.B., McCartney, N. & Sale, D.G. (1990) Positive adaptations to weight-lifting training in the elderly. *Journal of Applied Physiology* **69**(5), 1725–1733.

Charette, S.L., McEvoy, L., Pyka, G. *et al.* (1991) Muscle hypertrophy response to resistance training in older women. *Journal of Applied Physiology* **70**, 1912–1916.

Chakravati, S., Collins, W.P., Forecast, J.D., Newton, J.R., Oram, D.H. & Studd, J.W. (1976) Hormonal profiles after menopause. *British Medical Journal* **2**, 782–787.

Clarkson, P., Kroll, W. & Melchionda, A. (1981) Age, isometric strength, rate of tension development and fiber type composition. *Journals of Gerontology* **36**, 648.

Enoka, R.M. (1988) Muscle strength and its development: New perspectives. *Sports Medicine* **6**, 146–168.

Enoka, R., Fuglevand, A. & Barreto, P. (1992) Age does not impair the voluntary ability to maximal activate muscle. In: *The Proceedings of the Second North American Congress in Biomechanics* (eds L. Draganich, R. Wells & J. Bechtold), pp. 63–64. Chicago, IL.

Essen-Gustavsson, B. & Borges, O. (1986) Histochemical and metabolic characteristics of human skeletal muscle in relation to age. *Acta Physiologica Scandinavica* **126**, 107–114.

Fiatarone, M.A., Marks, E.C., Ryan, N.D., Meredith, C.N., Lipsitz, L.A. & Evans, W.J. (1990) High-intensity strength training in nonagenarians. *Journal of the American Medical Association* **263**, 3029–3034.

Fiatarone, M.A., O'Neill, E.F., Ryan, N.D. *et al.* (1994) Exercise training and nutritional supplementation for physical frailty in very elderly people. *New England Journal of Medicine* **330**, 1769–1775.

Frontera, W.R., Meredith, C.N., O'Reilly, K.P., Knuttgen, H.G. & Evans, W.J. (1988) Strength conditioning in older men; skeletal muscle hypertrophy and improved function. *Journal of Applied Physiology* **71**, 644–650.

Frontera, W.R., Hughes, V.A., Lutz, K.J. & Evans, W.J. (1991) A cross-sectional study of muscle strength and mass in 45- to 78-yr-old men and women. *Journal of Applied Physiology* **71**(2), 644–650.

Grimby, G., Aniansson, A., Hedberg, M., Henning, G.B., Grangard, U. & Kvist, H. (1992) Training can improve muscle strength and endurance in 78- to 84-yr-old men. *Journal of Applied Physiology* **73**(6), 2517–2523.

Hagberg, J.M., Graves, J.E., Limacher, M. *et al.* (1989) Cardiovascular responses of 70- to 79-yr-old men and women to exercise training. *Journal of Applied Physiology* **66**, 2589–2594.

Hagerman, F.C., Walsh, S.J., Staron, R.S. *et al.* (2000) Effects of high-intensity resistance training on untrained older men. I. Strength, cardiovascular, and metabolic responses. *Journals of Gerontology: Biological Sciences and Medical Sciences* **55**(7), B336–B346.

Häkkinen, K. (1994) Neuromuscular adaptation during strength training, aging, detraining, and immobilization. *Critical Reviews in Physical and Rehabilitation Medicine* **6**, 161–198.

Häkkinen, K. & Häkkinen, A. (1991) Muscle cross-sectional area, force production and relaxation characteristics in women at different ages. *European Journal of Applied Physiology* **62**, 410–414.

Häkkinen, K. & Häkkinen, A. (1995) Neuromuscular adaptations during intensive strength training in middle-aged and elderly males and females. *Electromyography and Clinical Neurophysiology* **35**, 137–147.

Häkkinen, K. & Pakarinen, A. (1993) Muscle strength and serum hormones in middle-aged and elderly men and women. *Acta Physiologica Scandinavica* **148**, 199–207.

Häkkinen, K. & Pakarinen, A. (1994) Serum hormones and strength development during strength training in middle-aged and elderly males and females. *Acta Physiologica Scandinavica* **150**, 211–219.

Häkkinen, K. & Pakarinen, A. (1995) Acute hormonal responses to heavy resistance loading in men and women at different ages. *International Journal of Sports Medicine* **16**, 507–513.

Häkkinen, K., Pastinen, U.-M., Karsikas, R. & Linnamo, V. (1995) Neuromuscular performance in voluntary bilateral and unilateral contraction and during electrical stimulation in men at different ages. *European Journal of Applied Physiology* **70**, 518–527.

Häkkinen, K., Kallinen, M., Linnamo, V., Pastinen, U.-M., Newton, R.U. & Kraemer, W.J. (1996a) Neuromuscular adaptations during bilateral versus unilateral strength training in middle aged and elderly men and women. *Acta Physiologica Scandinavica* **158**, 77–88.

Häkkinen, K., Kraemer, W.J., Kallinen, M., Linnamo, V., Pastinen, U.-M. & Newton, R.U. (1996b) Bilateral and unilateral neuromuscular function and muscle cross-sectional area in middle-aged and elderly men and women. *Journals of Gerontology: Biological Sciences and Medical Sciences* **51A**, 1, B21–B29.

Häkkinen, K., Alen, M., Kallinen, M. *et al.* (1998a) Muscle CSA, force production, and activation of leg extensors during isometric and dynamic actions in middle-aged and elderly men and women. *Journal of Aging and Physical Activity* **8**(6), 232–247.

Häkkinen, K., Kallinen, M., Izquierdo, M. *et al.* (1998b) Changes in agonist-antagonist EMG, muscle CSA and force during strength training in middle-aged and older people. *Journal of Applied Physiology* **84**(4), 1341–1349.

Häkkinen, K., Newton, R.U., Gordon, S. *et al.* (1998c) Changes in muscle morphology, electromyographic activity, and force production characteristics during progressive strength training in young and older men. *Journals of Gerontology: Biological Sciences and Medical Sciences* **53A**, 6, B415–B423.

Häkkinen, K., Alen, M., Kallinen, M., Newton, R.U. & Kraemer, W.J. (2000a) Neuromuscular adaptations during prolonged strength training, detraining and re-strength-training in middle-aged and elderly people. *European Journal of Applied Physiology* **83**, 51–62.

Häkkinen, K., Pakarinen, A., Kraemer, W.J., Newton, R.U. & Alen, M. (2000b) Basal concentrations and acute responses of serum hormones and strength development during heavy resistance training in middle-aged and elderly men and women. *Journals of Gerontology: Biological Sciences and Medical Sciences* **55A**, B95–B105.

Häkkinen, K., Kraemer, W.J., Newton, R.U. & Alen, M. (2001a) Changes in electromyographic activity, muscle fibre and force production characteristics during heavy resistance/power strength training in middle-aged and older men and women. *Acta Physiologica Scandinavica* **171**(1), 51–62.

Häkkinen, K., Pakarinen, A., Kraemer, W.J., Häkkinen, A., Valkeinen, H. & Alen, M. (2001b) Selective muscle hypertrophy, changes in EMG and force and serum hormones during strength training in older women. *Journal of Applied Physiology* **91**, 569–580.

Hammond, G., Kontturi, M., Vihko, P. & Vihko, R. (1978) Serum steroids in normal males and patients with prostatic diseases. *Clinical Endocrinology* **9**, 113–121.

Harridge, S., Kryger, A. & Steengaard, A. (1999) Knee extensor strength, activation, and size in very elderly people following strength training. *Muscle and Nerve* **22**, 831–839.

Hicks, A.L., Cupido, C.M., Martin, J. & Dent, J. (1991) Twitch potentiation during fatiguing exercise in the elderly: the effects of training. *European Journal of Applied Physiology and Occupational Physiology* **63**(3–4), 278–281.

Hikida, R.S., Staron, R.S., Hagerman, F.C. *et al.* (2000) Effects of high-intensity resistance training on untrained older men. II. Muscle fiber characteristics and nucleo-cytoplasmic relationships. *Journals of Gerontology: Biological Sciences and Medical Sciences* **55**(7), B347–B354.

Izquierdo, M., Aguado, X., Gonzalez, R., López, J.L. & Häkkinen, K. (1999) Maximal and explosive force production capacity and balance performance in men of different ages. *European Journal of Applied Physiology* **79**, 260–267.

Judge, J.O., Underwood, M. & Gennosa, T. (1993) Exercise to improve gait velocity in older persons. *Archives of Physical Medicine and Rehabilitation* **74**(4), 400–406.

Kamen, G., Sison, S., Du Duke, C. & Patten, C. (1995) Motor unit discharge behavior in older adults during maximal-effort contractions. *Journal of Applied Physiology* **79**(6), 1908–1913.

Kawakami, Y., Abe, T. & Fukunaga, T. (1993) Muscle-fibre pennation angles are greater in hypertrofied than in normal muscles. *Journal of Applied Physiology* **74**, 2470–2744.

Kent-Braun, J.A. & Ng, A.V. (1999) Specific strength and voluntary muscle activation in young and elderly women and men. *Journal of Applied Physiology* **87**(1), 22–29.

Komi, P.V. (1986) Training of muscle strength and power: interaction of neuromotoric, hypertrophic and mechanical factors. *International Journal of Sports Medicine (Suppl.)* **7**, 10–15.

Kraemer, W.J., Patton, J., Gordon, S.E. *et al.* (1995) Compatibility of high intensity strength and endurance training on hormonal and skeletal muscle adaptations. *Journal of Applied Physiology* **78**(3), 976–989.

Kraemer, W.J., Häkkinen, K., Newton, R. *et al.* (1998) Acute hormonal responses to heavy resistance exercise in younger and older men. *European Journal of Applied Physiology* **77**, 206–211.

Kraemer, W.J., Häkkinen, K., Newton, R. *et al.* (1999) Effects of heavy resistance training on hormonal response patterns in younger vs. older men. *Journal of Applied Physiology* **87**(3), 982–992.

Larsson, L., Sjödin, B. & Karsson. J. (1978) Histochemical and biochemical changes in human skeletal muscle with age in sedentary males age 22–65 years. *Acta Physiologica Scandinavica* **103**, 31–39.

Lexell, J., Taylor, C.C. & Sjöström, M. (1988) What is the cause of the ageing atrophy? *Journal of Neurological Science* **84**, 275–294.

McCartney, N., Hicks, A., Martin, J. & Webber, C. (1996) A longitudinal trial of weight training in the elderly: Continued improvements in year 2. *Journals of Gerontology: Biological Sciences and Medical Sciences* **51A**, 6, B425–B433.

Morganti, C., Nelson, M., Fiatarone, M. *et al.* (1995) Strength improvements with 1 year of progressive resistance training in older women. *Medicine and Science in Sports and Exercise* **27**(6), 906–912.

Moritani, T. & DeVries, H.A. (1980) Potential for gross muscle hypertrophy in older men. *Journals of Gerontology* **35**, 672–682.

Narici, M., Bordini, M. & Cerretelli, P. (1991) Effect of aging on human adductor pollicis muscle function. *Journal of Applied Physiology* **71**, 1227–1281.

Narici, M., Hoppeler, H., Kayser, B. *et al.* (1996) Human quadriceps cross-sectional area, torque, and neural activation during 6 months strength training. *Acta Physiologica Scandinavica* **157**, 175–186.

Nichols, J.F., Omizo, D.K., Peterson, K.K. & Nelson, K.F. (1993) Efficacy of heavy-resistance training for active women over sixty: muscular strength, body composition, and program adherence. *Journal of the American Geriatrics Society* **41**(3), 205–210.

Porter, M.M., Vandervoort, A.A. & Lexell, J. (1995) Aging of human muscle: structure, function and adaptability. *Scandinavian Journal of Medicine and Science in Sports* **5**, 129–142.

Pyka, G., Lindenberger, E., Charette, S. & Marcus, R. (1994) Muscle strength and fiber adaptations to a one year-long resistance training program in elderly men and women. *Journals of Gerontology: Biological Sciences and Medical Sciences* **45**(1), M22–M27.

Rice, C.L., Cunningham, D.A., Paterson, D.H. & Dickinson, J.R. (1993) Strength training alters contractile properties of the triceps brachii in men aged 65–78 years. *European Journal of Applied Physiology and Occupational Physiology* **66**(3), 275–280.

Roman, W.J., Fleckenstein, J., Stray-Gundersen, J.S., Alway, S.E., Peshock, R. & W.J.Gonyea (1993) Adaptation in the elbow flexors of elderly males after heavy-resistance training. *Journal of Applied Physiology* **74**, 750–754.

Roth, S.M., Martel, G.F., Ivey, F.M. *et al.* (2000) High-volume, heavy-resistance strength training and muscle damage in young and older women. *Journal of Applied Physiology* **88**(3), 1112–1118.

Sale, D.G. (1992) Neural adaptation to strength training. In: *Strength and Power in Sports. The Encyclopedia of Sports Medicine* (ed. P.V. Komi), pp. 249–165. Blackwell Scientific Publications, Oxford.

Staron, R.S., Leonardi, M.J., Karapondo, D.L. *et al.* (1991) Strength and skeletal muscle adaptations in heavy-resistance trained women after detraining and retraining. *Journal of Applied Physiology* **70**, 631–640.

Staron, R.S., Karapando, D.L., Kraemer, W.J. *et al.* (1994) Skeletal muscle adaptation during early phase of heavy resistance training in men and women. *Journal of Applied Physiology* **76**, 1247–1255.

Tracy, B., Ivey, F., Hurlbut. D. *et al.* (1999) Muscle quality. II. Effects of strength training in 65- to 75-yr-old men and women. *Journal of Applied Physiology* **86**(1), 15–201.

Van Cutsem, M., Duchateau, J. & Hainaut, K. (1998) Changes in single motor unit behaviour contribute to the increase in contraction speed after dynamic training in humans. *Journal of Physiology* **513**, 295–305.

Vermulen, A., Rubens, R. & Verdonck, L. (1972) Testosterone secretion and metabolism in male senescence. *Journal of Clinical Endocrinology* **34**, 730–735.

Viitasalo, J., Era, P., Leskinen, A. & Heikkinen, E. (1985) Muscular strength profiles and anthropometry in random samples of men aged 31–35, 51–55 and 71–75 years. *Ergonomics* **28**, 1503.

Yue, G.H., Ranganathan, V.K., Siemionow, V., Liu, J.Z. & Sahgal, V. (1999) Older adults exhibit a reduced ability to fully activate their biceps brachii muscle. *Journals of Gerontology: Biological Sciences and Medical Sciences* **54**(5), M249–M253.

Chapter 22

Use of Electrical Stimulation in Strength and Power Training

GARY A. DUDLEY AND SCOTT W. STEVENSON

Introduction

Transcutaneous electromyostimulation (EMS) has long been used by clinicians to aid in the rehabilitation of patients with limited motor function (Delitto & Robinson 1989). For example, it has been used in the treatment of knee joint injuries such as chondromalacia patellae (Johnson *et al.* 1977) because reflex inhibition and pain impair voluntary control. In postoperative patients with immobilized joints or a limited ability to generate force due to pain or neural inhibition, EMS has been shown to retard muscular atrophy and dysfunction (Eriksson & Häggmark 1979; Gould *et al.* 1983; Wigerstad-Lossing *et al.* 1988).

There has been a proliferation of EMS studies involving healthy subjects during the last three decades (for review see Kramer & Mendryk 1982). Likewise, EMS has received attention as a training method for athletes (Delitto *et al.* 1989). Much of this interest has arisen in response to reports of Jakov Kots' work in the former Soviet Union (Kots & Chwilon 1971). Kots has claimed that a brief programme of high-frequency EMS can produce marked strength gains in highly trained athletes. Several studies have since been conducted in an apparent effort to duplicate these results (e.g. Currier & Mann 1983; St Pierre *et al.* 1986).

In this chapter we will limit the discussion to the use of EMS in the conditioning of elite athletes. For the sake of simplicity, we will focus on the potential use of EMS by endurance and strength/power athletes such as marathon runners and Olympic weightlifters, respectively. These athletes represent the extremes of the spectrum of humans to develop muscular power. The marathon runner maintains an impressive steady-state energy expenditure for over 2 h, which is supported by aerobic metabolism. The Olympic weightlifter, in contrast, uses great muscular strength to develop as much as 15 times more power, but it is only sustained for milliseconds.

This chapter will be presented in four parts: methods of application of EMS; rationale for the use of EMS in conditioning athletes; data supporting the efficacy of EMS in conditioning athletes; and directions for future research. It is hoped that this approach will give some clarity to the plethora of concepts and ideas that presently exist concerning the use of EMS.

Methods of application of EMS

A variety of different stimulation protocols have been used to artificially activate skeletal muscle using EMS. The simplest approach has been to control the pulse duration and frequency and the duration and amplitude of activation. For example, 500-μs rectangular pulses at 20 Hz have been applied via a surface bipolar electrode configuration for 1 s (Hultman *et al.* 1983). The amplitude of stimulation can be set to induce a force equal to a given percentage of maximal voluntary isometric force (Currier & Mann 1983) or, as is generally done, to subject tolerance (e.g. Laughman *et al.* 1983).

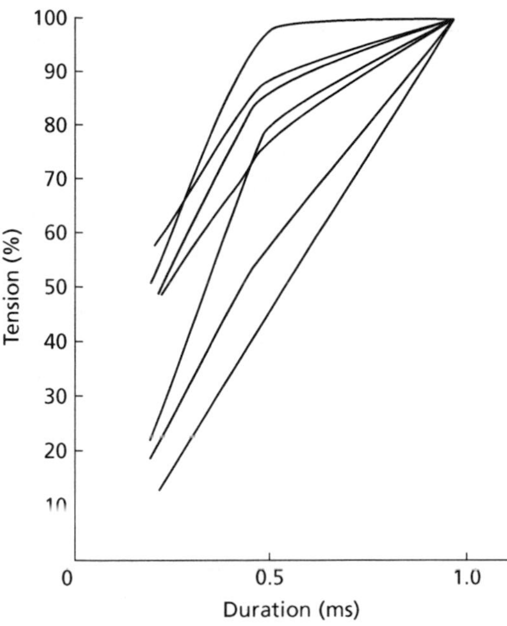

Fig. 22.1 The relationship between pulse duration and relative force during trancutaneous EMS of the knee extensor muscle group. Pulse duration was increased from 200 μs to 1 ms. Square pulses were delivered at 20 Hz and amplitude was held constant at a value that would elicit force up to 70% of maximal voluntary isometric action under optimal conditions. (From Hultman *et al.* 1983.)

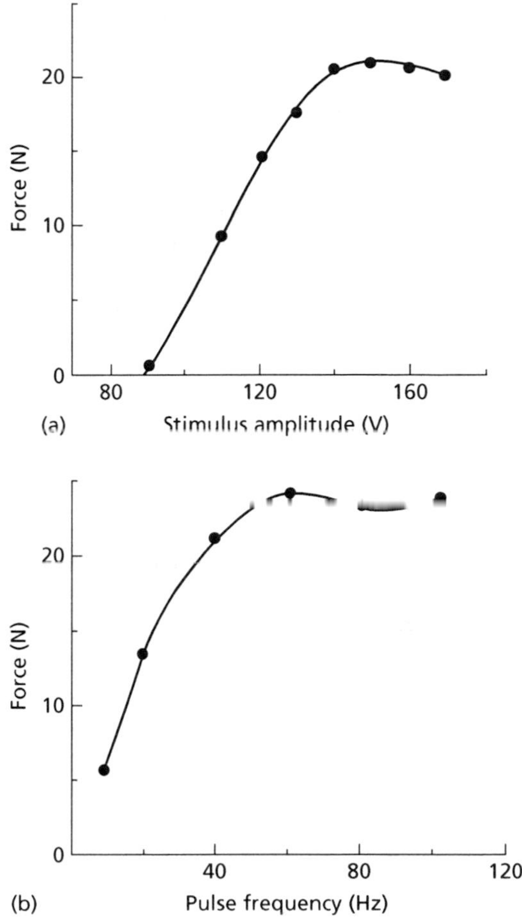

Fig. 22.2 The relationship between the amplitude of stimulation and tetanic force (a) and between pulse frequency and force (b) during transcutaneous EMS of the first dorsal interosseus muscle. Square pulses of 100 μs were used for a duration of 500 ms. The frequency of pulses was 40 Hz in (a). The amplitude of stimulation was supramaximal in (b). (From Davies *et al.* 1985.)

The influence of altering one of these factors on isometric force development while the others are held at a given value has received some attention. Increasing pulse duration from 200 to 500 μs during 20-Hz stimulation results in markedly increased force (Hultman *et al.* 1983) (Fig. 22.1). Further increases in pulse duration to 1000 μs have only a modest effect. The authors recommended that pulse durations between 500 and 1000 μs be used during EMS for optimal force development, although this has not always been appreciated (Enoka 1988). The relation between pulse frequency and isometric force is sigmoidal in nature, with tetanic force occurring at about 50 Hz in human skeletal muscle (Davies *et al.* 1985) (Fig. 22.2b). Likewise, the relation between isometric force and stimulation amplitude (current) is sigmoidal (Davies *et al.* 1985) (Fig. 22.2a). When amplitude is increased from the threshold of isometric force, rather large increases are required to induce modest increases in force, suggesting that much of the additional current is not activating muscle, but rather flowing through other structures. Thereafter, force increases abruptly with increases in amplitude until a plateau is realized (Fig. 22.2a). The plateau is not always attained at forces greater than maximal voluntary isometric force (MVIF). However, several studies have reported forces during stimulation that are greater than MVIF (e.g. Hultman *et al.* 1983; Delitto *et al.* 1989).

A major hindrance to force development during EMS appears to be subject intolerance to pain. Along these lines, high-frequency stimulation has been suggested to be more tolerable (Moreno-Aranda & Seireg 1981a,b). A carrier frequency of 10 000 Hz of a sinusoidal signal is used and modulated at 100 Hz. Moreover, the stimulation is applied with a duty cycle of 20%. The 10 000 Hz indicates that the pulse duration is 100 μs. The 100-Hz modulation indicates that the signal is given in 10-ms blocks. Finally, the duty cycle of 20% indicates that the stimulation is on for the first 2 ms of the 10-ms block. Thus, 20 sinusoidal 100-μs pulses are delivered continuously for the first 2 ms of each 10-ms block. The duration of the tetanic stimulation is around 1–2 s with 4–5 s rest. While this type of stimulation appears to be most tolerable, force development is not optimal, probably because of the short pulse duration. On the other hand, our experience suggests that many individuals can develop tolerance to high-amplitude EMS (> 70% MVIF) after several days of familiarization (Stevenson & Dudley 2001).

In an effort to refute or substantiate the work of Kots and Chwilon (1971), several investigators have used medium-frequency stimulation. The sinusoidal signal at 2500 Hz is modulated at 50 Hz. What is not obvious is that the signals are given with a 50% duty cycle. Thus, 400-μs pulses are delivered continuously for the first 10 ms of each 20-ms time period. The duration of the stimulation is usually a few seconds. Because the refractory period of motoneurones is around 3 ms (Miller *et al.* 1981), they are activated at most 3 times during each 10-ms period or 150 times per second for the 50 10-ms blocks. In essence, 400 μs signals excite the motoneurones 150 times per second. Likewise, during high-frequency stimulation, the motoneurones are essentially activated by 100-ms duration pulses 100 times per second.

In the few studies where the interest has been to increase the endurance capacity of skeletal muscle, a markedly different stimulation protocol has been used (Scott *et al.* 1985). Square wave 50-μs pulses were delivered at 5–10 Hz for 1 h, 3 times daily.

Electrodes of a variety of different materials, such as aluminium foil or carbon-conditioned, have been used, generally in the bipolar configuration, for the application of EMS. The negative electrode is generally placed over the motor point of a given muscle or muscle group of interest, while the positive one is placed distally. In the case of the knee extensors, it has been shown that greater force is developed as electrode size increases (Alon 1985) and that both electrodes need to be placed superficially to this muscle group (Ferguson *et al.* 1989).

The pain sensations associated with EMS arise due to the non-homogeneity of the electrode–skin interface (Mason & Mackay 1976). This results in localized areas of low resistance where current densities can become large enough to exceed the threshold for damage. Wetting the electrodes prior to application provides a more uniform resistance and reduces occurrence of these 'hot-spots' (Mason & Mackay 1976). Alternatively leaving the electrodes in place for 30 min prior to stimulation allows accumulation of insensible perspiration, which creates a more homogeneous electrode–skin interface. Using the largest electrodes possible may also reduce pain sensations by reducing current density, as well as distributing the current through a large volume of the muscle.

Rationale for the use of EMS in conditioning athletes

The practical use of EMS obviously requires that it provide some advantage over voluntary muscle activation. In this regard two lines of reasoning have been proposed. First, it is suggested that neural factors limit force during maximal voluntary efforts. Thus, EMS can provide a more intense contraction to the muscle that is stimulated, and thereby induce greater adaptive responses (Delitto & Snyder-Mackler 1990). How the EMS-trained muscle that could not be

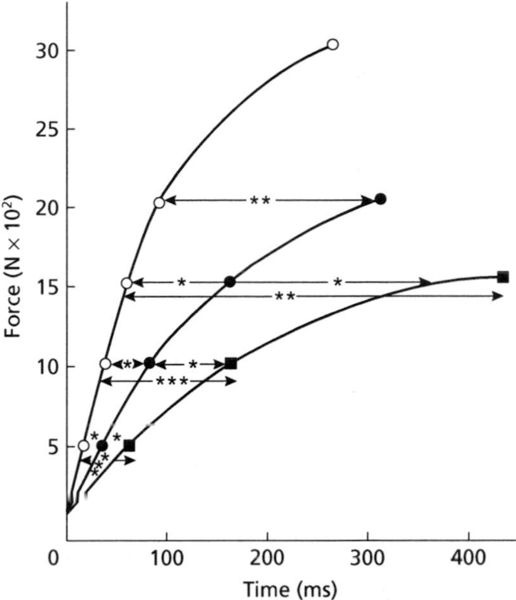

Fig. 22.3 Force plotted as a function of time during the bilateral isometric extension exercise that is similar to a leg press. Force is developed as rapidly as possible on auditory command. The male strength athletes were seven elite bodybuilders and power lifters (○). The physically active males (black spot ●) ($n = 9$) and females (black square ■) ($n = 10$) were not trained but engaged in different types of physical activities (e.g. jogging or weightlifting) 1–3 times per week. The symbol indicates a significant difference among groups in the time required to develop a given force. *, $P < 0.05$; **, $P < 0.01$; ***, $P < 0.001$. (From Ryushi *et al.* 1988.)

voluntarily activated before EMS is to be voluntarily activated after EMS is not clear (McDonagh & Davies 1984).

It is generally accepted that the intensity of training, judged by the magnitude of the training load, is the most important factor for inducing adaptive responses in strength/power athletes (Häkkinen & Keskinen 1989). It is not so obvious how EMS could provide a greater training stimulus for these individuals. An increased ability to maximally activate skeletal muscle is a fundamental adaptive response to strength training (Komi 1986). Moreover, strength training increases the rate of activation, and thereby the speed at which a given force can be developed (Fig. 22.3) (Ryushi *et al.* 1988). Finally, MVIF per unit cross-sectional area of skeletal muscle is markedly greater in strength/power-trained athletes than in active individuals (Ryushi *et al.* 1988; Häkkinen & Keskinen 1989). This has been attributed in part to greater activation in the trained athletes. If strength/power athletes have developed such an impressive ability to activate their trained skeletal muscle, it is not clear how EMS could augment this adaptive response. Thus, it is not obvious how EMS could increase their intensity of training and thereby induce greater strength. However, because EMS stimulates the motoneuronal axons distal to the spinal cord, inhibitory influences present during voluntary contractions are absent. This might be especially favourable if EMS were applied during eccentric contractions during which muscle-specific tension appears to be greater than during voluntary efforts (Dudley *et al.* 1990). EMS that evokes ~ 80–90% MVIF will result in force 20–30% greater than MVIF during eccentric actions. We have applied EMS in such a manner to evoke muscular growth that is superior to that observed during voluntary resistance training, at least in previously untrained individuals (Ruther *et al.* 1995). Whether such an effect may be possible in elite athletes already displaying significant muscle hypertrophy remains to be seen.

Secondly, the efficacy of EMS for enhancing strength training adaptations is based on the concept that fast-twitch fibres, which are difficult to activate during maximal voluntary isometric efforts, are preferentially stimulated by EMS (Delitto & Snyder-Mackler 1990). It is well known that as the force of voluntary isometric effort is progressively increased, motor units are recruited in a precise orderly manner (Henneman *et al.* 1965). There is considerable evidence suggesting that the difference in motoneurone size is the physiological basis for this orderly recruitment (for review see Burke 1981). According to Henneman's 'size principle' the input resistance and thus susceptibility to discharge is inversely related to motoneurone size. Motor units innervated by the smallest α motoneurones are comprised of slow-twitch muscle fibres, which are few in number and small in diameter. Conversely, larger motoneurones innervate larger motor units containing fast muscle fibres. This arrangement ensures that, for sustained low-intensity exercise, small fatigue-resistant motor units are preferentially recruited.

Hultman *et al.* (1983) demonstrated that EMS of the thigh muscles of curarized patients fails to elicit a contraction even when voltage is far in excess of that needed to evoke force before curarization. It is therefore apparent that EMS does not directly activate the muscle. Instead, the stimulation current is propagated along the more excitable terminal nerve branches within the muscle.

Since muscle activation via EMS involves excitation of peripheral nerves and not direct stimulation of the muscle (Hultman *et al.* 1983), the question arises as to whether motor units are activated in a specific order. It has been demonstrated that larger motoneurones have a lower threshold of electrical excitability (e.g. Solomonow *et al.* 1986). This apparently occurs as a result of lower resistance offered by larger motoneurones. The use of EMS via surface electrodes may thus be expected to activate the largest units at the lowest stimulation level. Indeed, two recent reviews have concluded that EMS preferentially activates the large fast-twitch motor units and thus occurs in reverse of the normal recruitment order (Enoka 1988; Delitto & Snyder-Mackler 1990). This preferential activation of fast motor units is thought (Enoka 1988; Delitto & Snyder-Mackler 1990) to be facilitated by afferent input from stimulation of cutaneous afferents, which inhibit motoneurones of slow motor units and excite motoneurones of fast motor units (Garnett & Stephens 1981). However, because EMS activates the distal motoneurone branches (Hultman *et al.* 1983), it is not clear how reflex inhibition of slow motoneurones via cutaneous afferent stimulation could override this distal motoneurone activation.

Indirect evidence to support this idea is provided by Cabric *et al.* (1988) who demonstrated that 19 days of EMS to the triceps surae for 10 min each day resulted in increases in myonuclei size and mitochondrial fraction. The greatest responses were suggested to occur in fast fibres. Unfortunately, muscle fibre types were differentiated by indirect morphometric measures. It has recently been suggested, in a case study, that EMS causes preferential glycogen depletion in fast-twitch Type IIA fibres (Sinacore *et al.* 1990). Thus, it was suggested that mainly this fibre type was stimulated. This was based on the observation that Type IIA fibres showed qualitatively less glycogen staining intensity after than before a single bout of EMS. This observation is difficult to reconcile with the fact that the glycogen content of the mixed fibre biopsy samples was the same before and after stimulation. Additionally, one might expect greater glycogen use in Type II fibres, which generally have greater glycogenolytic activity.

Evidence that EMS does not preferentially activate fast-twitch fibres has been presented by Knaflitz *et al.* (1990) and Kim *et al.* (1995). Motor unit recruitment order was assessed by measuring conduction velocity and mean and median power frequency at different relative levels of voluntary or EMS force in Knaflitz *et al.* (1990). Conduction velocity and mean and median power frequency increased with increasing force during voluntary efforts, indicating the recruitment of progressively larger fibres with higher conduction velocities. It was demonstrated that for both voluntary and EMS-evoked muscle actions conduction velocity and mean and median power frequency were less at lower force levels, suggesting activation of slower motor units. It was concluded that motor unit activation via EMS does not occur in reverse of the normal recruitment order. This may have occurred because large motor axons do not necessarily have large branches and/or because their motor branches may not have been orientated in the current field to favour activation (Feiereisen *et al.* 1997). This may explain why Kim *et al.* (1995) found marked glycogen loss as determined by the periodic acid–Schiff staining in slow and fast fibres after 60 min of 30-W dynamic knee extension exercise evoked by EMS.

The evidence is not clear, therefore, that EMS preferentially activates fast-twitch fibres. If this were the case, it would appear to be advantageous, as it has been suggested that the fast-twitch fibre composition of a given muscle may ultimately determine the magnitude of the adaptive responses to strength training (Häkkinen *et al.* 1985). It is also obvious, however, that strength/power-trained athletes have large, fast-twitch fibres (Tesch 1987). In fact, preferential fast-twitch fibre hypertrophy is a common adaptive response to strength training (Tesch 1987). This would suggest that these fibres are recruited during training, and that they respond accordingly. While the large fast-twitch motor units may be difficult to activate during isometric efforts, they appear to be preferentially recruited during voluntary eccentric actions (Romano & Schieppati 1987; Nardone & Schieppati 1988; Nardone *et al.* 1989). Thus, it is not difficult to envision their repeated use during the high-force repetitions of a weight training exercise where both eccentric and concentric muscle actions are performed. On the other hand, if EMS were to activate slow-twitch motor units not normally subjected to eccentric loading, it seems possible that a greater adaptive (hypertrophic) response in these motor units might result in performance enhancement.

It seems that low-frequency long-term EMS might be used to increase the resistance to fatigue in endurance-trained athletes. This type of stimulation in lower mammals has been shown to induce several well-documented changes including an almost complete fast- to slow-twitch muscle conversion, and a marked increase and decrease in oxidative and glycolytic enzymes, respectively (Pette & Vrbovä 1985), although fast-twitch fibre degeneration and fibre atrophy may also occur (Maier *et al.* 1986). While the latter two responses are not especially attractive, skeletal muscle composed mainly of slow-twitch fibres with a high aerobic capacity is characteristic of muscle tissue in endurance-trained athletes. The use of EMS to this end has received little attention. Three hours per day of 5–10-Hz EMS has been shown to increase the resistance to fatigue in tibialis anterior muscle of untrained females (Scott *et al.* 1985). It should be noted that the well-documented effects of low-frequency long-term stimulation of skeletal muscle of lower mammals has often been erroneously cited to support the use of artificial stimulation in EMS studies designed to increase muscle strength and size (see e.g. Delitto *et al.* 1989). However, we have recently observed that EMS-evoked, high-intensity, coupled concentric–eccentric actions can elicit improvements in both muscle size and fatigue resistance simultaneously (Stevenson & Dudley 2001).

Data to support the efficacy of EMS in conditioning athletes

There are few reports of the effects of EMS on strength and muscle size in athletes. The work of Kots and Chwilon (1971) appears to have generated interest in this area. Kots suggests that athletes can enjoy strength improvements of 30–40% after only 4–5 weeks of EMS. The stimulation protocol uses medium-frequency EMS like that described above. A sinusoidal 2500-Hz signal modulated at 50 Hz is applied for 10 ms with a 10-ms interval between trains. Ten 10-s contractions are performed per day, 5 days each week for 4–5 weeks. There was a 50-s rest interval between contractions. It is argued that frequencies at this level minimize the sensation of pain, while maximizing force development during the isometric actions (Kots & Chwilon 1971). It has been suggested elsewhere, however, that EMS at this frequency is in fact quite painful (Moreno-Aranda & Seireg 1981a,b). It was indicated, but the actual data were not reported, that such EMS allows force development that is 10–30% greater than MVIF.

Unfortunately, Kots and colleagues have not been able to duplicate these results. Strength and muscle size were unchanged or reduced in 10 athletes after seven sessions of EMS (St Pierre *et al.* 1986). The EMS protocol described above was applied to the knee extensor muscle group during 7 days of the 8-day experiment. The authors indicated that EMS induced an isometric force that was 80–100% of MVIF, but again the actual data for either variable were not reported.

Peak torque during isokinetic concentric muscle actions decreased on average by 10%. Interestingly, fast-twitch fibre size decreased significantly in the males and did not change in the females. Slow-twitch fibre size did not change for either group. These data do not seem to support the use of EMS in the conditioning of athletes, and suggest that liberal use of EMS can even result in overtraining.

Other studies of competitive swimmers (Pichon *et al.* 1995) and basketball players (Maffiuletti *et al.* 2000) have indicated that application of EMS during isometric actions of the latissimus dorsi and quadriceps femoris muscles, respectively, increases maximal voluntary eccentric and concentric isokinetic actions of these muscles. Pichon *et al.* (1995) found swimmers receiving EMS reduced 25-m and 50-m freestyle swim times, whereas no improvement was noted for the control group of swimmers. Similarly, Maffiuletti *et al.* (2000) found that 4 weeks of EMS increased squat-jump height 14%, and that the basketball players receiving EMS improved countermovement vertical jump by 17% 4 weeks after EMS was discontinued. Unfortunately, neither study controlled for the potential placebo effects of EMS or compared EMS to a programme of voluntary training. On the other hand, Wolf *et al.* (1986) found that EMS applied bilaterally to the quadriceps femoris of competitive tennis players during the 2nd half of a 6-week squat-based resistance training regime was not superior to voluntary training alone in enhancing squatting performance, 25-m sprint time or vertical jump.

To date, the most convincing data to support the use of EMS in the conditioning of athletes were reported in a case study (Delitto *et al.* 1989). A weightlifter who competed in the 1984 Olympic Games was studied over the course of 3.5 months. Electromyostimulation of the knee extensors during isometric actions was done 3 days per week in conjunction with his normal training during weeks 5–8 and weeks 13 and 14. A 2500-Hz triangular wave interrupted at 75 pulses·s^{-1} was used to induce 10 11-s muscle actions per day. Three minutes of rest separated the isometric actions. In essence, 400-μs signals were delivered continuously for about the first 7 ms of each 14 ms time period. Because the refractory period of motoneurones is about 3 ms (Miller *et al.* 1981), each 11-s isometric muscle action was induced using 400-μs signals delivered at 150 Hz. The amplitude of EMS was set to induce an isometric force on average equal to 112% of MVIF. As is usually the case, neither the stimulated nor voluntary isometric values were reported.

Most notable was that the one repetition maximum (1 RM) for the squat exercise increased about 20 kg during the periods of EMS. The 1 RM for the clean and jerk, and snatch also increased with EMS. The magnitude of these responses is impressive, especially in the squat, considering the level of the athlete. Elite weight trainees do not show such increases in strength over 2 years of training (Häkkinen *et al.* 1988). It is difficult to ascertain the mechanism(s) responsible for the increased weightlifting ability. Both fast- and slow-twitch fibre size decreased significantly, such that relative fibre area actually decreased by about 16%. The authors suggested that hyperplasia may have occurred and actually increased muscle mass. Hyperplasia of such an extent has not been reported for other models of muscle hypertrophy (Gollnick *et al.* 1981; see also Chapter 13). Electromyography was not conducted; thus it is not known whether increased neural activation occurred.

Directions for future research

The data to date are not convincing that EMS should be used by strength/power or endurance athletes to enhance performance. A well-controlled study to determine whether EMS can enhance performance in strength/power athletes is needed. A sufficient number of subjects needs to be used to ensure scientific validity of the data. Control subjects must be used and an effort should be made to delineate the potential placebo effect of EMS *per se*. Moreover, measures of muscular performance during EMS and the competitive sport must be made. Finally, measures of muscle size, muscle performance and neural activation should be made to establish the mechanisms responsible for the adaptive responses, if any, induced by EMS.

Studies also need to be conducted to examine the effect of EMS that is applied during dynamic muscle actions. It has long been known that skeletal muscle of lower mammals activated artificially *in situ* develops force that is markedly greater during eccentric than isometric actions (Katz 1939). Likewise, we have recently found that with EMS, force of the knee extensor muscle group is about 40% greater during eccentric than isometric muscle actions (Dudley *et al.* 1990). Eccentric torque developed by the knee extensors during maximal voluntary efforts, in contrast, is not appreciably greater than isometric, at least for untrained individuals (Westing *et al.* 1988). It should be possible therefore to elicit forces with EMS that are markedly greater than maximal voluntary force. Westing *et al.* (1989) have shown this to be the case. Electromyostimulation of the knee extensors was applied at an amplitude that resulted in an isometric torque (262 Nm) equal to about 85% of maximal voluntary isometric torque (306 Nm). The EMS torque (345 Nm) during eccentric actions was greater than maximal voluntary isometric (306 Nm) or eccentric (316 Nm) torque. Because the intensity of training, as judged by the magnitude of load acted against or the force developed during a given muscle action, is an important factor in inducing adaptive responses to strength/power training, EMS during eccentric actions warrants consideration as a training method for competitive athletes. Recently, we have demonstrated that EMS can be applied during coupled concentric–eccentric isokinetic actions to increase muscle size at a rapid rate (~ 10% in 8 weeks) in untrained (Ruther *et al.* 1995) and recreationally resistance-trained individuals (3+ years of training) (Stevenson & Dudley 2001).

It is well documented that long-term low-frequency stimulation of skeletal muscle in lower mammals results in mainly slow-twitch fibres with a high mitochondrial content (Pette & Vrbovä 1985). These characteristics of skeletal muscle appear to be important attributes for successful competition in endurance-type sports. It seems reasonable therefore that low-frequency, long-term EMS should be investigated as a conditioning method to enhance the performance ability of these athletes. As noted above, high-frequency (70-Hz) EMS that increases muscle size can also elicit improvements in muscular fatigue resistance (Stevenson & Dudley 2001).

Acknowledgements

The graphical assistance of Ms Susan Loffek is gratefully acknowledged. The research reported by the authors was supported under NASA contracts NAS10 10285 and NAS10 11624 and a National Strength and Conditioning Association Graduate Student Research Award (SWS).

References

Alon, C. (1985) High voltage stimulation: Effects of electrode size on basic excitatory responses. *Physical Therapy* **65**, 890–895.

Burke, R.E. (1981) Motor units. Anatomy, Physiology and Functional Organization. In: *Handbook of Physiology. The Nervous System*, Section 1, Vol. II (ed. V.B. Brooks), pp. 345–422. American Physiological Society, Bethesda.

Cabric, M., Appell, H.I. & Resic, A. (1988) Fine structural changes in electrostimulated human skeletal muscle. *European Journal of Applied Physiology* **57**, 1–5.

Currier, D.P. & Mann, R. (1983) Muscular strength development by electrical stimulation in healthy individuals. *Physical Therapy* **63**, 915–921.

Davies, C.T.M., Dooley, P., McDonagh, M.J.N. & White, Mi. (1985) Adaptation of mechanical properties of muscle to high force training in man. *Journal of Physiology* **365**, 277–284.

Delitto, A. & Robinson, A.J. (1989) Electrical stimulation of muscle: techniques and applications. In: *Clinical Electrophysiology: Electrotherapy and Electrophysiologic Testing* (eds L. Snyder-Mackler & A.J. Robinson), pp. 95–138. Williams & Wilkins, Baltimore.

Delitto, A. & Snyder-Mackler, L. (1990) Two theories of muscle strength augmentation using percutaneous electrical stimulation. *Physical Therapy* **70**, 158–164.

Delitto, A., Brown, M., Strube, M.I., Rose, S.I. & Lehman, R.C. (1989) Electrical stimulation of quadriceps femoris in an elite weight lifter: a single subject experiment. *International Journal of Sports Medicine* **10**, 187–191.

Dudley, G.A., Harris, R.T., Duvoisin, M.R., Hather, B.M. & Buchanan, P. (1990) Effect of voluntary vs. artificial activation on the relationship of muscle torque to speed. *Journal of Applied Physiology* **69**, 2215–2221.

Enoka, R.M. (1988) Muscle strength and its development, new perspectives. *Sports Medicine* **6**, 146–168.

Eriksson, F. & Häggmark, T. (1979) Comparison of isometric muscle training and electrical stimulation supplementing isometric muscle training in the recovery after major knee ligament surgery. *American Journal of Sports Medicine* **7**, 169–171.

Feiereisen, P., Duchateau, J. & Hainaut, K. (1997) Motor unit recruitment order during voluntary and electrically induced contractions in the tibialis anterior. *Experimental Brain Research* **114**, 117–123.

Ferguson, J.P., Blackley, M.W., Knight, R.D., Sutlive, T.G., Underwood, F.B. & Greathouse, D.C. (1989) Effects of varying electrode site placements on the torque output of an electrically stimulated involuntary quadriceps femoris muscle contraction. *Journal of Orthopaedic and Sports Physical Therapy* **11**, 24–29.

Garnett, R. & Stephens, J.A. (1981) Changes in the recruitment threshold of motor units produced by cutaneous stimulation in man. *Journal of Physiology* **311**, 463–473.

Gollnick, P.D., Timson, B.F., Moore, R.L. & Riedy, M. (1981) Muscular enlargement and number of muscle fibers in skeletal muscles of rats. *Journal of Applied Physiology* **50**, 936–943.

Gould, N., Donnermeyer, D., Gammon, C., Pope, M. & Ashikaga, T. (1983) Transcutaneous muscle stimulation to retard disuse atrophy after open meniscectomy. *Clinical Orthopaedics and Related Research* **178**, 190–197.

Häkkinen, K. & Keskinen, K.L. (1989) Muscle cross-sectional area and voluntary force production characteristics in elite strength- and endurance-trained athletes and sprinters. *European Journal of Applied Physiology and Occupational Physiology* **59**, 215–220.

Häkkinen, K., Komi, P.V. & Alon, M. (1985) Effect of explosive type strength training on isometric force- and relaxation-time, electromyographic and muscle fibre characteristics of leg extensor muscles. *Acta Physiologica Scandinavica* **125**, 587–600.

Häkkinen, K., Pakarinen, A., Akin, M., Kauhanen, H. & Komi, P.V. (1988) Neuromuscular and hormonal adaptations in athletes to strength training in two years. *Journal of Applied Physiology* **65**, 2406–2412.

Henneman, F., Somjen, C. & Carpenter, D.O. (1965) Functional significance of cell size in spinal motor neurones. *Journal of Neurophysiology* **28**, 560–580.

Hultman, E., Sjoholm, H., Jaderholm-Ek, I. & Krynicki, J. (1983) Evaluation of methods for electrical stimulation of human skeletal muscle in situ. *Pflügers Archiv* **398**, 139–141.

Johnson, D.H., Thurston, P. & Ashcroft, P.J. (1977) The Russian technique of faradism in the treatment of chondromalacia patellae. *Physiotherapy Canada* **29**, 266–268.

Katz, B. (1939) The relation between force and speed in muscular contraction. *Journal of Physiology* **96**, 45–64.

Kim, C.K., Bangsbo, J., Strange, S., Karpakka, J. & Saltin, B. (1995) Metabolic response and muscle glycogen depletion pattern during prolonged electrically induced dynamic exercise in man. *Scandinavian Journal of Rehabilitation Medicine* **27**, 51–58.

Knaflitz, M., Merletti, R. & DeLuca, C.J. (1990) Inference of motor unit recruitment order in voluntary and electrically elicited contractions. *Journal of Applied Physiology* **68**, 1657–1667.

Komi, P.V. (1986) Training of muscle strength and power: Interaction of neuromotoric, hypertrophic, and mechanical factors. *International Journal of Sports Medicine* **7**, 10–15.

Kots, Y. & Chwilon, W. (1971) Muscle training with the electrical stimulation method. *Teoriya i Prakitka Fizieheskoi Kultury*, USSR, 3/4.

Kramer, J.F. & Mendryk, S.W. (1982) Electrical stimulation as a strength improvement technique: a review. *Journal of Orthopaedic and Sports Physical Therapy* **4**, 91–98.

Laughman, R.K., Youdas, J.W., Garrett, T.R. & Chao, E.Y.S. (1983) Strength changes in the normal quadriceps femoris muscle as a result of electrical stimulation. *Physical Therapy* **63**, 494–499.

McDonagh, M.J.N. & Davies, C.T.M. (1984) Adaptive response of mammalian skeletal muscle to exercise with high loads. *European Journal of Applied Physiology* **52**, 139–155.

Maffiuletti, N.A., Cometti, G., Amiridis, I.G., Martin, A., Pousson, M. & Chatard, J.C. (2000) The effects of electromyostimulation training and basketball practice on muscle strength and jumping ability. *International Journal of Sports Medicine* **21**, 437–443.

Maier, A., Gambke, B. & Pette, D. (1986) Degeneration–regeneration as a mechanism contributing to the fast to slow conversion of chronically stimulated fast-twitch rabbit muscle. *Cell and Tissue Research* **244**, 635–643.

Mason, J.L. & Mackay, N.A.M. (1976) Pain sensations associated with electrocutaneous stimulation. *IEEE Transactions on Biomedical Engineering* **23**, 405–409.

Miller, R.G., Mirka, A. & Maxfield, M. (1981) Rate of tension development in isometric contractions of a human hand muscle. *Experimental Neurology* **73**, 267–285.

Moreno-Aranda, J. & Seireg, A. (1981a) Electrical parameters for over-the-skin muscle stimulation. *Journal of Biomechanics* **14**, 579–585.

Moreno-Aranda, J. & Seireg, A. (1981b) Investigation of over-the-skin electrical stimulation parameters for different normal muscles and subjects. *Journal of Biomechanics* **14**, 587–593.

Nardone, A. & Schieppati, M. (1988) Shift of activity from slow to fast muscle during voluntary lengthening contractions of the triceps surae muscles in humans. *Journal of Physiology* **395**, 363–381.

Nardone, A., Romano, C. & Schieppati, M. (1989) Selective recruitment of high-threshold human motor units during voluntary isotonic lengthening of active muscles. *Journal of Physiology* **409**, 451–471.

Pette, D. & Vrbovä, G. (1985) Invited review: Neural control of phenotypic expression in mammalian muscle fibers. *Muscle and Nerve* **8**, 676–689.

Pichon, F., Chatard, J.C., Martin, A. & Cometti, G. (1995) Electrical stimulation and swimming performance. *Medicine and Science in Sports and Exercise* **27**, 1671–1676.

Romano, C. & Schieppati, M. (1987) Reflex excitability of human soleus motoneurones during voluntary shortening or lengthening contractions. *Journal of Physiology* **390**, 271–284.

Ruther, C.L., Golden, C.L., Harris R.T. & Dudley, G.A. (1995) Hypertrophy, resistance training, and the nature of skeletal muscle activation. *Journal of Strength and Conditioning Research* **9**, 155–159.

Ryushi, T.H., Škkinen, K., Kauhanen, H. & Komi, P.V. (1988) Muscle fiber characteristics, muscle cross-sectional area and force production in strength athletes, physically active males and females. *Scandinavian Journal of Sports Science* **10**, 7–15.

Scott, O.M., Vrbova, C., Hyde, S.A. & Dubowitz, V. (1985) Effects of chronic low frequency electrical stimulation on normal human tibialis anterior muscle. *Journal of Neurology, Neurosurgery and Psychiatry* **48**, 774–781.

Sinacore, D.R., Delitto, A., King, D.S. & Rose, S.J. (1990) Type II fiber activation with electrical stimulation: a preliminary report. *Physical Therapy* **70**, 416–422.

Solomonow, M., Baratta, R., Shoji, H. & Ambrosia, R. (1986) The myoelectric signal of electrically stimulated muscle during recruitment: an inherent feedback parameter for a closed loop control scheme. *IEEE Transactions on Biomedical Engineering* **33**, 735–745.

St Pierre, D., Taylor, A.W., Lavoie, M., Sellers, W. & Kots, Y.M. (1986) Effects of 2500 Hz sinusoidal current on fibre area and strength of the quadriceps femoris. *Journal of Sports Medicine* **26**, 60–66.

Stevenson, S.W. & Dudley, G.A. (2001) Dietary creatine supplementation and muscular adaptation to resistive overload. *Medicine and Science in Sports and Exercise* **33**, 1304–1310.

Tesch, P.A. (1987) Acute and long-term metabolic changes consequent to heavy-resistance exercise. *Medicine and Sport Science* **26**, 67–89.

Westing, S.H., Seger, J.Y., Karlson, E. & Ekblom, B. (1988) Eccentric and concentric torque–velocity characteristics of the quadriceps femoris in man. *European Journal of Applied Physiology* **58**, 100–104.

Westing, S.H., Seger, J. & Thorstensson, A. (1989) Does neural inhibition suppress eccentric knee extension torque in man? *Medicine and Science in Sports and Exercise* **21**, S67.

Wigerstad-Lossing, I., Grimby, C., Jonsson, T., Morelli, B., Peterson, L. & Renstrom, P. (1988) Effects of electrical muscle stimulation combined with voluntary contractions after knee ligament surgery. *Medicine and Science in Sports and Exercise* **20**, 93–98.

Wolf, S.L., Ariel, G.B., Saar, D., Penny, M.A. & Railey, P. (1986) The effect of muscle stimulation during resistive training on performance parameters. *American Journal of Sports Medicine* **14**, 18–23.

PART 5

STRENGTH AND POWER TRAINING FOR SPORTS

Chapter 23

Biomechanics of Strength and Strength Training

VLADIMIR M. ZATSIORSKY

Of recent years physiologists have been so concerned with the efforts to delve deeper into the actual mechanism of a muscular contraction that they have largely lost sight of other interesting mechanical problems relating to the utilization of the muscle force after it has been developed. It is my purpose therefore, to discuss some of these mechanical aspects of muscular movements in humans in the hope of reviving some interest in this neglected subject. It should not be left solely to the attentions of the athletic director and the orthopaedic surgeon (W. O. Fenn 1938).

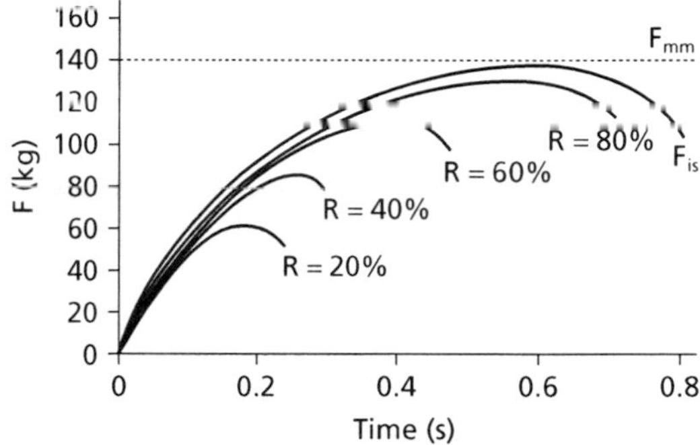

Fig. 23.1 Force–time histories of a leg extension against different levels of resistance. The subject was asked to perform the effort in an explosive way, i.e. as quickly and strongly as possible. The magnitude of weights, i.e. resistance (R), varied from 20% to 80% of F_{mm}. F_{mm} was determined in the isometric conditions without any restriction with respect to time. Force–time curve for an explosive isometric effort is also shown. (Adapted from Verchoshansky 1977.)

The term strength (or muscular strength) designates the ability of an athlete to exert maximal force on the environment. The terms maximal voluntary contraction (MVC) and maximal end-point force are also in use.

The magnitude of the force depends not only on the selected movement (e.g. leg extension) but also on numerous characteristics of the selected motor task (e.g. body posture, movement velocity, type and amount of resistance, etc.). For instance, when a subject performs maximum-effort leg extensions against various loads he or she generates different maximal forces (F_m in the trials (Fig. 23.1). The heavier the load, the larger the maximal force F_m. In this chapter, the symbol F_m will be used to designate a maximal force attained in a given movement under specified conditions (e.g. the maximal force during a leg extension at the load of 60% or the maximal force exerted on a 7-kg shot during a delivery phase of shot putting). Under one of the conditions, the F_m is the highest among all the maximal forces. The highest force value is termed the maximal maximorum force. The symbol F_{mm} is used to represent it. F_m may be much smaller than F_{mm}; as an example compare the F_m at the resistance of 20% with the F_{mm} (Fig. 23.1).

Strength and power athletes generate large F_m in their athletic movements, and to enhance performance they usually need to increase the force production. For instance, they are interested in exerting a maximal force of leg extension during take-off in the high jump or a maximal force of arm extension during shot putting. Similar to the example presented in Fig. 23.1, the F_ms can be quite different from the values of F_{mm} attained in the same movement, i.e. leg or arm extension, when performed in the most favourable conditions. While one of the main goals of training is the increasing of F_m, athletes also train to enhance F_{mm}, considering this enhancement a way of improving performance results. Questions arise about the relationship between the F_m and F_{mm}: what exactly determines the magnitude of F_m and F_{mm} and the difference between them? What prevents the athletes from generating F_{mm} in their athletic movement?

As follows from Fig. 23.1, the values of F_m exerted against various resistances are different. While several factors contribute to the differences (e.g. the body posture at the instant of the maximal force production, movement velocity, etc.), one factor is most evident—the time available for force development.

Time and rate of force development

The *maximal maximorum* muscular force F_{mm} cannot be developed instantly; it takes usually in excess of 0.3–0.4 s to generate the F_{mm}. In many athletic movements, the duration of the periods during which the maximal forces should be generated is less than 0.3 s (Table 23.1). In these

Table 23.1 The duration of the periods of the 'explosive' force production in some athletic movements (M, males; F, females).

Sport and motion	Time (s)	Athletes and performance	Reference
Take-off			
Sprint running	0.101 (M) 0.108 (F)	M: mean 100-m record 10.62 s F: mean 100-m record 12.22 s	Mero and Komi (1986)
Long jump	0.105–0.125 (M)	680–818 cm (a correlation coefficient between the take-off time and the performance results is −0.833; $n = 43$)	Zatsiorsky (1974)
High jump	0.15–0.23 (M) 0.14–0.18 (F)	Best world athletes; M: 234–238 cm; F: 196–205 cm	Dapena (2000)
Ski jumping	0.25–0.30	Experienced athletes	Komi and Virmavirta (2000)
Figure skating	0.17	Experienced athlete, single Axel	King (2000)
Platform diving	≈ 0.33 ≈ 0.15	Standing take-off Running dives	Miller (2000)
Running forward somersault	0.13 ± 0.02	University gymnasts	Brüggemann (1994)
Horse vaulting	0.11–0.12		
Somersault following a handspring	0.10 ± 0.02	Experienced gymnasts	Brüggemann (1994)
Push-off, vaulting	0.19–0.21	Experienced gymnasts	Brüggemann (1994)
Delivery			
Javelin	0.12	M: release velocity 30 m·s^{-1} (the equivalent performance result > 80 m)	Bartonietz (2000b)
Shot putting	0.22–0.27	M: 19.60–21.35 m	Lanka (2000)
Support time			
Hammer throwing, double support	0.18–0.22	Elite world athletes, 3rd turn	Bartonietz (2000a)

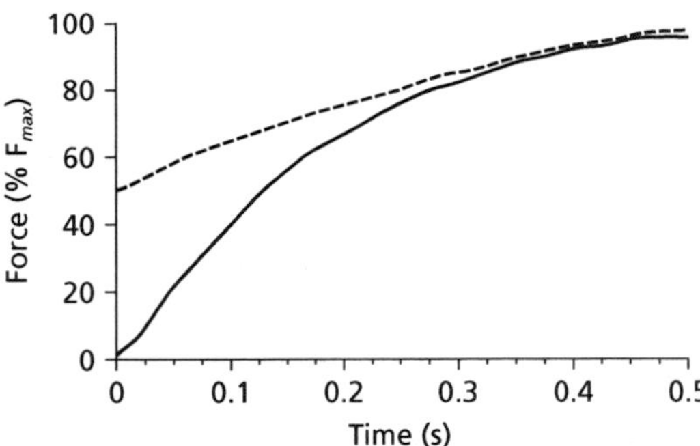

Fig. 23.2 Isometric force–time curves at varying initial tensions, at zero and 50% of the maximal force. The graph is based on the data from Godik and Zatsiorsky (1965).

activities, athletes do not have sufficient time to produce the F_{mm}.

The percentage difference between the F_{mm} and F_m attained during an explosive strength production is called the *explosive strength deficit* (ESD):

$$\text{ESD, \%} = \frac{F_{mm} - F_m}{F_{mm}} \times 100 \qquad (1)$$

ESD shows the percentage of an athlete's strength potential that was not used in a given trial. In many athletic movements, the ESD amounts to 50% of the F_{mm}. For instance, among the best shot-putters during throws of 20.0–21.0 m, the peak force F_m applied to the shot is 500–600 N. These athletes typically bench press 220–240 kg, thus exerting a force in excess of 1070–1176 N with each arm. Thus, in throwing, they exert only about 50% of F_{mm}. Typical force–time curves for different initial force levels F_{in} are presented in Fig. 23.2. The force–time history can be described by an empirical exponential equation (Clarke 1968):

$$F(t) = -a_1(1 - e^{-k_1 t}) + a_2(1 - e^{-k_2 t}) + a_3(1 - e^{-k_3 t}) \qquad (2)$$

where $F(t)$ is the force at any time t, e is the base of the natural logarithms (e = 2.7182), k_1, k_2 and k_3 are the rate constants and $F_{in} + a_2 + a_3 - a_1 = F_{mm}$ the steady state force when the maximum contraction has been attained. From Fig. 23.2, it follows that the time to peak force does not depend on the initial force level F_{in}.

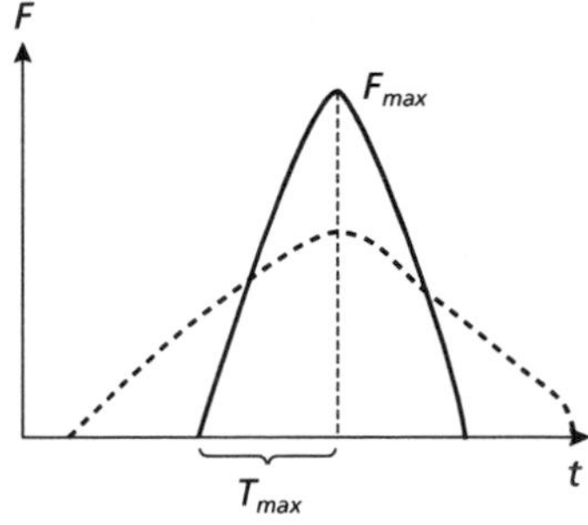

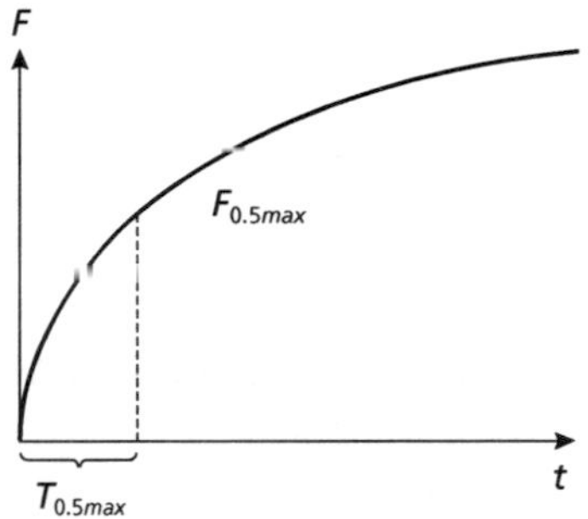

Fig. 23.3 Explosive strength (above) and S-gradient (below), a schematic. In the top panel, the solid line represents a force–time curve for a highly skilled athlete and the broken line represents a low-skilled athlete. The highly skilled athlete exerts a larger force in a smaller time. T_{max} is the *peak time,* the elapsed interval between the initiation of the force rise and the point at which peak force occurs. During the isokinetic strength testing, the *rise time,* i.e. the elapsed interval at which force or torque increases from 10% to 90% of the peak value, is also used (Weiss 2000).

The rate of force development (RFD) can be computed as the time derivative of eqn 2. For a single trial, the RFD is not constant; it is a function of time t. As an approximate estimate of the average RFD, the ratio F_{max}/T_{max}, where T_{max} is the time to peak force (Fig. 23.3, top panel), is often used. The ratio is termed the *explosive strength*. In applications, the explosive strength is commonly computed per 1 kg of body weight. Also, the *force gradient*, also called the S-gradient, is used: S signifies 'start' (Godik & Zatsiorsky 1965) (Fig. 23.3, bottom panel). The S-gradient characterizes the average RFD at the beginning

Table 23.2 Maximal frequency and 'theoretical acceleration' (maximal joint moment/moment of inertia) for some body parts (Fenn 1938).

Body part	Period at maximal frequency (s)	Theoretical acceleration (rad·s^{-2})
Whole leg	0.24	71
Lower leg	0.33	298
Forearm	0.15	775
First finger	0.18	42 500
Great toe	0.30	85 800

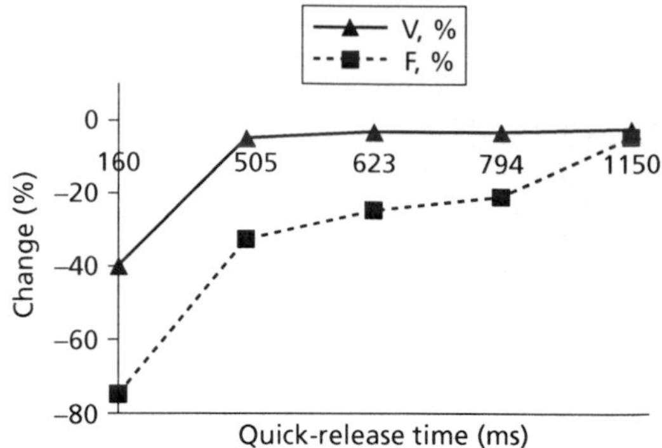

Fig. 23.4 The difference (%) in the values of the maximal velocity and the maximal force in the ordinary and quick release conditions. After the release, the resistance was provided by an inertia wheel of the various equivalent masses (up to 270 kg). The graph is based on the data from Zatsiorsky and Smirnov (1968).

phase of a muscular effort. It is computed as the ratio

$$S\text{-gradient} = F_{0.5max}/T_{0.5max} \quad (3)$$

where $F_{0.5max}$ is one half of the maximal force and $T_{0.5max}$ is the time to attain it.

The force $F_{0.5max}$ and the time to attain it $T_{0.5max}$ do not correlate with each other (Zatsiorsky 1966; 100 male athletes, $r = 0.11$). Hence, the ability to exert large forces (*muscular strength*) and the ability to exert the force quickly are independent. The ability to perform movements with large frequency also does not depend on the muscular strength (Fenn 1938). For instance, the ratio of the maximal joint moment (as measured statically) to the moment of inertia differs for the different body parts to a much larger extent than the maximal frequency (Table 23.2).

In research, the contribution of the RFD can be eliminated by employing the *quick-release method*: during testing, a subject exerts isometrically a certain magnitude of force, then a trigger is suddenly released and the movement is performed against a given resistance. Figure 23.4 illustrates the percentage difference in the maximal velocity V_m and F_m in the same movement (elbow flexion) performed under the ordinary and quick-release conditions. When movement was of a short duration, the difference exceeded 40% for the V_m and 75% for the F_m.

The time course of the force uptake is due to several factors: 'taking up of slack' in the subcutaneous soft tissues and the muscle–tendon–joint system (this factor is believed to account for the first term in eqn 2); the spreading of the excitation over the motoneurone pools that innervate the involved muscles (recruitment of the motor units); propagation of action potentials along and around the muscle fibres; the process of calcium release and reuptake from the sarcoplasmic reticulum (so called *activation dynamics*); the time for extending the serial elastic components of the muscle–tendon complexes; and some other factors. The relative contribution of these factors to the T_m in athletes remains unknown.

Some data indicate that the time expended for the extension of the series elastic components may be an important contributor to the time to peak force. The theory is based on the following observation: if during the period of force development the muscle is quickly stretched, as we may expect, for example, in drop landing, the muscle produces a much larger force (Fig. 23.5). This finding indicates that during the periods of force development the contractile components can bear large forces without lengthening. The muscle is said to be in the *active state*. During the active state, the contractile components generate a force in a very short period of time, about 20 ms in some animals. However, the lengthening of the series elastic components within the muscle

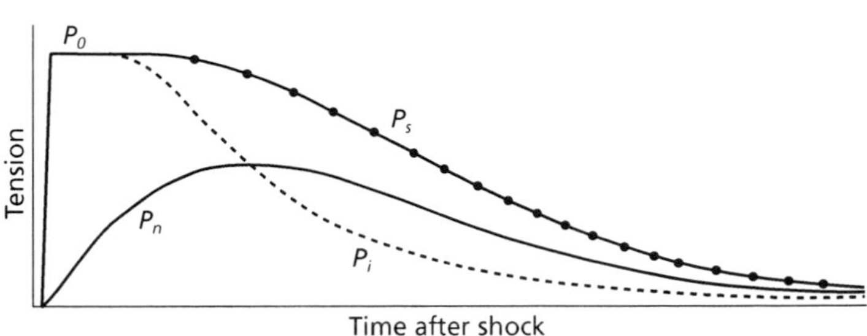

Fig. 23.5 Diagram of mechanical changes during a muscle contraction (twitch). P_n, tension at the muscle end; P_i, intrinsic strength of the contractile component of the muscle; P_s, tension in muscle stretched quickly after the latent period; P_0, initial value of P_i and P_s. (Reprinted by permission from Hill 1949.)

slows the rate at which tension rises at the muscle end. Even if the muscle is held isometrically, there is some shortening of the contractile component while the corresponding stretching of the series elastic component takes place. When the whole muscle–tendon unit length stays constant, the corresponding muscle fibres may shorten by up to 30% of their initial length (Kawakami *et al.* 1998). Due to the stretching of the series components, the force exerted by the tendon on the bone lags considerably behind the force of the contractile components (Wilkie 1956; Carlson & Wilkie 1974; for a discussion see also Zatsiorsky 1997). Unfortunately, this theory does not explain why T_m in some athletes is much shorter than in others.

One of the factors that seems to affect the rate of force development, as well as the relaxation time, is the muscle composition. Fast, glycolytic fibres have a shorter twitch rise time than slow, oxidative fibres (Burke *et al.* 1971; Gonyea *et al.* 1981). Most human muscles are composed of both slow and fast motor fibres. It is usually expected that athletes with a large percentage of fast muscle fibres can exert force faster than athletes with a low percentage of the fast fibres. The relationship, however, is not so straightforward. The rise and relaxation time depends not only on the muscle composition but also on the recruitment order. The recruitment follows the size principle (Hennemann *et al.* 1965). According to the principle, slow motor units (innervated by the small motoneurones) are recruited at low force levels and, with increasing force, increasingly faster motor units (innervated by larger motoneurones) are activated. In a mixed population of muscle fibres, both the onset and the end of force development are determined by the slowest muscle fibres (the 'weakest link in the chain' principle, Savelberg 2000). Hence, percentage of fast muscle fibres may not be a decisive factor for the time to peak force T_m. However, when smaller forces are produced, the dependence of the rise time on muscle composition is substantial (Viitasalo & Komi 1978, 1981). It seems that the force gradient, which is based on determining the $T_{0.5\ max}$, is more sensitive to muscle composition than the T_m. This issue deserves future research efforts.

Motor unit discharge rates are higher during ballistic movements (60–120 Hz) than in slow ramp tracking contractions (≤ 30 Hz) (Desmedt & Godaux 1977). This finding suggests that rate coding could be used to grade the RFD. If this hypothesis is correct one may expect that in quick athletes motoneurones will discharge at higher frequencies (see Chapters 3 and 10 in this volume).

Heavy-resistance training leads to enhancement of the F_{mm} but not the RFD (Fig. 23.6, top panel). The rate of force development increases after dynamic strength training (Fig. 23.6, bottom panel) and after training employing 'explosive' strength production—at the maximal rate of force development (Behm & Sale 1993a). The type of muscle action (isometric or concentric) appears to be of lesser importance. The increase of the RFD after dynamic (ballistic) training is associated with the change of the motor unit activity (Van Cutsem *et al.* 1998). In the latter study, the training consisted of fast joint movements against a load of 30–40% of the maximal muscle

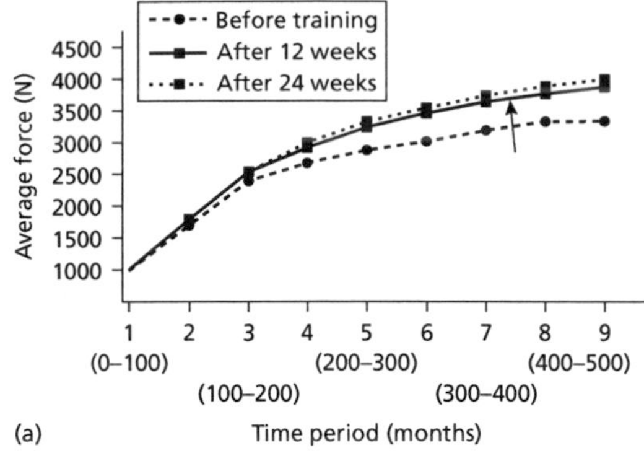

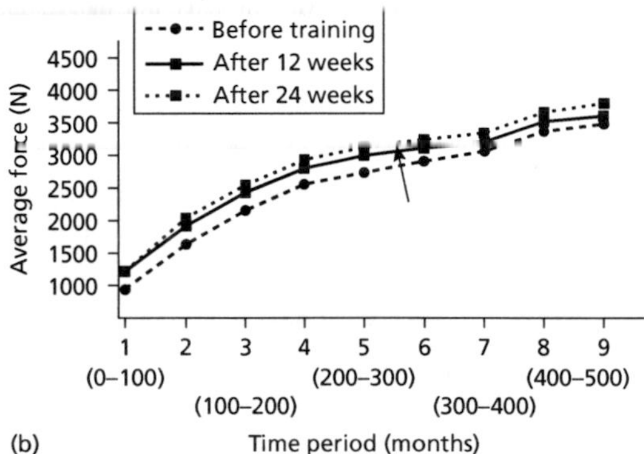

Fig. 23.6 The influence of heavy-resistance training (top) and dynamic (explosive) resistance training (bottom) on maximum strength and the rate of force development during an explosive maximal bilateral leg extension. After the heavy-resistance training, only F_{mm}, not the initial part of the force–time curve, is enhanced. The rate of force development, especially the *S*-gradient, is unchanged. (Adapted from Häkkinen & Komi 1985a,b.)

strength for 12 weeks. Brief (2–5-ms) interspike intervals of motor units were observed ('doublets'). Training increased the percentage of units firing doublets from 5.2 to 32.7% as well as the maximal firing frequency of the motor units.

For athletes and coaches, the following facts/conclusions are the most relevant.

1 In efforts of short duration, the rate of force development (explosive strength) may be more important than the maximal strength F_{mm}.

2 When testing athletes, characteristics such as the force gradient or the force exerted at 100 ms from the start of action are recommended. For instance, the single best correlate of the maximum sprinting speed was the force applied at 100 ms from the start of a loaded jumping action (Young 1995; Young *et al.* 1995).

3 If exercises are performed slowly, heavy-resistance training enhances F_{mm} but not the RFD (Fig. 23.6). Hence, special dynamic training is necessary. This recommendation is especially valid for experienced athletes.

Body posture

The strength that an athlete can generate in a given motion depends on body posture (joint angles). For instance, the maximal force that one can exert on a barbell depends on the height of the bar (Fig. 23.7). The maximal force F_{mm} is exerted when the bar is near knee height.

Figures 23.8 and 23.9 illustrate dependencies between joint configuration and muscle strength (an externally registered F_{mm}) in various single-joint and multijoint tasks. The curves, known as *human strength curves* (Darcus 1951; Darcus & Salter 1955), describe the maximum isometric force as a function of joint configuration. Note a large difference for force produced at different joint positions (Figs 23.8 & 23.9). An extensive review on human strength curves was published by Kulig *et al.* (1984).

For each joint movement, there are angular positions at which the maximal values of the F_{mm} can be reached. During elbow flexion, the maximal force is generated at an angle of 90° (Fig. 23.8a); for elbow extension, as well as for knee extension, the maximal values are obtained at an angle of 120° (Franke 1920; Carpenter 1938), etc. The maximum grip strength is attained when the metacarpophalangeal joint is at 30° of flexion and the proximal interphalangeal joint at 70° of flexion (Mundale 1970). The highest forces in leg or arm extension can be exerted when the extremity is almost completely extended (Fig. 23.9). The goal of the ensuing discussion is to shed some light on the cause of these findings.

Biomechanically, the F_{mm} is a function of muscle forces, or tensions, that undergo two transformations: the muscle forces transform into joint

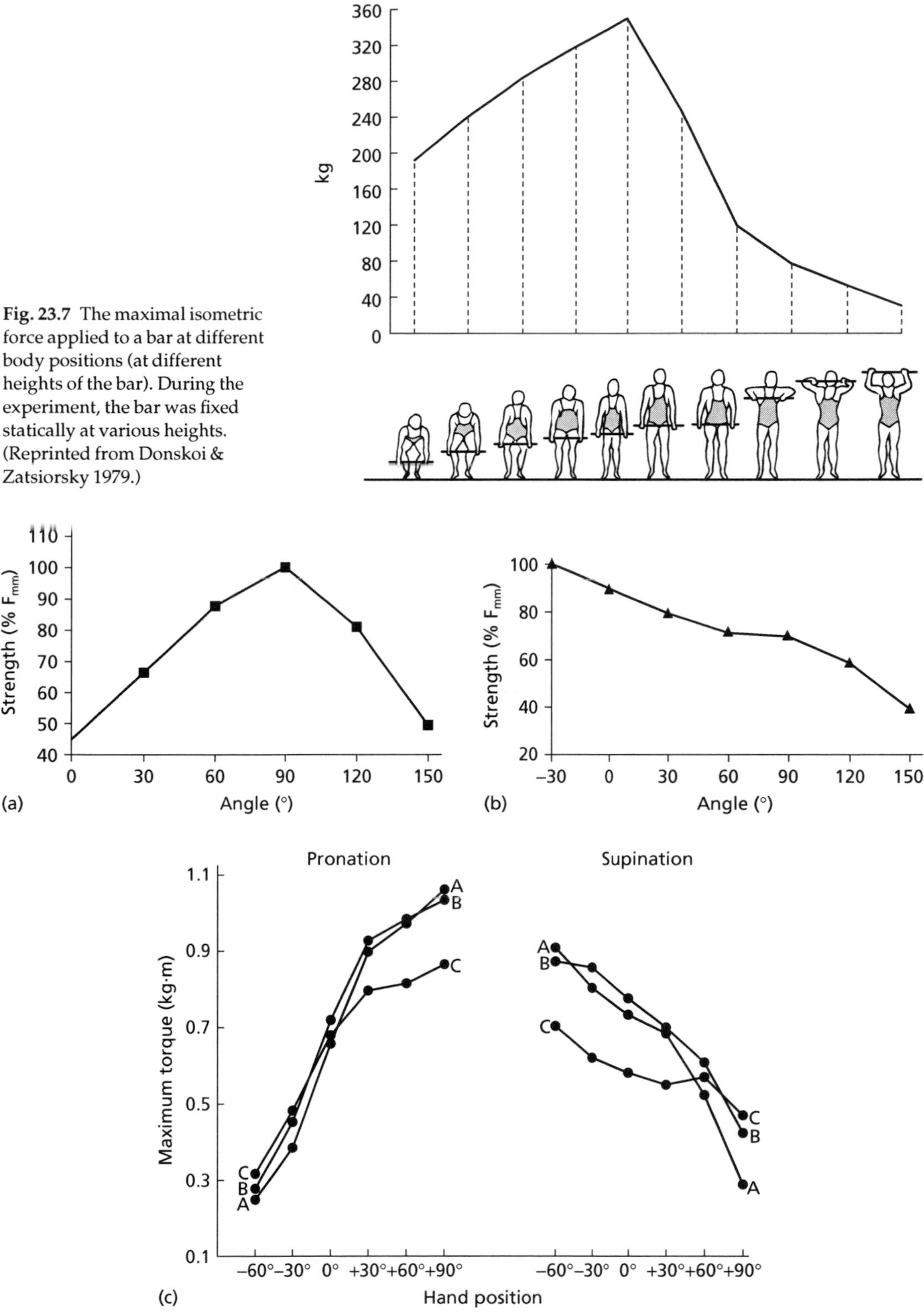

Fig. 23.7 The maximal isometric force applied to a bar at different body positions (at different heights of the bar). During the experiment, the bar was fixed statically at various heights. (Reprinted from Donskoi & Zatsiorsky 1979.)

Fig. 23.8 Strength curves in single-joint movements. (a) Elbow flexion (from Zatsiorsky 1995). (b) Shoulder flexion (from Zatsiorsky 1995). (c) Arm pronation and supination (from Salter & Darcus 1952); elbow flexed to (A) 150°; (B) 90°; (C) 30°.

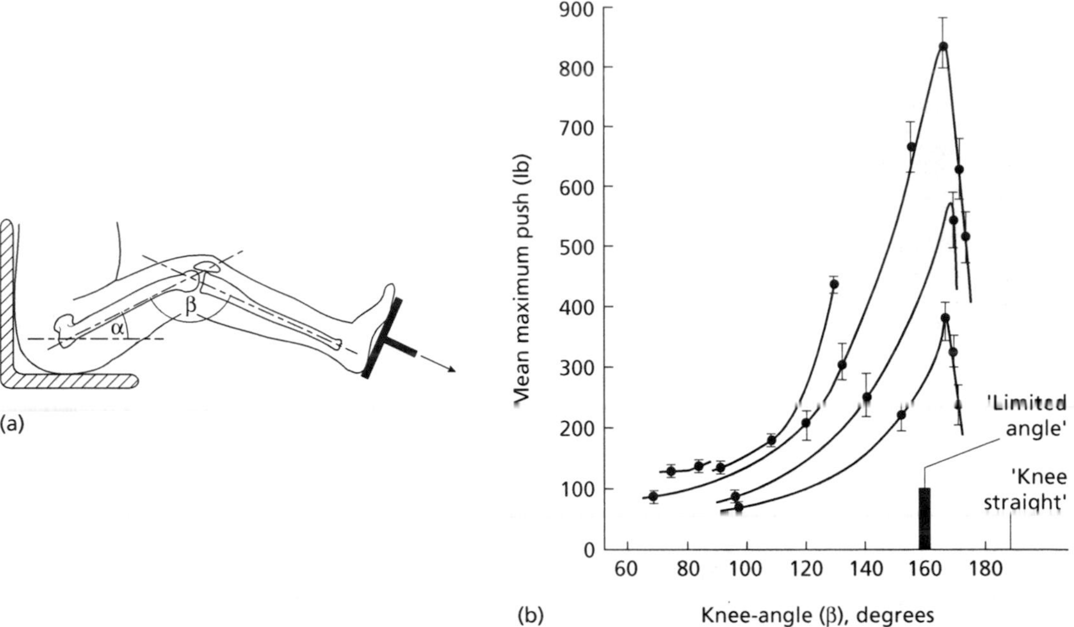

Fig. 23.9 Dependence of the pushing force on limb position in seated subjects. (a) Experimental set-up. (b) The mean maximum push (± 2 SD) exerted isometrically by six subjects on a pedal placed in different positions. For each of the five different angles of thigh to the horizontal (α), the knee angle (β) varied. Curve 1 represents the data for angle α between −15° and −6°; curve 2 between +5° and +10°; curve 3, 15–19°; curve 4, 33–36°; and curve 5 corresponds to the thigh angle α = 48–49°. Curves 4 and 5 necessarily stop as shown well before the limiting angle is reached. At these thigh positions, the knee cannot be extended further due to the limitation provided by the hamstring. (Adapted by permission from Hugh-Jones 1947.)

moments and the joint moments transform into external force:

muscle–tendon forces → joint moments → endpoint force (muscle strength, F_{mm}).

We consider these two transformations in sequence.

From muscle tension to joint moments

Muscle tension depends on the muscle length and, hence, on the joint angle. This fact was established in the 19th century by Blix (1891, 1893, 1894) who measured the maximal isometric tension that muscle exerts at different lengths. Because the muscle length–tension relations have been discussed previously (see Chapter 9), the current discussion is limited to the manifestation of these relations in athletic movements. The muscle length is understood as the distance from origin to insertion and not as the muscle fibre length. Length changes of muscle–tendon units during various athletic movements are discussed in a recent review (Hay 2000).

MUSCLE FORCE AT DIFFERENT BODY POSITIONS

For sport practitioners, two main questions attract interest:

1 Are athletic movements performed on the ascending or descending limbs of the muscle force–length curves?

2 What is the contribution of the passive forces, if any, at different body postures?

The answer to the second question is evident: when a joint approaches the limits of its range of motion the passive forces increase. For instance,

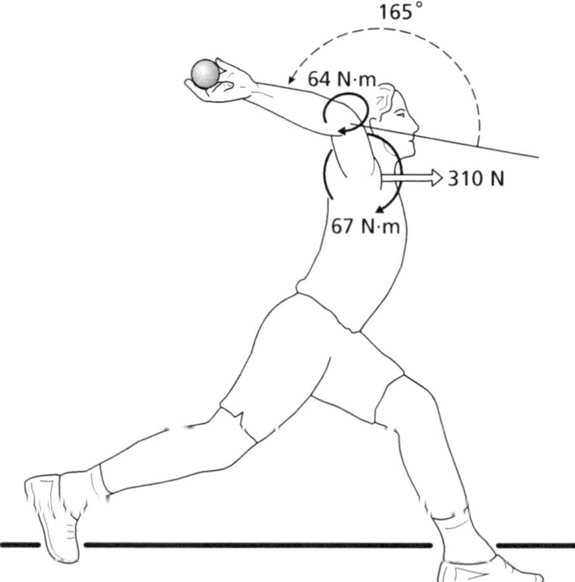

Fig. 23.10 The loading of the shoulder in pitching. At the instant shown, the arm was externally rotated 165°, and the elbow was flexed 95°. Among the loads generated at this time were 67 Nm of internal rotation torque and 310 N of anterior force at the shoulder, and 64 Nm of varus torque at the elbow. (Reprinted by permission from Fleisig *et al.* 1995.)

in pitching, during the arm cocking the external rotation of the shoulder approaches 180° (Fig. 23.10). At this angular position, the muscles and other soft anatomical tissues of the shoulder are deformed (Dillman 1994). Resisting the deformation, the tissues contribute to the joint torques that reach maximal values. With the exception of the finger joints, the passive resistance in the middle range of joint angular motion is small. For example, the contribution of the passive forces into the ankle joint torque in the sagittal plane during walking is less than 6% (Siegler *et al.* 1984). At the hip joint, the contribution of the passive moment is less than 10% (Vrahas *et al.* 1990).

The answer to the first question is much more difficult. While length–tension relations for animal muscles have been measured in abundance, the data on human muscles are scarce and nonsystematic. Direct measurements of the length–tension relations have been performed on amputees with cineplastic tunnels through the distal end of a muscle (Fig. 23.11). The subjects exerted maximal voluntary efforts. In isometric conditions, the human force–length curves were similar to those obtained on animals (see Chapter

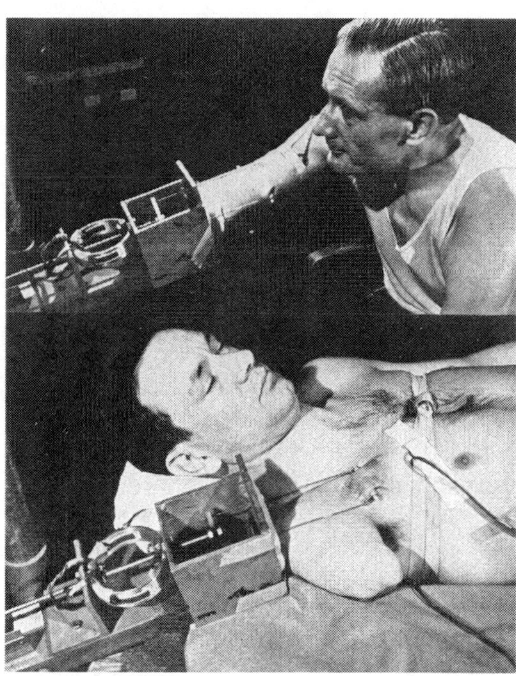

Fig. 23.11 Experiments with cineplastic amputees. During the force measurements the subjects exerted maximal efforts. (Reprinted by permission from Ralston *et al.* 1947.)

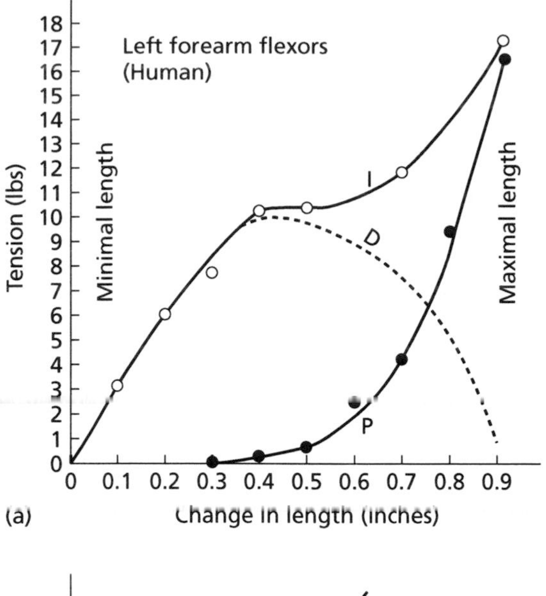

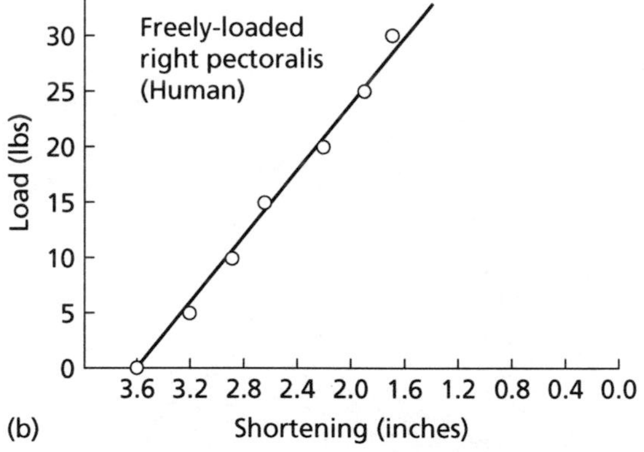

Fig. 23.12 (a) Force–length curves as measured isometrically. ●, measurements performed on passive (relaxed) muscles. ○, forces recorded during the maximal efforts. (b) Ability of a muscle (pectoralis major) to shorten from a given initial length under successive applications of increasing loads. (Reprinted by permission from Ralston *et al.* 1947.)

10). As the load was increased, the amount of shortening that the muscle achieved, was less (Fig. 23.12). It is not clear, however, to what extent the measurements performed on amputees are representative of able-bodied subjects.

When length–tension relations were computed from the values of the joint angles and joint torques, it was usually observed that when muscles shorten they generate smaller tension (Franke 1920; Reijs 1921; Darcus 1951; Clarke 1956). Hence, the muscles act mainly on the ascending limb of the length–tension curves. Unfortunately, the precise values of the individual muscle forces cannot be established from these experiments. Only 'lumped' length–tension relationships for groups of muscles can be determined (Fig. 23.13).

Some muscles, or perhaps some muscles in some people, may act on the descending limb of the length–tension curves. In particular, a substantial portion of the normal range of motion of some wrist extensors, e.g. extensor carpi radialis brevis, is on the descending limb of the length–tension curve (Lieber *et al.* 1994, 1997). This muscle generates maximum tension when the wrist is fully extended and the muscle is maximally shortened. Another wrist extensor, extensor carpi radialis longus, also operates on its descending limb but over a much narrower sarcomere length range. As the wrist flexes, the wrist torque

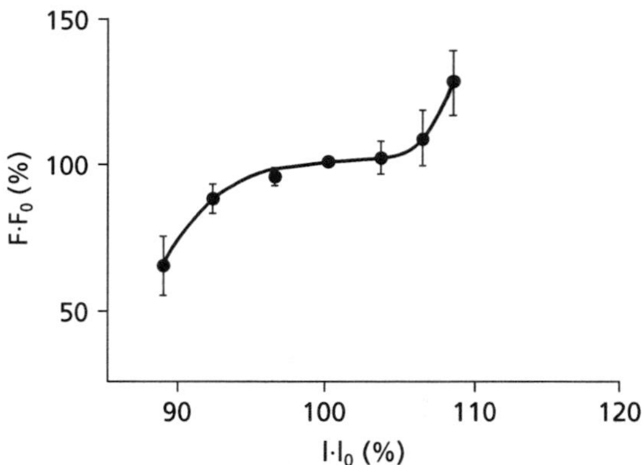

Fig. 23.13 Length–tension curve of the 'equivalent' elbow flexor for maximal isometric contractions. The four muscles that are prime movers for elbow flexion (long and short heads of the biceps, brachioradialis and brachialis) are mentally replaced by one equivalent muscle that has the same point of insertion as the biceps. Additional assumptions are: (a) the axis of rotation at the elbow joint is fixed; (b) the line of action of the 'equivalent' muscle is a straight line; (c) the muscle origin and insertion are considered at points rather than surfaces; and (d) the body segments are rigid.

Each point is the mean of 10 observations made on five subjects. Abscissa: lengths in per cent of standard length l_0 of the muscle equivalent. Ordinate: forces in per cent of the maximal force corresponding to this standard length. Standard deviation is also indicated. Note that the force at the minimal muscle length (after a maximal muscle shortening) is approximately 60% of the force at the standard length. (Reprinted from Bouisset 1990. The original figure is due to Pertuzon 1972 and Pertuzon & Bouisset 1971.)

decreases due to extensor lengthening along the descending limb of their length–tension curve and flexor shortening along the ascending limb of their length–tension curve. Overall, the wrist muscles appear to be designed for balance and control rather than for generating maximal torques (Lieber & Fridén 1998).

The length–tension curves are usually recorded for isometric contraction at discrete joint positions and/or at discrete muscle lengths. The curves do not represent precisely the force exerted during muscle stretching or shortening. For a stretch, the tension is larger and for shortening the tension is smaller than the tension exerted in the static conditions. The same is valid for the joint angle–moment relations (Fig. 23.14).

The length of a two-joint muscle depends on the angular positions at both the joints that the muscle crosses. In such joints, the F_{mm} values depend not only on the angular position at the joint being tested but also on the angular position of the second joint. For instance, isometric strength curves for elbow flexion, shoulder flexion and supination–pronation depend on the whole-arm configuration (Winters & Kleweno 1993). The contribution of the gastrocnemius, which is a two-joint muscle, to plantar flexion torque at the ankle joint is reduced as the knee is flexed and, consequently, the gastrocnemius is shortened (Fig. 23.15; see also Sale *et al.* 1982). When the knee is maximally flexed and the ankle is plantarflexed, the gastrocnemius muscle is not able to produce active force (Herzog *et al.* 1990). This leg position can be used for a selective training of the soleus muscle.

The knee strength curve depends on the position at the hip joint (Fig. 23.16; cf. the data for knee flexion). Because the rectus femoris muscle is extended in the supine position and is shortened in the seated position, it is expected that the strength of knee extension in the supine position should be larger than in the seated position. However, this is not true for all the subjects (see Fig. 23.16 where such a difference was evidently not observed). In particular, cyclists tend to be stronger at short compared

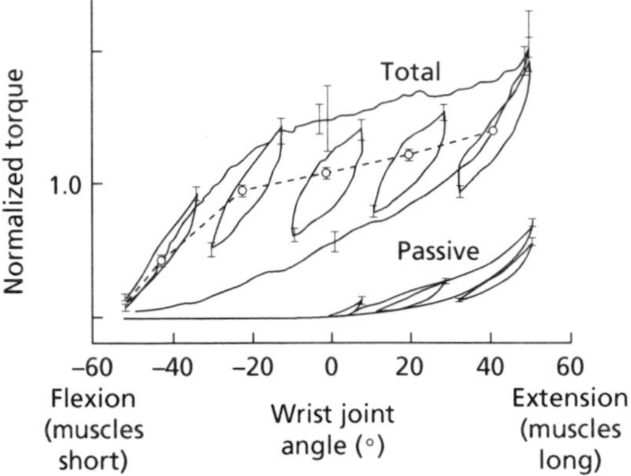

Fig. 23.14 Joint angle–joint torque curves for voluntary activation of wrist flexors. These are *not* the maximal torque data. During the experiment, the subjects were asked to maintain a constant level of EMG of a wrist flexor, the flexor carpi radialis. The EMG level was established at 10% of the maximal voluntary contraction. Joint torque was measured in three contraction conditions: (i) isometric (dotted line); (ii) ± 10° angular displacements centred at five different angles (small loops); and (iii) ± 50° angular displacements over full range of motion of the wrist joint (large loop). Narrow loops at bottom of the figure show angle–torque profiles with muscles completely relaxed. The torque values are normalized to mean torques of ± 10°angle–torque loops at 0° wrist angle. Note the difference between the values of the torques recorded in the static and dynamic conditions. The difference depends on the amplitude of the joint angular displacement. (Reproduced from Gillard *et al.* 2000.)

with long rectus femoris lengths, whereas the opposite is true for runners (Herzog *et al.* 1991). This finding was explained by the different range of the hip joint motion in cycling and running (Fig. 23.17). Cyclists use the rectus femoris at shorter lengths than runners in their respective sports. It is not clear whether the difference between the joint strength curves of the cyclists and runners is due to training or is inherited.

A take-home message for coaches and athletes is that, with a few exceptions mentioned previously (some wrist extensors, the rectus femoris muscle in some athletes), the muscles exert smaller tension at smaller lengths.

TRANSFORMATION OF MUSCLE FORCES INTO JOINT MOMENTS: MOMENT ARMS

Any force tends to rotate the body about any axis that does not intersect the line of force action. In particular, when a muscle exerts tension, the muscle tension generates a rotational effect at the joint. *Moment of force*, **M**, is a measure of the turning effect of the force. The effect is proportional to the distance of the line of force action from the axis of rotation. An extensive review on the moment arms of muscle forces is published by Pandy (1999). The present discussion is limited to the basic ideas.

In a planar case, the moment of a force **F** about a joint centre equals the product of the magnitude of the force F and the perpendicular distance, d, from the centre to the line of force action: $M = Fd$. The distance d is called a *moment arm*. The moment arm is equal to the moment of force produced by a unit force. Moments of force in a plane are scalars. An analysis of the muscle action can be reduced to two dimensions if, and only if, the line of muscle force action and the axis of rotation are perpendicular to each other. In this case, the muscle acts in the plane of joint movement. Table 23.3 contains the literature sources on the muscle moment arms at the main joints.

In humans, due to deformation of the soft tissues, including joint cartilages, moment arms during maximal force production may differ from the moment arms at rest (Aruin *et al.* 1987). For instance, the moment arm of the Achilles tendon during isometric plantarflexion MVC is 1.2–1.27 times larger than the resting moment arm (Maganaris *et al.* 1998, 2000). Similar facts are reported for the moment arm of the tibialis anterior (Maganaris *et al.* 1999, 2000). For this muscle, the moment arm at 0% MVC is significantly smaller than at 30 and 60% MVC (Ito *et al.* 2000).

When a joint angle varies, the moment arm of a muscle spanning the joint changes. For instance, at the elbow joint the flexion/extension moment arms vary by at least 30% over a 95° range of motion (Murray *et al.* 1995). Several computer

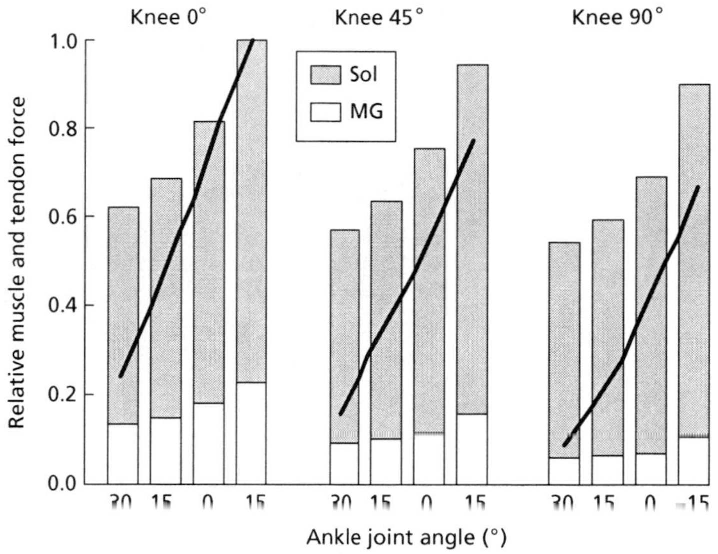

Fig. 23.15 Estimated relative tendon force of the medial gastrocnemius (MG) and soleus (Sol) (bars). Data are normalized to the maximal value when the knee is extended (0°) and the ankle is dorsiflexed at −15°. Lines in the bars are estimated Achilles tendon forces (also normalized to the maximal value). (Reprinted by permission from Kawakami *et al.* 2000.)

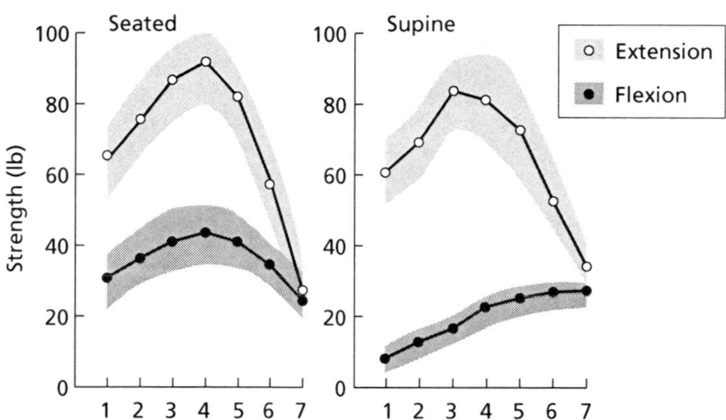

Fig. 23.16 Isometric strength recorded during knee extension and flexion in the seated and supine positions. (Reprinted by permission from Houtz *et al.* 1957.)

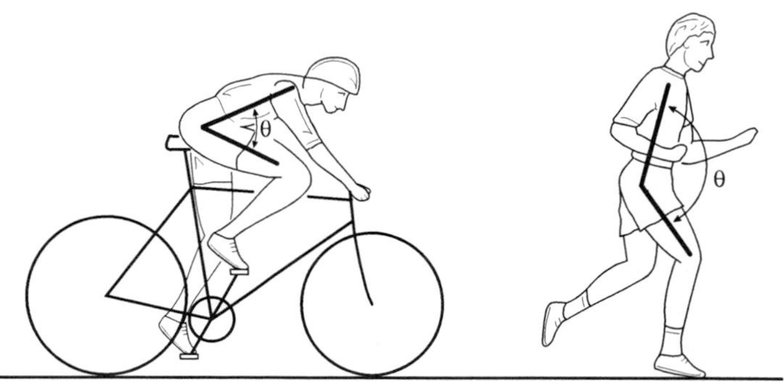

Fig. 23.17 Typical trunk–thigh angles (θ) for cycling and running. (Reprinted by permission from Herzog 1991.)

Table 23.3 Experimental studies of the moment arms of the muscles at the main joints.

Joints/muscles	References
Toe joints	Aper *et al.* (1996)
Ankle	Zatsiorsky *et al.* (1985); Aruin *et al.* (1987, 1988); Rugg *et al.* (1990); Klein *et al.* (1996); Maganaris *et al.* (1998, 1999, 2000); Maganaris (2000); Ito *et al.* (2000)
Knee	Smidt (1973); Grood *et al.* (1984); Nisell (1985); Nisell *et al.* (1986); Draganich *et al.* (1987); Mansour and Pereira (1987); Spoor *et al.* (1990, 1992); Visser *et al.* (1990); Herzog and Read (1993); Delp *et al.* (1994); Kellis and Baltzopoulos (1999)
Hip	Jensen and Davy (1975); Dostal and Andrews (1981); Nemeth and Olsen (1985); Mansour and Pereira (1987); Visser *et al.* (1990); Delp *et al.* (1994, 1999); Lengsfeld *et al.* (1997); Arnold and Delp (2001)
Trunk muscles	Nemeth and Olsen (1986, 1987) (erector spinae and rectus abdominis); Reid *et al.* (1994) (psoas muscle)
Shoulder	Poppen and Walker (1978); Wood *et al.* (1989); Bassett *et al.* (1990); Otis *et al.* (1994); Hughes *et al.* (1998); Nakajima *et al.* (1999); Kuechle *et al.* (2000)
Elbow	Amis *et al.* (1979); An *et al.* (1981); Gerbeaux *et al.* (1993); Murray *et al.* (1995, 2000); Lemay and Crago (1996); Ettema *et al.* (1998)
Wrist	Youm *et al.* (1976); Brand *et al.* (1981); Buchanan *et al.* (1993); Loren *et al.* (1996); Herrmann and Delp (1999)
Finger and thumb joints	Smith *et al.* (1964); Brand *et al.* (1975); Berme *et al.* (1977); Armstrong and Chaffin (1978); An *et al.* (1979, 1983); Chao *et al.* (1989); Lee and Rim (1990); Casolo and Lorenzi (1994); Smutz *et al.* (1998); Wilson *et al.* (1999); Brand and Hollister (1999); Omokawa *et al.* (2000); Fowler *et al.* (2001)

models for estimating moment arm lengths from the known values of the joint angles are available; the models are developed for the lower extremity (Hoy *et al.* 1990; Hawkins 1992) and the upper extremity (Pigeon *et al.* 1996).

At some joint configurations, the moment arms assume their maximal and minimal values. At these joint angular positions, the same muscle tension produces maximal and minimal moments of force about the joint centre, respectively. In general, a joint moment $M(\alpha)$ produced by a muscle at different joint angles α equals the product:

$$M(\alpha) = F(\alpha)d(\alpha) \quad (4)$$

Hence, when a joint angle varies, the externally registered force (strength) changes due to two reasons: (i) the muscles produce different tension; and (ii) the muscle forces act through different moment arms (Fig. 23.18).

A joint position at which maximal strength (maximal joint moment) is exerted may be different from the position where the muscles exert maximal tension. The relationships between the muscular strength (externally manifested moment or force) and the contributing factors—muscle tensions and moment arms—may be quite complex. The relationships are dissimilar for various joints as well as for different movements at the same joint. For instance, at the wrist joint the moment-angle profile in flexion is determined mainly by the dependence of muscle tension from the muscle length while the torque profile in extension is strongly influenced by the changes in the moment arms (Fig. 23.19).

A planar action of the muscle force can be compared to a pulling or pushing a door handle in a horizontal direction. The door hinges are orientated vertically and the force is at 90° to the

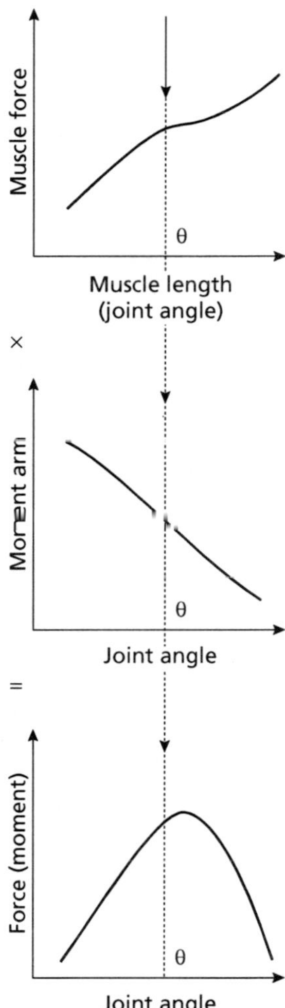

Fig. 23.18 Joint moment (strength) registered at joint angle θ is the product of muscle tension and muscle moment arm at this joint configuration, a schematic. (Reprinted from Zatsiorsky 1995.)

axis of rotation. Such a situation can be studied with the simple methods described previously (see eqn 4). A more complex situation would occur if the force to the handle were directed at a certain angle to the horizon. A three-dimensional analysis should be used. This is typical for the muscle action.

Many muscles produce moments about more than one joint axis. They have several functions. For instance, at the shoulder joint the short head of the biceps assists with flexion, adduction, inward rotation and horizontal flexion. At the elbow joint, the biceps flexes and supinates the forearm. The line of force action of such muscles is at an angle other than 90° to the axes of main anatomical movements at the joints (flexion/extension, abduction/adduction and internal/external rotation). In three dimensions, the moment arm of a muscle about a certain axis, e.g. flexion–extension, may depend not only on the configuration of the bones about this axis but also on the bones' position about other axes, e.g. the supination–pronation axis (Mansour & Pereira 1987; Murray *et al.* 1995; see also Klein *et al.* 1996).

Moments of force in the space are vectors. They have both magnitude and direction. In three dimensions, a moment of force can be determined about a point or about an axis. The moment of force $\mathbf{M}_O$ about a point O is defined as a cross-product of vectors **r** and **F**, where **r** is the position vector from O to the point of force application P (Fig. 23.20):

$$\mathbf{M}_O = \mathbf{r} \times \mathbf{F} \quad (5)$$

The moment $\mathbf{M}_O$ is a vector that possesses the following features.

1 The line of action of $\mathbf{M}_O$ is perpendicular to the plane containing vectors **r** and **F**. The line represents the axis about which the body tends to rotate at O when subjected to the force **F**.

2 The magnitude of moment is $\mathbf{M}_O = F(r \sin \theta) = Fd$, where θ is the angle between the vectors **r** and **F** and d is the shortest distance from O to the line of action of **F**, the *moment arm*. The moment arm is in the plane containing O and **F**. The magnitude of the moment of force does not depend upon the position of the point of force application along the line of force action. Only the moment arm is important. Hence, **r** is a vector from O to *any* point on the line of action of **F**.

3 The direction of the vector $\mathbf{M}_O$ is furnished by the right-hand rule in rotating from **r** to **F**: when the fingers curl in the direction of the induced rotation the vector is pointing in the direction of the thumb.

The expression 'rotation about a point O' really means 'rotation about an axis passing

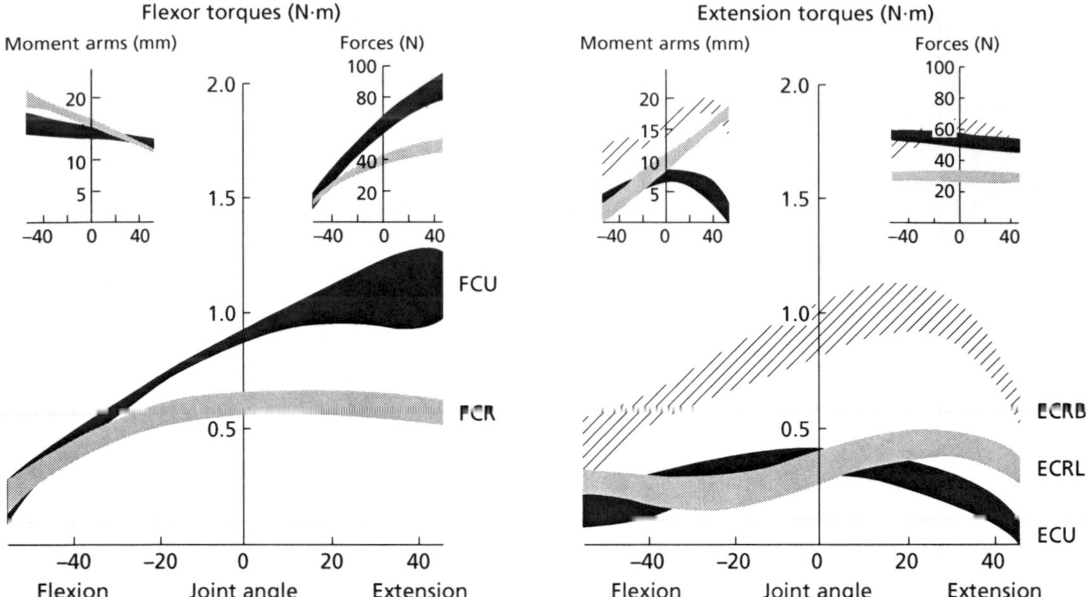

Fig. 23.19 Determinants of flexion torque (left panel) and extension torque (right panel) at the wrist joint. Torque profiles of muscle–tendon units are shown enlarged with moment arm–joint angle relations provided as insets. Note the considerable influence of muscle tension changes on the torque profiles in flexion and the large changes of the moment arms of wrist extensors. Abbreviations: ECBR, extensor carpi radialis brevis; ECRL, extensor carpi radialis longus; ECU, extensor carpi ulnaris; FCR, flexor carpi radialis; FCU, flexor carpi ulnaris. The data are for neutral forearm rotation. Shaded area represents mean ± 1 SD. (Reprinted by permission from Loren *et al*. 1996.)

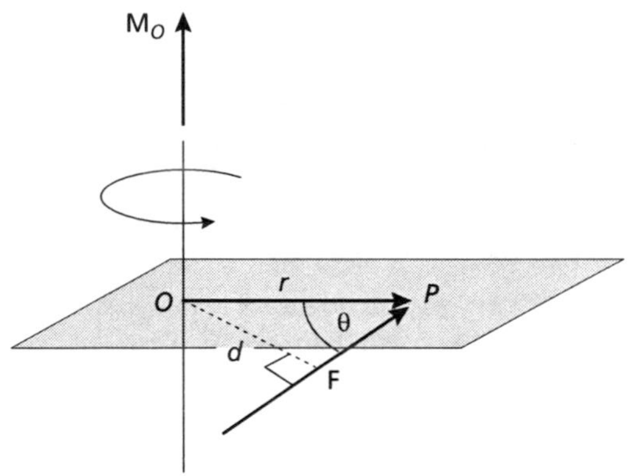

Fig. 23.20 Force **F** produces a moment of force $\mathbf{M}_O$ at a point O. See explanation in the text.

through O in a direction perpendicular to the plane containing O and the line of force action'. In two dimensions, the line of force action and the axis of rotation are always perpendicular to each other. In three directions, they may be at different angles.

The moment of force **F** about an axis is defined as a component of the moment along this axis. Consider again a force **F** acting on a rigid body (Fig. 23.21). The force exerts a moment $\mathbf{M}_B = \mathbf{r} \times \mathbf{F}$ about a point B where **r** is a position vector from B to A (the point of force application). Let O–O be an axis through B and $\boldsymbol{U}_{OO}$ be the unit vector along O–O. Then, the moment of force **F** about the axis O–O $\mathbf{M}_{OO}$ is defined as a component (or projection) of the moment $\mathbf{M}_B$ along this axis. The magnitude of the moment $\mathbf{M}_{OO}$ equals the dot product of the vectors $\boldsymbol{U}_{OO}$ and $\mathbf{M}_B$:

$$\mathbf{M}_{OO} = \mathbf{U}_{OO} \cdot \mathbf{M}_B \, \mathbf{U}_{OO} \cdot (\mathbf{r} \times \mathbf{F}) \quad (6)$$

Eqn 6 represents the so-called *mixed triple product of vectors*. Hence, the moment of force about an axis is a mixed triple product of three vectors: the unit vector along the axis of rotation, the position

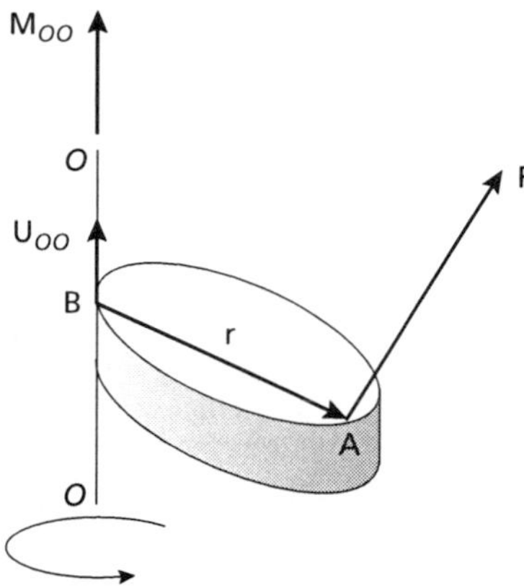

Fig. 23.21 Moment of force **F** about an axis O–O. See explanation in the text.

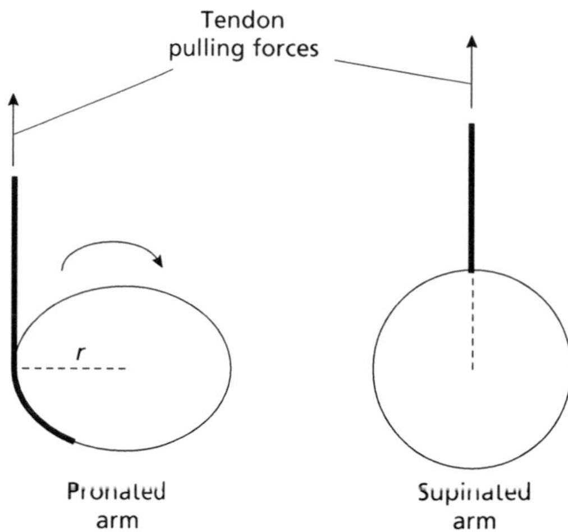

Fig. 23.22 Proximal view of the right arm, a schematic. For a fully pronated arm, the biceps acts as a supinator; it also produces a flexion moment (secondary moment). When the arm is supinated the biceps acts as a pure flexor.

vector from an arbitrary point on the axis to any point on the line of force action, and the force vector.

While the definition of the moment of force in three dimensions is mathematically involved, the consequences of the three-dimensional arrangement of muscles in the body are straightforward. We briefly discuss two effects that are important for practitioners.

Firstly, muscles produce not only moments of force in the desired direction (*primary moments*) but also moments in other directions (*secondary moments*—Mansour & Pereira 1987; Li *et al.* 1998a,b). To counterbalance the secondary moments, which are not necessary for the intended purpose, additional muscles are activated. The number of active muscles increases but the strength may decrease. Consider, for example, a forceful arm supination with the elbow flexed at a right angle, as in driving a screw with a screwdriver. During the supination effort, the triceps, even though it is not a supinator, is also active. A simple demonstration —and one suitable for class purposes—proves this: perform an attempted forceful supination against a resistance while placing the second hand on the biceps and triceps of the working arm. Both the biceps and the triceps spring into action simultaneously. The explanation is simple: when the biceps acts as a supinator, it also produces a flexion moment (secondary moment), Fig. 23.22. The flexion moment is counterbalanced by the extension moment exerted by the triceps.

When performing elbow flexion, pronation of the forearm decreases the strength of the elbow curl (Rasch 1956; Jørgensen & Bankov 1971). For instance, in the second study the following strength values have been observed (26 male subjects, elbow angle 90°): with the forearm in a supinated position 43.2 ± 8.4 lb, midposition 47.8 ± 8.9 lb, pronation 27.5 ± 4.4 lb. With the arm pronated, the biceps cannot generate its maximal tension because of the possible supination effect. Due to this anatomical fact, it is simpler to perform chin-ups on a high bar using an undergrasp than an overgrasp.

Secondly, athletes tend to perform forceful movements in such a way as to minimize secondary moments. For instance, when pull-ups are performed on gymnastic rings, the performers always supinate the arms while flexing the elbow joints. Nobody teaches them to do that. This movement pattern is simply more convenient for the performers. In throwing, athletes tend to

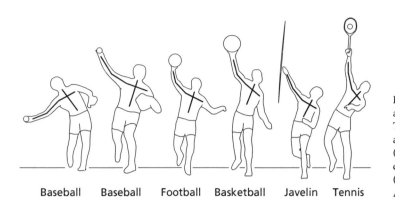

Fig. 23.23 Position of the athletes at the instant of release or hitting. To exert maximal forces, the athletes keep the upper arm (almost) collinear with the line connecting the shoulder centres. (Reprinted by permission from Atwater 1979.)

move the arm in parallel with the shoulder line (Fig. 23.23). When maximal efforts are required, the throwers prefer bending the trunk rather than lifting the arm above the shoulder.

Some muscles have large attachment sites; individual bundles of such muscles may have different moment arms with respect to different axes of rotation. For instance, 200 individual bundles have been counted in the muscles of the shoulder (Van der Helm & Veenbaas 1991). Mechanical analysis of their action is a complicated task.

In summary, selection of a proper body position affects the joint torque production.

From joint moments to muscle strength (endpoint force)

This section addresses a relation between joint moments/torques and forces exerted at an end effector (*muscle strength*). In a single-joint task, the transformation is described by eqn 5. The magnitude of the strength (the force exerted at the end effector) equals the ratio *joint moment/moment arm of the external force*. In multilink chains the transformation of the joint moments into the endpoint force is more complex. The analysis is straightforward but, unfortunately, not trivial. It is based on the matrix algebra.

Consider an open kinematic chain such as an arm or leg. An isometric force **F** is exerted at the end effector. The joints are assumed frictionless. Gravity is neglected. The following theorem is valid (for a proof and detailed discussion see Zatsiorsky 2002):

$$\mathbf{T} = \mathbf{J}^T\mathbf{F} \tag{7a}$$

where **T** is the vector of the joint torques ($\mathbf{T} = T_1, T_2 \ldots T_n)^T$ and $\mathbf{J}^T$ is the transpose of the Jacobian matrix that relates infinitesimal joint displacement $d\boldsymbol{\alpha}$ to infinitesimal end-effector displacement $d\mathbf{P}$. The Jacobian is a $6 \times n$ matrix, where n is the number of joints (in a planar case) or the kinematic degrees of freedom (in a three-dimensional case). The Jacobians are explained in Zatsiorsky (1998). According to eqn 7a the equilibrating joint torques in a given chain configuration are uniquely defined by the external force. If the magnitude and direction of the endpoint force are constant, the torques in all the joints are fixed. The endpoint force depends on the joint torques in the following manner:

$$\mathbf{F} = (\mathbf{J}^T)^{-1}\mathbf{T} \tag{7b}$$

where $(\mathbf{J}^T)^{-1}$ is the inverse of the transverse Jacobian matrix. The equation is valid when the chain is a non-singular configuration, i.e. if it is not completely extended or flexed.

Eqns 7a and 7b provide a convenient tool for establishing a relation between the joint moments and the endpoint force exerted or resisted by an athlete (muscle strength). The equation is universal; it can be used for studying complex three-dimensional multijoint movements. We limit our discussion to simple planar cases.

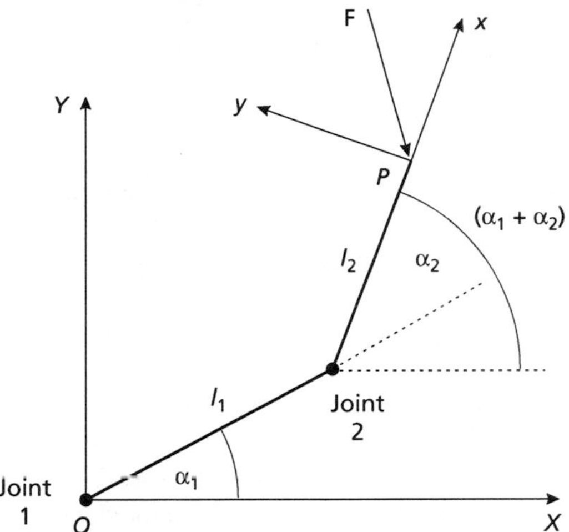

Fig. 23.24 A planar two-link chain. Force **F** is exerted at the endpoint **P**. The task is to establish a relationship between **F** and the torques at joints 1 and 2. Length of the segments 1 and 2 is l_1 and l_2, respectively. The global system of coordinates is *O-XY* and the local system of coordinates at the endpoint is *P-xy*.

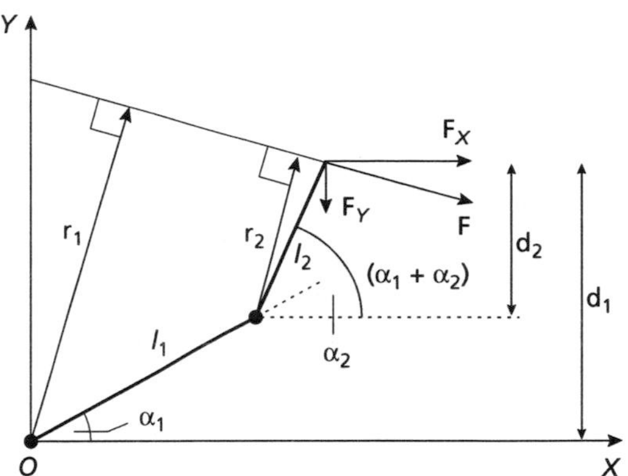

Fig. 23.25 The correspondence between the moment arms of the external force **F** and the rows of the transpose Jacobian. The equivalent joint torques $\mathbf{T}_1$ and $\mathbf{T}_2$ to the external force **F** have the magnitude $T_1 = Fr_1$ and $T_2 = Fr_2$ where r_1 and r_2 are the perpendicular distance from the corresponding joint to the line of **F**. When the equations are written in scalar form, in the projections on the axes of the system of coordinates, they can be conveniently represented by using the transposed Jacobian of the chain. (Adapted by permission from Zatsiorsky 2002.)

END FORCE–JOINT TORQUE RELATIONS FOR SIMPLE KINEMATIC CHAINS

Consider a two-link chain presented in Fig. 23.24. If the vector **F** is expressed in the global system *O-XY*, with respect to the environment, eqn 7 can be applied immediately.

The chain Jacobian (equation 3.16 in Zatsiorsky 1998) is:

$$\mathbf{J} = \begin{bmatrix} -l_1S_1 - l_2S_{12} & -l_2S_{12} \\ l_1C_1 + l_2C_{12} & l_2C_{12} \end{bmatrix} \tag{8}$$

where the subscripts 1 and 2 refer to the angles α_1 and α_2, correspondingly, and the subscript 12 refers to the sum of the two angles $(\alpha_1 + \alpha_2)$. *S* and *C* stand for the sine and cosine, respectively. Transposing the Jacobian and applying eqn 7, we have:

$$\begin{bmatrix} T_1 \\ T_2 \end{bmatrix} = \begin{bmatrix} -l_1S_1 - l_2S_{12} & l_1C_1 + l_2C_{12} \\ -l_2S_{12} & l_2C_{12} \end{bmatrix} \begin{bmatrix} F_X \\ F_Y \end{bmatrix} \tag{9}$$

The elements of the transposed Jacobian represent the moment arms of the external force **F** with respect to the individual joints 1 and 2 when the external force is written in projections on the *X* and *Y* axes (Fig. 23.25). For instance, the horizontal component of the external force F_X exerts a moment about joint 2 that equals $-M_2 = F_Xd_2$, where the moment arm $d_2 = -l_2S_{12}$. The moment is negative, in the clockwise direction. The moment of F_X about joint 1 is $-M_2 = F_Xd_1$, where $d_1 = -(l_1S_1 + l_2S_{12})$. Hence, the joint torque in joint 1 is:

$$T_1 = -(l_1S_1 + l_2S_{12})F_X + (l_1C_1 + l_2C_{12})F_Y \tag{10}$$

If the joint torques T_1 and T_2 are known, the external force can be calculated by inverting the transposed Jacobian matrix, $\mathbf{J}^T$. For a planar two-link chain, the inverse exists in all joint configurations except for singular ones. (The singular chain configurations are explained in Zatsiorsky 1998, section 3.1.1.1.4.) The inverse of the transposed Jacobian is:

$$(\mathbf{J}^T)^{-1} = \frac{1}{l_1l_2S_2} \begin{bmatrix} l_2C_{12} & -l_1C_1 - l_2C_{12} \\ l_2S_{12} & -l_1S_1 - l_2S_{12} \end{bmatrix} \tag{11}$$

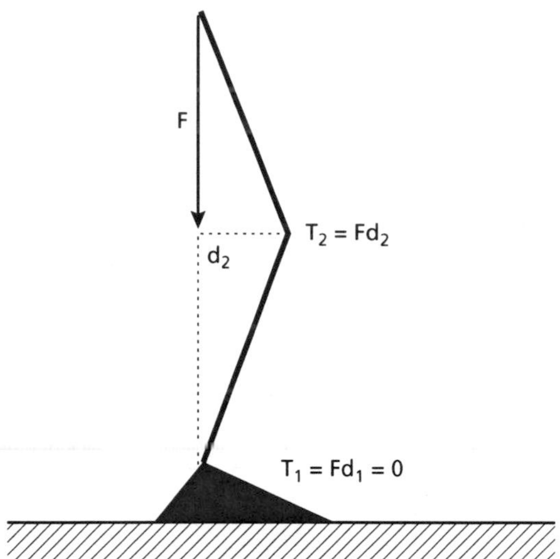

Fig. 23.26 The closer the leg to full extension the smaller the knee joint moment required to bear the force **F**. This explains why the heaviest loads can be borne when the legs are (almost) completely extended. When the line of force action passes through the joint centre, the equivalent joint moment is zero. When the leg/arm is nearly outstretched, large external forces can be exerted with low joint moments. Compare with Fig. 23.9. (Reprinted by permission from Zatsiorsky 2002.)

Singular joint configurations are observed when α_2 equals either zero or π. In this case $S_2 = 0$ and eqn 11 cannot be solved. If a two-link chain represents an arm or a leg, the singular position corresponds to complete arm/leg extension when the included elbow/knee angle is 180° (complete flexion is impossible for human body links). At a singular joint configuration, the distal segment is an extension of the proximal body segment. At this particular joint posture, the force component that is acting along the distal link does not influence the joint torques; its line of force action intersects the joint axes of rotation. The external load is taken by the skeleton.

When the chain, e.g. the leg, approaches a singular joint configuration—a complete extension—the chain can bear large forces in the direction of the extension from the endpoint to the proximal joint (Fig. 23.26). However at this chain configuration, the transfer of joint angular velocity into the velocity of the leg extension is minimal (see Zatsiorsky 1998, section 3.1.1.1.7).

Control of external contact forces

To move, people exert forces on the ground. To manipulate objects, people exert forces on them. In all cases, the force magnitude and direction should correspond to the requirement of the motor task. This section concentrates on the problems associated with the exertion of an intended contact force on the environment. In general, the external contact force may be generated in two ways, dynamically and/or statically. Dynamic force exertion involves accelerated movement of the body parts that may be located far away from the point of force application. For instance, if a person standing in an upright posture with the legs extended performs a fast arm swing or trunk flexion, the ground reaction force (GRF) changes. In this case, the legs serve as force transmitters. They do not generate the force; they just transmit it. Force transmission is seen in many movements, especially in those where the body passes quickly over the supporting leg giving only a short time for the leg flexion and extension, e.g. during the take-off in long jumps. In this case, the direction and magnitude of the GRF are highly influenced by the acceleration of the body parts other than the grounded leg, for instance by the swinging motion of the arms and the free leg. The supporting leg resists a thrust from the upper parts of the body and transmits it to the ground. It also exerts a force and a moment on the torso that results in the acceleration of the entire upper body. In static conditions, the situation is simpler. At a given joint configuration, the external contact force is controlled by the joint torques of the involved body limb, the arm or leg. We will limit the discussion to the simple kinematic chains.

Two-link chains

Consider a planar two-link chain in a non-singular configuration (Fig. 23.27). The axis X of the global system of coordinates is along link l. The endpoint force **F** is characterized by its

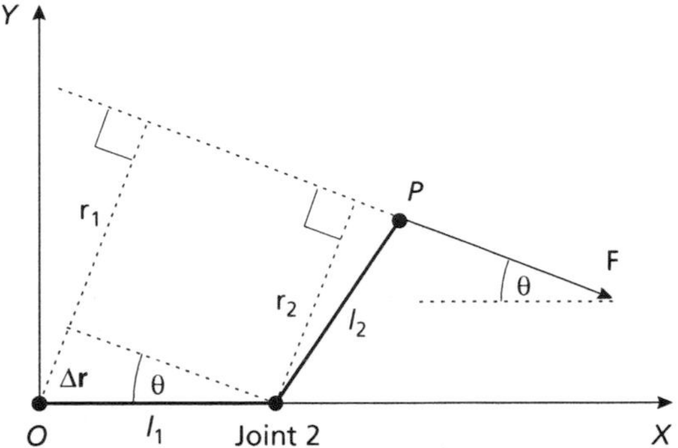

Fig. 23.27 The direction of the endpoint force as a function of the difference in the moment arms r_1 and r_2. For convenience, the coordinate X-axis is along the first link. See explanation in the text.

magnitude and direction. The magnitude is $F = T_1/r_1$ or $F = T_2/r_2$. Consequently, for a given joint configuration and a given force direction (r_1 and r_2 are constant) the magnitude of the endpoint force is determined by the joint torques T_1 and T_2. Note that in order to produce a larger (smaller) endpoint force in the same direction the joint torques must change proportionally. For instance, to exert a $2F$ force the joint torques must be $2T_1$ and $2T_2$. Hence, to alter the magnitude of the external force the central nervous system (CNS) should change the level of muscle activation in all the involved joints proportionally (metaphorically speaking, the CNS should 'multiply the muscle activity level by the same coefficient').

To characterize the force direction, consider the difference $\Delta T = T_1 - T_2$:

$$\Delta T = Fr_1 - Fr_2 = F(r_1 - r_2) = F\Delta r \tag{12}$$

where $\Delta r = (r_1 - r_2)$. From Fig. 23.27 it follows that $\Delta r = l_1 \sin\theta$, where θ is the angle of the line of force with the X axis. Therefore, the direction of the endpoint force is characterized by the trigonometric function:

$$\sin\theta = \frac{1}{Fl_1}(T_1 - T_2) \tag{13}$$

According to eqn 13, for an endpoint force of a constant magnitude F, the force direction is controlled by the difference in the joint torques. An example of exerting force of a given magnitude in different directions is presented in Fig. 23.28.

It is convenient to analyse the relationship between the endpoint force and the joint torques in a polar system of coordinates. For a two-link model of the human arm, the following angles with respect to the axis X are defined: (i) the *polar angle* θ for the axis connecting the shoulder S with the endpoint, the *radial axis*; and (ii) the *pointing angle* ϕ for the line drawn from the elbow E along the forearm, the *pointing axis* (Fig. 23.29).

The radial and pointing axes define four sectors marked in Fig. 23.29. The flexion at the shoulder joint and extension at the elbow joint produce an endpoint force exerted in sector 1. This effort corresponds to *arm* extension. In sector 2, the endpoint force is due to flexion in the two involved joints. In sector 3 the force is due to S extension and E flexion, and in sector 4 the endpoint force is a result of combined extension torques in the shoulder and elbow joints.

For the leg, contrary to the arm, the hip and the knee flexion (extension) correspond to opposite angular directions, i.e. if the flexion at the hip joint is defined in a clockwise direction it is counterclockwise for the knee. Therefore, a force exertion in sector 1, which is typical for take-offs, corresponds to simultaneous hip and knee extension. The reader is invited to find the hip/knee flexion/extension correspondence in sectors 2–4.

The endpoint force may be resolved into two contributing force components that are due to individual joint torques. Such decomposition allows for the determination of the relative contribution of each joint torque to the endpoint force. To find the contributing forces consider cases when the line of force action is either along the radial or along the pointing axis. When the endpoint force is exerted along the radial axis, the torque at the proximal joint equals zero (see Fig. 23.29). In the distal joint, the torque is zero when the endpoint force is exerted along the pointing axis. In both cases, the line of force action crosses the joint centre and the corresponding moment arm is zero. Thus, in the

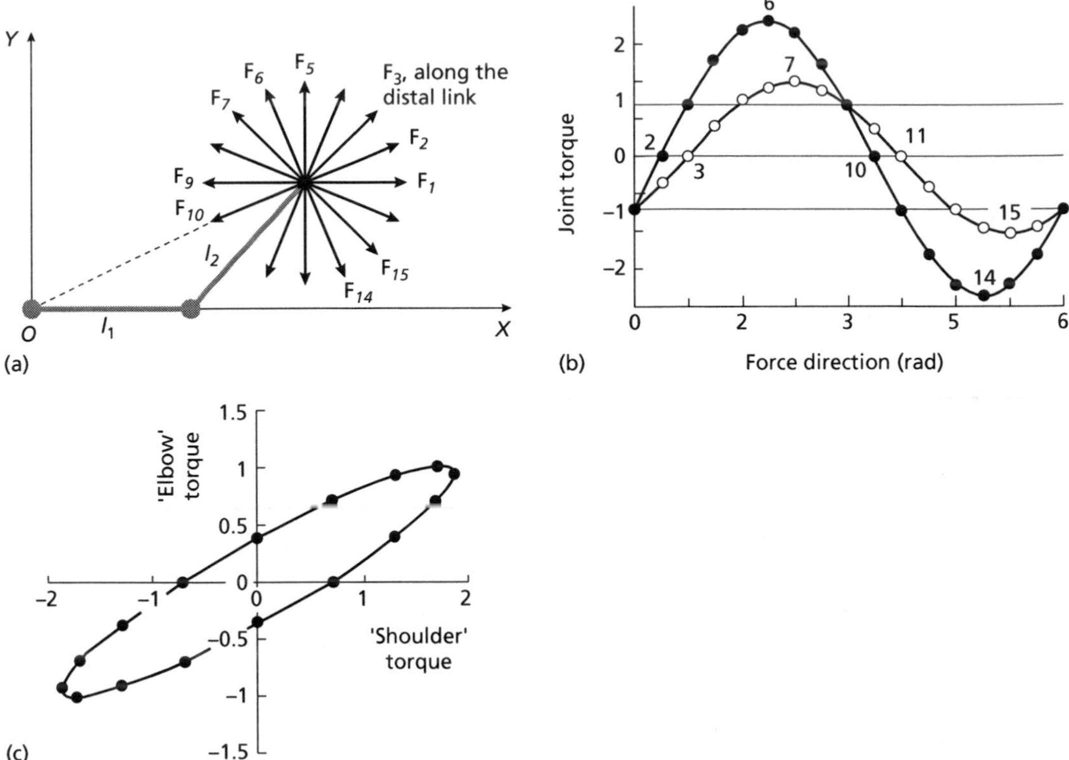

Fig. 23.28 The joint torques that generate an endpoint force of the same magnitude in various directions. (a) A two-link planar chain. The axis X of the global reference system is along the proximal link. An endpoint exerts a force with a magnitude of 1 on the environment in 16 various directions. The angular distance between the neighbouring forces is 22.5°. The forces are numbered in a counterclockwise sequence. The forces are due to the torques T_1 and T_2 acting at joints 1 and 2, respectively. The link lengths, l_1 and l_2, equal 1. Joint angle α_2 is 45°. Force F_{11} is along the distal link, opposite to force $\mathbf{F}_3$, and is not shown. (b) Joint torques that produce an endpoint force of unit magnitude in various directions. The numbers in the graph correspond to the force directions shown in (a). Black rectangles represent the torques at joint 1 ('shoulder') and crosses represent the torques at joint 2 ('elbow'). The joint torques are maximal when the force direction is perpendicular to the corresponding moment arms: for the proximal joint in directions 6 and 14, and for the distal joint in directions 7 and 15. The joint torques are zero when the line of force action passes through the joint centre. In particular, the torque at the proximal joint is zero when the endpoint force is exerted in directions 2 or 10, and the torque at the distal joint is zero when the endpoint force is in directions 3 or 11. (c) Torque vs. torque values for the different directions of the endpoint force of unit magnitude. (Panels a and b reprinted by permission from Zatsiorsky 2002.)

described conditions the endpoint force is due to the activity in solely one joint. It can be said that the distal joint produces the endpoint force along the radial axis and the proximal joint produces the endpoint force along the pointing axis.

For a purpose of illustration, consider a simple model of a static force exertion in leg extension presented in Fig. 23.30. The weight of the legs as well as the ankle joint torque is neglected. The hip joint axis does not displace. In the model, the force on the ground is exerted by the combined hip and knee extension torques. The force that is due to knee torque F_K acts along the axis from the hip H to the ankle joint A (Fig. 23.30a). Hip joint extension generates force F_H along the shank (Fig. 23.30b). The resultant force exerted on the ground is the vector sum of these two force components (Fig. 23.30c). Note that extension at the

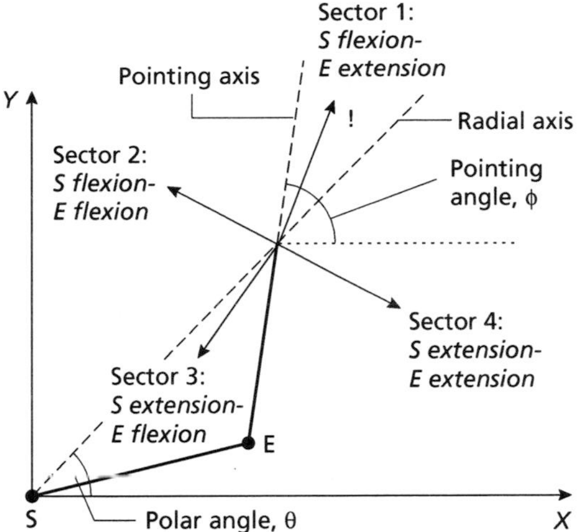

Fig. 23.29 The polar and pointing angles of a two-link arm and the sectors that define the shoulder (S) and elbow (E) flexion or extension. Flexion is a counterclockwise rotation and extension is a clockwise rotation of the corresponding link. (Reprinted by permission from Zatsiorsky 2002.)

knee can be prevented by a cord linking H and A, and the hip extension can be prevented by a cord along the line KB. The cords would behave as struts and maintain a constant direction.

From the foregoing discussion, it follows that when force is generated along the shank ('in the pointing direction'), we should expect a zero or minimal activity of the muscles serving the knee joint. Similarly, when the force is exerted in the radial direction the activity of the muscles serving the hip joint is expected to be close to zero. The largest torques are required when force vector is perpendicular to the radius from the joint to the point of force application.

Three-link chains

For a three-link chain, the force exerted on the environment by a performer can be resolved into the components associated with the individual joint torques. Consider a planar three-link chain in a non-singular configuration (Fig. 23.31). An external force is exerted on the end link of the chain at a point P. It is not necessary for P to be at the endpoint of the distal link (unlike ballet dancers, who can stand on their toes, most people stand on the entire plantar surface of the foot). To find the contributing forces, we introduce lines passing through the joint centres, L_{23}, L_{13}, and L_{12}, where the subscripts refer to the corresponding joint centres. The following rule exists: individually applied joint torques, T_1, T_2 and T_3, cause the end effector to apply forces to the environment along the lines L_{23}, L_{13}, and L_{12}, respectively.

The three-link systems allow not only for exerting push–pull forces on the environment but also for producing rotation effects. In particular, both a force and a force couple (free moment) can be exerted on working tools. In the absence of sticking, the moment (couple) exerted on the environment is manifested as a displacement of a point of application of the resultant force along the end link of the chain (Fig. 23.32).

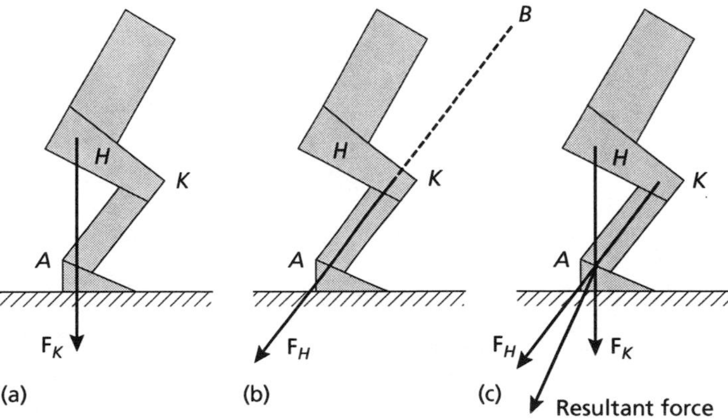

Fig. 23.30 Resultant force exerted on the ground is a sum of the force components that are due to the torques at the hip and knee joints. In this example, the ankle joint torque is zero. The force vectors are scaled to the figure. (Reprinted by permission from Zatsiorsky 2002.)

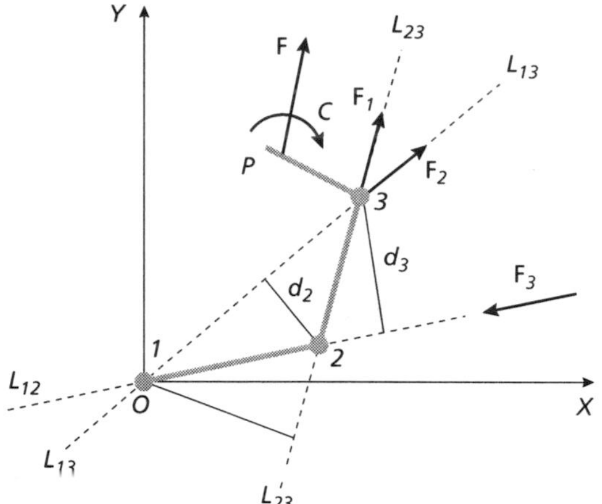

Fig. 23.31 Joint torque–endpoint force analysis of a planar three-link chain. The torques at joints 1, 2 and 3 contribute to the end-effector force **F**. The torque T_1 acting at joint 1 develops a contributing force $\mathbf{F}_1$ along the line L_{23}. The magnitude of F_1 is equal to the ratio T_1/d_1 where d_1 is the moment arm. The magnitudes of the contributing forces from the other joints can be computed in a similar way as the quotients $F_2 = T_2/d_2$ and $F_3 = T_3/d_3$. These forces are acting along the lines L_{13} and L_{12}, correspondingly. Forces $\mathbf{F}_1$ and $\mathbf{F}_2$ are shown with their tails at joint 3. Force F_3 is shown along the line of its action. A couple (free moment) C represented in the figure by a curved arrow is also exerted on the environment. (Reprinted by permission from Zatsiorsky 2002.)

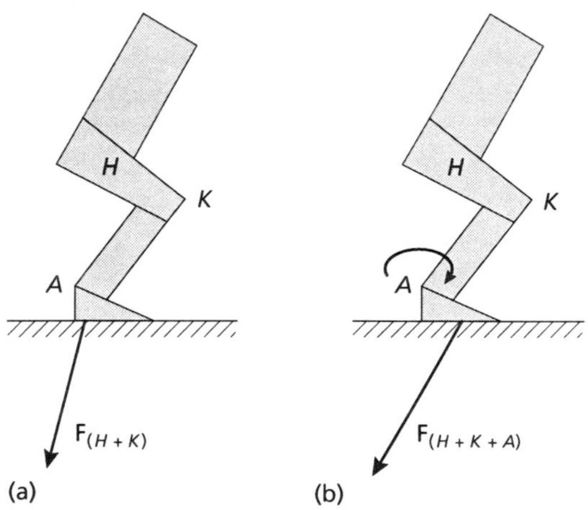

Fig. 23.32 Exertion of a force on the ground. (a) The force is exerted by the hip and knee torques. The ankle torque is zero. (b) The force is exerted by the hip, knee and ankle torques. Note the displacement of the point of force application.

In summary, control of a multijoint chain is different from that of a single-joint system. In the single-joint case, the endpoint force is proportional to the joint torque. In the multilink chains, the endpoint force depends on both torque magnitudes and chain configuration. The same joint torques at variable body postures would generate different endpoint forces at different directions.

Exerting force in various directions: force ellipsoids

The endpoint force depends on the joint torques and the chain configuration. To separate these factors, it is convenient to analyse endpoint forces produced by the joint torques of the constant magnitude. A set of a joint torques $T_1, T_2 \ldots T_n$ can be viewed as a vector $\mathbf{T} = [T_1, T_2 \ldots T_n]$. The magnitude of a vector is described by its *norm*. For a vector $\mathbf{T}$ the norm is $\sqrt{T_1^2 + T_2^2 + \ldots + T_n^2}$, where $T_1, T_2 \ldots T_n$ are the magnitudes of the torque in the individual joints (vector components). Consider a case when the norm of the vector $\mathbf{T}$ is constant and is equal to 1. The following equation is valid (for the proof and the detailed discussion see Zatsiorsky 2002):

$$\mathbf{F}^T\mathbf{J}\mathbf{J}^T\mathbf{F} = 1 \qquad (14)$$

In the planar case, the equation represents an ellipse. In three dimensions, eqn 14 represents a three-dimensional ellipsoid with the principal axes along the eigenvectors of the matrix $\mathbf{J}\mathbf{J}^T$. The length of a principal axis i is given by $1/\sqrt{\lambda_i}$ where λ_i is an eigenvalue associated with eigenvector i. The largest eigenvalue corresponds to the minor axis of the ellipsoid and the smallest value to the major axis (Fig. 23.33). When the magnitude of the total torque vector is constant, maximal force can be exerted along the major axis. Therefore, efforts are most effective when they are directed along this axis: a unit torque is converted into the largest endpoint force. The minor axis indicates the direction in which the endpoint force is minimal.

Because eqn 14 includes the Jacobian, the shape and orientation of the force ellipsoid depends

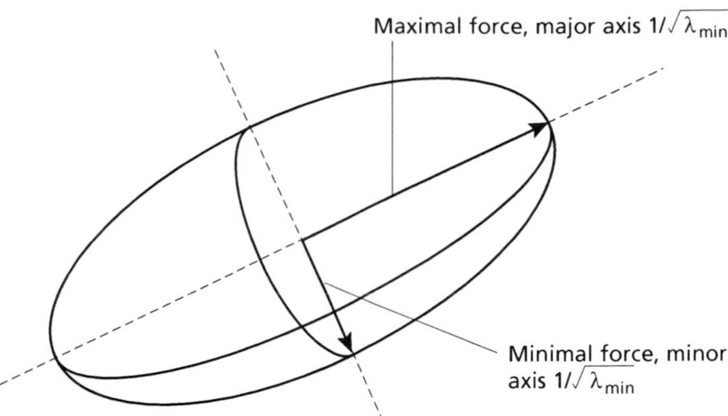

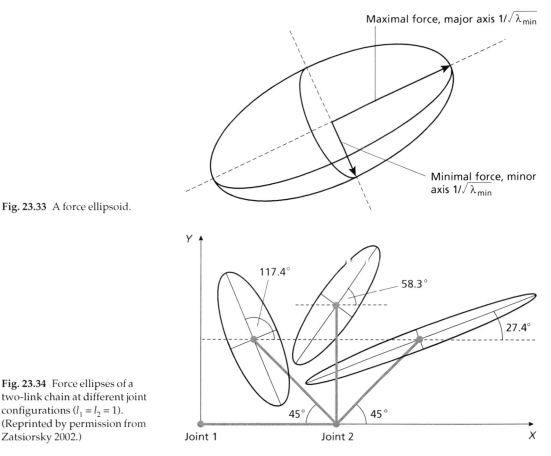

Fig. 23.33 A force ellipsoid.

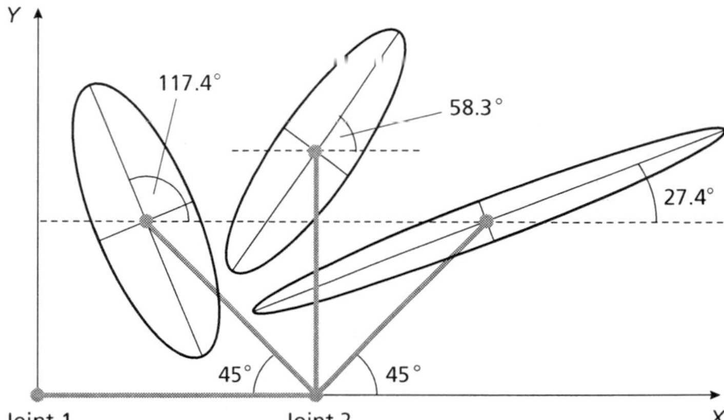

Fig. 23.34 Force ellipses of a two-link chain at different joint configurations ($l_1 = l_2 = 1$). (Reprinted by permission from Zatsiorsky 2002.)

on the chain configuration. As the end effector moves from one location to another, the force ellipsoid also changes accordingly. Figure 23.34 illustrates the force ellipses for a two-link chain with $l_1 = l_2 = 1$ at different joint configurations.

The force ellipsoids in the above discussion were computed under an assumption that the magnitude of the vector of the joint torques is constant. In real life, the magnitude may depend on the force direction and actual forces exerted in various directions may deviate from an ellipse. However, the available evidence suggests that this deviation is relatively small (Fig. 23.35).

Effects of geometric constraints

Geometric, or *holonomic*, constraints restrict movement in certain directions. Examples include opening a door, pushing a bobsled, pedalling on a bicycle and exercising on strength exercise machines. When the end effector is constrained, the performer may exert force in a direction different from the direction of motion and still perform the task. The actual constraints—the tangible physical obstacles to movement—may completely change joint torques. Consequently, different muscle groups may act when body motion is free or is actually (physically) constrained. In particular, when working on strength exercise machines, the direction of the endpoint force and the joint torques may be quite distinct from what is observed in lifting or holding free weights.

When performers in addition to exerting force on an object stabilize it in space, the force production drops. For instance, in one of the

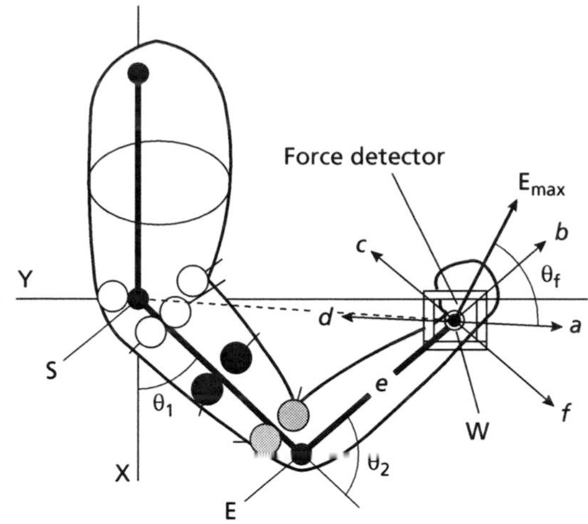

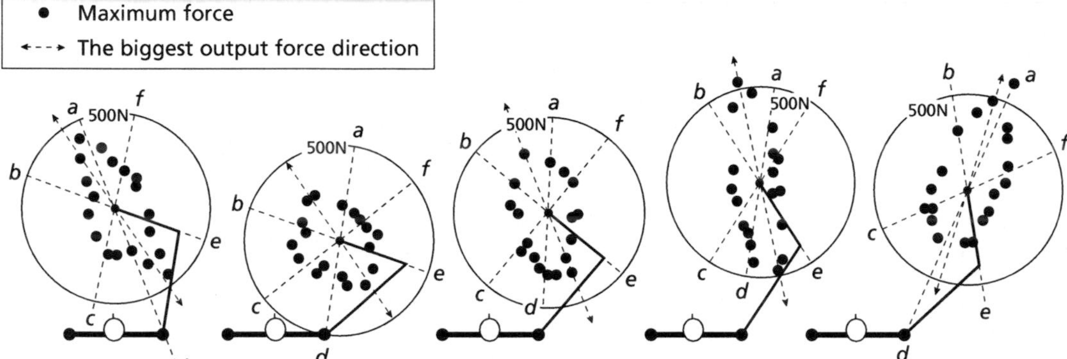

Fig. 23.35 Distribution of the maximal endpoint forces. Upper panel, subject position and the measuring device. S, E and H stand for the shoulder, elbow and wrist, respectively. Line *a–d* is along the radius to the shoulder, line *b–e* is along the pointing axis, and line *c–f* is perpendicular to the forearm. White, black and grey circles designate the electrode placement (the EMG data are not described here). Bottom panel, distribution of the maximal force at the different arm configurations. a: $\theta_1 = 80°$, $\theta_2 = 80°$; b: $\theta_1 = 37°$, $\theta_2 = 120°$; c: $\theta_1 = 50°$, $\theta_2 = 90°$; d: $\theta_1 = 60°$, $\theta_2 = 60°$; e: $\theta_1 = 42°$, $\theta_2 = 57°$. The force envelopes resemble ellipses (the authors, who developed a model with six muscles, suggest that the envelopes are hexagons). (Adapted by permission from Fujikawa *et al.* 1997.)

experiments the subjects pushed maximally a handle that was either fixed or free to rotate with respect to one or two axes (Bober *et al.* 1982). When the handle was not fixed, the peak force was on average equal to 76% of the force exerted against the stationary handle. The percentage did not change after special training and did not depend on athletic mastership (athletes including World Champions in various sports were compared with students not practising sports). The force loss was a price all the subjects paid to stabilize the arm and the handle.

Preferred directions for the exertion of endpoint forces

As previously mentioned, when people exert forces on objects with geometric constraints, the exerted forces may not be exactly in the direction of the desired movement. For instance, during pedalling on a bicycle, even professional athletes wearing toe-clips do not exert force perpendicularly to the crank throughout the complete circular cycle. In some leg positions, large force components are exerted along the crank thus tending to compress or extend it (Fig. 23.36). Mechanically, these force components are losses; they do not produce useful effect. Formally, the effectiveness of force action may be computed as a projection of the force on the direction of movement. However, such a measure may be misleading. The following example illustrates the problem. Assume that one is asked to push horizontally a cart whose handlebar is located very low, at the knee level. One has two choices, either to push the handlebar strictly forward or to push it in the oblique direction, forward and down. In the first case, there will be no force loss due to pushing in an incorrect direction but the body posture will be awkward and the exerted force will not be very large. With the second technique, the vertical component of force will be lost to friction and cart deformation. However, the generated force will be larger. A similar question arises in bobsledding. After the start, the athletes push the bob. What is the optimal angle of the push?

In some cases the maximal force in a desired direction may be achieved by directing force efforts in another direction. The projection of the exerted force on the desired direction may exceed the force intentionally exerted in this direction (Fig. 23.37). This conclusion follows from the analysis of the force ellipsoids.

When large efforts are required people are prone to exert forces in the direction of larger force production (along the major axis of the force ellipsoid), rather than in the 'useful' direction. For instance, wheelchair users do not typically exert forces tangentially to the hand rims. They tend to extend the arm, thus compressing the rims (Fig. 23.38).

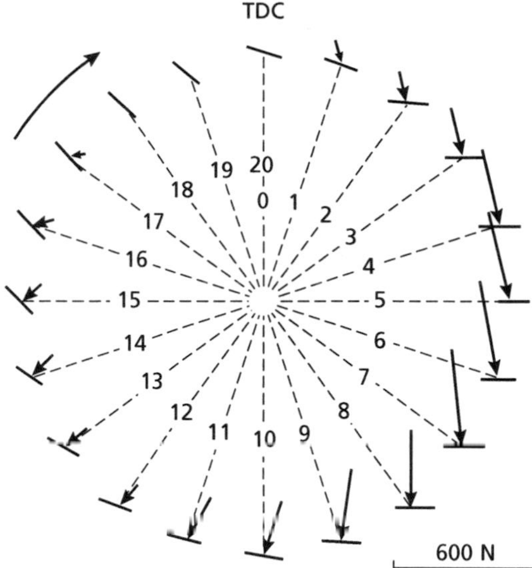

Fig. 23.36 Forces applied to a pedal during bicycling. Average data for elite pursuit riders at 100 r.p.m. and 400 W. The orientation of the pedal and the resultant force vector are shown at 20 positions of the crank. The force acting on the crank can be decomposed into tangential and normal components. Positive tangential force advances the crank and positive normal force is directed toward the crank centre. Mechanically, the normal force can be considered a loss. In position 4, the force is perpendicular to the crank and is close to being 100% effective. At the bottom dead centre, a large force exists, but—as one can see from its orientation—it is not very effective. In positions 11 to 17, a force still pushes down on the pedals and, hence, produces a countertorque opposing forward movement. (Reprinted by permission from Cavanagh *et al.* 1986.)

Exertion of maximal force: limiting joints

According to eqn 7, when a subject exerts a static force on the environment and the body posture and force direction do not change, the torques in the involved joints are defined in a unique way. Any increase in the endpoint force requires simultaneous proportional increase of all the joint torques.

During maximal force exertion, the torques in some joints reach their maximal value (for the given body posture) while other joints are taxed only submaximally. The endpoint force cannot be increased further because of the insufficient torque in one (or two or three) of several joints involved in the task. Such joints are known as *limiting joints* (for a given performer, in a given task and for a given body posture). Limiting

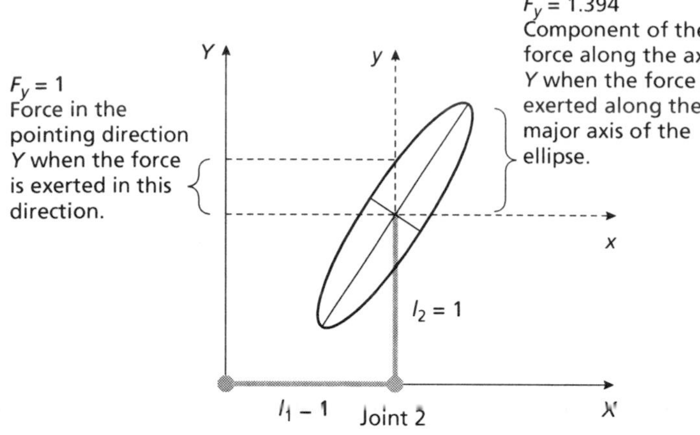

Fig. 23.37 Force intentionally exerted in a given direction *Y* may be smaller than the component along *Y* of the force exerted in a more beneficial direction.

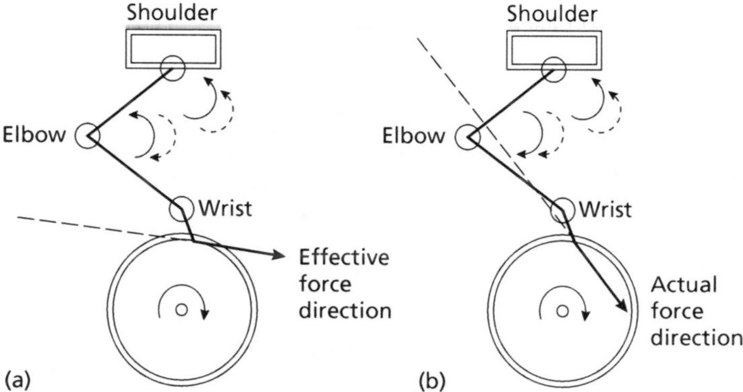

Fig. 23.38 The tangential force direction (a) and the actual force direction in wheelchair users (b). The solid lines indicate the joint torques at the shoulder and elbow. The dashed lines indicate the rotation direction at those joints. (Reprinted by permission from van der Woude *et al.* 2000.)

joints can differ in various athletes. For example, two athletes who are able to lift from the floor a 100-kg barbell and cannot lift 105 kg may have different limiting joints (e.g. knee extension in one athlete and spine extension in the second). Evidently, these athletes should be trained in a different way.

Some strength coaches believe that the value of maximal joint torque depends on whether the joint *generates* the torque or *transmits* it. A popular opinion among practitioners is that the joint can transmit a larger torque that it can generate. This issue is not a purely mechanical one and eqn 7 cannot solve it. The problem should be resolved by experiments. At this time, experimental evidence is not sufficient to make a decisive conclusion. Available scientific evidence speaks against the hypothesis: it seems that the maximal values of joint torque do not depend on whether the joint generates or transmits the torque (Fig. 23.39).

Body posture and strength training

If the body posture is changed, muscle activity can vary substantially. It is quite common in sport practice that coaches and athletes assume that they train a certain muscle group, e.g. the knee extensors, but in reality this muscle group is not loaded and, consequently, not trained. It is even possible that the antagonistic muscles, e.g. the knee flexors instead of the extensors, are mainly loaded (Fig. 23.40).

Effects of strength training are posture specific (Gardner 1963; Zatsiorsky & Raitsin 1974; Wilson *et al.* 1996). They depend on the range of joint

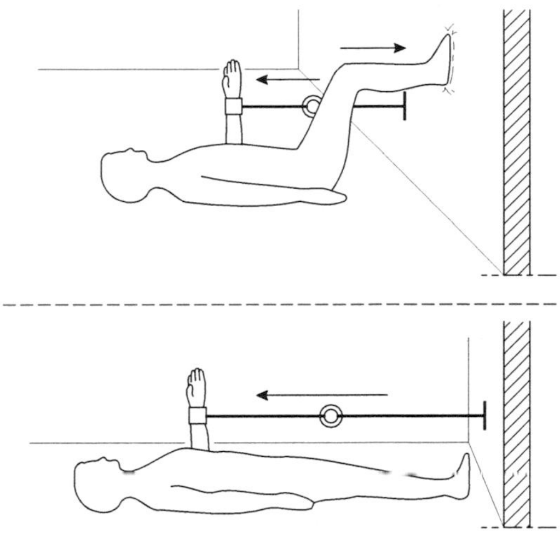

Fig. 23.39 Measurement of elbow flexion strength when supine. During the experiments, the elbow joint acted either as a force transmitter (upper panel) or as a force generator (bottom panel). In the first case, the subjects lay on a free-wheeling dolly which enabled the push-off force exerted with the legs to be freely transmitted to the elbow. The strength test results in both the tests were similar. (Reprinted by permission from Andersson & Schultz 1979.)

motion and, in the case of isometric exercises, on the joint position used in training (Fig. 23.41).

In the practice of sport training, three approaches/principles are used to manage the force–posture paradigm (the fourth 'solution' is not to pay attention to this issue at all). They are

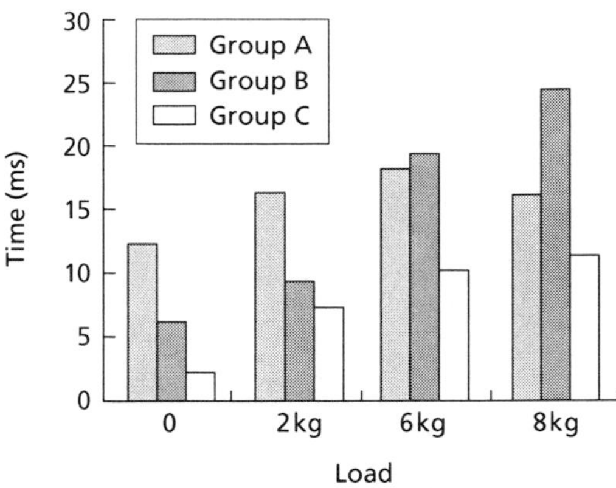

Fig. 23.41 Effects of isometric training at the different joint positions on the time of the maximally fast arm movement (the difference between the movement time before and after the training). Starting from the dependent posture the subjects ($n = 32$) performed a maximally fast shoulder flexion with a barbell in the hand. The mass of the barbells was 2, 6 and 8 kg. The subjects were beginner weightlifters (age 17 ± 1.2 years). In addition to the main training routine that was the same for all the subjects, group A (11 subjects) performed isometric training of the shoulder flexors at an angle of 0–5°. Group B trained at a shoulder angle of 90°. Group C (10 subjects) served as a control. The isometric training consisted of 3 sets of 3 maximal efforts in a session, 3 times a week for 24 weeks. The rest intervals were 10 s between the trials and 60 s between the sets. Training at the angle of 90° was beneficial for the lifting of a heavy 8-kg barbell, while training at the starting position was advantageous for the lifting of a 2-kg barbell and the movement of the unloaded arm. (Data from Zatsiorsky *et al.* 1967.)

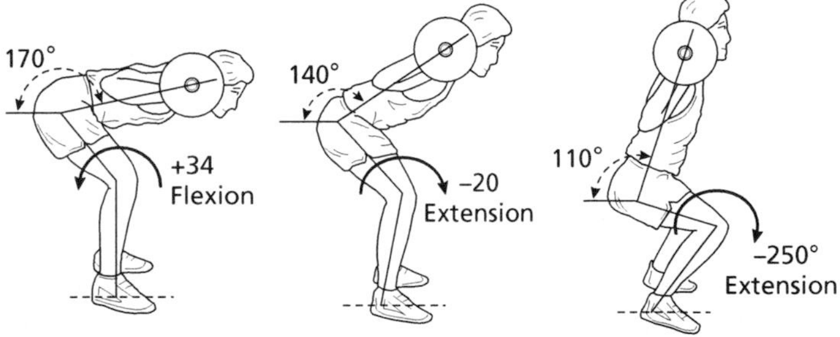

Fig. 23.40 Moments of force in the knee joints (Nm) during squatting with an 80-kg barbell. Both the magnitude and direction (flexion or extension) of the moment are altered when the athlete's posture is changed. When the squatting is performed with the tilted trunk (leftmost figure), the knee extensors are not activated and the knee flexors are active. The knee extensors are loaded maximally when the trunk is upright (rightmost figure). (Reprinted by permission from Zatsiorsky 1995.)

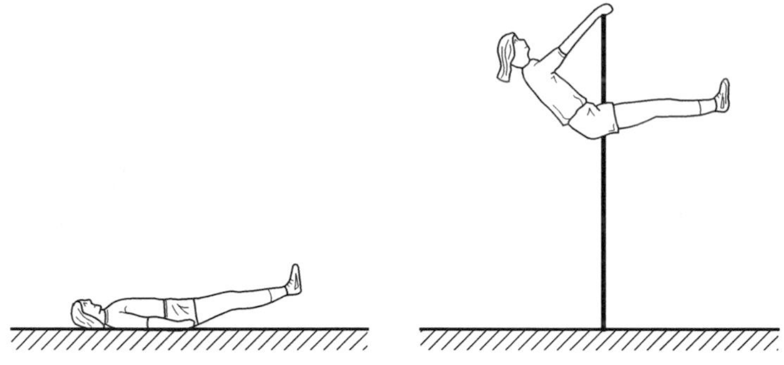

Fig. 23.42 Leg raising from two starting positions. The load is higher in leg raising performed on a horizontal bar than in leg raising from a supine position. (Reprinted by permission from Zatsiorsky 1995.)

the *peak-contraction principle*, *accommodating resistance* and *accentuation*. The techniques are described in detail in Zatsiorsky (1995). A brief account only is given here.

The *peak-contraction principle* is based on the idea of targeting the *weakest* points of the human strength curve. The principle is realized, if 'the worst comes to the worst', when the external resistance, e.g. moment of gravity force, is maximal at the joint position where strength F_m is minimal. The strength is smallest at the position where (i) muscle tension is the lowest, i.e. when the muscles are shortened, and (ii) the muscle moment arms are small. As an example, compare a leg raising from two starting body positions: lying supine and hanging on a horizontal bar (Fig. 23.42). The second exercise imposes a much greater demand that the first. In both the exercises, the moment arm of gravity force acting on the legs is maximal when the legs are placed horizontally. However, when the legs are raised in the recumbent position, the maximal resistance coincides with the strongest points of the force–angle curve (the hip flexors are not shortened). When the leg raising is performed on the horizontal bar, the hip flexor muscles are shortened at the instant the legs cross the horizontal line. Thus, the position of maximal resistance coincides with the minimal (weakest) point on the force–position curve ('the worst comes to the worst').

To implement the peak-contraction principle, special training devices can be used (Fig. 23.43).

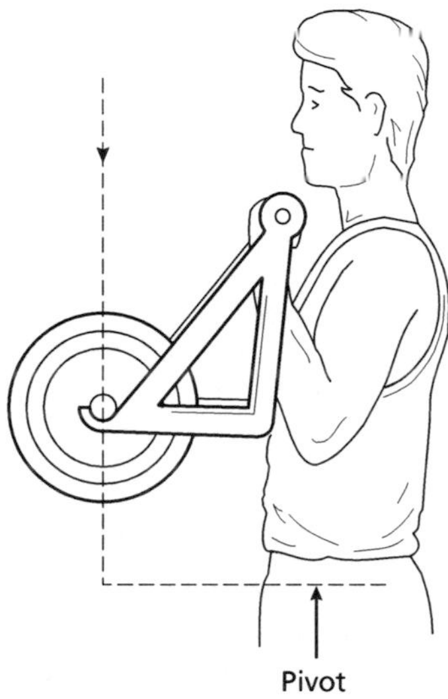

Fig. 23.43 A device used for implementing the peak-contraction principle. The device is employed to perform the arm curl. With the device, the highest resistance is provided at the end of the movement. When the elbow is maximally flexed, the athlete's strength potential is minimal (see Fig. 23.8a) and the resistance is the greatest ('the worst comes to the worst'). (Reprinted by permission from Zatsiorsky 1995.)

Contrary to the peak-contraction principle, the idea of *accommodating resistance* is to develop maximal tension throughout the complete range of motion rather than at a particular, e.g. the weakest, point. The accommodating resistance can be achieved in two ways, either by isokinetic machines or by varying resistance in concert with the human strength curve (Nautilus-type equipment). The idea was suggested in the 19th century by Zander (1879) who developed many strength exercise machines based on this principle

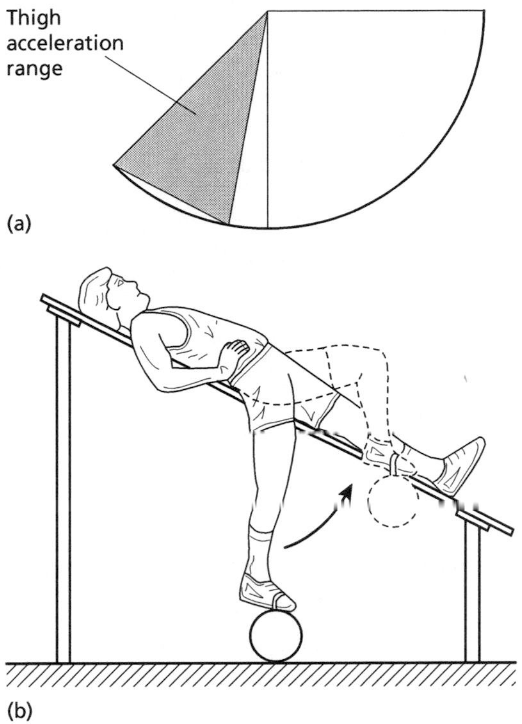

Fig. 23.44 (a) 'Accentuated' range of motion in swing movement of the leg. (b) An exercise designed to satisfy the requirement for 'accentuated' muscular efforts. (Reprinted by permission from Zatsiorsky 1995.)

(for the history of the problem see Levertin 1893, and for the first scientific review on the topic see Reijs 1921). The accommodating resistance is the cornerstone of the *medicomechanical gymnastics* that were popular before World War I. Today, some of the Zander equipment can be seen at the Smithsonian Institution in Washington, DC. Numerous attempts to compare the effectiveness of isokinetic strength training with varying-resistance training and free-weight training were not successful due to the specificity of the training gains, i.e. isokinetic training resulted in greater increases in isokinetic strength while the free-weight training resulted in greater increases in the magnitude of the lifted load (see Kraemer *et al.* 1996, 2000, for a review). It seems that for athletes the accommodating resistance should not be a first-choice training technique (with the possible exception of aquatic sports, such as swimming and rowing).

The main idea of *accentuation* is to be maximally specific: to train strength in the range of the main sport movement where the demand for high force production is maximal. According to this idea, there is no need for athletes to train strength over the entire range of motion if the maximal force is required in only a small part of the range. For instance, if the training objective is to increase strength of the hip flexor muscles to improve velocity of the swing movement, there is no reason to increase the strength of these muscles in a range beyond the range this activity requires. An exercise shown in Fig. 23.44 satisfies the requirement for specificity of the range of force application.

The mechanisms of the joint-position specificity of strength training are not clear. It may be due to unknown mechanisms of neural coordination or specific adaptation of the muscles themselves, e.g. through the change in the number of sarcomeres in series in muscle fibres (Herzog *et al.* 1991).

Type and amount of resistance

The force exerted by an athlete on an external object depends on the resistance provided by the object. For instance, as previously mentioned (see Figs 23.9 & 23.26), the isometric strength in leg extension is maximal when the leg is close to full extension. However, in running jumps exactly opposite is happening: the peak active force during take-offs is exerted when the leg is maximally flexed. At this instant the acceleration of the athlete's body is maximal and because the resistance is provided by the body's inertia (plus its weight) the force is also maximal. Hence, the dependence of the force exerted by an athlete on the body posture is not absolute; it depends on the type of the resistance. The muscle activity also depends on the resistance provided to movement (Fig. 23.45).

When resistance based on *elasticity*, the magnitude of force increases with the range of motion. The force is maximal at the end of movement,

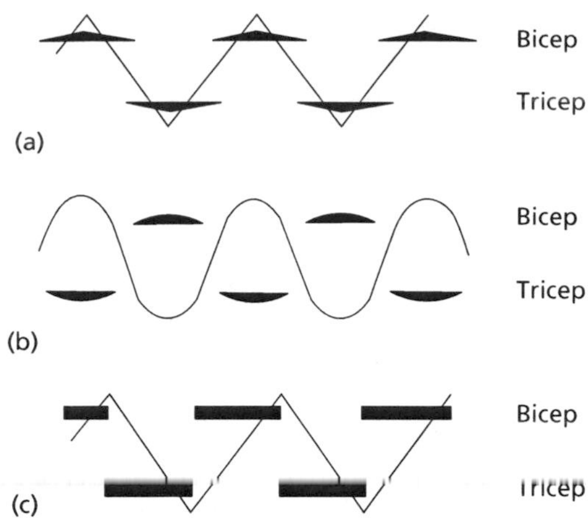

Fig. 23.45 The periods of muscle activity during rhythmic elbow flexion and extension against various resistances. The duration of one flexion or extension is about 1 s; the range of motion is 90°. Ascending curves, elbow flexion; descending curves, elbow extension. (a) Elastic forces (the resistance is provided by two springs). During the maximal flexion (extension) the elbow flexors (extensors) are active. (b) Inertia (horizontal movement with a mass added to the forearm). The muscle activity is exactly opposite to the previous case: during maximal flexion the extensor muscles are active and during maximal extension the elbow flexors are maximally activated. This pattern of muscle activation is necessitated by the mechanics: at the instant of maximal elbow flexion the acceleration is directed toward extension and is maximal. (c) Viscous forces (the arm moves in thick dough). The muscles are maximally active when the elbow is at an intermediate position and joint angular velocity is maximal. (Adapted from Wagner 1925.)

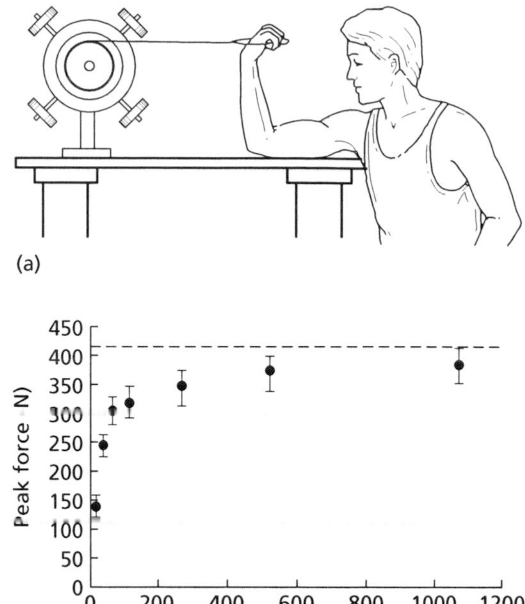

Fig. 23.46 (a) Inertia wheel. A rope is wound repeatedly around the pulley and a subject then pulls the rope. The inertial resistance (equivalent mass) is changed by varying the moment of inertia of the wheel (locating the attached loads closer to or further from the axis of rotation) and by winding the rope around the tubes of different diameters. The inertia wheel was first suggested by Hill in 1922 (the paper was reprinted in 2001). (Reprinted from Zatsiorsky 1995.) (b) Dependence of the peak force on the moving mass. The horizontal dotted line represents the F_{mm}, the maximal isometric force at an elbow angle of 90°. The subjects were experienced weightlifters and wrestlers. (Data from Zatsiorsky *et al.* 1968.)

when a resisting object (rubber band, stretch cord, spring, etc.) is maximally extended. In some exercise machines the resistance is provided by *viscosity*: during the movement viscous oil is squeezed through the narrow openings. When working on such machines, the resistance is proportional to velocity and the peak force is exerted at the instant when the velocity is maximal. *Hydrodynamic resistance* in water sports depends on the velocity squared.

When resistance is provided by *inertia*, a movement follows Newton's second law of motion: the force is proportional to the mass (inertia) of the accelerated body and its acceleration. Movement against inertial resistance is usually studied by using an *inertia wheel* (Fig. 23.46a). When the mass of an accelerated object is small, the maximal force exerted by an athlete on the object depends on the amount of mass (Fig. 23.46b). It is impossible to exert a large F_m against a body of small mass. For instance, it is unrealistic to apply a great force to a coin. However, if the mass of an object is large the F_m depends mainly on the athlete's strength.

The strength gains resulting from training with different resistance are modality specific.

For instance, the subjects who trained on a device that provided a hydraulic resistance experienced significant increases in peak force when the force was measured on this device; the peak force exerted on an isokinetic device changed only slightly (O'Hagan *et al.* 1995).

Force–velocity relations

The relations between the force and velocity in athletic movements have attracted considerable interest among researchers.

Types of force–velocity relations

Several force–velocity relations are explored in the biomechanics literature.

1 Relation between force acting on a human body and the body's velocity. The ratio 'force/velocity' is called *mechanical impedance* (see Encyclopaedia of Science & Technology 1977). The impedance characterizes the total resistance of the human body to external forces (Weis & Primiano 1966; Winters *et al.* 1988; Hogan 1990; Batman & Seliktar 1993; Tsuji *et al.* 1995; Cornu *et al.* 1997; Tsuji 1997) and is especially important when the body collides with an external object or is undergoing vibration. The impedance includes elastic, damping and inertial components. We will not discuss it here.

2 Submaximal force–velocity curves which are obtained in the following way: an athlete performs several trials of the same movement, e.g. standing vertical jump. The trials are performed with different efforts, from low to maximal. In each trial force and velocity are measured, e.g. peak force exerted on the ground and the take-off velocity. Then, the values of the force and velocity are plotted against each other. The relation is usually positive: the higher the force the larger the velocity. This relation is considered trivial and has not attracted much attention in the literature.

3 Relation between the force and velocity registered in a single movement. The force and velocity are registered continuously and then plotted against each other. The examples are rhythmic to-and-fro oscillations of the forearm (Fig. 23.47a) and running (Fig. 23.47b). In the first example, the angular velocity of the forearm is plotted against angular acceleration and force (force is proportional to acceleration). In the second, the relation between the Achilles tendon tension and its speed of shortening and lengthening is presented. Such single-trial force–velocity curves are different from the force–velocity curves registered in multitrial experiments described below (with an exception of the case described later; see Fig. 23.50).

Another two relations are obtained when the athletes put forth maximal efforts to produce highest possible force and/or speed.

4 Relation between the *maximum maximorum* force F_{mm} and the maximal movement speed V_m. For sport practitioners, this relation is important because it helps in answering the question as to whether the increasing of F_{mm} is helpful for the improvement of movement speed. An example is the relation between the F_{mm} in a leg extension and the take-off velocity (or the height) of a standing vertical jump. The question is whether stronger athletes jump higher. Such relations were coined *non-parametric relations* (Zatsiorsky *et al.* 1968–1969). The reason behind this terminology will be explained later in the text.

The non-parametric relations are either positive (the larger F_{mm} the larger V_m) or zero. The relation depends on the amount of resistance: the larger the resistance, e.g. mass of an implement, the higher the correlation between the F_{mm} and V_m (Fig. 23.48). There is no correlation between F_{mm} and V_{mm} (*maximal maximorum* velocity) obtained at a zero resistance: the ability to produce maximal force (i.e. muscular strength) and the ability to achieve great velocity in the same movement are independent motor abilities (Rasch 1954; Henry 1960; Clarke & Henry 1961).

5 *Parametric relations* between maximal force and velocity. The term *parametric relation* is used for designating the force–velocity relations obtained in the following way (Zatsiorsky *et al.* 1968–1969).

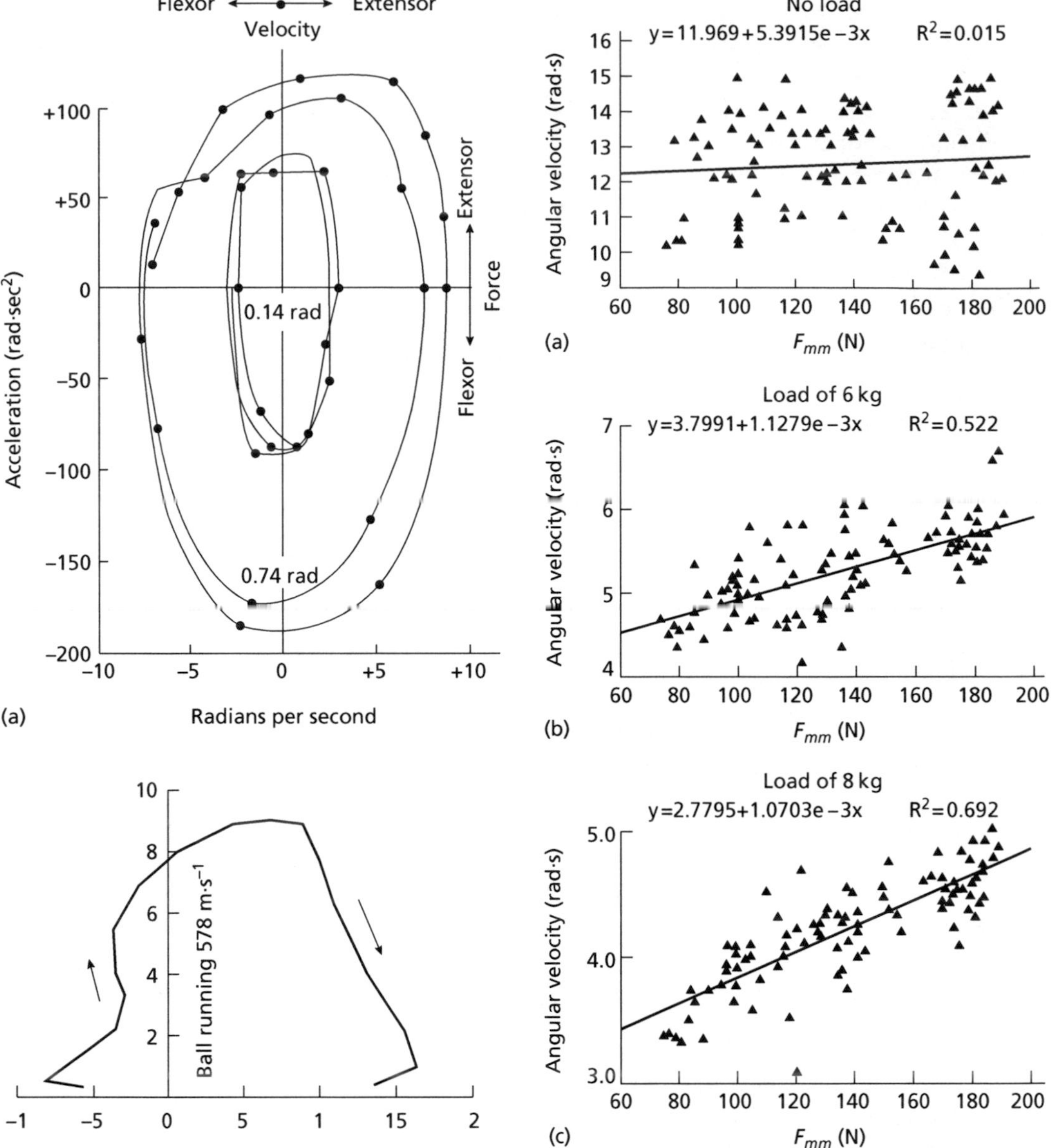

Fig. 23.47 Force–velocity curves obtained in single trials. The task parameters are constant. (a) Successive changes of force and velocity during to-and-fro movements of the forearm at amplitudes of 0.14 and 0.74 radians. The movement progresses in a clockwise direction. The moment of inertia of the arm is about 5.6×10^5 g·cm^{-2}. (Reprinted by permission from Fenn 1938.) (b) The force–velocity profile of the human triceps surae muscles during ball of the foot contact running at 5.78 m·s^{-1} (bottom). Forces represent Achilles tendon forces while velocities represent the rate of the muscle–tendon length changes for the gastrocnemius muscle. (Adapted from Komi 1990.)

Fig. 23.48 Non-parametric relationships between the *maximum maximorum* force F_{mm} and the velocity of shoulder flexion V_m with arm extended; 100 subjects. Bottom panel, load (a dumbbell) of 8 kg in the hand; there is a high correlation between F_{mm} and V_m. Middle panel, load of 6 kg. Upper panel, no load; there is no significant correlation between F_{mm} and V_m. (Adapted from Zatsiorsky 1995.)

(a) The subjects perform several trials with maximal efforts.

(b) A certain parameter of the task, e.g. weight of an implement, varies in a systematic way from trial to trial.

(c) In each trial, both the force and velocity are measured, F_m and V_m. Each F_m–V_m pair corresponds to a certain value of the parameter. (Isokinetic devices allow for fixing movement velocity and registering the exerted force.)

(d) The values of F_m and V_m are plotted against each other.

To distinguish this relationship from the F_{mm}–V_m relation described above, the former was called the non-parametric relation. The following discussion is limited to concentric muscle action. Eccentric muscle action is addressed in Chapter 10 of this volume.

Parametric force–velocity relations

This relation attracted the most interest in the literature where it is frequently called simply the *force–velocity relation* or, especially when speaking about individual muscles, *Hill's curve* (see Fig. 9.xx in Chapter 9). The latter term is in reference to the A.V. Hill work (1938). Some examples of the parametric relations encountered in sport practice are presented in Table 23.4 and the examples of the force–velocity curve are given in Fig. 23.49. In field conditions, instead of velocity its approximate estimates are often used (panels b and c in Fig. 23.49). The parametric force–velocity relationships are negative: the larger the velocity the smaller the force. The curves are concave upward.

Force–velocity curves that may look *similar in appearance* to the Hill curve can be recorded in a single trial (case **3** above). This happens if the velocity increases monotonically to a certain saturation level and, consequently, the acceleration monotonically decreases (Fig. 23.50, panel a). When the resistance is provided by inertia, the relation between the force and acceleration is given by Newton's second law $F = ma$. If the mass is constant, the force–velocity relation is in essence the 'acceleration–velocity' relation. In such a case, the observed force–velocity relation is a consequence of the velocity saturation: when velocity increases the acceleration decreases. This relation is not a parametric relation (all parameters of the task are constant). The corresponding curve can be called the *pseudo-Hill curve* (the word *pseudo* does not have any negative connotation; it simply indicates that the curve was obtained in a different way). The pseudo-Hill curves should be distinguished from the real Hill curves described previously. The pseudo-Hill curves are usually straight lines.

Some coaches that I have met have regarded parametric force–velocity relations as trivial: obviously, heavy objects cannot be lifted or moved

Table 23.4 Parametric force–velocity relations in athletic movements.

Activity (parameter)	Variable factor	Force	Velocity
Cycling frequency (or velocity)	Gear ratio	Force applied to the pedal	Pedalling
Rowing, kayaking, canoeing	Blade area of an oar or a paddle	Applied to the oar or to the paddle	The blade with respect to the water
Uphill/downhill ambulation	Incline/decline	At take-off	Ambulation
Throwing	Mass of the implement	Exerted upon the implement	Implement at the release
Standing vertical jump	Modified body weight. Weight added (waist belt) or deduced (suspension system)	At take-off	Body at the end of take-off

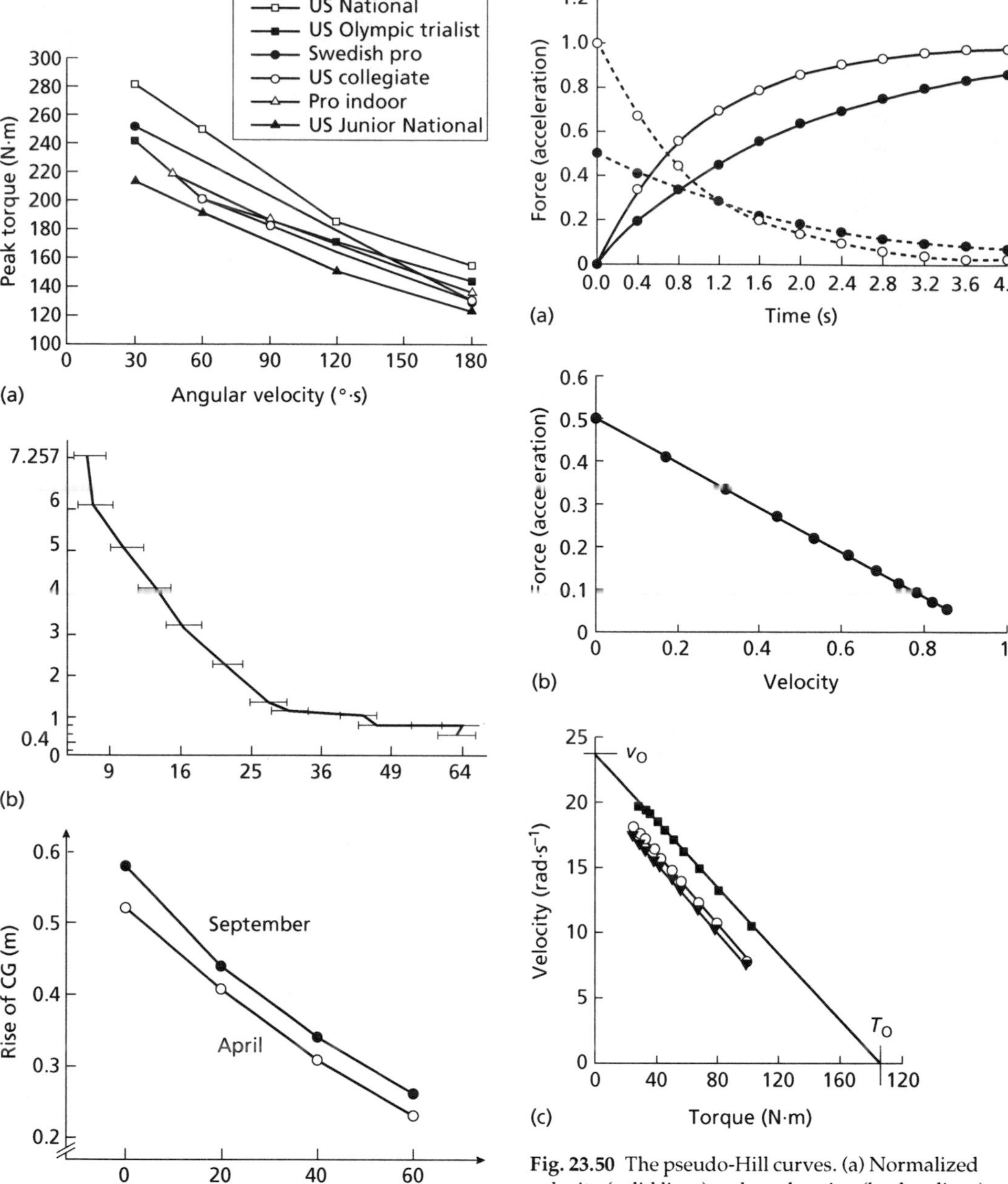

Fig. 23.49 Force–velocity curves obtained in various movements. (a) Knee extension in soccer players of different skill levels, joint angular velocity vs. joint moment. (Reprinted from Kirkendall 1985.) (b) Mass of the implement (ordinate) vs. square root of the throwing distance abscisse. The square root of the distance approximates the release velocity. (Reprinted from Zatsiorsky *et al.* 1964.) (c) Jumping height vs. extra loads in standing vertical jumps. The jumping height is used as an approximate estimate of the take-off velocity. (Reprinted from Viitasalo 1985.)

Fig. 23.50 The pseudo-Hill curves. (a) Normalized velocity (solid lines) and acceleration (broken lines) in a single trial. If intracycle velocity fluctuations are neglected or filtered, such curves are registered at the beginning of the sprint running and cycling. The velocity curve $V(t)$ can be described by an equation (Henry & Trafton 1951; Zatsiorsky & Primakov 1969) $V(t) = V_{max}\,(1 - e^{-kt})$ where V_{max} is the maximal velocity and k is an acceleration constant (the magnitude of acceleration at the start, $t = 0$). The acceleration equals $a(t) = V_{max}\,ke^{-kt}$. The velocity and acceleration curves are normalized with respect to the V_{max} and correspond to $k = 0.5$ (black circles) and $k = 1.0$ (open circles). When velocity increases the acceleration decreases. When velocity is maximal, the acceleration is zero.

continued opposite

with the same high speed as light objects. This is equally valid for inanimate objects: the speed of a car decreases when it is towing a trailer. So what is all this fuss about?

On the other hand, scientists have focused on the parametric force–velocity relations at length. The reason is that force–velocity relations in whole-body movements epitomize the force–velocity relations for muscles, the famous Hill's curve discussed previously in Chapter 9. The fundamental importance of the muscle force–velocity curve is well grounded: the force–velocity curve is nicely explained by the cross-bridge theory of muscle contraction (Huxley 1957) and is closely related to the total amount of energy (mechanical work + heat) liberated during muscle contraction: more energy is liberated when shortening is permitted (for short reviews see Zatsiorsky 1998; Huxley 2000). In an influential paper by Hill (1938), the force–velocity curve was derived from the heat measurements. Direct measurements of the force-velocity curve on isolated muscles in humans are extremely rare (Ralston *et al.* 1949).

The relationship between the force–velocity curves for individual muscles and the analogous curve for a whole-body movement is anything but simple. The problem starts from selecting values of force and velocity for the analysis. In experiments performed on isolated muscle fibres or muscles, there is a significant period of constant force and velocity during the movement (Wilkie 1967; Fig. 23.51). In these cases, the specific time at which the variables are measured is not critical.

During natural human movements, both force and velocity vary over time. Even if the velocity or force is kept constant as an independent variable, the dependent variable is not constant. The dependent variable(s) are measured at a specific point in time, e.g. at an instant when the maximal force or velocity occurs, or at a specific body position, e.g. at an angle of 90°. Choices are numerous. The choice made by a researcher affects the results.

Fig. 23.50 (*cont'd*) (b) The plot of acceleration (force) vs. velocity for $k = 0.5$. (c) Relationship between the pedal velocity and torque in three cyclists. In the experiment, the subjects performed a single all-out sprint on a cycle ergometer. The crank angle–torque curves were recorded during the first 10 revolutions. Each point corresponds to the average velocity and torque during one revolution. (c is from Butelli *et al.* 1996.)

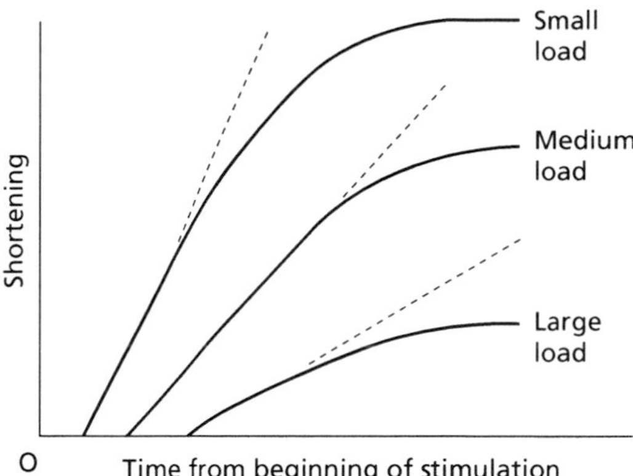

Fig. 23.51 Diagram to show how an isolated muscle shortens when lifting various loads from a fixed initial length. The slope of the interrupted lines gives the speed of shortening. With the increasing loads, the maximum speed of shortening decreases. Also, as larger loads are lifted, the following changes are seen. (i) The interval before the load begins to move increases. This time is mainly spent in building up isometric tension to a level equal that to of the load. (ii) The total amount of shortening decreases. (Reprinted from Carlson & Wilkie 1974.)

SINGLE-JOINT MOVEMENTS

In single-joint movements, the force–velocity (or torque–angular velocity) relations have been studied mainly in two joints: the elbow (Dern *et al.* 1947; Wilkie 1950; Komi 1973; Jørgensen 1976; de Koning *et al.* 1985, 1986; Kojima 1991; Martin *et al.* 1995; Thomis *et al.* 1998) and the knee (Thorstensson *et al.* 1976; Lesmes *et al.* 1978; Perrine & Edgerton 1978; Gregor *et al.* 1979; Johansson *et al.* 1987; Westing *et al.* 1988; Prietto & Caiozzo 1989; Marshall *et al.* 1990; Kanehisa *et al.* 1997; Chow *et al.* 1999; Rahmani *et al.* 1999; Seger *et al.* 1999; Seger & Thorstensson 2000). Other joints, in particular the wrist (Chow & Darling

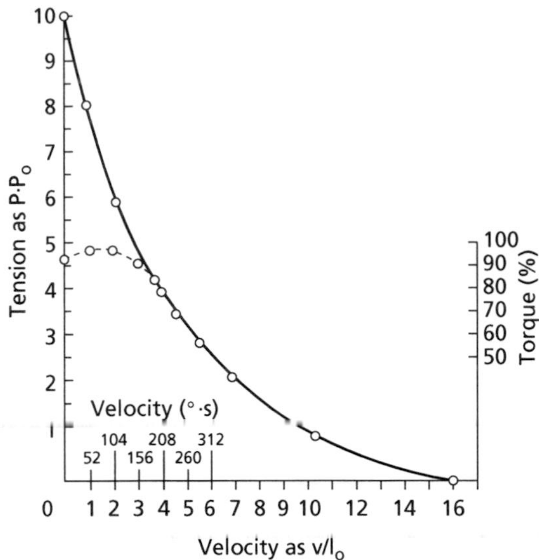

Fig. 23.52 Force–velocity relation in isokinetic knee extension. (Reprinted from Perrine & Edgerton 1978.)

1999), the finger joints (Cook & McDonagh 1996), the thumb (De Ruiter *et al.* 1999), the hip (Hawkins & Smeudlers 1999) and the ankle (Fugl-Meyer *et al.* 1982; Bobbert & van Ingen Schenau 1990), have been studied to a lesser extent. The most common approach has been isokinetic flexion and extension but other protocols have been also used: hanging weights (Wilkie 1950; Kojima 1991), elastic resistance (Hawkins & Smeudlers 1999), a constant force spring (de Koning *et al.* 1985) and the moment of inertia provided by an inertia wheel (Tihanyi *et al.* 1982).

Force–velocity and torque–angular velocity curves for single-joint movements are not identical to analogous curves of single muscles because they are a result of the superposition of the force outcome of several muscles possessing different features. Nevertheless, they are similar in shape to the single-fibre/muscle force–velocity plots. The most important exception is that in some movements, most notably in knee extension, the torque values in the high-torque range of the torque–angular velocity curves are smaller than would be expected from the Hill force–velocity equation (Fig. 23.52) (Perrine *et al.* 1978; Kojima 1991). This was hypothesized to be due to a central nervous system inhibition aimed at preventing injuries at high forces.

In athletes with higher percentages of fast-twitch fibres, the force–velocity curves have less curvature (Gregor *et al.* 1979; Tihanyi *et al.* 1982; Froese & Houston 1985). Similar results were obtained when comparing sprinters and distance runners (Johansson *et al.* 1987; Wakayama *et al.* 1995). When the Hill equation (see eqn x in Chapter 9) is used, the curvature of the force–velocity curve can be described by the ratio a/F_{mm}. The larger the ratio the smaller the curvature. On average, the ratio equals 0.39 for elbow flexion (Kojima 1991) and 0.4 for knee extension (Tihanyi *et al.* 1982). In elbow flexion, the ratio varies from approximately 0.10 to 0.60 (Zatsiorsky 1966). Athletes in power sports usually have a ratio higher than 0.30 while endurance athletes have a ratio that is lower. When the curvature of the force–velocity is small, the curve may be satisfactorily approximated by a linear equation (Fugl-Meyer *et al.* 1982; Kues & Mayhew 1996).

Fatigue shifts the force–velocity curve downward (De Ruiter *et al.* 1999) while an increased training level shifts it upward (Jorgensen 1976; de Koning *et al.* 1985; Dudley & Djamil 1985; Ameredes *et al.* 1995; Martin *et al.* 1995).

MULTIJOINT MOVEMENTS

On the whole, the parametric force–velocity relations recorded in multijoint movements preserve the main features of the muscle force–velocity curves: the relations are negative (the higher the force the smaller the velocity—what else can be expected?) and (in many cases) the curves are concave upward. The details depend, however, on how the force and velocity were recorded (maximal, average, at a certain joint position, etc.).

In multijoint movements the end-effector force and velocity depend on body posture even when joint moments and joint angular velocities do not change. When the magnitude of the joint torque vector **T** is constant ($T = 1$), the possible force vectors at the endpoint of the chain satisfy eqn 14: $\mathbf{F}^T\mathbf{J}\mathbf{J}^T\mathbf{F} = 1$, which is an equation of an ellipse. The joint angular velocities $\boldsymbol{\omega}$ are related to the endpoint velocity **V** by the Jacobian matrix **J**,

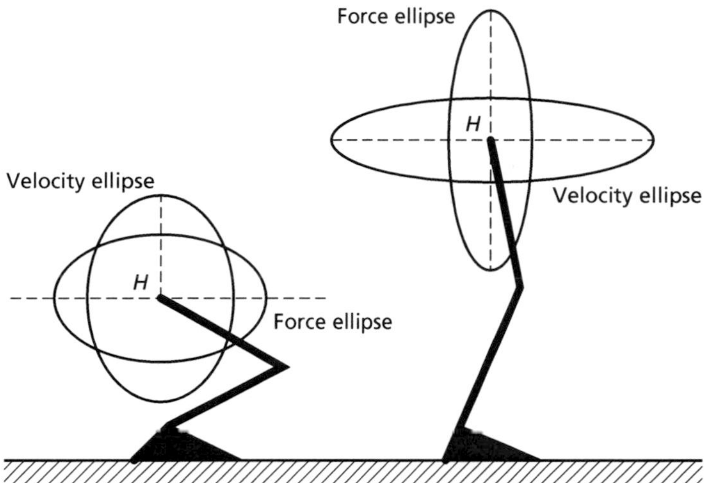

Fig. 23.53 Force and velocity ellipses in the two leg positions during a take-off (a schematic). By an assumption, the joint velocity vector and the joint torque vector are of a constant magnitude throughout the entire movement. The endpoint of the chain is at the hip joint, *H*. When the magnitudes of the vectors **T** and **ω** are constant, the endpoint velocity and force depend solely on the leg position (chain Jacobian). The force and velocity ellipses change in the opposite directions during the movement. In a squatting position (left figure), the vertical velocity of *H* is large but the force of leg extension is small. When the leg is close to complete extension, the vertical velocity of *H* is small but a large force of the leg extension can be generated. The ellipses are not to scale.

$\mathbf{V} = \mathbf{J}\boldsymbol{\omega}$ (for a detailed explanation see Zatsiorsky 1998). When the Jacobian is invertible (the Jacobian is of a full rank and the chain is not in a singular configuration), the joint angular velocity vector can be found from the vector of the endpoint velocity as $\boldsymbol{\omega} = \mathbf{J}^{-1}\mathbf{V}$. The requirement for the magnitude of the angular velocity vector to be constant ($\omega = 1$), can be written as a dot product of the vectors: $\boldsymbol{\omega}^T\boldsymbol{\omega} = 1$. Substitution gives:

$$\mathbf{V}^T(\mathbf{J}^{-1})^T(\mathbf{J}^{-1})\mathbf{V} = 1 \quad (15)$$

The equation represents the ellipse of the endpoint velocities for a given magnitude of the vector of joint angular velocities. The force and velocity ellipses for two leg positions are illustrated in Fig. 23.53. When the leg approaches complete extension the transfer of the joint angular velocities into the leg extension velocity decreases (for a nice discussion of this subject see van Ingen Schenau 1989) and the transfer of the joint torques into the endpoint force increases. Therefore, even when the magnitudes of the vectors of joint torques and joint angular velocities are constant, the endpoint force and velocity change during the leg extension in the opposite directions. The force–velocity curve, if it were determined by continuously measuring the force and velocity values at the different leg positions, would be hyperbolic. This conclusion follows from the following consideration. Although the force F and velocity V along the leg extension change, their product FV = power remains constant. Hence, the F–V relation is a hyperbole. However, the curve only characterizes the change in the chain Jacobian. This is certainly not a Hill's curve.

In multijoint movements, the involved joints and muscles do not act in the same way at the same time. This sharply deviates from the classical experiments on force–velocity relationships. Therefore, the force–velocity curves registered in multijoint movements may not conform to the classical form of Hill's curve (Hardyk 2000). In particular, linear relationships between force and velocity are repeatedly reported (Sargeant *et al.* 1981; Driss *et al.* 1998; Rahmani *et al.* 2001). The relationship still remains negative: the higher the velocity the smaller the force.

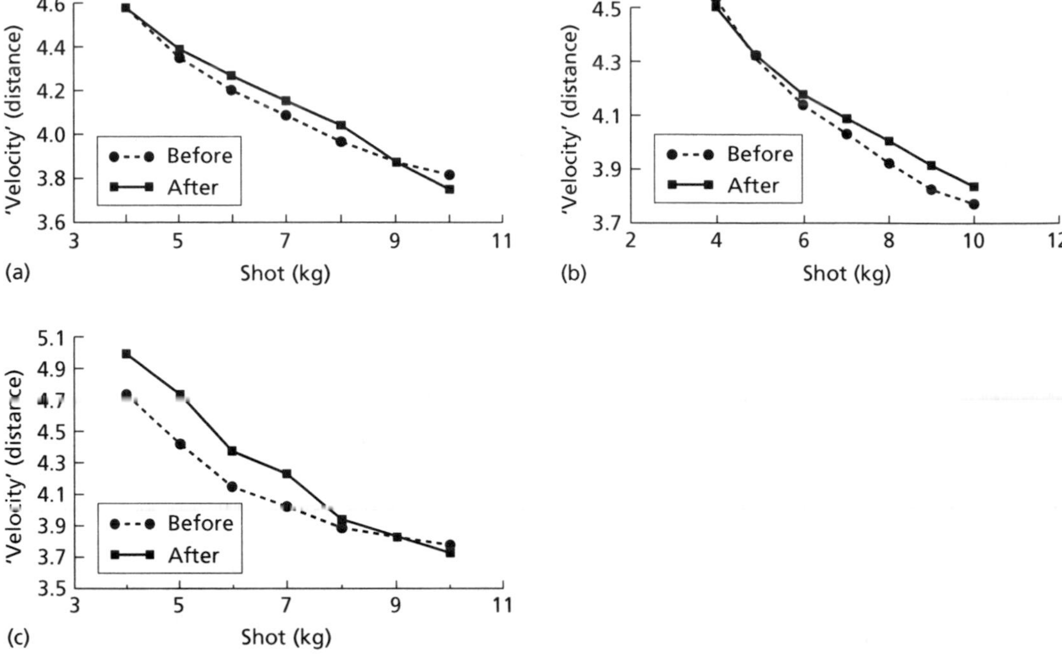

Fig. 23.54 Performance results in standing shot putting before and after 7-week training with different shots; 4–10-kg shots were used for testing. The subjects were among the best athletes in the country. (a) Standard shots; only 7.257-g shots were used ($n = 4$). (b) Heavy shots (8–10 kg); a throwing routine consisting of heavy shots (70% of all the puts) and standard shots (7.257 kg, 30%). (c) Light shots (4.5–6.0 kg); the puts of light shots comprised 70% of all efforts ($n = 3$). In shot putting, the throwing distance D is the function of the release velocity (v), angle of release (α) and the height of release (h):

$$D = \frac{v^2}{g}\cos\alpha\left(\sin\alpha + \sqrt{\sin^2\alpha + \frac{2gh}{v^2}}\right)$$

where g is the acceleration due to gravity. As the distance is the quadratic function of release velocity, the square root of distance plotted along the ordinate axis represents (approximately) the velocity at release. While such an approximation may not be accurate enough for a scientific research, sport practitioners use it due to its simplicity. (Reprinted from Zatsiorsky 1995; data from Zatsiorsky & Karasiov 1978.)

SOME PRACTICAL ISSUES

Parametric force–velocity relations have several applications in sport practice. Because force–velocity relation is difficult to study, instead of this relation the 'load–jumping height' or 'mass of an implement–square root of throwing distance' relations are frequently investigated (the throwing distance is a function of the release velocity squared). These relations approximately represent the force–velocity curve.

Effects of strength training are velocity specific (Rutherford & Jones 1986; Behm & Sale 1993b; Almåsbakk & Hoff 1996; Hortobágyi *et al.* 1996). Training in a certain range of the force and velocity improves the performance results mainly in the trained span of the curve (Fig. 23.54). In training, the athletes can target either the 'high force–low velocity' or the 'low force–high velocity' ranges of the entire force–velocity curve. Heavy-resistance exercises mainly affect the 'force end' of the curve, while dynamic exercises with high movement velocity have an effect on the 'velocity end' of the curve (Ikai & Fukunaga 1970; Thorstensson 1977; Lesmes *et al.* 1978; Caiozzo *et al.* 1981; de Koning *et al.* 1985; Kanehisa & Miyashita 1983).

When force F and velocity V are in the same direction, the mechanical power P equals the product of the instant values of force and velocity: $P = F \times V$. One practical consequence of the force–velocity relation is that muscles generate maximal mechanical power when the muscle tension and its speed of shortening have about one-third of their maximal values (see Chapter 9). By manipulating such parameters as a gear ratio on a bicycle or a blade area of an oar in rowing, it is possible, at least in principle, to match load and speed to the muscle properties. However, for multilink movements, for example bicycle pedalling, this task is not trivial: many variables interact in a complex manner (Davies & Young 1984a,b, 1985; Hull & Gonzalez 1988; Gonzalez & Hull 1989; Hautier *et al.* 1996; Yoshihuku & Herzog 1996; Baron *et al.* 1999; MacIntosh *et al.* 2000; Marsh *et al.* 2000; Zoladz *et al.* 2000). It seems that the pedalling rate that maximizes mechanical power output in sprint cycling follows from the interaction between Hill's power–velocity relationship and 'activation dynamics', the time course of the muscle tension rise and relaxation (van Soest & Casius 2000).

References

Almåsbakk, B. & Hoff, J. (1996) Coordination, the determinant of velocity specificity? *Journal of Applied Physiology* **81**, 2046–2052.

Ameredes, B.T., Brechue, W.F., Andrew, G.M. & Stainsby, W.N. (1992) Force–velocity shifts with repetitive isometric and isotonic contractions of canine gastrocnemius in situ. *Journal of Applied Physiology* **73**(5), 2105–2111.

Amis, A.A., Dowson, D. & Wright, V. (1979) Muscle strengths and musculo-skeletal geometry of the upper arm. *Engineering in Medicine* **8**(1), 41–48.

An, K.N., Chao, E.Y., Cooney, W.P. & Linscheid, R.L. (1979) Normative model of human hand for biomechanical analysis. *Journal of Biomechanics* **12**, 775–788.

An, K.N., Hui, F.C., Morrey, B.F., Linscheid, R.L. & Chao, E.Y. (1981) Muscles across the elbow joint: a biomechanical analysis. *Journal of Biomechanics* **14**, 659–669.

An, K.N., Ueba, Y., Chao, E.Y., Cooney, W.P. & Linscheid, R.L. (1983) Tendon excursion and moment arm of index finger muscles. *Journal of Biomechanics* **16**(6), 419–425.

Andersson, G.B.J. & Schultz, A.B. (1979) Transmission of moments across the elbow joint and the lumbar spine. *Journal of Biomechanics* **12**, 747–755.

Aper, R.L., Saltzman, C.L. & Brown, T.D. (1996) The effect of hallux sesamoid excision on the flexor hallucis longus moment arm. *Clinical Orthopaedics* **325**, 209–217.

Armstrong, T.J. & Chaffin, D.B. (1978) An investigation of the relationship between displacements of the finger and wrist joints and the extrinsic finger flexor tendons. *Journal of Biomechanics* **11**, 119–128.

Arnold, A.S. & Delp, S.L. (2001) Rotational moment arms of the medial hamstrings and adductors vary with femoral geometry and limb position: implications for the treatment of internally rotated gait. *Journal of Biomechanics* **34**(4), 437–447.

Aruin, A.S., Zatsiorsky, V.M., Prilutsky, B.I. & Shakhnazarov, A.I. (1987) Biomechanical method used for determining the arms of muscular force. In: *Biomechanics* X-B (ed. B. Jonson), pp. 1117–1121. Human Kinetics, Champaign, IL.

Aruin, A.S., Zatsiorsky, V.M. & Prilutsky, B.I. (1988) Moment arms and elongations of muscles of lower extremities under various values of joint angles. *Archives of Anatomy, Histology and Embryology* **94**(6), 52–55.

Atwater, A.E. (1979) Biomechanics of overarm throwing movements and of throwing injuries. *Exercise and Sport Sciences Reviews* **7**, 43–85.

Baron, R., Bachl, N., Petschnig, R., Tschan, H., Smekal, G. & Pokan, R. (1999) Measurement of maximal power output in isokinetic and non-isokinetic cycling. A comparison of two methods. *International Journal of Sports Medicine* **20**(8), 532–537.

Bartonietz, K. (2000a) Hammer throwing: Problems and prospects. In: *Biomechanics in Sport: Performance Enhancement and Injury Prevention* (ed. V.M. Zatsiorsky), pp. 458–486. Blackwell Science, Oxford.

Bartonietz, K. (2000b) Javelin throwing: an approach to performance development. In: *Biomechanics in Sport: Performance Enhancement and Injury Prevention* (ed. V.M. Zatsiorsky), pp. 401–434. Blackwell Science, Oxford.

Bassett, R.W., Browne, A.O., Morrey, B.F. & An, K.N. (1990) Glenohumeral muscle force and moment mechanics in a position of shoulder instability. *Journal of Biomechanics* **23**, 405–415.

Batman, M. & Seliktar, R. (1993) Characterization of human joint impedance during impulsive motion. *Journal of Electromyography and Kinesiology* **3**(4), 221–230.

Behm, D.G. & Sale, D.G. (1993a) Intended rather than actual movement velocity determines velocity-specific training response. *Journal of Applied Physiology* **74**(1), 359–368.

Behm, D.G. & Sale, D.G. (1993b) Velocity specificity of resistance training. *Sports Medicine* **15**(6), 374–388.

Berme, N., Paul, J.P. & Purves, W.K. (1977) A biomechanical analysis of the metacarpophalangeal joint. *Journal of Biomechanics* **10**(7), 409–412.

Blix, M. (1891) Die Lange und die Spannung des Muskels. *Scandinavian Archives of Physiology* **3**, 295–318.

Blix, M. (1893) Die Lange und die Spannung des Muskels. *Scandinavian Archives of Physiology* **4**, 399–409.

Blix, M. (1894) Die Lange und die Spannung des Muskels. *Scandinavian Archives of Physiology* **5**, 149–206.

Bobbert, M.F. & van Ingen Schenau, G.J. (1990) Isokinetic plantar flexion: Experimental results and model calculation. *Journal of Biomechanics* **23**, 105–120.

Bober, T., Kornecki, S., Lehr, R.P., Jr & Zawadski, J. (1982) Biomechanical analysis of human arm stabilization during force production. *Journal of Biomechanics* **15**(11), 825–830.

Bouisset, S. (1990) Mechanical properties of human muscle. In: *Biomechanics of Human Movement: Applications in Rehabilitation, Sports and Ergonomics* (eds N. Berme & A. Cappozzo), pp. 10–19. Bertec Corporation, Worthington, OH.

Brand, P.W. & Hollister, A.M. (eds) (1999) *Clinical Biomechanics of the Hand*. Mosby, Chicago.

Brand, P.W., Cranor, K.C. & Ellis, J.C. (1975) Tendon and pulleys at the metacarpophalangeal joint of a finger. *Journal of Bone and Joint Surgery* **57-A**, 779–784.

Brand, P.N., Beach, R.B. & Thompson, D.E. (1981) Relative tension and potential excursion of muscles in the forearm and hand. *Journal of Hand Surgery* **3**, 209–219.

Brüggemann, G.P. (1994) Biomechanics of gymnastic techniques. In: *Sport Biomechanics* (eds R.C. Nelson & V.M. Zatsiorsky), pp. 79–120. Human Kinetics, Champaign, IL.

Buchanan, T.S., Moniz, M.J., Dewald, J.P.A. & Rymer, W.Z. (1993) Estimation of muscle forces about the wrist joint during isometric tasks using an EMG coefficient method. *Journal of Biomechanics* **26**, 547–560.

Burke, R.E., Levine, D.N. & Zajac, F.E. (1971) Mammalian motor units: physiological–histochemical correlation in three types in cat gastrocnemius. *Science* **174**(10), 709–712.

Buttelli, O., Vandewalle, H. & Peres, G. (1996) The relationship between maximal power and maximal torque-velocity using an electronic ergometer. *European Journal of Applied Physiology* **73**(5), 479–483.

Caiozzo, V.J., Perrine, J.J. & Edgerton, V.R. (1981) Training-induced alterations of the in vivo force–velocity relationship of human muscle. *Journal of Applied Physiology* **51**(3), 750–754.

Carlson, F.D. & Wilkie, D.R. (1974) *Muscle Physiology*. Prentice Hall, Englewood, NJ.

Carpenter, A. (1938) A study of angles in the measurement of the leg lift. *Research Quarterly* **9**(3), 70–72.

Casolo, F. & Lorenzi, V. (1994) Finger mathematical modeling and rehabilitation. In: *Advances in the Biomechanics of the Hand and Wrist* (eds F. Shuind, K. An, U.P. Cooney & M. Garcia-Elias), pp. 197–224. Plenum Press, New York.

Cavanagh, P.R. & Sanderson, D.J. (1986) The biomechanics of cycling. Studies on the pedaling mechanics of elite pursuit riders. In: *The Science of Cycling* (ed. E.R. Burke), pp. 91–122. Human Kinetics, Champaign, IL.

Chao, E.Y.S., An, K.N., Cooney, W.P. & Linscheid, R.L. (1989) Normative model of human hand. In: *Biomechanics of the Hand: a Basic Research Study* (eds E.Y.S. Chao, K.-N. An, W.P. Cooney & R.L. Linscheid), pp. 121–139. World Scientific Publishing Co., Singapore.

Chow, J.W. & Darling, W.G. (1999) The maximum shortening velocity of muscle should be scaled with activation. *Journal of Applied Physiology* **86**(3), 1025–1031.

Chow, J.W., Darling, W.D. & Ehrhardt, J.C. (1999) Determining the force–length–velocity relations of the quadriceps muscles: 1. Anatomical and geometric parameters. *Journal of Applied Biomechanics* **15**, 182–190.

Clarke, H.H. (1956) Recent advances in measurement and understanding of volitional muscle strength. *Research Quarterly* **27**(3), 263–275.

Clarke, D.H. (1968) Force–time curves of voluntary muscular contraction at varying tensions. *Research Quarterly* **39**(4), 900–907.

Clarke, D.H. & Henry, F.M. (1961) Neuromotor specificity and increased speed from strength development. *Research Quarterly* **32**(3), 315–325.

Cook, C.S. & McDonagh, M.J. (1996) Force responses to constant-velocity shortening of electrically stimulated human muscle–tendon complex. *Journal of Applied Physiology* **81**(1), 384–392.

Cornu, C., Almeida Silveira, M.I. & Goubel, F. (1997) Influence of plyometric training on the mechanical impedance of the human ankle joint. *European Journal of Applied Physiology* **76**(3), 282–288.

Dapena, J. (2000) The high jump. In: *Biomechanics in Sport: Performance Enhancement and Injury Prevention* (ed. V.M. Zatsiorsky), pp. 284–311. Blackwell Science, Oxford.

Darcus, H.D. (1951) The maximum torques developed in pronation and supination of the right hand. *Journal of Anatomy (London)* **85**, 55–67.

Darcus, H.D. & Salter, N. (1955) The effect of repeated muscular exertion on muscle strength. *Journal of Physiology (London)* **129**, 325–336.

Davies, C.T. & Young, K. (1984) Effects of external loading on short term power output in children and young male adults. *European Journal of Applied Physiology and Occupational Physiology* **52**(3), 351–354.

Davies, C.T. & Young, K. (1985) Mechanical power output in children aged 11 and 14 years. *Acta Paediatrica Scandinavica* **74**(5), 760–764.

Davies, C.T., Wemyss-Holden, J. & Young, K. (1984) Measurement of short term power output: comparison between cycling and jumping. *Ergonomics* **27**(3), 285–296.

De Ruiter, C.J., Jones, D.A., Sargeant, A.J. & De Haan, A. (1999) The measurement of force/velocity relationships of fresh and fatigued human adductor pollicis muscle. *European Journal of Applied Physiology* **80**(4), 386–393.

Delp, S.L., Ringwelski, D.A. & Carroll, N.C. (1994) Transfer of the rectus femoris: effects of transfer site on moment arms about the knee and hip. *Journal of Biomechanics* **27**(10), 1201–1211.

Delp, S.L., Hess, W.E., Hungerford, D.S. & Jones, L.C. (1999) Variation of rotation moment arms with hip flexion. *Journal of Biomechanics* **32**(5), 493–501.

Dern, R.J., Levene, J.M. & Blair, H.A. (1947) Forces exerted at different velocities in human arm movements. *American Journal of Physiology* **151**, 415–437.

Desmedt, J.E. & Godaux, E. (1977) Ballistic contractions in man: Characteristic recruitment pattern of single motor units of the tibialis anterior muscle. *Journal of Physiology (London)* **264**, 673–693.

Dillman, C.J. (1994) Biomechanical contributions to the science of rehabilitation in sports. In: *Sport Biomechanics* (eds R.C. Nelson & V.M. Zatsiorsky), pp. 70–78. Human Kinetics, Champaign, IL.

Donskoi, D.D. & Zatsiorsky, V.M. (eds) (1979) *Biomechanics*. Fizkultura i Sport, Moscow.

Dostal, W.F. & Andrews, J.G. (1981) A three-dimensional biomechanical model of hip musculature. *Journal of Biomechanics* **14**(11), 803–812.

Draganich, L.F., Andriacchi, T.P. & Andersson, G.B. (1987) Interaction between intrinsic knee mechanics and the knee extensor mechanism. *Journal of Orthopaedic Research* **5**, 539–547.

Driss, T., Vandewalle, H. & Monod, H. (1998) Maximal power and force–velocity relationships during cycling and cranking exercises in volleyball players. Correlation with the vertical jump test. *Journal of Sports Medicine and Physical Fitness* **38**(4), 286–293.

Dudley, G.A. & Djamil, R. (1985) Incompatibility of endurance- and strength-training modes of exercise. *Journal of Applied Physiology* **59**(5), 1446–1451.

Encyclopaedia of Science and Technology. (1977) *Impedance, Mechanical*, p. 44. McGraw-Hill, New York.

Ettema, G.J.C., Styles, G. & Kippers, V. (1998) The moment arms of 23 muscle segments of the upper limb with varying elbow and forearm positions: Implications for motor control. *Human Movement Science* **17**(2), 201–220.

Fenn, W.O. (1938) The mechanics of muscular contraction in man. *Journal of Applied Physics* **19**, 165–177.

Fleisig, G.S., Andrews, J.R., Dillman, C.J. & Escamilla, R.F. (1995) Kinetics of baseball pitching with implications about injury mechanisms. *American Journal of Sports Medicine* **23**(7), 223–239.

Fowler, N.K., Nicol, A.C., Condon, B. & Hadley, D. (2001) Method of determination of three dimensional index finger moment arms and tendon lines of action using high resolution MRI scans. *Journal of Biomechanics* **34**(6), 791–797.

Franke, F. (1920) Die Kraftkurve menschlichen Muskeln bei willkürlichen Innnervation und die Frage der absoluten Muskelkraft. *Pflügers Archiv* **184**, 300–323.

Froese, E.A. & Houston, M.E. (1985) Torque-velocity characteristics and muscle fiber type in human vastus lateralis. *Journal of Applied Physiology* **59**, 309–314.

Fugl-Meyer, A.R., Mild, K.H. & Hornsten, J. (1982) Output of skeletal muscle contractions. a study of isokinetic plantar flexion in athletes. *Acta Physiologica Scandinavica* **115**(2), 193–199.

Fujikawa, T., Oshima, T., Kumamoto, M. & Yokoi, N. (1997) Functional coordination control of pairs of antagonistic muscles. *Transactions of the Japanese Society of Mechanical Engineers* **63**(607), 769–776.

Gardner, G. (1963) Specificity of strength changes of the exercised and nonexercised limbs following isometric training. *Research Quarterly* **34**(1), 98–101.

Gerbeaux, M., Pertuzon, E., Turpin, E. & Lensel-Corbeil, G. (1993) Determination of the length of the lever arm of the triceps brachii. *Journal of Biomechanics* **26**, 795–801.

Gillard, D.M., Yakovenko, S., Cameron, T. & Prochazka, A. (2000) Isometric muscle length–tension curves do not predict angle–torque curves of human wrist in continuous active movements. *Journal of Biomechanics* **33**(11), 1341–1348.

Godik, M.A. & Zatsiorsky, V.M. (1965) Method and the first results of the measurements of the explosive strength of the athletes. *Theory and Practice of Physical Culture* **28**(7), 22–24 [in Russian].

Gonyea, W.J., Marushia, S.A. & Dixon, J.A. (1981) Morphological organization and contractile properties of the wrist flexor muscles in the cat. *Anatomical Record* **199**(3), 321–339.

Gonzalez, H. & Hull, M.L. (1989) Multivariable optimization of cycling biomechanics. *Journal of Biomechanics* **22**(11–12), 1151–1161.

Gregor, R.J., Edgerton, V.R., Perrine, J.J., Campion, D.S. & de Bus, C. (1979) Torque–velocity relationships and muscle fiber composition in elite female athletes. *Journal of Applied Physiology* **47**, 388–392.

Grood, E.S., Suntay, W.J., Noyes, F.R. & Butler, D.L. (1984) Biomechanics of the knee-extension exercise. Effect of cutting the anterior cruciate ligament. *Journal of Bone and Joint Surgery (American)* **66**(5), 725–734.

Häkkinen, K. & Komi, P. (1985a) Changes in electrical and mechanical behavior of leg extensor muscles during heavy resistance strength training. *Scandinavian Journal of Sports Sciences* **7**, 55–64.

Häkkinen, K. & Komi, P. (1985b) Effect of explosive type strength training on electromyographic and force production characteristics of leg extensor muscles during concentric and various stretch-shortening cycle exercise. *Scandinavian Journal of Sports Sciences* **7**, 65–75.

Hardyk, A.T. (2000) Force– and power–velocity relationships in a multi-joint movement. PhD dissertation The Pennsylvania State University.

Hautier, C.A., Linossier, M.T., Belli, A., Lacour, J.R. & Arsac, L.M. (1996) Optimal velocity for maximal power production in non-isokinetic cycling is related to muscle fibre type composition. *European Journal of Applied Physiology* **74**(1–2), 114–118.

Hawkins, D. (1992) Software for determining lower extremity muscle–tendon kinematics and moment arm lengths during flexion/extension movements. *Computers in Biology and Medicine* **22**(1–2), 59–71.

Hawkins, D. & Smeudlers, M. (1999) An investigation of the relationship between hip extension torque, hip extension velocity, and muscle activation. *Journal of Applied Biomechanics* **15**(3), 253–269.

Hay, J.G. (2000) Length changes of muscle–tendon units during athletic movements. In: *Biomechanics and Biology of Movement* (eds B.M. Nigg, B.R. Macintosh & J. Mester), pp. 31–47. Human Kinetics, Champaign, IL.

Hennemann, E., Somjen, G. & Carpenter, D.O. (1965) Functional significance of cell size in spinal motoneurons. *Journal of Physiology* **28**, 560–580.

Henry, F.M. (1960) Factorial structure of speed and static strength in a lateral arm movement. *Research Quarterly* **31**(3), pp. 221–228.

Henry, F.M. & Trafton, I.R. (1951) The velocity curve of sprint running with some observation on the muscle viscosity factor. *Research Quarterly* **22**(4), 409–422.

Herrmann, A.M. & Delp, S.L. (1999) Moment arm and force-generating capacity of the extensor carpi ulnaris after transfer to the extensor carpi radialis brevis. *Journal of Hand Surgery (American)* **24**(5), 1083–1090.

Herzog, W. & Read, L. (1993) Lines of action and moment arms of the major force carrying structures crossing the human knee joint. *Journal of Anatomy* **182**, 213–230.

Herzog, W., Abrahamse, S.K. & ter Keurs, H.E. (1990) Theoretical determination of force–length relations of intact human skeletal muscles using the cross-bridge model. *Pflügers Archiv* **416**(1–2), 113–119.

Herzog, W., Guimaraes, A.C., Anton, M.G. & Carter-Erdman, K.A. (1991) Moment–length relations of rectus femoris muscles of speed skaters/cyclists and runners. *Medicine and Science in Sports and Exercise* **23**(11), 1289–1296.

Hill, A.V. (1922) The maximum work and mechanical efficiency of human muscles, and their most economical speed. *Journal of Physiology* **56**, 19–41. [Note. The paper is reprinted in Latash, M.L. & Zatsiorsky, V.M. (eds) (2001) *Classics in Movement Science.* Human Kinetics, Champaign, IL.]

Hill, A.V. (1938) The heat of shortening and the dynamic constants of muscle. *Proceedings of the Royal Society of London* **126-B**, 136–195.

Hill, A.V. (1949) The abrupt transition from rest to activity in muscle. *Proceedings of the Royal Society of London* **136-B**, 405–420.

Hogan, N. (1990) Mechanical impedance of single- and multi-articular systems. In: *Multiple Muscle Systems* (eds J.M. Winters & S.L.Y. Woo), pp. 149–164. Springer-Verlag, New York.

Hortobágyi, T., Hill, J.P., Houmard, J.A., Fraser, D.D., Lambert, N.J. & Israel, R.G. (1996) Adaptive responses to muscle lengthening and shortening in humans. *Journal of Applied Physiology* **80**(3), 765–772.

Houtz, S.J., Lebow, M.J. & Beyer, F.R. (1957) Effect of posture on strength of the knee flexor and extensor muscles. *Journal of Applied Physiology* **11**(3), 475–480.

Hoy, M.G., Zajac, F.E. & Gordon, M.E. (1990) A musculoskeletal model of the human lower extremity: the effect of muscle, tendon, and moment arm on the moment–angle relationship of musculotendon actuators at the hip, knee, and ankle. *Journal of Biomechanics* **23**(2), 157–169.

Hughes, R.E., Niebur, G., Liu, J. & An, K.N. (1998) Comparison of two methods for computing abduction moment arms of the rotator cuff. *Journal of Biomechanics* **31**(2), 157–160.

Hugh-Jones, P. (1947) The effect of limb position in seated subjects on their ability to utilize the maximum contractile force of the limb muscles. *Journal of Physiology (London)* **105**, 332–344.

Hull, M.L. & Gonzalez, H. (1988) Bivariate optimization of pedalling rate and crank arm length in cycling. *Journal of Biomechanics* **21**(10), 839–849.

Huxley, A.F. (1957) Muscle structure and theories of contraction. *Progress in Biophysics and Biophysical Chemistry* **7**, 255–318.

Huxley, A.F. (2000) Cross-bridge action: Present views, prospects and unknowns. In: *Skeletal Muscle Mechanics: from Mechanisms to Function* (ed. W. Herzog), pp. 7–32. John Wiley & Sons, Chichester.

Ikai, M. & Fukunaga, T. (1970) A study on training effect on strength per unit cross-sectional area of muscle by means of ultrasonic measurement. *Internationale Zeitschrift für Angewandte Physiologie* **28**(3), 173–180.

van Ingen Schenau, G.J. (1989) From rotation to translation: Constraints on multi-joint movements and the unique action of bi-articular muscles. *Human Movement Science* **8**, 301–337.

Ito, M., Akima, H. & Fukunaga, T. (2000) In vivo moment arm determination using B-mode ultrasonography. *Journal of Biomechanics* **33**(2), 215–218.

Jensen, R.H. & Davy, D.T. (1975) An investigation of muscle lines of action about the hip: a centroid line approach vs. straight line approach. *Journal of Biomechanics* **8**, 103–110.

Johansson, C., Lorentzon, R., Sjostrom, M., Fagerlund, M. & Fugl-Meyer, A.R. (1987) Sprinters and marathon runners. Does isokinetic knee extensor performance reflect muscle size and structure? *Acta Physiologica Scandinavica* **130**(4), 663–669.

Jørgensen, K. (1976) Force–velocity relationships in human elbow flexors and extensors. In: *Biomechanics* V-A (ed. P. Komi), pp. 145–151. University Park Press, Baltimore.

Jørgensen, K. & Bankov, S. (1971) Maximum strength of elbow flexors with pronated and supinated forearm. In: *Biomechanics* II (eds J. Vredenbregt & J. Wartenweiler), pp. 174–180. Karger, Basel.

Kanehisa, H. & Miyashita, M. (1983) Specificity of velocity in strength training. *European Journal of Applied Physiology and Occupational Physiology* **52**(1), 104–106.

Kanehisa, H., Ikegawa, S. & Fukunaga, T. (1997) Force–velocity relationships and fatiguability of strength and endurance-trained subjects. *International Journal of Sports Medicine* **18**(2), 106–112.

Kawakami, Y., Ichinose, Y. & Fukunaga, T. (1998) Architectural and functional features of human triceps surae muscles during contraction. *Journal of Applied Physiology* **85**(2), 398–404.

Kawakami, Y., Kumagai, K., Huijing, P.A., Hijikata, T. & Fukunaga, T. (2000) The length–force characteristics of human gastrocnemius and soleus muscles in vivo. In: *Skeletal Muscle Mechanics: from Mechanisms to Function* (ed. W. Herzog), pp. 327–341. John Wiley & Sons, Chichester.

Kellis, E. & Baltzopoulos, V. (1999) In vivo determination of the patella tendon and hamstrings moment arms in adult males using videofluoroscopy during submaximal knee extension and flexion [in process citation]. *Clinical Biomechanics* **14**(2), 118–124.

King, D.L. (2000) Jumping in figure skating. In: *Biomechanics in Sport* (ed. V.M. Zatsiorsky), pp. 312–325. Blackwell Science, Oxford.

Kirkendall, D.T. (1985) The applied sport science of soccer. *Physician and Sports Medicine* **134**, 53–59.

Klein, P., Mattys, S. & Rooze, M. (1996) Moment arm length variations of selected muscles acting on talocrural and subtalar joints during movement: an *in vitro* study. *Journal of Biomechanics* **29**(1), 21–30.

Kojima, T. (1991) Force–velocity relationship of human elbow flexors in voluntary isotonic contraction under heavy loads. *International Journal of Sports Medicine* **12**(2), 208–213.

Komi, P.V. (1973) Relationship between muscle tension, EMG, and velocity of contraction under concentric and eccentric work. In: *New Developments in Electromyography and Clinical Neurophysiology* (ed. J.E. Desmedt), pp. 596–606. Karger, Basel.

Komi, P.V. (1990) Relevance of in vivo force measurements to human biomechanics. *Journal of Biomechanics* **23** (Suppl. 1), 23–34.

Komi, P.V. & Virmavirta, M. (2000) Determinants of successful ski-jumping performance. In: *Biomechanics in Sport* (ed. V.M. Zatsiorsky), pp. 349–362. Blackwell Science, Oxford.

de Koning, F.L., Binkhorst, R.A., Vos, J.A. & van't Hof, M.A. (1985) The force–velocity relationship of arm flexion in untrained males and females and arm-trained athletes. *European Journal of Applied Physiology and Occupational Physiology* **54**(1), 89–94.

de Koning, F.L., van't Hof, M.A., Binkhorst, R.A. & Vos, J.A. (1986) Parameters of the force–velocity curve of human muscle in relation to body dimensions. *Human Biology* **58**(2), 221–238.

Kraemer, W.J., Fleck, S.J. & Evans, W.J. (1996) Strength and power training: physiological mechanisms of adaptation. *Exercise and Sport Sciences Reviews* **24**, 363–398.

Kraemer, W.J., Mazetti, S.A., Ratamess, N.A. & Fleck, S.J. (2000) Specificity of training modes. In: *Isokinetics in Human Performance* (ed. L.E. Brown), pp. 25–41. Human Kinetics, Champaign, IL.

Kuechle, D.K., Newman, S.R., Itoi, E., Niebur, G.L., Morrey, B.F. & An, K.N. (2000) The relevance of the moment arm of shoulder muscles with respect to axial rotation of the glenohumeral joint in four positions. *Clinical Biomechanics (Bristol, Avon)* **15**(5), 322–329.

Kues, J.M. & Mayhew, T.P. (1996) Concentric and eccentric force–velocity relationships during electrically induced submaximal contractions. *Physiotherapy Research International* **1**(3), 195–204.

Kulig, K., Andrews, J.G. & Hay, J.G. (1984) Human strength curves. *Exercise and Sport Sciences Reviews* **12**, 417–466.

Lanka, J. (2000) Shot putting. In: *Biomechanics in Sport* (ed. V.M. Zatsiorsky), pp. 435–457. Blackwell Science, Oxford.

Lemay, M.A. & Crago, P.E. (1996) A dynamic model for simulating movements of the elbow, forearm and wrist. *Journal of Biomechanics* **29**(10), 1319–1330.

Lengsfeld, M., Pressel, T. & Stammberger, U. (1997) Lengths and lever arms of hip joint muscles: geometrical analyses using a human multibody model. *Gait and Posture* **6**, 18–26.

Lesmes, G.R., Costill, D.L., Coyle, E.F. & Fink, W.J. (1978) Muscle strength and power changes during maximal isokinetic training. *Medicine and Science in Sports* **10**(4), 266–269.

Levertin, A. (ed.) (1893) *Dr Gustav Zander's Medico-Mechanical Gymnastics*. Stockholm.

Li, Z.M., Latash, M.L. & Zatsiorsky, V.M. (1998a) Force sharing among fingers as a model of the redundancy problem. *Experimental Brain Research* **119**(3), 276–286.

Li, Z.M., Latash, M.L., Newell, K.M. & Zatsiorsky, V.M. (1998b) Motor redundancy during maximal voluntary contraction in four-finger tasks. *Experimental Brain Research* **122**(1), 71–77.

Lieber, R.L. & Fridén, J. (1998) Musculoskeletal balance of the human wrist elucidated using intraoperative laser diffraction. *Journal of Electromyography and Kinesiology* **8**(2), 93–100.

Lieber, R.L., Loren, G.L. & Fridén, J. (1994) *In vivo* measurement of human wrist extensor muscle sarcomere length changes. *Journal of Neurophysiology* **71**, 874–881.

Lieber, R.L., Ljung, B.O. & Fridén, J. (1997) Intraoperative sarcomere length measurements reveal differential design of human wrist extensor muscles. *Journal of Experimental Biology* **200**(1), 19–25.

Loren, G.J., Shoemaker, S.D., Burkholder, T.J., Jacobson, M.D., Friden, J. & Lieber, R.L. (1996) Human wrist motors: biomechanical design and application to tendon transfers. *Journal of Biomechanics* **29**(3), 331–342.

MacIntosh, B.R., Neptune, R.R. & Horton, J.F. (2000) Cadence, power, and muscle activation in cycle ergometry. *Medicine and Science in Sports and Exercise* **32**(7), 1281–1287.

Maganaris, C.N. (2000) In vivo measurement-based estimations of the moment arm in the human tibialis anterior muscle–tendon unit. *Journal of Biomechanics* **33**(3), 375–379.

Maganaris, C.N., Baltzopoulos, V. & Sargeant, A.J. (1998) Changes in Achilles tendon moment arm from rest to maximum isometric plantarflexion: in vivo observations in man. *Journal of Physiology* **510**(3), 977–985.

Maganaris, C.N., Baltzopoulos, V. & Sargeant, A.J. (1999) Changes in the tibialis anterior tendon moment arm from rest to maximum isometric dorsiflexion: in vivo observations in man. *Clinical Biomechanics* **14**(9), 661–666.

Maganaris, C.N., Baltzopoulos, V. & Sargeant, A.J. (2000) In vivo measurement-based estimations of the human Achilles tendon moment arm. *European Journal of Applied Physiology* **83**(4–5), 363–369.

Mansour, J.M. & Pereira, J.M. (1987) Quantitative functional anatomy of the lower limb with application to human gait. *Journal of Biomechanics* **20**(1), 51–58.

Marsh, A.P., Martin, P.E. & Sanderson, D.J. (2000) Is a joint moment-based cost function associated with preferred cycling cadence? *Journal of Biomechanics* **33**(2), 173–180.

Marshall, R.N., Mazur, S.M. & Taylor, N.A. (1990) Three-dimensional surfaces for human muscle kinetics. *European Journal of Applied Physiology* **61**(3–4), 263–270.

Martin, A., Martin, L. & Morlon, B. (1995) Changes induced by eccentric training on force–velocity relationships of the elbow flexor muscles. *European Journal of Applied Physiology and Occupational Physiology* **72**(1–2), 183–185.

Mero, A. & Komi, P.V. (1986) Force–, EMG–, and elasticity–velocity relationships at submaximal, maximal and supramaximal running speeds in sprinters. *European Journal of Applied Physiology* **55**, 553–561.

Miller, D.I. (2000) Springboard and platform diving. In: *Biomechanics in Sport* (ed. V.M. Zatsiorsky), pp. 326–348. Blackwell Science, Oxford.

Mundale, M.O. (1970) The relationship of intermittent isometric exercise to fatigue of hand grip. *Archives of Physical Medicine and Rehabilitation* **51**, 532–539.

Murray, W.M., Delp, S.L. & Buchanan, T.S. (1995) Variation of muscle moment arms with elbow and forearm position. *Journal of Biomechanics* **28**(5), 513–525.

Murray, W.M., Buchanan, T.S. & Delp, S.L. (2000) The isometric functional capacity of muscles that cross the elbow. *Journal of Biomechanics* **33**(8), 943–952.

Nakajima, T., Liu, J., Hughes, R.E., O'Driscoll, S. & An, K.N. (1999) Abduction moment arm of transposed subscapularis tendon. *Clinical Biomechanics* **14**(4), 265–270.

Nemeth, G. & Ohlsen, H. (1985) In vivo moment arm lengths for hip extensor muscles at different angles of hip flexion. *Journal of Biomechanics* **18**(2), 129–140.

Nemeth, G. & Ohlsen, H. (1986) Moment arm lengths of trunk muscles to the lumbosacral joint obtained in vivo with computed tomography. *Spine* **11**(2), 158–160.

Nemeth, G. & Ohlsen, H. (1987) Moment arm lengths of the erector spinae and rectus abdominis muscles obtained *in vivo* with computed tomography. In: *Biomechanics* X-A (ed. B. Jonsson), pp. 189–194. Human Kinetics, Champaign, IL.

Nisell, R. (1985) Mechanics of the knee. *Acta Orthopaedica Scandinavica* **56** (Suppl. 216), 5–41.

Nisell, R., Nemeth, G. & Ohlsen, H. (1986) Joint forces in extension of the knee. *Acta Orthopaedica Scandinavica* **57**, 41–46.

O'Hagan, F.T., Sale, D.G., MacDougall, J.D. & Garner, S.H. (1995) Response to resistance training in young women and men. *International Journal of Sports Medicine* **16**(5), 314–321.

Omokawa, S., Ryu, J., Tang, J.B., Han, J. & Kish, V.L. (2000) Trapeziometacarpal joint instability affects the moment arms of thumb motor tendons. *Clinical Orthopaedics* **372**, 262–271.

Otis, J.C., Jiang, C.C., Wickiewicz, T.L., Peterson, M.G., Warren, R.F. & Santner, T.J. (1994) Changes in the moment arms of the rotator cuff and deltoid muscles with abduction and rotation. *Journal of Bone and Joint Surgery (American)* **76**(5), 667–676.

Pandy, M.G. (1999) Moment arm of a muscle force. *Exercise and Sport Sciences Reviews* **27**, 79–118.

Perrine, J.J. & Edgerton, V.R. (1978) Muscle force–velocity and power–velocity relationships under isokinetic loading. *Medicine and Science in Sports* **10**(3), 159–166.

Pertuzon, E. (1972) *La contraction musculaire dans le mouvement volontaire maximal*. PhD thesis, Lille.

Pertuzon, E. & Bouisset, S. (1971) Maximum velocity of movement and maximum velocity of muscle shortening. In: *Biomechanics* II (eds J. Vredenbregt & J. Wartenweiler), pp. 170–173. Karger, Basel.

Pigeon, P., Yahia, L. & Feldman, A.G. (1996) Moment arms and lengths of human upper limb muscles as functions of joint angles. *Journal of Biomechanics* **29**(10), 1365–1370.

Poppen, N.K. & Walker, P.S. (1978) Forces at the glenohumeral joint in abduction. *Clinical Orthopaedics and Related Research* **135**, 165–170.

Prietto, C.A. & Caiozzo, V.J. (1989) The in vivo force–velocity relationship of the knee flexors and extensors. *American Journal of Sports Medicine* **17**(5), 607–611.

Rahmani, A., Belli, A., Kostka, T., Dalleau, G., Bonnefoy, M. & Lacour, J.R. (1999) Evaluation of knee extensor muscles under non-isokinetic conditions in elderly subjects. *Journal of Applied Biomechanics* **15**(3), 337–344.

Rahmani, A., Viale, F., Dalleau, G. & Lacour, J.R. (2001) Force/velocity and power/velocity relationships in squat exercise. *European Journal of Applied Physiology* **84**(3), 227–232.

Ralston, H.J., Inman, V.T., Strait, L.A. & Shaffrath, M.D. (1947) Mechanics of human isolated voluntary muscle. *American Journal of Physiology* **151**, 612–620.

Ralston, H.J., Polossar, M.J., Inman, V.T., Close, J.R. & Feinstein, B. (1949) Dynamic features of human isolated voluntary muscle in isometric and free contractions. *Journal of Applied Physiology* **1**, 526–533.

Rasch, P.J. (1954) Relationship of arm strength, weight and length to speed of arm movement. *Research Quarterly* **25**(3), 333–337.

Rasch, P.J. (1956) Effect of position of forearm on strength of elbow flexion. *Research Quarterly* **27**(3), 333–337.

Reid, J.G., Livingston, L.A. & Pearsall, D.J. (1994) The geometry of the psoas muscle as determined by magnetic resonance imaging. *Archives of Physical Medicine and Rehabilitation* **75**(6), 703–708.

Reijs, J.H.O. (1921) Über die Veränderung der Kraff wärend der Bewegung. *Pflügers Archiv* **191**, 234–257.

Rugg, S.G., Gregor, R.J., Mandelbaum, B.R. & Chiu, L. (1990) In vivo moment arm calculations at the ankle using magnetic resonance imaging (MRI). *Journal of Biomechanics* **23**(5), 495–501.

Rutherford, O.M. & Jones, D.A. (1986) The role of learning and coordination in strength training. *European Journal of Applied Physiology and Occupational Physiology* **55**(1), 100–105.

Sale, D., Quinlan, J., Marsh, E., McComas, A.J. & Belanger, A.Y. (1982) Influence of joint position on ankle plantarflexion in humans. *Journal of Applied Physiology* **52**(6), 1636–1642.

Salter, N. & Darcus, H.D. (1952) The effect of the degree of elbow flexion on the maximum torques developed in pronation and supination of the right hand. *Journal of Anatomy (London)* **86**, 197–202.

Sargeant, A.J., Hoinville, E. & Young, A. (1981) Maximum leg force and power output during short-term dynamic exercise. *Journal of Applied Physiology* **51**(5), 1175–1182.

Savelberg, H.H.C.M. (2000) Rise and relaxation times of twitches and tetani in submaximally recruited, mixed muscle: A computer model. In: *Skeletal Muscle Mechanics: from Mechanisms to Function* (ed. W. Herzog), pp. 225–240. John Wiley & Sons, Ltd., Chichester.

Seger, J.Y. & Thorstensson, A. (2000) Muscle strength and electromyogram in boys and girls followed through puberty. *European Journal of Applied Physiology* **81**(1–2), 54–61.

Seger, J.Y., Ovendal, A. & Thortstensson, A. (1999) Voluntary and electrically evoked torque–velocity curves are not congruent. *Journal of Sports Sciences* **17**(7), 533–535.

Siegler, S., Moskowitz, G.D. & Freedman, W. (1984) Passive and active components of the internal moment developed about the ankle joint during human ambulation. *Journal of Biomechanics* **17**, 647–652.

Smidt, G.L. (1973) Biomechanical analysis of knee flexion and extension. *Journal of Biomechanics* **6**, 79–92.

Smith, E.M., Juvinall, R.C., Bender, L.F. & Pearson, J.R. (1964) Role of the finger flexors in rheumatoid deformities of the metacarpophalangeal joints. *Arthritis and Rheumatism* **7**, 467–480.

Smutz, W.P., Kongsayreepong, A., Hughes, R.E., Niebur, G., Cooney, W.P. & An, K.N. (1998) Mechanical advantage of the thumb muscles. *Journal of Biomechanics* **31**(6), 565–570.

van Soest, O. & Casius, L.J. (2000) Which factors determine the optimal pedaling rate in sprint cycling? *Medicine and Science in Sports and Exercise* **32**(11), 1927–1934.

Spoor, C.W. & van Leeuwen, J.L. (1992) Knee muscle moment arms from MRI and from tendon travel. *Journal of Biomechanics* **25**(2), 201–206.

Spoor, C.W., van Leeuwen, J.L., Meskers, C.G., Titulaer, A.F. & Huson, A. (1990) Estimation of instantaneous moment arms of lower-leg muscles. *Journal of Biomechanics* **23**(12), 1247–1259. [Note: Comment in *Journal of Biomechanics* (1991) **24**(9), 870.]

Thomis, M.A., Beunen, G.P., Van Leemputte, M. *et al.* (1998) Inheritance of static and dynamic arm strength and some of its determinants. *Acta Physiologica Scandinavica* **163**(1), 59–71.

Thorstensson, A. (1977) Observations on strength training and detraining. *Acta Physiologica Scandinavica* **100**(4), 491–493.

Thorstensson, A., Grimby, G. & Karlsson, J. (1976) Force–velocity relations and fiber composition in human knee extensor muscles. *Journal of Applied Physiology* **40**(1), 12–16.

Tihanyi, J., Apor, P. & Fekete, G. (1982) Force–velocity–power characteristics and fiber composition in human knee extensor muscles. *European Journal of Applied Physiology* **48**(3), 331–343.

Tsuji, T. (1997) Human arm impedance in multi-joint movement. In: *Self-Organization, Computational Maps, and Motor Control* (eds P. Morasso & V. Sanguineti), pp. 357–382. Elsevier Science B.V., Amsterdam.

Tsuji, T., Morasso, P.G., Goto, K. & Ito, K. (1995) Human arm impedance characteristics during maintained posture. *Biological Cybernetics* **72**, 475–485.

Van Cutsem, M., Duchateau, J. & Hainaut, K. (1998) Changes in single motor unit behaviour contribute to the increase in contraction speed after dynamic training in humans. *Journal of Physiology* **513**(1), 295–305.

Van der Helm, F.C. & Veenbaas, R. (1991) Modelling the mechanical effect of muscles with large attachment sites: application to the shoulder mechanism. *Journal of Biomechanics* **24**(12), 1151–1163.

Verchoshansky, Y.V. (ed.) (1977) *Special Strength Training in Sport*. Fizkultura i Sport, Moscow.

Viitasalo, J.T. (1985) Effects of training on force–velocity characteristics. In: *Biomechanics* IX-A (ed. D.A. Winter, R.W. Norman, R.P. Wells, L.C. Hayes & A.E. Patla), pp. 91–95. Human Kinetics, Champaign, IL.

Viitasalo, J.T. & Komi, P.V. (1978) Force–time characteristics and fiber composition in human leg extensor muscles. *European Journal of Applied Physiology and Occupational Physiology* **40**(1), 7–15.

Viitasalo, J.T. & Komi, P.V. (1981) Interrelationships between electromyographic, mechanical, muscle structure and reflex time measurements in man. *Acta Physiologica Scandinavica* **111**(1), 97–103.

Visser, J.J., Hoogkamer, J.E., Bobbert, M.F. & Huijing, P.A. (1990) Length and moment arm of human leg muscles as a function of knee and hip-joint angles. *European Journal of Applied Physiology and Occupational Physiology* **61**(5–6), 453–460.

Vrahas, M.S., Brand, R.A., Brown, T.D. & Andrews, J.G. (1990) Contribution of passive tissues to the intersegmental moments at the hip. *Journal of Biomechanics* **23**(4), 357–362.

Wagner, R. (1925) Über die Zusammenarbeit der Antagonisten bei der Wilkürbewegung. I. Abhängigkeit von mechanischen Bedingungen. *Zeitschrift für Biologie* **83**, 59.

Wakayama, A., Yanagi, H., Matsui, H., Sugita, M. & Fukashiro, S. (1995) Force–velocity curves of knee extensor and flexor in elite runners. In: *XVth Congress of the International Society of Biomechanics* (eds K. Häkkinen, K.L. Kekkinen, P.V. Komi & A. Mero), pp. 978–979. Juvaskyla, Finland.

Weis, E.B., Jr & Primiano, F.P. (1966) The motion of the human center of mass and its relationship to mechanical impedance. *Human Factors* **8**, 399–406.

Weiss, L.W. (2000) Multiple-joint performance over a velocity spectrum. In: *Isokinetics in Human Performance* (ed. L.E. Brown), pp. 196–208. Human Kinetics, Champaign, IL.

Westing, S.H., Seger, J.Y., Karlson, E. & Ekblom, B. (1988) Eccentric and concentric torque-velocity characteristics of the quadriceps femoris in man. *European Journal of Applied Physiology* **58**, 100–104.

Wilkie, D.R. (1950) The relation between force and velocity in human muscle. *Journal of Physiology (London)* **110**, 249–280.

Wilkie, D.R. (1956) The mechanical properties of muscle. *British Medical Bulletin* **12**(3), 177–182.

Wilkie, D.R. (1967) *Muscle*. Edward Arnold Ltd, London.

Wilson, G.J., Murphy, A.J. & Walshe, A. (1996) The specificity of strength training: the effect of posture. *European Journal of Applied Physiology and Occupational Physiology* **73**(3–4), 346–352.

Wilson, D.L., Zhu, Q., Duerk, J.L., Mansour, J.M., Kilgore, K. & Crago, P.E. (1999) Estimation of tendon moment arms from three-dimensional magnetic resonance images. *Annals of Biomedical Engineering* **27**(2), 247–256.

Winters, J.M. & Kleweno, D.G. (1993) Effect of initial upper-limb alignment on muscle contributions to isometric strength curves. *Journal of Biomechanics* **26**(2), 143–153.

Winters, J.M., Stark, L. & Seif-Naraghi, A.H. (1988) An analysis of the sources of muscle–joint impedance. *Journal of Biomechanics* **21**, 1011–1025.

Wood, J.E., Meek, S.G. & Jacobsen, S.G. (1989) Quantitation of human shoulder anatomy for prosthetic arm control—II. Anatomy matrices. *Journal of Biomechanics* **22**, 309–325.

van der Woude, L.H.V., Veeger, H.E.J. & Dallmeijer, A.J. (2000) Manual wheelchair propulsion. In: *Biomechanics in Sport: Performance Enhancement and Injury Prevention* (ed. V.M. Zatsiorsky), pp. 609–636. Blackwell Science, Oxford.

Yoshihuku, Y. & Herzog, W. (1996) Maximal muscle power output in cycling: a modelling approach. *Journal of Sports Science* **14**(2), 139–157.

Young, W. (1995) Laboratory strength assessment of athletes. *New Studies in Athletics* **10**, 89–96.

Young, W., McLean, B. & Ardagna, J. (1995) Relationship between strength qualities and sprinting performance. *Journal of Sports Medicine and Physical Fitness* **35**(1), 13–19.

Zander, G. (1879) *L'Etablissement de Gymnastique Médicale Méchanique*. Paris.

Zatsiorsky, V.M. (ed.) (1966) *Motor Abilities of Athletes*. Fizkultura i Sport, Moscow. [The book is also available in German, Italian, Japanese and other languages.]

Zatsiorsky, V.M. (1974) Studies of motion and motor abilities of sportsmen. In: *Biomechanics* IV (eds R.C. Nelson & C.A. Morehouse), pp. 273–275. University Park Press, Baltimore.

Zatsiorsky, V.M. (1995) *Science and Practice of Strength Training*, 1st edn. Human Kinetics, Champaign, IL.

Zatsiorsky, V.M. (1997) The review is nice. I disagree with it. *Journal of Applied Biomechanics* **13**(4), 479–483.

Zatsiorsky, V.M. (1998) *Kinematics of Human Motion*. Human Kinetics, Champaign, IL.

Zatsiorsky, V.M. (2002) *Kinetics of Human Motion*. Human Kinetics, Champaign, IL.

Zatsiorsky, V.M. & Matveev, E.N. (1964) Force–velocity relations in throwing. *Theory and Practice of Physical Culture* **27**(8), 24–28.

Zatsiorsky, V.M. & Primakov, Y.N. (1969) Dynamics of start acceleration phase in sprint running and determining factors. *Theory and Practice of Physical Culture* **32**(7), 5–11 [in Russian]. [The paper was also translated and published in French: Zaciorski, W.M. & Primakov, Y.N. (1970) Dinamique de l'acceleration de deport du course et ses facteurs leur determination. *Kinanthropologie* **2**(1), 69–85.]

Zatsiorsky, V.M. & Raitsin, L.M. (1974) Transfer of the results of training in strength exercises. *Theory and Practice of Physical Culture* **6**, 8–14 [in Russian]. [The paper is also available in German: Zaciorskij, W.M. & Raitsin, L.M. (1975) Die Ubertragung des kumulativen Trainingseffects bei Kraftubungen. *Theorie und Praxis der Korperkultur* **24**(9), S826–834.]

Zatsiorsky, V.M. & Smirnov, Y.I. (1968) The effect of force gradient on the performance in speed–strength tasks. *Theory and Practice of Physical Culture* **31**(7), 63–68 [in Russian].

Zatsiorsky, V.M., Smirnov, Y.I. & Micheev, A.I. (1967) The effects of the isometric training at the various joint angles on the strength and velocity of movements. *Theory and Practice of Physical Culture* **30**(11), 24–27 [in Russian].

Zatsiorsky, V.M., Kulik, N.G. & Smirnov, Y.I. (1968–1969). The study of the relationships between the motor abilities. *Theory and Practice of Physical Culture*, Part 1 1968, **31**(12), 35–48; Part 2 1969, **32**(1), 2–8; Part 3 1969, **2**, 28–33. [The paper is also available in German: (1) Saciorskij, W.M., Kulik, N.G. & Smirnov, Ju. I. Die Wechselbeziehungen zwischen der korperlichen Eigenschaften. *Theorie und Praxis der Korperkultur* **19**(2), S141–159; (2) Saciorskij, W.M., Kulik, N.G. & Smirnov, Ju. I. (1977) Wechselbeziehungen zwischen den motorishen Fahigkeiten. In: *Bewegungslehre Des Sports* (ed. H. Rieder). Karl Hoffmann Verlag, Schorndorf; and in Italian: Zaciorskij, W.M., Kulik, N.G. & Smirnov Ju. I. (1971) Dependenze resiproche tra la capacita del fizico umano. Atletica Leggera, Gennaio, 137.]

Zatsiorsky, V.M., Aruin, A.S., Prilutsky, B.I. & Schakhnazarov, A. (1985) Determination of the arms of forces of the ankle joint muscles (m. triceps surae) by the 'biomechanical' method. *Human Physiology* **4**, 616–622.

Zoladz, J.A., Rademaker, A.C. & Sargeant, A.J. (2000) Human muscle power generating capability during cycling at different pedalling rates. *Experimental Physiology* **85**(1), 117–124.

Chapter 24

Vibration Loads: Potential for Strength and Power Development

JOACHIM MESTER, PETER SPITZENPFEIL AND ZENGYUAN YUE

Introduction

For a very long time mechanical vibration has been considered to be of influence on human well-being. In the 17th century some attention was paid to the back pain of coachmen that was attributed to the vibration of horse coaches in those days. In modern life with all its technical devices many sources of vibration on the human body can be identified. These sources range from hand-held machines such as motor-saws, which exert vibration stimuli on the hands and body, to whole-body vibration in certain transportation devices. Here a great number of different devices can be observed, for example cars, motor cycles, tractors, boats, trains, aircraft, helicopters and many more. As vibration input can be severely detrimental to health, strict rules for the chronic vibration input at various workplaces have been elaborated by work science. These rules are put down in international conventions such as in those from the International Organization for Standardization (ISO 2631).

In sport none of these rules exist, although in many sports remarkable vibration load occurs, such as in sailing, surfing, alpine skiing, inline skating, off-road biking and horseback riding. As the potential dangers of vibration must also be taken into consideration in sports, it seems strange that this field has not been very much in the focus of scientific interest so far. The amount or the intensity of vibration exposure is as unknown as potential effects of training in these sports. Recently, however, the significance of mechanical vibration for equilibrium control and strength training in sport became an issue in the scientific discussion. As in sport there is, of course, a great interest in improving performance, e.g. muscular strength and power, various studies have been carried out dealing with the effects of vibration stimuli in strength training. In this context it is important to understand better the phenomena of biomechanical and neurophysiological aspects of human vibration in order to identify potential benefits for strength and power training but at the same time to consider and prevent potential dangers.

Categories of vibration

Vibration in terms of oscillatory motion can occur in various forms. The motion is, by definition, not constant but alternately greater and less than some average value (Griffin 1994). The main categories are listed below (see Fig. 24.1). It is important to state that the description of these pure forms of categories is necessary to understand the phenomenon. While handling technical devices, the pure forms, such as a periodic, sinusoidal oscillatory motion, can be measured. In many sports, however, other forms than these occur and the whole range of various categories can be covered. In this definition shocks or impacts are also regarded as 'transient vibrations, often of a fairly random nature' (Cole 1982).

There are various possibilities for measuring vibration. For large-amplitude and low-frequency motion the simple displacement between the

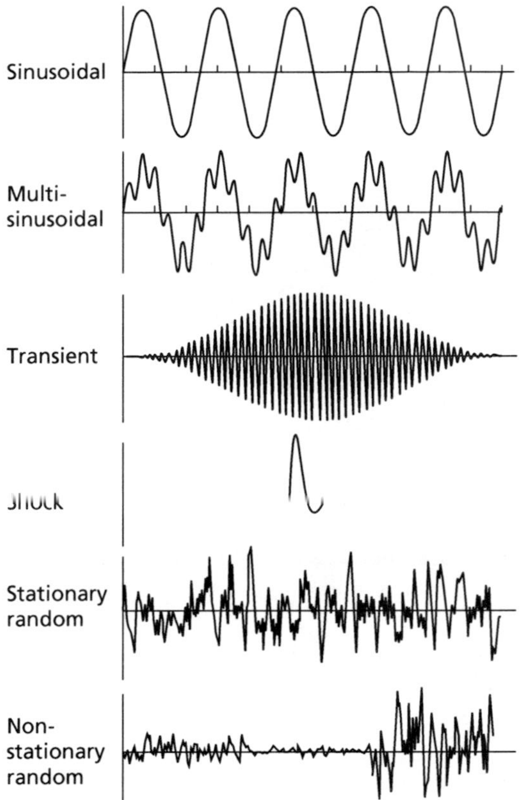

Fig. 24.1 Categories of vibration. (From Griffin 1994, with permission from Academic Press Ltd.)

two-directional peaks is used. The magnitude is normally indicated by means of the velocity or, most commonly, by the acceleration that can be expressed in terms of the peak-to-peak acceleration. As in many situations involving vibration load in sports a complex motion must be assumed where unrepresentative peaks occur, the measure of greatest use in engineering is the root mean square (r.m.s.) value (Griffin 1994). Here the root mean square acceleration ($m \cdot s^{-2}$ r.m.s.) is especially suitable for expressing the severity of human vibration exposures.

Response to vibration load

The human response to vibrations involves not only biomechanical but also physiological processes. Biomechanical considerations determine how the vibrations reach the body and propagate through the body, how each part of the body moves under given external vibration conditions, etc., while physiological approaches determine how the body reacts to these motions caused by the source of vibration. Although a tremendous amount of experimental data concerning the seat-to-head or foot-to-head transmission are available in the literature (e.g. Griffin 1994), the propagation of the vibration through the body is still poorly understood. As one example, the complexity of the topic can be seen by the fact that the frequency range of resonance, where the vibration is amplified rather than dampened, depends upon not only the part of the body, but also the position of the body and the direction of the vibration (Dupuis *et al.* 1972, 1976). It covers a range between 8 and 20 Hz depending on the organ involved.

Biomechanical response

The biomechanical response to vibration load itself is complicated because the body, of course, consists of both rigid masses and wobbling masses.

Theoretical approaches have been various spring-damper-mass models which were designed to simulate either whole-body vibration (Roberts *et al.* 1966; Anon 1971, 1978; von Gierke 1971; Sandover 1971; King 1975; Cole 1978; AGARD 1979; Ghista 1982) or running and hopping (Ferris & Farley 1977; Ito *et al.* 1983; Alexander 1988; Cavagna *et al.* 1988; Thompson & Raibert 1989; McMahon & Cheng 1990; Kim *et al.* 1994; Nigg & Anton 1994; Farley & Gonzalez 1996; Nigg & Liu 1999; Liu & Nigg 2000). These models help in the understanding of the propagation process of vibration or shock wave caused by an impact through the body. Some of the models are designed to fit certain data.

Special attention in the present section will be paid to the effects of wobbling masses on the whole-body vibration in terms of model analysis and physical reasoning. Thus it should help to contribute from a mainly theoretical background

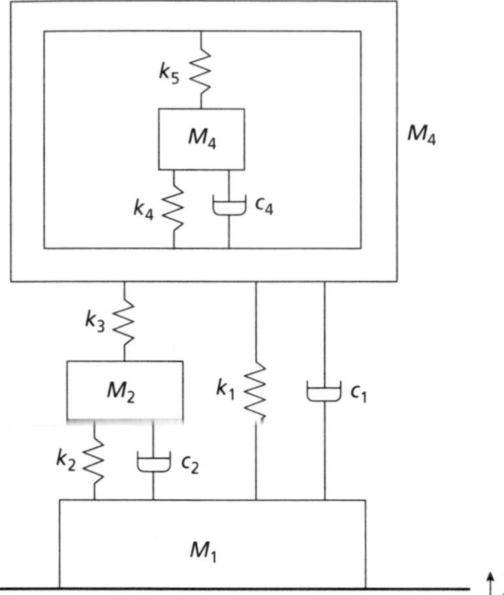

Fig. 24.2 Model A: The spring-damper-mass model used to simulate the whole-body vibrations in the present study. This model as well as the parameters in Table 24.1 are essentially the same as those used in Liu and Nigg (2000) except that the part under M_1 to simulate the ground reaction in their paper is now replaced by a vibrator to which M_1 is assumed to be fixed. M_1 and M_2 simulate the rigid and the wobbling masses of the lower body, while M_3 and M_4 simulate the rigid and the wobbling masses of the upper body. (From Liu & Nigg 2000, with permission from Elsevier Science.)

Table 24.1 The parameters (masses, spring constants and damping coefficients) of the system. (From Liu & Nigg 2000, with permission from Elsevier Science.)

M_1 (kg)	6.15
M_2 (kg)	6
M_3 (kg)	12.58
M_4 (kg)	50.34
k_1 (kN·m^{-1})	6
k_2 (kN·m^{-1})	6
k_3 (kN·m^{-1})	10
k_4 (kN·m^{-1})	10
k_5 (kN·m^{-1})	18
c_1 (kg·s^{-1})	300
c_2 (kg·s^{-1})	650
c_4 (kg·s^{-1})	1900

to the understanding of vibration and the transmission of shock waves through the body affecting the skeletal muscle and inducing adaptation stimuli (Yue *et al.* 2001).

A slightly varied version of the model of Liu and Nigg (2000) (Fig. 24.2 & Table 24.1) as a starting point is used because this model includes wobbling masses and was developed to study the effects of wobbling masses on running. Equally important is that this model was not designed just to fit existing data. Instead, the spring constants and damping coefficients in this model were determined based on the consideration of some muscle–tendon properties (Liu & Nigg 2000). Our model is used to study the effects of wobbling masses on whole-body vibrations in the situation where the subject stands on the vibrating platform with one foot, because the model was originally designed to simulate the impact during running as one foot touches the ground.

The only modification to the original model is that the part under M_1 in the original model for the simulation of the ground reaction during running is now replaced by the platform of the vibrator. We denote the vertical coordinate of the equilibrium position of the centre of mass of M_j when the system is at rest by Z_{j0}, and the vertical coordinate of the centre of mass of M_j as the system is vibrating by Z_j (t) (j = 1,2,3,4). Thus, the deviations of the centres of mass of M_j (j = 1,2,3,4) from their equilibrium positions

$$\zeta_j = Z_j - Z_{j0} \quad (j = 1,2,3,4) \tag{1}$$

satisfy the following equations:

$$M_1\ddot{\zeta}_1 = F - k_2(\zeta_1 - \zeta_2) - c_2(\dot{\zeta}_1 - \dot{\zeta}_2) - k_1(\zeta_1 - \zeta_3) - c_1(\dot{\zeta}_1 - \dot{\zeta}_3) \tag{2}$$

$$M_2\ddot{\zeta}_2 = - k_2(\zeta_2 - \zeta_1) - c_2(\dot{\zeta}_2 - \dot{\zeta}_1) - k_3(\zeta_2 - \zeta_3) \tag{3}$$

$$M_3\ddot{\zeta}_3 = - k_1(\zeta_3 - \zeta_1) - c_1(\dot{\zeta}_3 - \dot{\zeta}_1) - k_3(\zeta_3 - \zeta_2) - (k_4 + k_5)(\zeta_3 - \zeta_4) - c_4(\dot{\zeta}_3 - \dot{\zeta}_4) \tag{4}$$

$$M_4\ddot{\zeta}_4 = - (k_4 + k_5)(\zeta_4 - \zeta_3) - c_4(\dot{\zeta}_4 - \dot{\zeta}_3) \tag{5}$$

where $\dot{}$ stands for the time derivative d/dt, and

$$F = F_p - F_{p0} = F_p - (M_1 + M_2 + M_3 + M_4)g \tag{6}$$

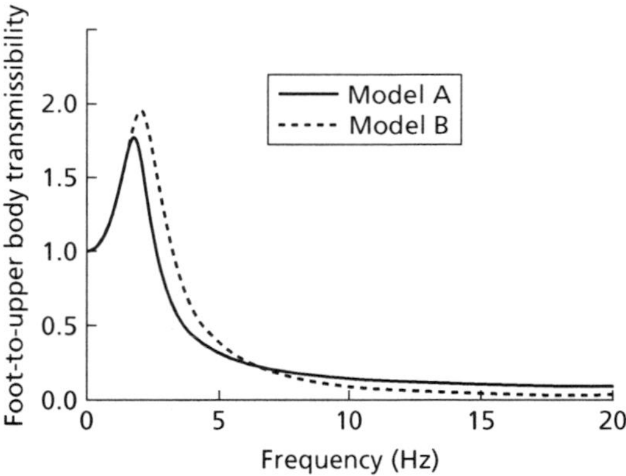

Fig. 24.3 The comparison of the foot-to-upper body transmissibility between Model A and Model B. (Figs 24.3–24.7 after Yue *et al.* 2001.)

is the total external force acting on the system, in which F_p is the pressure the platform gives to the system, $F_{p0} = (M_1 + M_2 + M_3 + M_4)g$ is the pressure of the platform in equilibrium state, g is the acceleration of gravity, and the masses M_j, spring constants k_j and damping coefficients c_j are given in Table 24.1.

Detailed vibration behaviour of this model, referred to as Model A, has been calculated and compared with the vibration behaviour of Model B, which is identical to Model A except that the wobbling mass M_4 is removed and merged into the rigid mass M_3. Some effects of wobbling mass can then be seen by the comparison between the two models.

From Fig. 24.3 it is seen that the foot-to-upper body transmissibility is reduced due to the wobbling mass for the frequency range in which the transmission is important. This reduction can be understood in terms of the power analysis as follows. It is easy to show that the average power which the wobbling mass M_4 gives to the rigid mass M_3 is

$$<P_{43}> = \tfrac{1}{2}\omega(k_4 + k_5)\,|A_3|\,|A_4|\,\sin(\varphi_4 - \varphi_3) \qquad (7)$$

Since φ_4 is smaller than φ_3 (see Fig. 24.4b), $<P_{43}>$ is negative. This explains why the amplitude of the oscillation of M_3 is reduced by the wobbling mass M_4. The fact that the phase of the wobbling

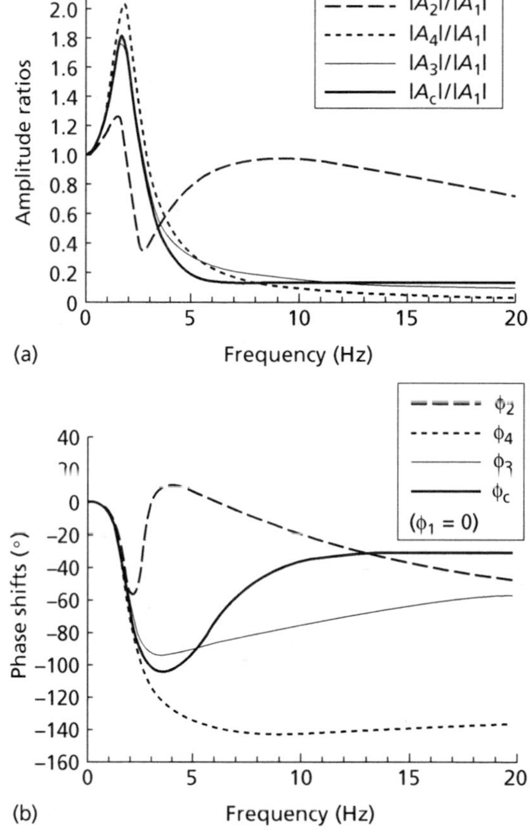

Fig. 24.4 (a) The amplitude ratios for Model A. (b) The phase shifts for Model A.

mass M_4 lags behind the phase of the rigid mass M_3 can also be seen in Fig. 24.5(a,b) where ζ_4 (t), the displacement of M_4, reaches the peak always later than ζ_3 (t), the displacement of M_3, does. The physical reason is that the vibration of the wobbling mass M_4 is carried by the vibration of the rigid mass M_3. This is also true for the real human body, in which all the internal organs and the skeletal muscles are carried by the skeleton of the body and therefore the phase of the wobbling mass lags behind the phase of the corresponding rigid mass during the whole-body vibration. Thus, we expect that the effects of the wobbling mass on the whole-body vibration we get from the present model analysis are also true for the

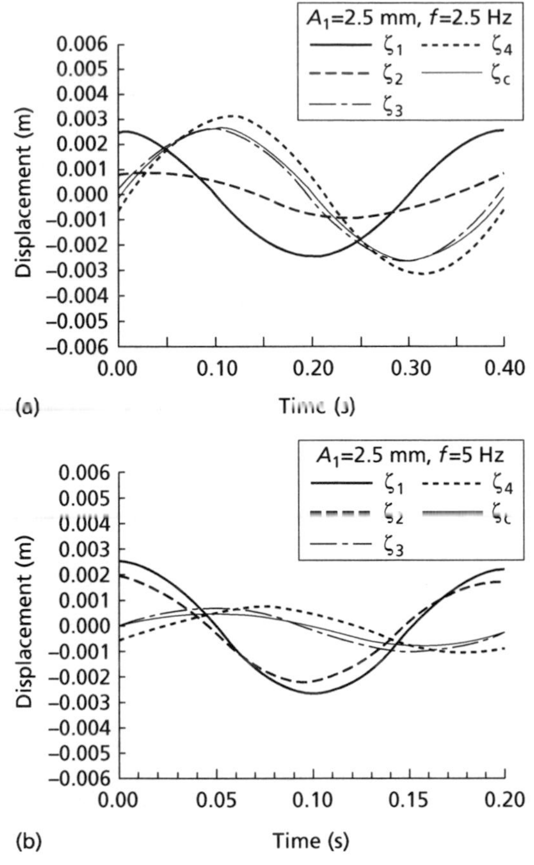

Fig. 24.5 Displacements vs. time at different frequencies for Model A: (a) $f = 2.5$ Hz; (b) $f = 5$ Hz.

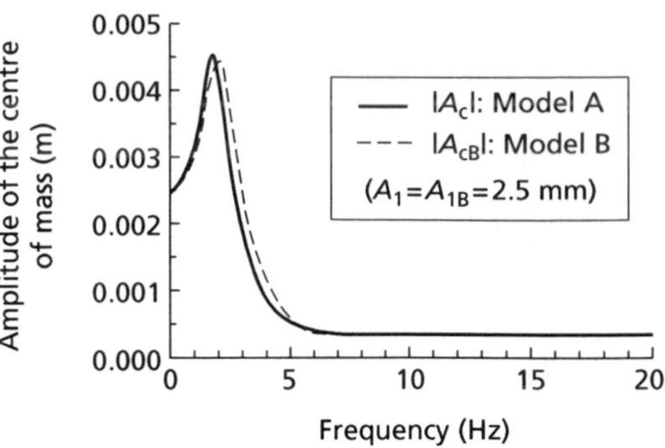

Fig. 24.6 Comparison of the amplitude of the centre of mass between Model A and Model B.

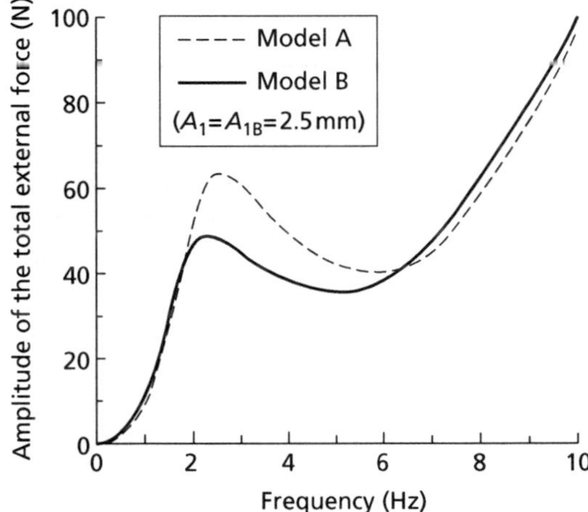

Fig. 24.7 Comparison of the amplitudes of the total external forces of Model A and Model B.

real human body, although the frequency range for large transmission is higher in the real human body (Griffin 1994) than in the present model analysis. From Fig. 24.6 it is seen that the amplitude of the oscillation of the centre of mass of the system is reduced by the wobbling mass for the frequency range where the transmission is important. This explains why the amplitude of the oscillation of the external force is reduced by the wobbling mass in the same frequency range (see Fig. 24.7). Actually, from the centre of mass theorem, the amplitude of external force must be reduced if the amplitude of the centre of mass of the system is reduced, provided that the frequency and the total mass of the system remain the same.

In summary, the present model analysis reveals the following effects of wobbling mass on the whole-body vibration. For the frequency range where the foot-to-upper body transmission is important, the wobbling mass is able to reduce the transmission, to reduce the amplitude of the oscillation of the centre of mass of the body, and therefore to reduce the amplitude of the fluctuation of the external force from the source of vibration. Since the oscillation of the wobbling mass in the upper body is carried by the oscillation of the rigid mass of the upper body, the phase of the wobbling mass lags behind the phase of the rigid mass. For this reason, the average power which the wobbling mass in the upper body gives to the rigid mass of the upper body is negative. This is the basic mechanism for the above-stated effects of the wobbling mass in the present model.

Neurophysiological response to vibration load

Several physiological studies show that the human response to vibration load depends mainly on three factors: amplitude, frequency, and muscle or joint stiffness (e.g. Hagbarth & Eklund 1966; Martin & Park 1997). The ranges of amplitude and frequency determine the intensity of load, whereas the reflex interaction together with the muscle tension and stiffness parameters can be regarded as the neuromuscular response to vibration stimulus.

The effects of vibration, which are known from a great number of studies in work science, are manifold. Some of them are really dramatic and thus range from severely destructive to potentially beneficial (Fritton *et al.* 1997). If people are exposed chronically over a long period of time to vibration, effects such as cognitive changes, vertigo, motion sickness, low back pain with or without degenerative changes in the lumbar spine, visual impairment, epilepsy, cerebrovascular diseases, haemodynamic alterations and changes of the mRNA expression in osteoblasts have been observed (von Gierke & Parker 1994; Bovenzi & Griffin 1997; Fritz 1997; Tjandrawinata *et al.* 1997; Pope *et al.* 1998; Martinho Pimenta & Castelo Branco 1999a,b). Moreover even genotoxic effects in terms of sister chromatid exchanges in lymphocytes have been demonstrated (Silva *et al.* 1999). Many reasons for these dangerous effects are due to the resonance areas of the human body (see Fig. 24.8).

In summary it can be stated that almost every biological system and subsystem may be affected by vibration input, especially if it is chronic and longlasting, as appears under certain working conditions. As these effects are due to a mechanical input that together with the biological reaction creates these consequences, generally speaking these long-term effects must be assumed in sport, also. There are, however, no empirical data proving or disproving this hypothesis. Compared to the findings in work science there are only very few studies in sport sciences dealing with biological reaction to vibration load. In sport the muscular reaction—and perhaps—adaptation plays a major role. Moreover the musculature with its various reflex mechanisms is by far the greatest biological human subsystem responding to vibration.

So it is likely that the Ia system could account for the entire stretch reflex under vibration. This was investigated in the context of the exceptional sensitivity of the spindle primary afferent terminals to tendon vibration, where short changes of stretch occur. As long ago as Matthews (1966a,b, 1967) it was shown that a vibratory stimulus which displaces the soleus muscle only by 10 μm activates the Ia fibre selectively. The high sensitivity of the Ia fibres can cause the activation of all fibres of this type if the amplitude and the frequency of the vibration are large enough. The spindle response can even be clamped and thus saturated at the vibration frequency making the spindle unresponsive to normal muscle stretch (Carew *et al.* 1983). The primary afferent terminals provide a steady excitatory contribution to the stretch reflex. It is very important to note that this Ia activity is not or only very little submitted to the so-called central fatigue, which has interesting consequences for the activation and the training of the muscles involved.

By the mid-1960s experiments were showing that the so-called 'tonic vibration reflex' (TVR) occurring in the muscle when the respective tendon was stimulated is complemented by a synchronous relaxation of the antagonist (e.g. Hagbarth & Eklund 1966). The TVR is also mainly induced via the activation of Ia fibres of the muscle spindle. There are results showing that the skin receptors and the afferent Type II fibres can also contribute to the TVR (Romaiguère *et al.* 1991; Park & Martin 1993).

When using vibrations as a method in strength and power training it is important to note that the TVR can be actively influenced by higher cortical centres of motor control. It has not been fully investigated whether the mono- and/or the

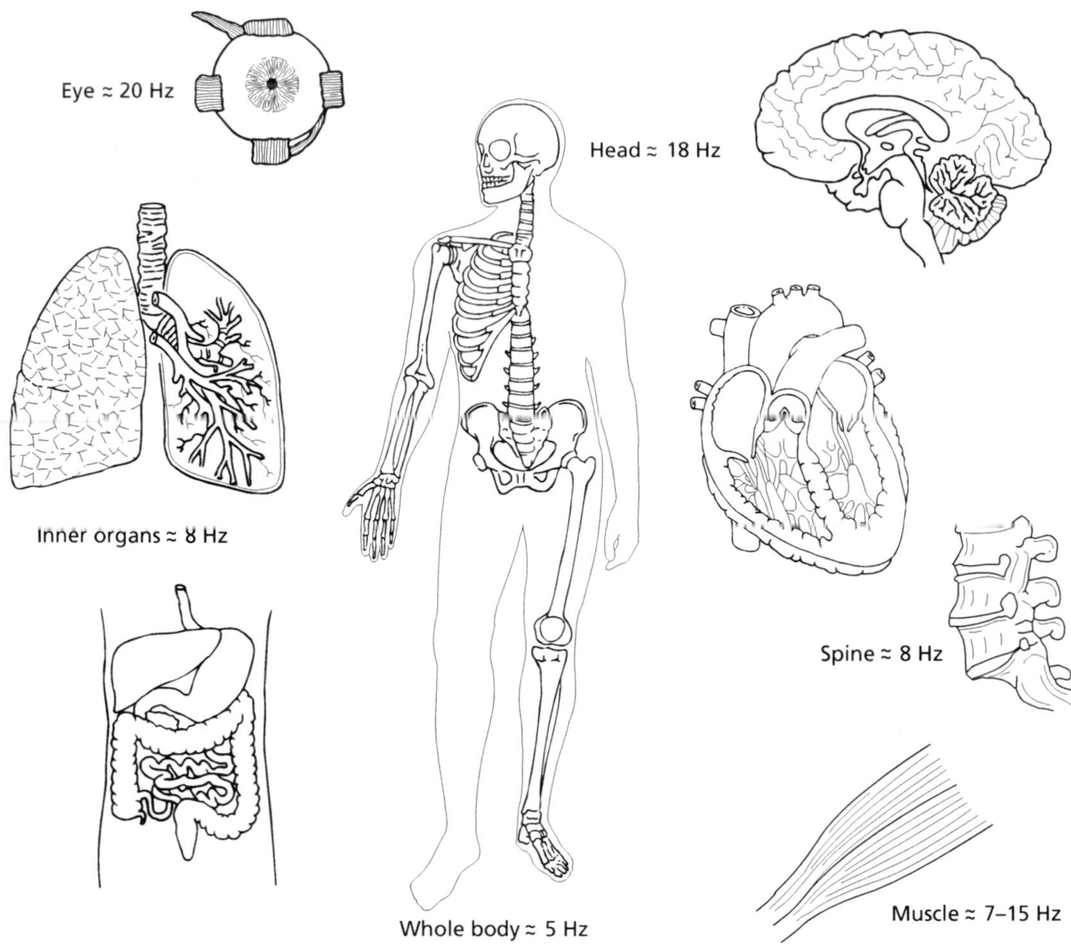

Fig. 24.8 Resonance frequencies for various parts of the body.

polysynaptic pathways are dominantly used for the signal transmission during vibration. In the same way it has not been experimentally proven that the TVR occurs in connection with whole-body vibration. As has been shown above, there is physical evidence for the involvement of the muscle as wobbling mass. Thus it can be assumed that a phase-locked or phase-lagged mechanical stimulation not only of the muscle spindles but also of Golgi organs takes place.

It is well known that vibration applied to a muscle or its tendon elicits reflex contractions in that muscle which lead to an increase in muscle activity, provided that a certain initial contraction level before and during vibration is available. This increase in muscle activity, measured in EMG recordings, does not necessarily evoke an increase in force as Park and Martin were able to show (1993), if the level of initial contraction is set e.g. to 10% or 20% maximal voluntary contraction. These findings are not inconsistent because the higher muscle activity due to the TVR is not necessarily linked to the control of muscle force by supraspinal centres.

On the other hand most of the stimulus frequencies are below the frequency that is associated with the fused tetanus, and the TVR response is increased only up to a certain limit with the stimulus frequency. At lower frequencies through the first harmonic synchronization the magnitude of the TVR increases with vibration frequency, and it was Romaiguère *et al.* (1991) who showed that the polysynaptic elements of the TVR can even be phase-locked to the cycle of vibration. This suggests that the increase in TVR in a range of ≤ 100-Hz stimulus frequency is due to an increase in motoneurone depolarization and a recruitment of motor units with higher thresholds. Although Martin and Park (1997) demonstrated that average muscle force does not necessarily boost with the TVR over a given period of time, via the reflex recruitment a cycle-dependent increase in muscle force may very well occur. So it is reasonable that muscle fatigue rises at higher levels of vibration. It can be argued that this effect is also triggered by the reduced pool of additional available motor units because vibration in general demands more motor units for a given production of muscle force. From these findings it can be deduced that both a direct muscle fibre-induced Ia activation and a tendon-induced TVR must be taken into account.

Strength and power development

The findings in literature concerning strength and power development associated with whole-body or segment-focused vibration training are not new. There were mainly results in Russian literature that brought these methods into discussion. Results in modern Western publications were presented by Nazarov and Spivak (1985) who discussed 'rhythmic neuromuscular stimulation' or 'biomechanical muscular stimulation' in order to improve strength and flexibility assuming that repetitive, eccentric vibration loads with small amplitudes would be effective due to a better synchronization of motor units. Künnemeyer and Schmidtbleicher (1997) tried to evaluate this approach by vibrating the stretched knee extensors and using contact time and jumping height in drop jumps for investigating the effects. They found a reduction in jumping height, an extension of contact time and signs of lower EMG activation which, of course, cannot be interpreted as positive effects for strength and power. For interpretation of the results it has to be taken into account that muscle stretching was the main topic of the study and the respective muscles were relaxed.

Compared with this various other publications, where a pre-enervation of the muscles was set, found remarkable enhancements in strength and power. Issurin *et al.* (1989, 1994; Issurin & Tenenbaum 1999) used the term 'vibratory stimulus training' and studied the effects of strength/power and flexibility training using a 'sitting-bench-pull-apparatus' (Issurin *et al.* 1994) (see Fig. 24.9) with 44-Hz vibration frequency and 3-mm amplitude for a training period of 3 weeks (experimental group). A control group carried out conventional strength and flexibility training. The experimental group showed an increase

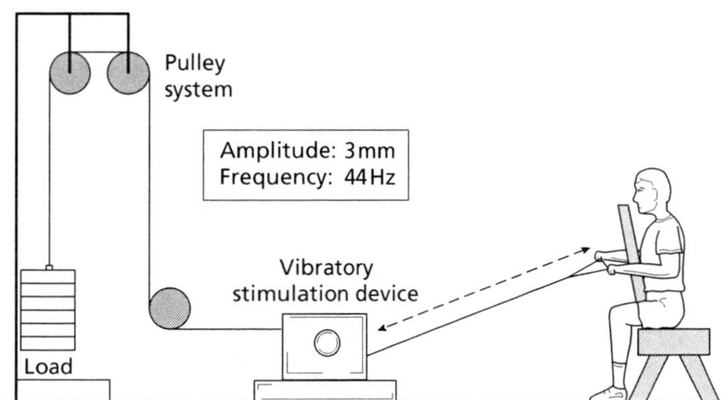

Fig. 24.9 Experimental set-up of the 'vibratory stimulus training' (Issurin *et al.* 1994).

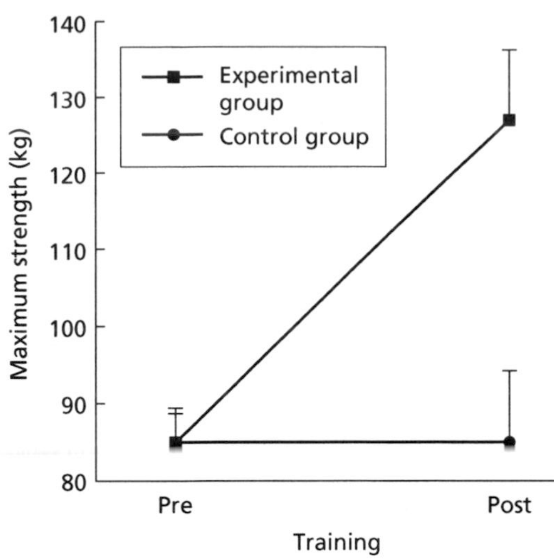

Fig. 24.10 Effects of 'vibratory stimulus training' (Issurin 1994).

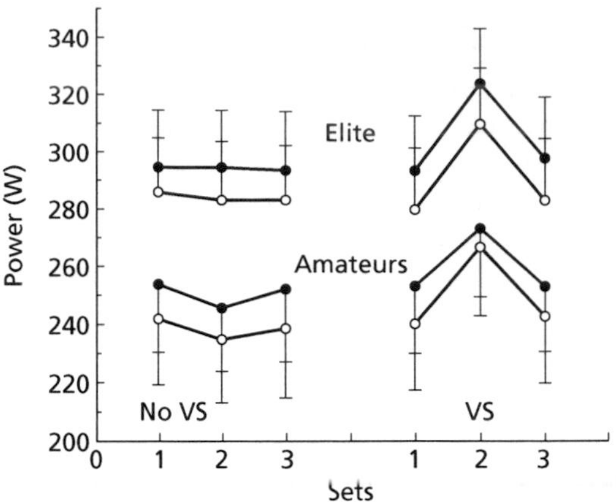

Fig. 24.11 Maximum (•) and average (○) power in two periods of strength training; VS, vibratory stimulation (Issurin *et al.* 1999).

in maximum strength of 49.8% whereas the traditional strength training without vibration led to an improvement of 16.1% (see Fig. 24.10). The results in flexibility were similar (increase in experimental group 8.7%, control group 2.4%).

The authors associate the remarkable enhancement of strength with a higher recruitment of motor units, referring to the studies of TVR in the literature. In a recent study Issurin *et al.* (1999) studied the acute response to vibration training comparing a group of subjects in elite sport with a group of subjects in mass sports. Using a load of 65–70% of one repetition maximum (1 RM) the subjects underwent two training sessions in random order with 3 series and 3 repetitions each and 2–3 min rest. In one session a normal strength training without vibration was carried out and in the other session a vibration load of 44 Hz with an amplitude of 1.5 mm was applied. Power output served as the criterion variable. Results show a significant increase of power under the influence of vibration (approximately 10%) in the second set (Fig. 24.11). The enhancement of power was significantly higher in the group of elite sport subjects. The reduction of power output in the 3rd set was explained by fatigue.

Investigations of a similar kind were also carried out by Weber (1997) who studied the effect of vibration training in elite gymnasts. After a training period of 12 weeks with vibration strength training twice a week in single cases an increase in maximum strength of 24–34% was found. The author stressed the fact that these enhancements could be found although a relatively low weight load was used.

The group of Bosco (Bosco *et al.* 1999a,b) carried out various studies in terms of vibration-associated strength training. In one study the subjects had to perform a training session under vibration load by standing for 60 s on the toes of one leg. They carried out 10 repetitions with 60 s rest. The other leg did the same exercise and served as the control group. Several strength tests before and after the training showed significant improvement of the vibrated leg.

Another study of this group showed a significant increase of power performance in arm muscles of boxing athletes. Similar to the above-mentioned study, the boxers performed with one arm 5 repetitions of 60 s isometric contraction under vibration load each followed by 60 s rest. The other arm again served as the control group, performing the same training but without vibration. This arm showed no significant increase in power performance (Fig. 24.12).

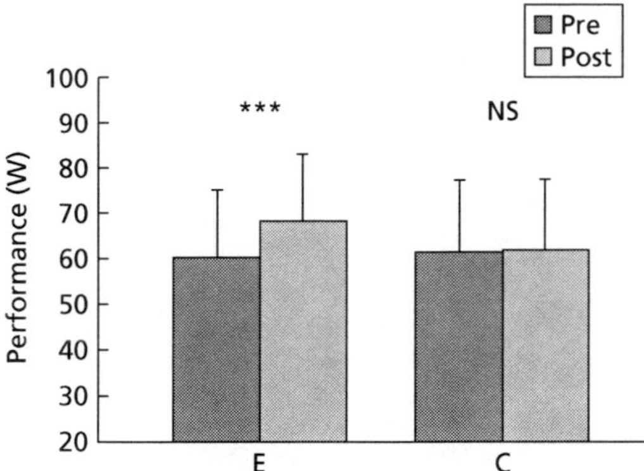

Fig. 24.12 Mean power performance during arm flexor training with (E) and without (C) vibration load. (Modified from Bosco *et al.* 1999a, with permission from Springer Verlag GmbH & Co.)

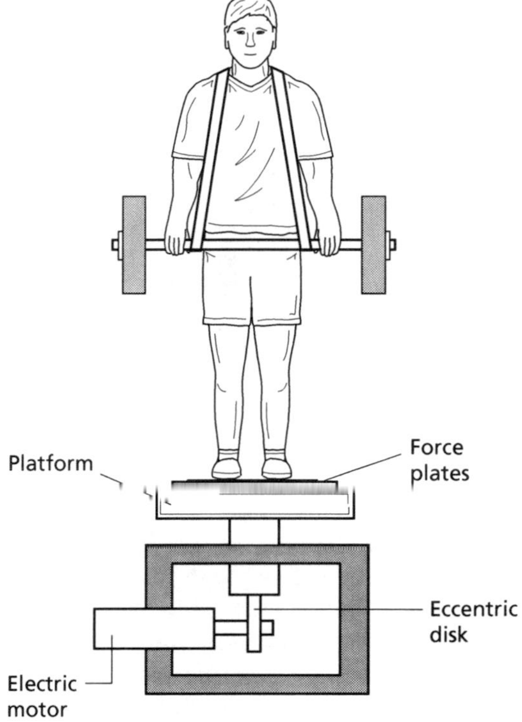

Fig. 24.13 Mechanical vibration generator.

Bosco and his group attributed the increases in strength to an improvement in neuromuscular regulation and referred to the results of Burke *et al.* (1976) and Hagbarth and Eklund (1966) by making the reflex action of muscle spindles (TVR) responsible for the increase of strength. Furthermore they take the vibratory stimulation of muscle tension by skin receptors into account.

Summing up the main findings in the literature, most of the results indicate remarkable effects from strength and power training associated with vibration load. Becerra Motta and Becker (2001) summarize results of various studies where improvements in strength and power of around 50% were found. Contradictory results seem to be related to the pretension of the muscle.

This effect could also be observed in our own studies. In single case studies on various vibration devices, EMG results showed a synchronous behaviour of muscle tension and relaxation to the vibration input. But by increasing the acceleration the biological system increases more and more its tonic activation (TVR) of the involved muscles. At its best this increased muscle and joint stiffness leads to an optimum damping behaviour of the body by reducing the transmission of the amplitude of the force of vibration to the rigid mass and thus to the wobbling mass of the body. By increasing the acceleration more the damping system of the body is overloaded, muscle tension increases further and the transmission of the amplitude exceeds biologically acceptable areas.

In a longitudinal study over 21 days, 36 training sessions with a well-trained athlete (28 years, height 193 cm, weight 93 kg) were performed (Mester *et al.* 1999). The training phase was divided into six periods each consisting of the same training content. In the 1st, 3rd and 5th period during exercise vibration stimuli were applied (vibration period) consisting of a sinusoidal oscillation with an amplitude of 2.5 mm and 24 Hz. The vibration load was generated by a training and diagnostic device, using an electrically driven eccentric cam, generating maximum frequencies up to 24 Hz with amplitudes up to ± 6 mm (see Fig. 24.13).

In the other periods the training was done without the vibration stimulus (non-vibration

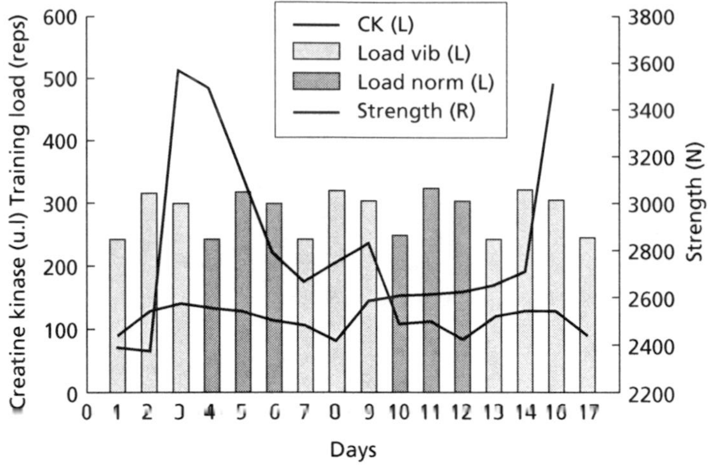

Fig. 24.14 Whole-body vibration strength training and muscular response. CK, creatine kinase; Load vib, training load under vibration (no. of repetitions of one-leg knee bends); Load norm, training load without vibration (no. of repetitions of one-leg knee bends).

period). The training consisted of exercises common in strength training for alpine skiing: knee bends (one-legged) with 70% of 1 RM, lunges (both with dumbbell), astride jumps, ankle jumps, drop jumps, step-ups, etc. For diagnostics the following tests were used: static leg press for static maximal strength; drop jump and squat-jump on force plate for dynamic maximal strength; vibration step test for regulative abilities under vibration load. For these tests the parameters heart rate, lactate, EMG, creatine kinase, urea, transmission factors and force were measured. The tests were performed on every day of the vibration period; creatine kinase and urea were taken on each day of training.

The results (see Fig. 24.14) show at the beginning of the experiment a dramatic increase of creatine kinase during each vibration period, indicating the high strain compared to the non-vibration period. According to this the performance of strength in the static leg press first decreases at the beginning of the training but increases at the end by about 43% of the initial value. The descriptive analysis of the jumps also shows an increase in the height of squat-jumps from 38.9 cm at the beginning up to the maximum value of 47.8 cm after 14 days of training. These results correspond very well to those findings in literature (see above) where significant effects of vibration strength and power training could be observed.

As also discussed above, some results suggest that vibration stimuli result in a relaxation of the muscle and decrease of strength and power parameters rather than in an improvement (Mester 1999). In order to study possible effects of this kind a group with 20 subjects comprising 14 males and 6 females (25.2 ± 4.7 years, height 179 ± 8 cm, weight 73.9 ± 9.9 kg) served to investigate the behaviour and adaptation associated with different vibration frequencies. All subjects executed 8 sessions of training consisting of knee bends with the above-shown weight bar with low loads (< 40% 1 RM). In contrast to the control group, the vibration group had to carry out their training under vibration load.

Motor control-related results showed that damping was significantly better ($P < 0.05$) at the higher frequencies (20 and 24 Hz) than at the lower ones (5, 9, 12 and 16 Hz) (Fig. 24.15) which is obviously attributable to an increase in muscle activity (Fig. 24.16). The increased muscle activity at higher frequencies is also related to a decrease of intermuscular coordination.

However the high standard deviations even at higher muscular activity indicate—besides the well-known methodological aspects of EMG—the individual responses to the vibration loads.

The results in adaptation of strength showed significant results neither in the control group nor in the experimental group, which can be mainly attributed to the low additional load.

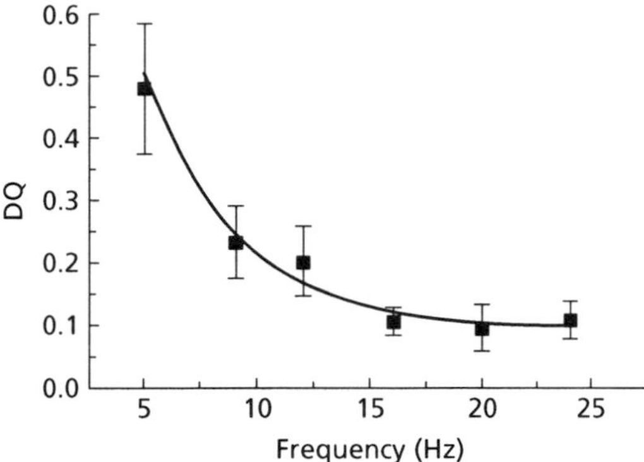

Fig. 24.15 Mean, SD and exponential fitting of damping quotient (DQ) at all frequency steps.

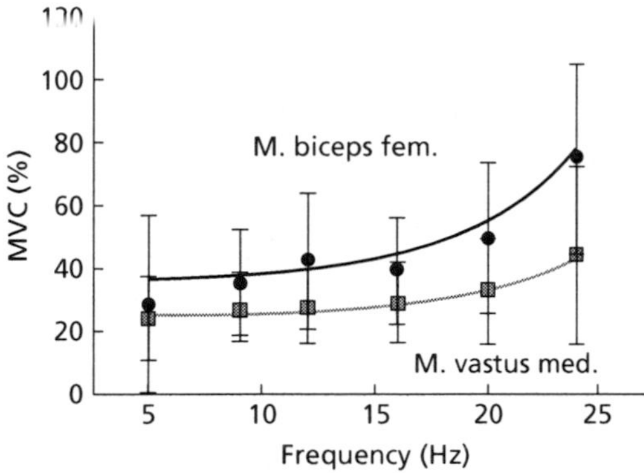

Fig. 24.16 Mean, SD and exponential fitting of muscle activity of biceps femoris and vastus medialis muscles at all frequency steps.

Discussion

Biomechanical considerations show the effects of wobbling masses such as the muscles under vibration. Besides the active damping effects due to the contractile tendomuscular system, a mechanical damping effect can be demonstrated that is associated with a phase lag of the wobbling mass compared to the rigid mass. This leads to a transformation of energy that directly affects the tendomuscular system. The high sensitivity of the Ia fibres to vibration suggests that this system could account for stretch-reflex activities under vibration. These activities are due not only to the vibration energy that mechanically affects the muscle but also to small changes in muscle length that can be observed in the respective joints, e.g. the knee and ankle, under vibration and what can be considered as an active damping. This movement, however, is effectively coordinated only at lower frequencies such as < 10 Hz. At higher frequencies (> 20 Hz) where vibration strength and power training normally should be located in order to avoid the biological resonance areas, a phase-locked coordination of the joints to the frequency of the vibration stimulus is no longer possible and thus a phase-lagged or even chaotic movement occurs. The reflex activity in this regard must be considered as extraordinarily high so that an increasing stiffness can be observed. If the muscle stiffness, however, is increasing a loop is induced which then in its turn results in a higher biomechanical and neurophysiological load on the tendomuscular system. In our own studies for vibration strength training a whole-body vibration generator was used where subjects carried out drop-jumps onto the platform. Hence it follows that in the contact phase of e.g. 300 ms at a vibration frequency of 25 Hz six to eight vibration-induced microcontractions occur which, together with a reduced fatigue sensation through the rerecruitment of motoneurones, seems to be highly effective. It is important to put emphasis on the level of pre-enervation/contraction of the muscles involved. If the pre-enervation is low a massage-like effect of the wobbling masses can be expected that leads to relaxation rather than an improvement in strength and power.

References

AGARD (Advisory Group for Aerospace Research and Development). (1979) Models and analogues for the evaluation of human biodynamic response, performance and protection. In: *Aerospace Medical Panel's Specialists' Meeting* (ed. H. E. von Gierke), Paris, 6–10 November 1978, Conference Proceedings CP-253. AGARD, Neuilly-sur-Seine.

Alexander, R.M. (1988) *Elastic Mechanisms in Animal Movement*. Cambridge University Press, Cambridge.

Anonymous. (1971) *Symposium on Biodynamic Models and Their Applications*. Technical Report no. 21–29, Aerospace Medical Research Laboratories.

Anonymous. (1978) Proceedings of Symposium on Biodynamic Models and Their Applications, 15–17 February 1977, Dayton, Ohio. *Aviation, Space and Environmental Medicine* **49** Section II.

Becerra Motta, J.A. & Becker, R.R. (2001) Die Wirksamkeit der Biomechanischen Stimulation (BMS) in Verbindung mit traditionellen Methoden der Kraftausdauerentwicklung im Schwimmsport. *Leistungssport* **31** no. 2, 29–35.

Bosco, C., Cardinale, M. & Tsarpela, O. (1999a) Influence of vibration on mechanical power and electromyogram activity in human arm flexor muscles. *European Journal of Applied Physiology* **79**, 306–311.

Bosco, C., Colli, R., Introni, E. *et al.* (1999b) Adaptive responses of human skeletal muscle to vibration exposure. *Journal of Clinical Physiology* **19**, 183–187.

Bovenzi, M. & Griffin, M.J. (1997) Haemodynamic changes in ipsilateral and contralateral fingers caused by acute exposures to hand transmitted vibration. *Occupational and Environmental Medicine* **54**, 566–576.

Burke, D., Hagbarth, K.-E., Löfstedt, L. & Wallin, B.G. (1976) The response of human muscle spindle endings to vibration during isometric contraction. *Journal of Physiology* **261**, 695–611.

Carew, T.J., Hawkins, R.D. & Kandel, E.R. (1983) Differential classical conditioning of a defensive withdrawal reflex in Aplysia california. *Science* **219**, 397–400.

Cavagna, G.A., Franzetti, P., Heglund, N.C. & Willems, P. (1988) The determinants of step frequency in running, trotting, and hopping in man and other vertebrates. *Journal of Physiology (London)* **399**, 81–92.

Cole, S.H. (1978) *The vertical transmission of impulsive energy through the seated human.* PhD thesis, Loughborough University of Technology.

Cole, S. (1982) Vibration and linear acceleration. In: *The Body at Work* (ed. W. T. Singleton), pp. 201–233. Cambridge University Press, Cambridge.

Dupuis, H., Hartung, E. & Louda, L. (1972) Vergleich regelloser Schwingungen einesbegrenzten Frequenzbereiches mit sinusförmigen Schwingungen hinsichtlich der Einwirkung auf den Menschen. *Ergonomics* **15**, 237–265.

Dupuis, H., Hartung, E. & Hammer, W. (1976) Biomechanisches Verhalten, Muskelreaktion und subjektive Wahrnehmung bei Schwingungserregung der oberen Extremitäten zwischen 8 und 80 Hz. *Internationales Archiv für Arbeits und Umweltmedizin* **37**, 9–34.

Farley, C.T. & Gonzalez, O. (1996) Leg stiffness and stride frequency in human running. *Journal of Biomechanics* **29**, 181–186.

Ferris, D.P. & Farley, C.T. (1977) Interaction of leg stiffness and surface stiffness during human hopping. *Journal of Applied Physiology* **82**, 15–22.

Fritton, J.C., Rubin, C.T., Qin, Y.X. & McLeod, K.J. (1997) Whole-body vibration in the skeleton: development of a resonance-based testing device. *Annals of Biomedical Engineering* **25**, 831–839.

Fritz, M. (1997) Estimation of spine forces under whole-body vibration by means of a biomechanical model and transfer functions. *Aviation, Space, and Environmental Medicine* **68**, 512–519.

Ghista, D.N. (1982) *Human Body Dynamics: Impact, Occupational, and Athletic Aspects.* Clarendon Press, Oxford.

von Gierke, H.E. (1971) Biodynamic models and their applications. *The Journal of the Acoustical Society of America* **50**, 1397–1413.

von Gierke, H.E. & Parker, D.E. (1994) Differences in otolith and abdominal viscera graviceptor dynamics: implications for motion sickness and perceived body position. *Aviation, Space, and Environmental Medicine* **65**, 747–751.

Griffin, M.J. (1994) *Handbook of Human Vibration.* Academic Press Limited, London.

Hagbarth, K.-E. & Eklund, G. (1966) Motor effects of vibratory muscle stimuli in man. In: *Proceedings of the First Nobel Symposium. Stockholm 1965* (ed. R. Granit), pp. 177–186. Stockholm.

ISO, 2631–1 (1997) *Mechanical Vibration and Shock—Evaluation of Human Exposure to Whole Body Vibration,* Part 1. *General Requirements.* International Organization of Standardization.

Issurin, V.B. & Tenenbaum, G. (1999) Acute and residual effects of vibratory stimulation on explosive strength in elite and amateur athletes. *Journal of Sport Science* **17**, 177–182.

Issurin, V.B., Kuksa, S.V. & Temnov, P.N. (1989) Effectiveness of different vibrostimulational regimes during speed–strength exercises. In: *Proceedings of the Conference 'Speed-Strength Training in Top-Level Athletes'*, Moscow.

Issurin, V.B., Liebermann, D.G. & Tenenbaum, G. (1994) Effect of vibratory stimulation training on maximal force and flexibility. *Journal of Sport Science* **12**, 561–566.

Ito, A., Komi, P.V., Sjodin, B., Bosco, C. & Karlsson, J. (1983) Mechanical efficiency of positive work in running at different speeds. *Medicine and Science in Sports and Exercise* **15**, 299–309.

Kim, W., Voloshin, A.S. & Johnson, S.F. (1994) Modelling of heal strike transients during running. *Human Movement Science* **13**, 221–244.

King, A.I. (1975) Survey of the state of the art of human biodynamic response. In: *Aircraft Crashworthiness* (eds K. Saczalski, G.T. Singley III, W.D. Pilkey & R.L. Husten), pp. 83–120. University Press of Virginia.

Künnemeyer, J. & Schmidtbleicher, D. (1997) Die neuromuskuläre Stimulation (RNS). *Leistungssport* **2**, 39–42.

Liu, W. & Nigg, B.M. (2000) A mechanical model to determine the influence of masses and mass distribution on the impact force during running. *Journal of Biomechanics* **33**, 219–224.

McMahon, T.A. & Cheng, G.C. (1990) The mechanics of running: how does stiffness couple with speed? *Journal of Biomechanics* **23** (Suppl.), 65–78.

Martin, B.J. & Park, H.-S. (1997) Analysis of the tonic vibration reflex: influence of vibration variables on motor unit synchronisation and fatigue. *European Journal of Applied Physiology* **75**, 504–511.

Martinho Pimenta, A.J. & Castelo Branco, N.A. (1999a) Neurological aspects of vibroacoustic disease. *Aviation, Space, and Environmental Medicine* **70**(3 Part 2), A91–A95.

Martinho Pimenta, A.J. & Castelo Branco, N.A. (1999b) Epilepsy in the vibroacoustic disease. *Aviation, Space, and Environmental Medicine* **70**(3 Part 2), A122–A127.

Matthews, P.B. (1966a) Reflex activation of the soleus muscle of the decerebrate cat by vibration. *Nature* **209**, 204–205.

Matthews, P.B. (1966b) The reflex excitation of the soleus muscle of the decerebrate cat caused by vibration applied to its tendon. *Journal of Physiology (London)* **184**, 450–472.

Matthews, P.B. (1967) The reflex response to muscle vibration in the decerebrate cat. *Journal of Physiology (London)* **192**, 18P–19P.

Mester, J. (1999) Biological response to vibration load. In: *International Society of Biomechanics XVIIth Congress* (eds W. Herzog & A. Jinha), Calgary, 1999. Book of Abstracts, p. 32.

Mester, J., Spitzenpfeil, P., Schwarzer, J. & Seifriz, F. (1999) Biological reaction to vibration—implications for sport. *Journal of Science and Medicine in Sport* **2**, 211–226.

Nazarov, V. & Spivak, G. (1985) Development of athlete's strength abilities by means of biomechanical stimulation method. *Theory and Practice of Physical Culture* **12**, 445–450.

Nigg, B.M. & Anton, M.G. (1994) Energy aspect for elastic and viscous shoe soles and playing surfaces. *Medicine and Science in Sports and Exercise* **27**, 92–97.

Nigg, B.M. & Liu, W. (1999) The effect of muscle stiffness and damping on simulated impact force peaks during running. *Journal of Biomechanics* **32**, 849–856.

Park, H.-S. & Martin, B.J. (1993) Contribution of the tonic vibration reflex to muscle stress and muscle fatigue. *Scandinavian Journal of Work Environment and Health* **19**, 35–42.

Pope, M.H., Magnusson, M. & Wilder, D.G. (1998) Kappa Delta Award. Low back pain and whole body vibration. *Clinical Orthopaedics* **354**, 241–248.

Roberts, V.N., Terry, C.T. & Stech, E.L. (1966) Review of mathematical models which describe human response to acceleration. In: *American Society of Mechanical Engineers* 66-WA/BHF-13, pp. 2–12. American Society of Mechanical Engineers.

Romaiguère, P., Vedel, J.-P., Azulay, J.-P. & Pagni, S. (1991) Differential activation of motor units in the wrist extensor muscles during the tonic vibration reflex in man. *Journal of Physiology* **444**, 645–667.

Sandover, J. (1971) *Study of Human Analogues*, Part 1. *A Survey of the Literature*. Department of Ergonomics and Cybernetics, Loughborough University of Technology.

Silva, M.J., Carothers, A., Castelo Branco, N.A., Dias, A. & Boavida, M.G. (1999) Sister chromatid exchange analysis in workers exposed to noise and vibration. *Aviation, Space, and Environmental Medicine* **70**(3 Part 2), A40–A45.

Thompson, C. & Raibert, M. (1989) *Passive Dynamic Running*. In: *International Symposium of Experimental Robotics* (eds V. Hayward & O. Khatib), Springer, New York, pp. 74–83.

Tjandrawinata, R.R., Vincent, V.L. & Hughes-Fulford, M. (1997) Vibrational force alters mRNA expression in osteoblasts. *FASEB Journal* **11**, 493–497.

Weber, R. (1997) Muskelstimulation durch Vibration. *Leistungssport* **1**, 53–56.

Yue, Z., Kleinoeder, H. & Mester, J. (2001) A model analysis of the effects of wobbling mass on the whole-body vibration. *European Journal of Sport Science* **1**, no. 1.

Chapter 25

Training for Weightlifting

JOHN GARHAMMER AND BOB TAKANO

Introduction

Since 1972 two overhead lifts have been contested in the sport of weightlifting, the snatch and the clean and jerk. The sport is often referred to as Olympic (style) weightlifting since it is contested in the Olympic Games. In the snatch lift, the barbell is lifted in one continuous motion from the competition platform to arms' length overhead. The athlete catches the barbell overhead in a deep squat position, and then stands with the barbell in control until a 'down' signal is received from the officials (Fig. 25.1).

The 'clean' phase of the clean and jerk lift is similar to the snatch except that the barbell is first lifted to the shoulders rather than overhead, and a narrower hand spacing is used on the bar. When the athlete stands from the squat position to finish the clean lift he or she must then 'jerk' the barbell overhead to complete this two-part lift. The jerk is performed starting with the barbell held firmly on the shoulders. The knee and hip joints are then slightly flexed and then rapidly extended in a jumping action (rising onto the balls of the feet) to thrust the barbell upward. The lifter then either splits the feet forward and backward, or again quickly flexes the knee and hip joints, to lower the body and catch the barbell at arms' length overhead. The feet are then brought together and the legs straightened to hold the barbell under control overhead until the 'down' signal is given by the officials (Fig. 25.2). The above three lifting movements are performed very rapidly, with the major lifting forces applied to the bar for about 0.8 s in the snatch and clean, and about 0.2 s in the jerk.

The training programmes followed by athletes who compete in weightlifting are based primarily on three principles: specificity of exercise, overload, and variability. Specificity implies the use of training lifts similar to the competitive lifts, performed for a low number of repetitions with near-maximal loads, since in competition the goal is to lift the heaviest weight possible in the snatch and clean and jerk for one repetition. Overload relates to lifting heavier and/or more total weight in workouts than a given athlete is accustomed to. Variability relates to changes and variety in the composition of the training programme in order to avoid physiological and psychological maladaptation problems commonly referred to as 'overtraining' (Stone *et al.* 1990). As the following discussion emphasizes, the variability principle leads to some training programme designs that seem to violate the principles of specificity and overload. Before proceeding with a more detailed presentation of training methods for weightlifting, it must be stated that details of training programme design and content may vary considerably based on: (i) the ability level and years of training and competition experience of a given athlete; (ii) whether or not the athlete can train full time due to employment or educational responsibilities; and (iii) the supervising coach's training philosophy. Many national-level athletes in the USA cannot train as professionals

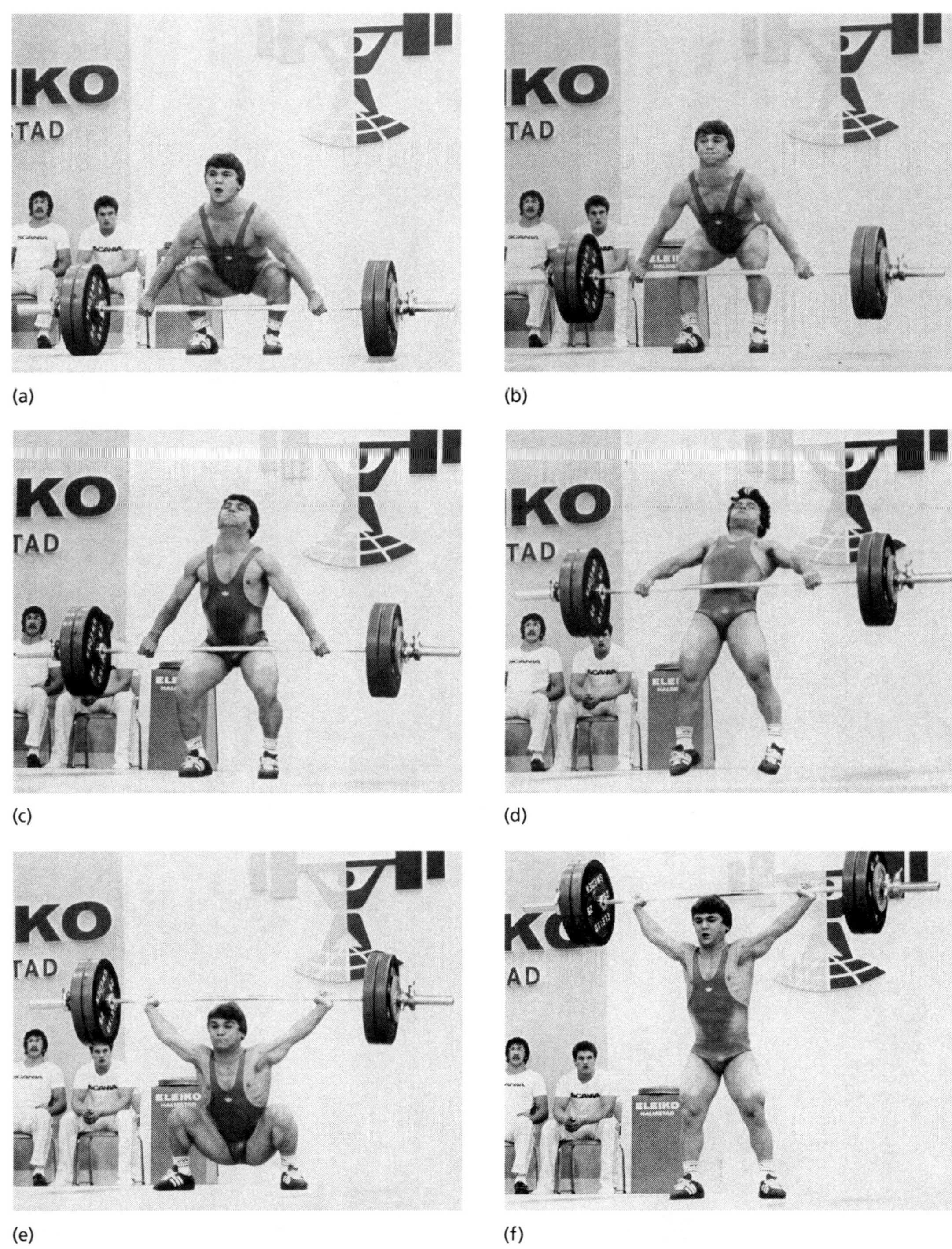

Fig. 25.1 The snatch lift. (a) Start position; (b) end of first pull; (c) start of second pull (power position) after transition from the first pull (note rebending of knees); (d) end of second pull (jump phase); (e) catch position; (f) finish of the lift. (Courtesy of B. Klemens Photos.)

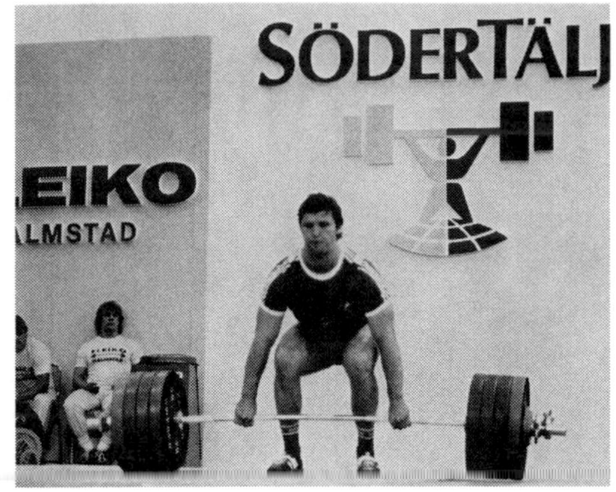
SÖDERTÄLJ
EIKO
LMSTAD
(a)

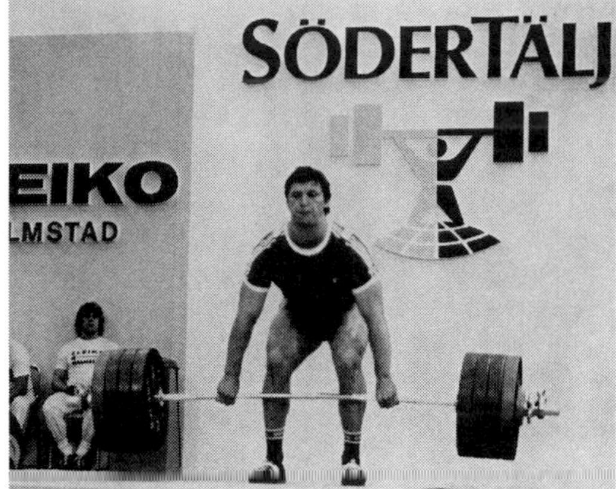
SÖDERTÄLJ
EIKO
LMSTAD
(b)

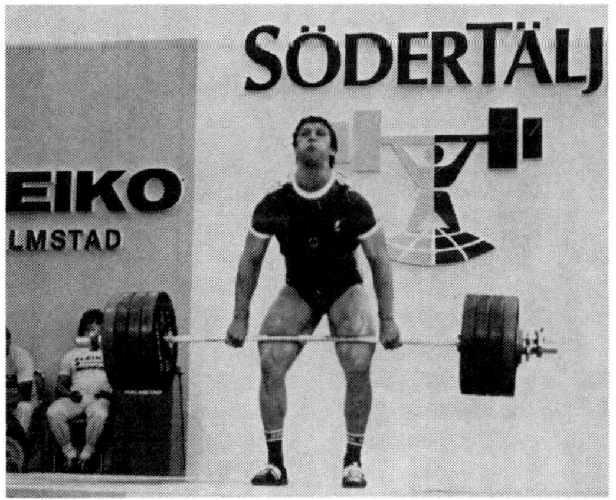
SÖDERTÄLJ
EIKO
LMSTAD
(c)

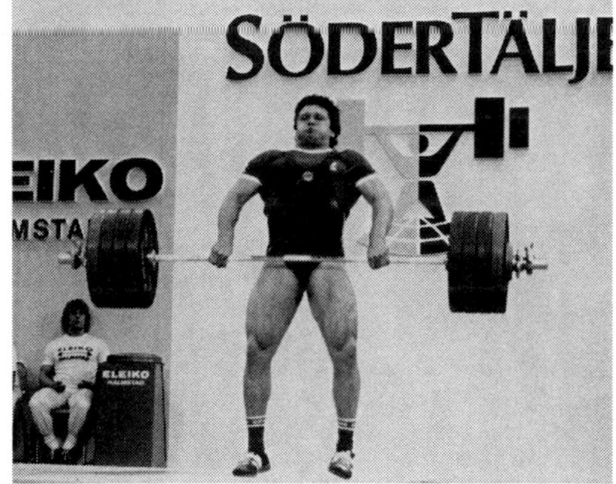
SÖDERTÄLJE
EIKO
MSTA
ELEIKO
(d)

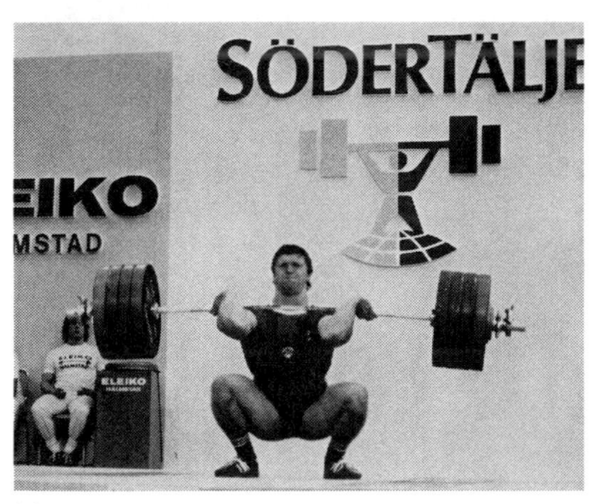
SÖDERTÄLJE
EIKO
MSTAD
ELEIKO
(e)

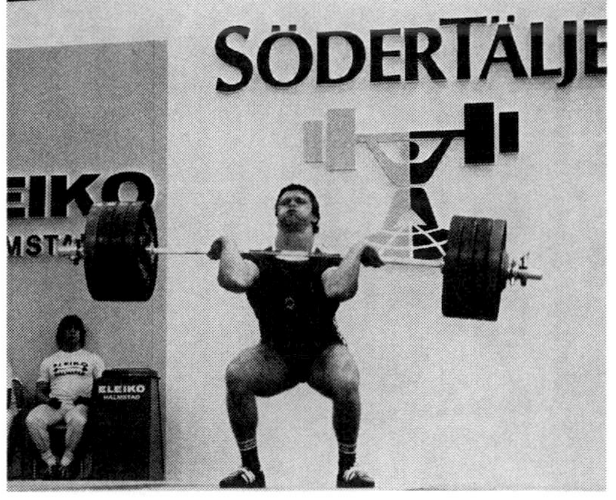
SÖDERTÄLJE
ELEIKO
(f)

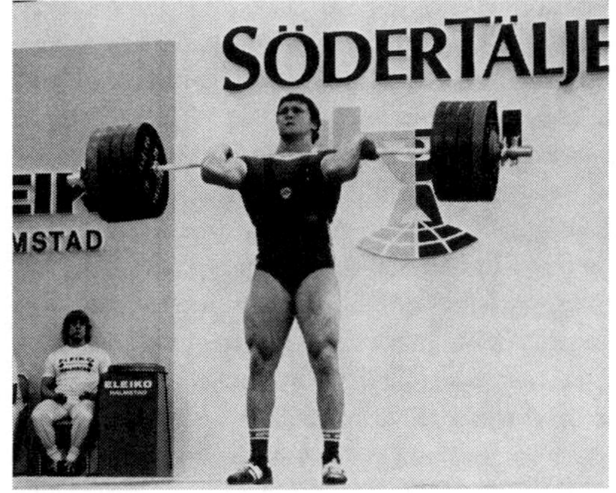

(g)

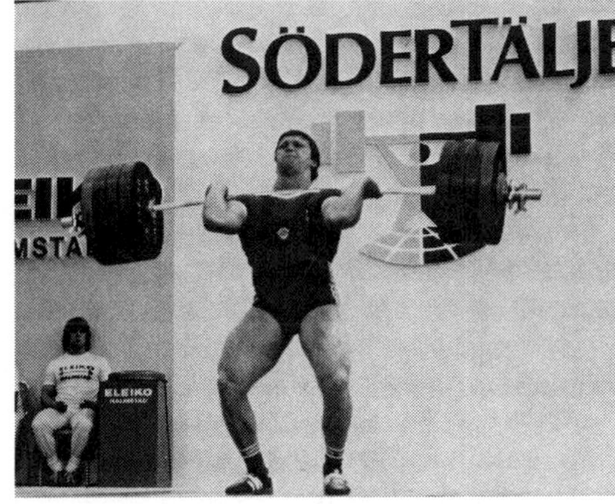

(h)

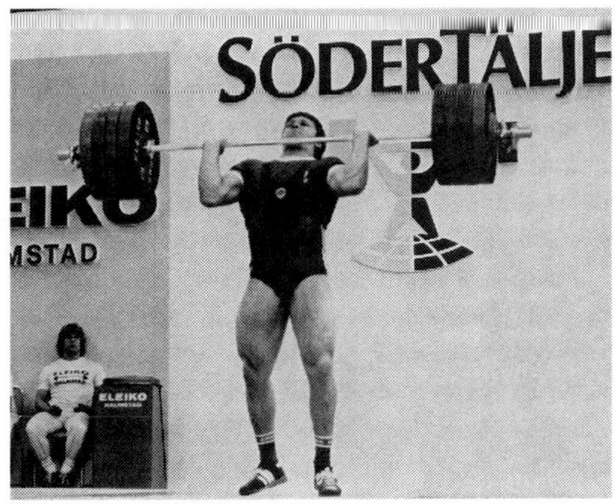

(i)

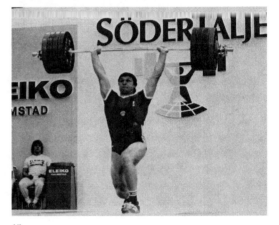

(j)

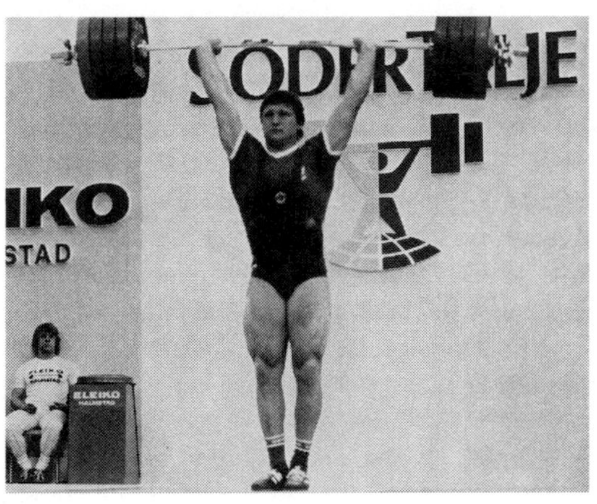

(k)

Fig. 25.2 The clean and jerk lift. (a) Start ('lift-off'); (b) middle of first pull; (c) near the start of the second pull; (d) end of the second pull (jump phase); (e) catch position; (f) standing from the catch position (front squat movement); (g) start position for the jerk; (h) bottom of the 'dip' prior to the upward thrust; (i) end of the thrust phase (jump) of the jerk; (j) 'split' catch position; (k) finish of the lift. (Courtesy of B. Klemens Photos.)

and must adjust their programme accordingly. Examples of such programmes have been published (Jones 1993; Drechsler 1998). The remainder of this chapter will relate primarily to elite-level weightlifters who have trained for the sport for 3 or more years and who compete at the national and international level. Since the initial publication of this chapter in 1992, considerable additional information about the training of elite weightlifters, including female athletes, has been published in the form of books, articles and interviews. Of particular interest are articles contained in the proceedings of the weightlifting symposia held in Ancient Olympia, Greece in 1993 and 1997, and published by the International Weightlifting Federation (IWF), Budapest. Some individual articles from these symposia will be referenced later in this chapter.

Variability as the key training principle

If specificity and overload were dominant and/or exclusive principles of training, the design of a weightlifter's exercise programme would be fairly simple: (i) perform the competitive lifts in low repetitions with maximal weights; and (ii) add a few 'assistance' exercises to emphasize and improve physical qualities associated with proper execution of the competitive lifts, such as speed, strength and flexibility. Practical experience, however, shows that such a plan fails if followed for any prolonged period of time (several days to several weeks). The reason for failure of such an approach to training is summarized by the term 'overtraining'. Overtraining can involve psychological factors, such as loss of motivation, and/or physiological factors related to muscle fatigue or injury, as well as neural and hormonal changes (Nilsson 1986; Kuipers & Keizer 1988; Stone *et al.* 1990). Sale (1988) and Enoka (1988) have discussed the importance of neural adaptations for increases in strength, particularly in the early stages of a resistance training programme.

Kraemer (1988, 2000) has reviewed the responses of the endocrine system to resistive exercise and has pointed out the conflicting research results, likely due to variables such as exercise volume (total number of lifts performed) and intensity (average weight lifted relative to maximum possible), rest intervals and training status of subjects. As discussed below, Häkkinen and colleagues have performed considerable research on the neural and hormonal responses that occur in elite weightlifters during typical training programmes. In studies of 1–2 years' duration Häkkinen *et al.* (1987, 1988a) found that increases in performance correlated to increases in leg extensor isometric force and integrated electromyogram (IEMG) activity (neural activation levels), serum testosterone levels and anabolic/catabolic (A/C) hormone ratios (endocrine responses). Short-duration studies (Häkkinen *et al.* 1988b, 1988c) showed that such responses were sensitive to acute intense workout sessions, with IEMG activity and leg extensor isometric force decreasing. Testosterone was found to increase during the second workout session in one day but decreased gradually after several days of intense workouts. A single rest day was sufficient to reverse this trend. Results of such research indicate the importance of neural adaptations, even in experienced strength and power athletes, and that neural fatigue (decreased IEMG levels) does occur with intense exercise. Also, endocrine responses could be monitored in elite strength and power athletes during important training periods in order to adjust training intensity to optimal levels, that is, without causing decreases in serum testo-sterone levels and A/C ratios which likely relate to reduced adaptability levels and the possibility of overtraining. An additional article (Häkkinen *et al.* 1990) suggests that these conclusions are applicable for both male and female athletes. Thus, variability in well designed training programmes for weightlifters can reduce the possibility of overtraining while maintaining reasonable, if not optimal, progress for the athlete. This is possible via periodic oscillations in overload, meaning planned underload or 'unload' training sessions and training weeks, and strategically placed rest days.

Variability vs. biomechanical specificity

A variety of lifting exercises, beyond the competition lifts, are regularly used in the training programme of weightlifters (for an extensive discussion of them see Vorobyev 1978). This permits not only emphasis on the development of various physical qualities needed to execute the competition lifts optimally, such as strength, speed and flexibility, but also a biomechanical variation which may help avoid overtraining symptoms caused by movement pattern monotony. The weightlifting coach, however, needs to be aware of how the movement properties of a given 'assistance' exercise differ from those of the actual competition lifts. That is, how do the applied force pattern, bar movement velocity and trajectory profile, range of motion of involved body joints and mechanical power output of the exercise relate to the physical qualities that are to be developed by the exercise? Also, how do these factors change as the weight of the barbell changes? In a review article Garhammer (1989) points out that several sport scientists have published data indicating that as barbell weight increases the height to which it is lifted, maximal vertical bar velocity, peak applied vertical force and/or power output decrease (e.g. Häkkinen *et al.* 1984; Garhammer 1985; Garhammer & Gregor 1979, 1992). Thus, for example, an athlete who needs to be faster should emphasize lower-intensity lifts (70–85%) while one who needs to improve strength should emphasize higher-intensity lifts (85 + %). For a given weight, the same trends in the above parameters have been noted for later repetitions in a multiple repetition sequence (set) (Häkkinen 1988). Numerous reports have been published comparing the biomechanical properties of various assistance exercises with the competition lifts; for example, for snatch-related exercises: Häkkinen (1988), Häkkinen and Kauhanen (1986) and Frolov *et al.* (1977); for clean-related exercises: Häkkinen and Kauhanen (1986) and Medvedjev *et al.* (1981); and for jerk-related exercises: Medvedjev *et al.* (1982). The most common snatch-related assistance exercises are: (i) power snatch—very similar to the competition snatch lift but caught overhead with only slight knee and hip flexion rather than in a deep squat position; (ii) snatch pull —similar to the competition snatch lift but the barbell is only pulled to the height of the abdominal to chest area and no attempt is made to catch the weight overhead; (iii) snatch or snatch pull from the hang–initial barbell position is not on the floor but rather held just above the floor to just above the knees; and (iv) snatch or snatch pull from blocks–initial barbell position is above the floor resting on blocks, usually positioning the bar at about knee height. It is difficult to make general statements about the results of biomechanical comparisons between these assistance exercises and the competition lifts due to the dependence of measured parameters on the weight of the barbell used in any given exercise. However, some specific cases can be discussed. The maximal weight that can be used in the power snatch by a given athlete is about 80% of the weight of that athlete's maximal competition snatch lift. With this load the barbell will be pulled higher, reach a greater maximum vertical velocity, result in a greater peak applied vertical propulsion force, elicit slightly different IEMG activity from leg extensor muscles, include a higher peak knee angular velocity and greater range of motion at the knee, and result in greater mechanical power output when compared to the competition snatch lift. Power snatches are therefore a useful assistance exercise for an athlete who needs to improve speed of movement and speed–strength (power).

Conversely, a snatch pull from the floor may be performed with 5–10% above an athlete's maximum competition snatch weight. With a load on the barbell equal to or greater than the maximum competition snatch, it will be pulled to a lower height, reach a lesser maximum vertical velocity, result in a smaller peak applied vertical propulsion force, elicit slightly different IEMG activity from leg extensor muscles, and result in lower mechanical power output when compared to the competition snatch lift. Snatch pulls are therefore useful for an athlete who needs to improve strength in the snatch movement pattern. Biomechanical characteristics of snatch assistance exercises from the hang or from blocks depend on the exact starting position of the bar, such as above or below knee level, as well as on load. In general, if the starting position is above knee level the exercise will emphasize the development of speed–strength in the final phase of the snatch pull (upper or top pull). If the starting position is closer to the floor the biomechanical characteristics will be more similar to the snatch pull from the floor. Essentially identical statements to those for the snatch assistance exercises can be made regarding the clean assistance exercises; namely, the power clean, clean pull, and clean or clean pulls from the hang or from boxes.

The primary assistance exercises for improving the jerk are: (i) jerk—weight taken from supports rather than cleaned from the floor; (ii) jerk from behind the neck (taken from supports); (iii) push or power jerk—barbell thrust upward as in the competition jerk but caught overhead with only slight flexion at the knees and hips; and (iv) half-jerk—barbell is thrust upward as in the competition jerk but only to approximately head height; it then falls back to the athlete's shoulders. Medvedjev *et al.*'s work (1982) indicates that the most important variables related to success in the jerk are the maximum force generated against the ground, time interval to reach maximum force, and the time interval for 'breaking' or stopping the initial decent phase of the movement. The jerk and jerk from behind the neck were determined to be most effective in perfecting jerk technique, while the half-jerk and depth (drop) jumps were best for developing speed–strength. It was also recommended that no more than five to seven jerks be performed per workout with 90% or more of the maximum jerk (the higher the lifter's classification the lower the number of heavy jerks).

General concepts in the training plan for weightlifters

The above discussion presented information that can be helpful to a weightlifting coach when making specific decisions about the content of a training plan. Before detailed examples of actual training programmes used by weightlifters can be presented a few general concepts in training theory need to be explained.

Matveyev (1972) presented the basic ideas of periodized training programmes. A programme is periodized when it is divided into phases, each of which has primary and secondary goals. In his original model Matveyev suggested the initial phase of a strength–power programme (preparation phase) contain a high volume (many repetitions) with lower intensity (low average weight lifted relative to maximum possible in each movement). As weeks pass the volume decreases and intensity increases. The resulting higher intensity and lower volume represent the characteristics of a competitive phase of training, which leads up to an actual competition.

Typical high-volume (preparatory) phases for weightlifters contain more training sessions per week (6–15), more exercises per workout session (3–6), more sets per exercise (4–8), and more repetitions per set (4–6). Typical high-intensity (competition) phases for weightlifters contain fewer training sessions per week (5–12), fewer exercises per workout session (1–4), fewer sets per exercise (3–5), and fewer repetitions per set (1–3). The duration of each phase may be several weeks to several months in length. Two or more complete cycles (preparatory + competition) may fit into a training year. Stone *et al.* (1981) have proposed and successfully tested a periodized model of strength–power training with sequential phases that change rather drastically. For example, a phase to increase muscle size (5 sets of 10 repetitions in squat and pulling exercises), a phase to improve basic strength (3–5 sets of 5 repetitions), a phase to improve speed–strength (3–5 sets of 3 repetitions), and a phase to 'peak' for competition (1–3 sets of 1–3 repetitions). The use of 10 repetitions per set is higher than typically recommended in the early preparation phase but has proved to be successful in a number of studies (e.g. Stone *et al.* 1982).

The training programme for a weightlifter is generally planned in terms of a training year.

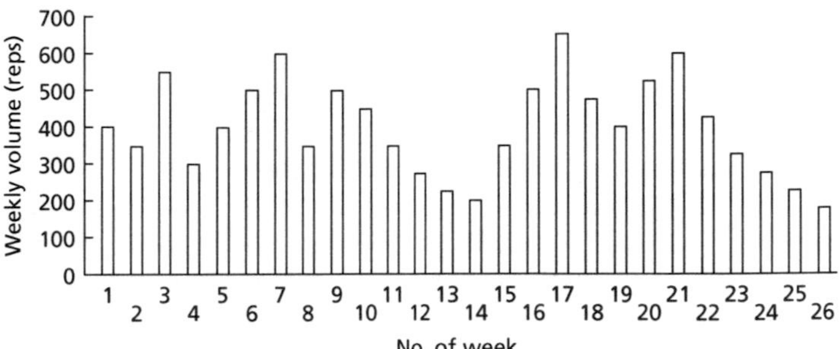

Fig. 25.3 Weekly training volume in repetitions for the first 26 weeks of a 52-week training year for an elite weightlifter. Total volume shown is 10 500 repetitions.

Modifications are made as the actual training year progresses based on specific observed needs of an athlete. The plan begins with a judgement as to how many total lifts (counting all major exercises) should be performed during the year. As an example, 20 000 is a reasonable number for an elite athlete. This total yearly 'volume' is then divided unequally into 12 4-week training months, some of which will be more than double the volume of other months. Each training month then has its volume divided unequally into four weekly volumes. The highest-volume week in a given month may have more than twice the lifts of the lowest-volume week. Each week then has its volume divided amongst an appropriate number of training sessions such that no session has an unreasonably large or small number of lifts. Multiple workout sessions per day are now common among elite weightlifters. A lifter may work out 5 or 6 days per week, with one to three sessions per day common. Each session must then be assigned specific lifting exercises based on the particular athlete's strengths and weaknesses. This approach to training programme development provides for extensive variation, which can stimulate progress while minimizing the chances of overtraining. Details related to the above overview of training plan development are discussed by Vorobyev (1978).

Figure 25.3 illustrates one possible division of repetitions for the first 6 months (26 weeks) of a training year based on a yearly volume of 20 000 repetitions. These 26 weeks contain two complete macrocycles (weeks 1–14 and 15–26), each composed of a preparation phase (10- and 8-week mesocycles) and a competition phase (4-week mesocycle each). It can be seen that in both macrocycles the preparation phase includes much higher volume than does the following competition phase. Also, the second macrocycle contains fewer total repetitions than the first. Competitions occur at the end of weeks 14 and 26. The second 6 months of this training year would follow a similar pattern but with fewer total repetitions (9500 vs. 10 500). This type of weekly (microcycle) training volume variation is typical for elite weightlifters. The following section describes examples of training weeks during preparatory and competition phases that are representative of two different national programme philosophies.

Training methods

Most of the world's weightlifting training programmes are variations of the models established by the weightlifting federations of Bulgaria and the former Soviet Union, the top two programmes in the sport for much of the three decades of the biathlon. In recent years both nations have allowed foreign coaches and athletes to participate in their training programmes, thus making this information available to students of the sport. These two programmes and their philosophies were strongly affected by geopolitical factors.

The former Soviet Union benefited from the diversity of human types that inhabited the vast geopolitical complex. The geographical distances between training centres created problems that inhibited strict monitoring of training, and allowed for a greater degree of variation from the established national philosophies. This also inhibited the frequency of collective training by national team members. During the final decade of the Soviet Union there was some discontinuity in the development of a standardized training methodology as the position of national coach, a largely administrative office, was filled by four different coaches. With the breakdown of the Union into 15 separate republics, each with different economic and funding problems, many coaches have continued developing weightlifters using the methods that correspond closely with the old Soviet programme.

The Bulgarian programme involves a smaller number of carefully selected athletes occupying a much smaller geographical area than the Soviet Union. The nearly 30-year term of service of national coach Ivan Abadjiev provided great continuity with little opportunity for variation. The relatively small size of the country allows the national junior and senior teams to train collectively for a majority of the time under strict oversight from Coach Abadjiev. Several smaller countries that have recently excelled in weightlifting at the world level, such as Greece, Turkey and Iran, follow training concepts that can be traced to the Bulgarian system.

The above two programmes differed philosophically in the longevity expected of the careers of their top performers. The Bulgarians expect an athlete to mature quickly, produce high results at a single Olympics and then, in all probability, to be replaced before the next renewal of the Games. Hence, double Olympic gold medallists are rare. The Soviets expected a lengthier career from their top performers.

Both programmes are designed to train talented athletes with no serious limitations in joint mobility. The technique learned by the athlete during the first year of training is not altered significantly, except to account for increases in body weight. The larger battery of exercises employed during the earlier developmental years of training should minimize any imbalances in the development of musculoskeletal anatomy. Those athletes involved in these training programmes must be in sufficiently fit condition to endure the stresses generated. An individual returning from injury rehabilitation or any other lay-off should employ a more diversified, less intense regimen before undertaking elite-level training.

The *K*-value is a derived parameter that is used to monitor the intensity of training programmes. The *K*-value can be defined as the average weight lifted per repetition in a complete training cycle divided by the two-lift total performed at the end of the competition phase. Empirical results indicate that the optimal range of average weight lifted per repetition lies between 38 and 42% of the competitive total (Takano 1990).

Restoration is a necessity for an athlete to train in these types of regimens. Jacuzzi, steam baths, sauna or massage must be employed and cycled several times weekly. Nutritional supplementation is also required.

Bulgarian training

The Bulgarian training approach is unique in that it does not deal with percentages of maximum or expected maximum lifts, a procedure common to weightlifting training for at least the last four decades. The battery of primary exercises is limited to only six (snatch, clean and jerk, power snatch, power clean and jerk, front squat and back squat). Training sessions are limited to 45-min periods. This time limit is to ensure that athletes are training only during the period during which the body can maintain elevated blood testosterone levels (Abadjiev 1989). Two 45-min sessions are combined into a complex around a 30-min rest period during which testosterone levels can be restored.

To begin a snatch complex (Table 25.1), the athlete warms up with snatch singles towards a weight near the maximum expected for that day. If the first lift is successful, more weight is added. This procedure is continued through the six attempts. As an alternative, the athlete may take singles at 15, 10 or 5 kg below maximum between

Table 25.1 Bulgarian preparation week.

Monday	
Morning	
Session 1	Snatch—singles to 6 maximum efforts Rest 30 min
Session 2	Clean and jerk—singles to 6 maximum efforts Front squat—singles to 1–6 maximum efforts
Afternoon	
Repeat morning complex	
Evening	
Repeat morning complex	
Tuesday	
Repeat Monday's training schedule	
Wednesday	
Session 1	Power snatch—singles to 6 maximum efforts Rest 30 min
Session 2	Power clean and jerk—singles to 6 maximum efforts Back squat—singles to 1–6 maximum efforts
Thursday	
Repeat Monday's training schedule	
Friday	
Repeat Monday's training schedule	
Saturday	
Repeat Wednesday's training schedule	
Sunday	
Morning	
Session 1	Less formally structured training

the six maximum attempts. Lifting is terminated at the 45-min limitation. The athlete then may recline while listening to music for 30 min. The second session of the complex involves the clean and jerk performed in the same progression pattern. Less time is required since less warm-up is necessary. Front squats with several maximum singles follow the clean and jerks. Training is terminated at 45 min. The same progression pattern is employed for the power snatch, power clean and jerk and back squat during the Wednesday and Saturday morning complexes (Table 25.1).

Variation seems limited on first inspection, but the following variants are available at the discretion of the supervising coach: (i) number of maximum lifts per session, per day and per week; and (ii) number of complexes per day. In addition, the maximum weights for each day will vary with the condition of the athlete. These weights are utilized as indicators for the planning of future training by the supervising coach. This system requires close supervision. Consequently, the ratio of athletes to coaches must be small. Three coaches are assigned to the 20-man senior team, with the periodic assistance of personal coaches. These coaches must be able to identify characteristics of each phase and make appropriate adjustments to the training.

In the competitive phase the same exercises are used on the same day as in the preparatory weeks. The number of times that the complexes may be performed is reduced to 1 or 2 times per day on Monday, Tuesday, Thursday and Friday. The number of times that the weights are reduced and then reloaded to maximum may also be varied during a workout in this phase.

Soviet-derived training

The Soviet-derived system may be even more diversified than it appears to be on the surface due to the aforementioned geopolitical factors. The widely dispersed elite-level coaches tended to develop and emphasize the successes of their own training methods, albeit within fairly narrow limits. This situation may lead to more variation in training programme design, especially when considering the lack of prolonged strong leadership that Bulgaria has enjoyed under former national coach Ivan Abadjiev.

The Soviet system utilizes a greater variety of exercises, more variation of these exercises, and fewer training sessions per day and week. All movements designated as 'hang' may be performed from three different heights above the floor. The issue of percentages is discussed in the next section.

The Soviet system also utilized diversified non-weightlifting activities in what is collectively termed active rest. Active rest normally involves calisthenics, running and jumping

Table 25.2 Reference maxima to determine weights for each exercise.

Exercises	Reference lift for 100% weight
Snatch, snatch pull, power snatch, snatch deadlift	Snatch
Clean and jerk, clean pull, power clean, clean deadlift, front squat	Clean and jerk
Press	Press
Good morning	*
Back squat	At least 125% of clean and jerk

* The style of performance will dictate the maximum weight.

drills, swimming, competitive games and similar activities that encourage the development of competitiveness, anaerobic endurance, motive qualities and increased localized circulation.

The notation of the accompanying training programmes (Tables 25.3 & 25.4) is (70%/3)3, where the numerator is the percentage of maximum, the denominator is the number of repetitions per set, the number following the parentheses is the number of sets, and a lack of parentheses indicates a single set.

The determination of the 100% weight

In order to determine the various intensities used in the exercises, the 100% weight must be determined. At various times some systems have used the maximum weight attained at the end of the previous competitive year as that figure. Other systems use selected goal weights for the upcoming season as the 100% figures. There is now some agreement that the 100% figure is a temporal one and based on the existing circumstances. The Romanians, who only utilize figures of 80% or higher, realize that the figure must be determined by the current training conditions (Ajan *et al.* 1988) although they provide no definitive methods of making this determination. The Greeks use the heaviest weight lifted in the previous session as the 100% figure for the current session (Iliou 1993). The Nigerians work up to 100% maxima each morning before the formalized training sessions begin (Ganev 2000). This approach places somewhat of a burden on the coach to select an appropriate means by which to determine the 100% weights, and in all probability will require some adjustments during the course of the training.

The training of women

Women's weightlifting, officially inaugurated in 1987 by the first Women's World's Championships, is rapidly passing through developmental stages. It is now an Olympic medal sport and had seven different weight classes contested for the first time at the 2000 Games of Sydney. The training of female lifters apparently varies little from the training of males since the intensities are commonly based on personal maxima. Blood testosterone levels and the ability of the female body to maintain them as training load drops before competition appear to be the main physiological factors in the designing of training.

The Chinese are the dominant nation in the sport, having won the team title at every Women's World Championship. Some anecdotal information has come forth regarding the effects of the menstrual cycle on training. Some female athletes were found to train most effectively during postovulation and postmenstrual periods while others seemed to experience little variation with respect to their menstrual cycles. As of 1993 the Chinese considered menstruation to have some effect on training (Cao 1993), but by 2000 it was not considered to merit any serious variation in the training program (Ma 2000).

Two variations employed in the training of Chinese women are the employment of more

Table 25.3 Soviet preparation week.

Day 1
Morning
1 Press: (60%/3)2, (70%/3)2
2 Snatch: (60%/3)2, (70%/3)3, (80%/2)2
3 Front squat: (60%/4)2, (70%/4)23, (80%/4)2
Afternoon
4 Hang clean and jerk: (60%/3 + 1)3, (70%/3 + 1)2, (80%/3 + 1)3
5 Clean pull: 70%/4, (80%/4)2, (85%/4)2
6 Good morning: (X/8)4

Day 2
Morning
1 Power snatch: (65%/3)3, (75%/3)2, (80%/2)2
2 Power clean and jerk: (60%/3 + 1)2, (70%/3 + 1)2, (80%/2 + 1)3
3 Jerk: (70%/3)2, (80%/2)2
4 Eccentric snatch deadlift: (80%/3)6–20 s descent
5 Eccentric clean deadlift: (90%/3)6–20 s descent

Day 3
Active rest

Day 4
Morning
1 Press: 60%/4, 70%/4, (80%/3)2
2 Clean and jerk: (60%/3 + 1)2, (70%/3 + 1)2, (80%/3 + 1)2
3 Back squat: (60%/5)2, (70%/5)2, (80%/5)2
Afternoon
4 Hang snatch: (60%/3)2, (70%/3)2, (75%/2)3
5 Snatch pull: (70%/4)2, 80%/4, (90%/4)2
6 Good morning: (X/8)4

Day 5
Morning
1 Snatch: (60%/3)3, (70%/3)2, (80%/2)2
2 Hang clean and jerk: (60%/3 + 1)3, (70%/3 + 1)2, (80%/2 + 1)2
3 Snatch pull: (70%/4)2, (80%/4)2, (90%/3)2
4 Front squat: (70%/5)2, (80%/4)2, (90%/3)2

Day 6
Morning
1 Power clean and jerk: (60%/3 + 1)2, (70%/3 + 1)2, (80%/2 + 1)2
2 Jerk: 70%/3, (80%/3)2, (90%/2)2
3 Back squat: (70%/5)2, (80%/5)2, (90%/3)2
Afternoon
4 Hang snatch: (60%/3)3, (70%/3)2, (80%/2)2
5 Snatch pull: (60%/4)2, (70%/4)2, 80%/3
6 Slow snatch deadlift: (80%/3)6–10 s

Day 7
Complete rest

Total repetitions: 582

X, an extremely variable weight from one individual to another with a varied relationship to either of the two competitive lifts (see also Table 25.2).

Table 25.4 Soviet competitive week.

Day 1
Morning
1 Snatch: (70%/3)3, (80%/2)2, (90%/1)2
2 Clean and jerk: (70%/2 + 1)3, (80%/2 + 1)2, (90%/1 + 1)2, (100%/1 + 1)2
3 Jerk: 70%/2, 80%/2, 90%/2, 100%/2
Afternoon
4 Front squat: (70%/3)3, (80%/3)2, (90%/3)2
5 Snatch pull: 60%/3, 70%/3, 80%/3, 90%/2
6 Good morning: (X/8)4

Day 2
1 Power snatch: (60%/3)2, (70%/3)2, (80%/2)2
2 Power clean: (60%/3)2, (70%/3)2, (80%/2)2
3 Clean pull: (80%/3)3, 90%/3, (100%/2)2
4 Back squat: 70%/3, (80%/3)2, 90%/3
5 Press: 60%/3, (70%/3)2

Day 3
Active rest

Day 4
Morning
1 Snatch: (70%/2)2, (80%/2)2, 90%/1
2 Clean and jerk: (70%/2 + 1)3, (80%/2 + 1)3, (90%/1 + 1)2
3 Jerk: 70%/3, 80%/2, (90%/1)2
Afternoon
4 Back squat: 70%/3, (80%/2)2, (90%/2)3
5 Snatch pull: 60%/4, (70%/3)2, (80%/3)2
6 Good morning: (X/8)4

Day 5
1 Hang snatch: 60%/3, (70%/2)2, (80%/2)2, (90%/1)2
2 Clean and jerk: 60%/3 + 1, (70%/2 + 1)2, (80%/2 + 1)2
3 Clean pull: 70%/3, (80%/3)2, (90%/3)2
4 Back squat: (70%/3)2, (80%/3)2, (90%/3)2
5 Press: (70%/3)2

Total repetitions: 324

X, see note to Table 25.3.

sets at high intensities for women (10 for women, 6 for men) and longer 'work' cycles between unload weeks (3 weeks for women and 2 for men) (Cao 1993; Ma 2000). There is also some variation between men and women in the frequencies with which specific movements are programmed into the training, although this could also be attributed to individual differences rather than those of gender.

References

Abadjiev, I. (1989) *The Bulgarian Training System* (lecture). National Strength and Conditioning Association study tour, Sophia, Bulgaria.

Ajan, T. & Baroga, L. (1988) *Weightlifting Fitness For All Sports*. International Weightlifting Federation, Budapest.

Cao, W. (1993) Training differences between males and females. In: *Proceedings of the Weightlifting Symposium*, Olympia, Greece, pp. 97–101. International Weightlifting Federation, Budapest.

Drechsler, A. (1998) *The Weightlifting Encyclopedia*. A Is A Communications, Whitestone, NY.

Enoka, R.M. (1988) Muscle strength and its development. *Sports Medicine* **6**, 146–168.

Frolov, V., Efimov, N. & Vanagas, M. (1977) Training weights for snatch pulls. *Tyazhelaya Atletika*, 65–67. In: *Soviet Sports Review* **18**(2), 58–61, 1983.

Ganev, I. (2000) *Weightlifting in Nigeria* (lecture). U.S. Weightlifting International Coaching Symposium, Colorado Springs, USA.

Garhammer, J. (1985) Biomechanical analysis of weightlifting at the 1984 Olympic Games. *International Journal of Sport Biomechanics* **1**(2), 122–130.

Garhammer, J. (1989) Weight lifting and training. In: *Biomechanics of Sport* (ed. C. L. Vaughan), pp. 169–211. CRC Publishers, Boca Raton, FL.

Garhammer, J. & Gregor, R. (1979) Force plate evaluations of weightlifting and vertical jumping. *Medicine and Science in Sports and Exercise* **11**(1), 106 (abstract).

Garhammer, J. & Gregor, R. (1992) Propulsive forces as a function of intensity for weightlifting and vertical jumping. *Journal of Applied Sports Science Research* **6**(3), 129–134.

Häkkinen, K. (1988) A biomechanical analysis of various combinations of the snatch pull exercises. *Journal of Human Movement Studies* **15**, 229–243.

Häkkinen, K. & Kauhanen, H. (1986) A biomechanical analysis of selected assistance exercises of weightlifting. *Journal of Human Movement Studies* **12**, 271–288.

Häkkinen, K., Kauhanen, H. & Komi, P.V. (1984) Biomechanical changes in the Olympic weightlifting technique of the snatch and clean & jerk from submaximal to maximal loads. *Scandinavian Journal of Sports Sciences* **6**(2), 57–66.

Häkkinen, K., Pakarinen, A., Alen, M., Kauhanen, H. & Komi, P.V. (1987) Relationships between training volume, physical performance capacity, and serum hormone concentrations during prolonged training in elite weight lifters. *International Journal of Sports Medicine* **8** (Suppl.), 61–65.

Häkkinen, K., Pakarinen, A., Alen, M., Kauhanen, H. & Komi, P.V. (1988a) Neuromuscular and hormonal adaptations in athletes to strength training in two years. *Journal of Applied Physiology* **65**(6), 2406–2412.

Häkkinen, K., Pakarinen, A., Alen, M., Kauhanen, H. & Komi, P.V. (1988b) Daily hormonal and neuromuscular responses to intensive strength training in 1 week. *International Journal of Sports Medicine* **9**(6), 422–428.

Häkkinen, K., Pakarinen, A., Alen, M., Kauhanen, H. & Komi, P.V. (1988c) Neuromuscular and hormonal responses in elite athletes to two successive strength training sessions in one day. *European Journal of Applied Physiology* **57**, 133–139.

Häkkinen, K., Pakarinen, A., Kyrolainen, H., Cheng, S., Kim, D.H. & Komi, P.V. (1990) Neuromuscular adaptations and serum hormones in females during prolonged power training. *International Journal of Sports Medicine* **11**(2), 91–98.

Iliou, G. (1993) Annual competition program for juniors. In: *Proceedings of the Weightlifting Symposium*, Olympia, Greece, pp. 51–62. International Weightlifting Federation, Budapest.

Jones, L. (1993) Training programs for the athletes unable to train full time. In: *Proceedings of the Weightlifting Symposium*, Olympia, Greece, pp. 77–88. International Weightlifting Federation, Budapest.

Kraemer, W.J. (1988) Endocrine responses to resistance exercise. *Medicine and Science in Sports and Exercise* **20**(5) (Suppl.), S152–S157.

Kraemer, W.J. (2000) Endocrine responses to resistance exercise. In: *Essentials of Strength Training and Conditioning* (T. R. Baechle & R. W. Earle), pp. 91–114. Human Kinetics, Champaign, IL.

Kuipers, H. & Keizer, H.A. (1988) Overtraining in elite athletes. *Sports Medicine* **6**, 79–92.

Ma, J. (2000) *Weightlifting in China* (lecture). U.S. Weightlifting International Coaching Symposium, Colorado Springs, USA.

Matveyev, L.P. (1972) *Periodisienang das Sportlichen Training* (translated into German by P. Tschiene with a chapter by A. Kruger). Beles and Wernitz, Berlin.

Medvedjev, A., Frolov, V., Lukashev, A. & Krasov, E. (1981) A comparative analysis of the clean and clean pull technique with various weights. *Tyazhelaya Atletika* **10**, 33–35. In *Soviet Sports Review* **18**(1), 17–19, 1983.

Medvedjev, A.S., Masalgin, N.A., Herrera, A.G. & Frolov, V.I. (1982) Classification of jerk exercises and methods of their use depending upon weightlifters qualification. In: *1982 Weightlifting Yearbook*, Fizkultura i Sport, Moscow. (Translated by Andrew Charniga, Sportivny Press, Livonia, Michigan, pp. 4–9.)

Nilsson, S. (1986) Overtraining. In: *An Update on Sports Medicine* (eds S. Maehium, S. Nilsson & P. Renstrom), pp. 97–104. *Proceedings of the Second Scandinavian Conference on Sports Medicine*, March 1986, Soria Moria, Oslo, Norway.

Sale, D.G. (1988) Neural adaptation to resistance training. *Medicine and Science in Sports and Exercise* **20**(5) (Suppl.), S135–S145.

Stone, M., O'Bryant, H. & Garhammer, J. (1981) A hypothetical model for strength training. *Journal of Sports Medicine and Physical Fitness* **21**(4), 342–351.

Stone, M., O'Bryant, H., Garhammer, J., McMillan, J. & Rozenek, R. (1982) A theoretical model of strength training. *National Strength and Conditioning Association Journal* **4**(4), 36–39.

Stone, M.H., Keith, R.E., Kearney, J.T., Fleck, S.J., Wilson, G.D. & Triplett, N.T. (1990) Overtraining: a review of the signs, symptoms and possible causes. *Journal of Applied Sports Science Research* **5**, 35–50.

Takano, B. (1990) K-Value: a tool for determining training intensity. *National Strength and Conditioning Association Journal* **12**(4), 60–61.

Vorobyev, A.N. (1978) *A Textbook on Weightlifting* (translated by J. Brice). International Weightlifting Federation, Budapest.

Index

Lightning Source UK Ltd.
Milton Keynes UK
178691UK00001B/18/P